AF711623

Pediatric Fundamental Critical Care Support

Society of Critical Care Medicine
Headquarters
500 Midway Drive
Mount Prospect, IL 60056 USA
Phone +1 (847)827-6869
Fax +1 (847)827-6886
www.sccm.org
International Standard Book Number: 978-0-936145-50-1

Fundamental Critical Care Contributors

Editor:

Rodrigo Mejía, MD, FAAP, FCCM
Associate Professor of Pediatrics and Critical Care Medicine
Center Medical Director for the Child and Adolescent Center
Associate Director of Pediatric Critical Care Services
Children's Cancer Hospital at
The University of Texas M. D. Anderson Cancer Center
Houston, Texas
Financial Disclosure: No financial disclosures

Co-Editors:

Alan Fields, MD, FCCM, FAAP
Professor of Pediatrics, Anesthesiology and Critical Care Medicine
Director of Pediatric Critical Care Services
Children's Cancer Hospital at
The University of Texas M.D. Anderson Cancer Center
Houston, Texas
Financial Disclosure: No financial disclosures

Bruce M. Greenwald, MD, FCCM, FAAP
Professor of Clinical Pediatrics
Director, Division of Pediatric Critical Care Medicine
Weill Cornell Medical College
New York Presbyterian Hospital
New York, New York
Financial Disclosure: No financial disclosures

Fernando Stein, MD, FAAP
Associate Professor
Medical Director of Progressive Care
Deputy Director of Pediatric Intensive Care
Texas Children's Hospital
Baylor College of Medicine
Houston, Texas
Financial Disclosure: No financial disclosures

Contributors:

Naomi B. Bishop, MD
Assistant Professor of Pediatrics
Weill Cornell Medical College
New York Presbyterian Hospital
New York, New York
Financial Disclosure: No financial disclosures

Gregory H. Botz, MD
Associate Professor of Anesthesiology and Critical Care
Medical Director, Medical Emergency Rapid Intervention Team
University of Texas M.D. Anderson Cancer Center
Houston, Texas
Financial Disclosure: No financial disclosures

Susanna R. Burkhead, MD
Medical Co-Director
Pediatric Intensive Care Unit
St. John Hospital and Medical Center
Detroit, Michigan
Financial Disclosure: No financial disclosures

Joseph Carcillo, MD
Associate Professor of Critical Care Medicine and Pediatrics
University of Pittsburgh School of Medicine
Department of Critical Care Medicine
Children's Hospital of Pittsburgh
Pittsburgh, Pennsylvania
Financial Disclosure: No financial disclosures

Edward E. Conway, Jr., MS, MD, FCCM
Professor of Clinical Pediatrics
Chairman of the Milton and Bernice Stern
Department of Pediatrics
Chief, Pediatric Critical Care
Beth Israel Medical Center
New York, New York
Financial Disclosure: No financial disclosures

Jose A. Cortes, MD, FAAP
Assistant Professor
Children's Cancer Hospital
The University of Texas
M. D. Anderson Cancer Center
Houston, Texas
Financial Disclosure: No financial disclosures

Alan L. Davis, MD, MPH, FCCM, FAAP
Director, Pediatric Critical Care
Associate Clinical Professor of Pediatrics, UMDNJ
Saint Barnabas Medical Center
Livingston, New Jersey
Financial Disclosure: No financial disclosures

Guillermo DeAngulo, MD
Attending
Cancer Center of Miami Children's Hospital
Miami, Florida
Financial Disclosure: No financial disclosures

Karen Farst, MD
Assistant Professor
Department of Pediatrics
Section for Children at Risk
University of Arkansas for Medical Sciences
College of Medicine
Arkansas Children's Hospital
Little Rock, Arkansas
Financial Disclosure: No financial disclosures

Kathryn A. Felmet, MD
Assistant Professor of Critical Care Medicine and Pediatrics
University of Pittsburgh School of Medicine
Department of Critical Care Medicine
Children's Hospital of Pittsburgh
Pittsburgh, Pennsylvania
Financial Disclosure: No financial disclosures

Jonathan D. Feldman, MD
Director, Pediatric ICU and Inpatient Services
Medical Director, Pediatric/Neonatal Transport Services
Kaiser Santa Clara Medical Center
Santa Clara, California
Clinical Associate Professor (Affiliated),
Department of Pediatrics
Stanford University School of Medicine
Stanford, California
Financial Disclosure: No financial disclosures

Joy D. Howell, MD, FAAP
Associate Professor of Clinical Pediatrics
Weill Cornell Medical College
New York Presbyterian Hospital
New York, New York
Financial Disclosure: No financial disclosures

Thomas Iolster, MD
Lecturer in Pediatrics, FCBM, Universidad Austral
Head Pediatric Intensive Care Unit Hospital Universitario Austral
Buenos Aires, Argentina
Financial Disclosure: No financial disclosures

Chhavi Katyal, MD
Assistant Professor of Pediatrics
Division of Critical Care Medicine
The Children's Hospital at Montefiore
Albert Einstein College of Medicine
Bronx, New York
Financial Disclosure: No financial disclosures

Carroll J. King, MD
Attending Pediatric Critical Care Unit
UTMB Children's Hospital
Galveston, Texas
Financial Disclosures: No financial disclosures

Keith C. Kocis, MD, MS
Professor of Pediatrics
Pediatric Cardiology
The University of North Carolina at Chapel Hill
Chapel Hill, North Carolina
Financial Disclosure: No financial disclosures

Martha C. Kutko, MD, FAAP
Associate Professor of Clinical Pediatrics
Weill Cornell Medical College
New York Presbyterian Hospital
New York, New York
Financial Disclosure: No financial disclosures

Maureen A. Madden, MSN, PNP-AC, CCRN, FCCM
Assistant Professor of Pediatrics
UMDNJ- Robert Wood Johnson Medical School
Pediatric Critical Care Nurse Practitioner
Bristol-Myers Squibb Children's Hospital
New Brunswick, New Jersey
Financial Disclosure: No financial disclosures

David Markenson, MD
Director, Center for Disaster Medicine
Associate Professor of Public Health
New York Medical College School of Public Health
Chief, Pediatric Emergency Medicine
Associate Professor of Pediatrics
Maria Fareri Children's Hospital
New York Medical College
Valhalla, New York
Financial Disclosure: No financial disclosures

Riza V. Mauricio, MSN, RN, CCRN, CPNP-AC
Pediatric Critical Care Nurse Practitioner
Children's Cancer Hospital at
The University of Texas M.D. Anderson Cancer Center
Houston, Texas
Financial Disclosure: No financial disclosures

Marilyn C. Morris, MD, MPH
Assistant Professor of Clinical Pediatrics
Columbia University
The Children's Hospital of New York Presbyterian
New York, New York
Financial Disclosure: No financial disclosures

Mohan R. Mysore, MBBS, FAAP, FCCM
Clinical Director, PICU
Children's Hospital
Omaha, Nebraska
Financial Disclosure: No financial disclosures

Regina Okhuysen-Cawley, MD
Associate Professor of Pediatrics
Children's Cancer Hospital at The University of Texas MD Anderson Cancer Center
Houston, Texas
Financial Disclosure: No financial disclosures

Michele C. Papo, MD, MPH
Medical Director, PICU
Medical City Children's Hospital
Pediatric Acute Care Associates of North Texas, PA
Dallas, Texas
Financial Disclosures: No financial disclosures

Jack M. Percelay, MD, MPH, FAAP
E.L.M.O. Pediatrics
New York, New York
Financial Disclosure: No financial disclosures

Steven Pon, MD, FCCM, FAAP
Associate Professor of Clinical Pediatrics
Associate Director, Pediatric Intensive Care Unit
Weill Cornell Medical College
New York Presbyterian Hospital
New York, New York
Financial Disclosure: No financial disclosures

Ellen Jane Pringle, RT
University of Texas MD Anderson Cancer Center
Acute Care Training Center
Houston, Texas
Financial Disclosure:

Parthak Prodhan, MD
Assistant Professor of Pediatrics
Sections of Pediatric Critical Care Medicine and Pediatric Cardiology
University of Arkansas for Medical Sciences College of Medicine
Arkansas Children's Hospital
Little Rock, Arkansas
Financial Disclosure: No financial disclosures

Gerardo Quezada, MD
Methodist Children's Hospital
San Antonio, Texas
Financial Disclosures:

Ramon Rivera, MD
Assistant Professor of Anesthesiology and Critical Care
University of Texas Medical Branch at Galveston
Driscoll Children's Hospital
Corpus Christi, Texas
Financial Disclosure: No financial disclosures

Alexandre Tellechea Rotta, MD, FAAP
Associate Professor of Anesthesiology
University of Texas Medical Branch
Department of Anesthesiology and Critical Care
Driscoll Children's Hospital
Corpus Christi, Texas
Financial Disclosure: No financial disclosures

Michael E. Rytting, MD
Assistant Professor, Pediatrics-Patient Care
Children's Cancer Hospital at
The University of Texas M. D. Anderson Cancer Center
Houston, Texas
Financial Disclosure: No financial disclosures

Charles L. Schleien, MD, MBA, FCCM, FAAP, FAHA
Professor of Pediatrics & Anesthesiology
Vice Chair, Department of Pediatrics
Director, Pediatric Critical Care Medicine
Columbia University College of Physicians & Surgeons
New York, New York
Financial Disclosure: No financial disclosures

Eduardo Julio Schnitzler, MD
Associate Professor, Pediatrics, FCBM, Universidad Austral
Consultant Pediatric Intensivist, Hospital Universitario Austral
Medical Director Hospital Universitario Austral
Buenos Aires, Argentina
Financial Disclosure: No financial disclosures

Steven M. Schwartz, MD
Associate Professor of Pediatrics
Head, Division of Cardiac Critical Care Medicine
The Labatt Family Heart Centre
Departments of Critical Care Medicine and Paediatrics,
The Hospital for Sick Children
Toronto, Canada
Financial Disclosure: No financial disclosures

Karl Serrao, MD, FAAP
Associate Professor of Anesthesiology
University of Texas Medical Branch at Galveston
Driscoll Children's Hospital
Corpus Christi, Texas
Financial Disclosure: No financial disclosures

Linda Snelling, MD
Associate Professor of Pediatrics & Surgery
Chief, Division of Pediatric Critical Care Medicine
The Warren Alpert Medical School at Brown University
Providence, Rhode Island
Financial Disclosure: No financial disclosures

Todd M. Sweberg, MD, FAAP
Assistant Professor of Pediatrics
Albert Einstein College of Medicine
Division of Critical Care Medicine
The Children's Hospital at Montefiore
Bronx, New York
Financial Disclosure: No financial disclosures

Gregory H. Tatum, MD
Assistant Professor of Pediatrics
Pediatric Cardiology
The University of North Carolina at Chapel Hill
Department of Pediatrics
The University of North Carolina at Chapel Hill
Chapel Hill, North Carolina
Financial Disclosure: No financial disclosures

Ann E. Thompson, MD, FCCM
Professor, Department of Critical Care Medicine
University of Pittsburgh School of Medicine
Director, Pediatric CCM
Children's Hospital of Pittsburgh
Pittsburgh, Pennsylvania
Financial Disclosure: No financial disclosures

H. Michael Ushay, MD, PhD, FCCM
Associate Professor of Clinical Pediatrics
Albert Einstein College of Medicine
Medical Director, Pediatric Critical Care Unit
The Children's Hospital at Montefiore
Bronx, New York
Financial Disclosure: No financial disclosures

Michael M. Wilhelm, MD
Assistant Professor of Pediatrics
Columbia University
New York, New York
Financial Disclosure: No financial disclosures

Jacqueline Williams-Phillips, MD, FAAP
Associate Professor of Pediatrics
UMDNJ—Robert Wood Johnson Medical School
Director, Pediatric Critical Care
Bristol-Myers Squibb Children's Hospital
New Brunswick, New Jersey
Financial Disclosure: No financial disclosures

Recognition is due to the Acute Care Training Center at the University of Texas MD Anderson Cancer Center in Houston, Texas, Medical City Children's Hospital in Dallas, Texas, and Presbyterian Hospital of Plano in Plano, Texas for their continued support throughout this project.

PEDIATRIC FUNDAMENTAL CRITICAL CARE SUPPORT

The Society of Critical Care Medicine (SCCM) has continued to offer the Fundamental Critical Care Support (FCCS) course to global audiences since the mid-1990s. The goal of this curriculum is to introduce principles important in the initial care of critically ill or injured patients to physicians, nurses, and other healthcare providers who are not skilled in critical care but who must care for such a patient in anticipation of the arrival of an intensivist or pending transfer of the patient to a more suitable facility. While FCCS addresses both adult and pediatric populations, the major focus has been on the critically ill/injured adult. Therefore, the need for a specific course to address the pediatric population special needs has been developed: P-FCCS.

This first edition has been developed as a result of the determination and dedication of the SCCM staff especially Lynn Retford and Gervaise Nicklas, MS, RN; a diverse group of multiprofessional chapter contributors; the invaluable guidance provided by Barbara McLean, MN, CCRN, CCNP, FCCM, and the commitment of the co-editors Alan Fields, MD, FCCM, and Bruce Greenwald, MD, FCCM, and the P-FCCS work group: Maureen Madden, MSN, PNP-AC, CCRN, FCCM; Karl Serrao, MD; Ellen Pringle, RT; Edward E. Conway, Jr., MD, MS, FCCM; Gregory H. Botz, MD, FCCM, and Mohan R. Mysore, MB, FCCM, MBBS, for offering many ideas to improve the text and course that helped reach this ambitious goal.

The chapters in the first edition have been carefully written, reviewed, and organized to reflect the most current guidelines and practices and are evidence based where applicable. Each chapter and major section begins with learning objectives and a case study that focuses attention on key clinical findings and patient presentation. The majority of these chapters are unique to the pediatric population while covering a broad range of pediatric-related topics. In addressing the diversity of healthcare professionals who may take this course, we realize that some may find the information provided in this first edition overly comprehensive. For those who may want a more rapid, less extensive review, information boxes in the margins provide essential principles and emphasize clinical cautions. This format maximizes learning and flow of information. In addition, for those who desire an even more complete review of the literature, many sections offer additional electronic resources for suggested readings.

It is hoped that this first edition of P-FCCS will help establish a tradition of offering educational content to those caring for critically ill children, thus promoting the mission of SCCM: Right Care Right Now.

Rodrigo Mejía, MD, FAAP, FCCM

Table of Contents

Table of Contents

Chapter 1:

Assessment of the Critically Ill Child

Objectives

- Explain how anatomic and physiologic differences between pediatric and adult patients affect fundamental critical care.
- Identify which aspects of the physical exam should be included in the rapid assessment of the critically ill child.
- Explain the importance of early recognition of respiratory failure and shock.
- Describe the clinical features of the different types of shock.
- Discuss the role of ancillary tests in the cardiopulmonary evaluation of a child.
- Explain how to do a rapid evaluation of a child's neurological status.
- Discuss the early recognition of sepsis.

Case Study

A 3-month-old girl with a history of prematurity is brought to the emergency department (ED) following a 1-week history of nasal congestion, cough, wheezing, posttussive emesis, tachypnea, and fever. On arrival in the ED the patient's vital signs are heart rate 182/min, respiratory rate 72/min, pulse oximetry 87% in room air, and temperature 38.7° C (101.7° F). She is tachypneic, grunting, retracting, and cyanotic. She is given an albuterol nebulizer treatment with 100% oxygen by the ED staff.

- What is this child's physiologic status?

- How should this patient be positioned during your exam?

- Does this patient exhibit signs of impending respiratory arrest?

I. INTRODUCTION

The evaluation and assessment of the critically ill child is the essential foundation upon which the rest of this course is built. Only after a patient has been evaluated can their physiologic status be ascertained. This, in turn, determines what the next appropriate intervention should be. After every intervention, the patient must be carefully reevaluated until he/she has been adequately resuscitated and stabilized. If important aspects of the exam are missed or ignored, appropriate treatment will be delayed, which may result in disastrous consequences for the patient. We often think of children as little adults, but because their physiology and anatomy can vary greatly, there are differences in the way they present when critically ill. This chapter approaches the pediatric evaluation by organ system to emphasize issues related to maturation, habitus, anatomy, and physiology. Many hospitals are using medical emergency teams (METS) to identify patients at risk and begin early treatment. (See **Appendix 1**)

II. THE GENERAL EXAMINATION

The general examination is probably the most important part of the physical exam. In the case study at the beginning of the chapter, ED personnel should recognize on sight that the infant is in respiratory failure and possibly in shock, necessitating immediate action.

A question that should be asked and answered in every healthcare provider's mind is, "Does this child look sick?" Because young children are unable to verbalize specific complaints, evaluation by the healthcare provider depends upon general and specific features of the examination in addition to information obtained from a parent or guardian. Although many of the early signs of distress are subtle, their recognition can increase the likelihood that interventions will be successful and that more serious progression will be prevented. If healthcare providers initially miss the more elusive signs of illness, they may later assume that a child's condition has suddenly deteriorated when, in fact, a seemingly abrupt change reflects an advanced point along a continuum of physiologic compromise. Important aspects to be considered in the general examination of a pediatric patient are listed in **Table 1-1.**

> **!** *A child's general appearance will immediately help the observer discern the presence of serious illness.* **!**

Table 1-1. General Examination

Skin

Loss of normal pink coloration of mucosa and nail beds

Mottling

Skin warmth or coolness

Prolonged capillary refill, determined with the extremity above the level of the patient's heart to prevent the mistaken assessment of venous refill

continued next page...

Table 1-1. General Examination (Continued)

Signs of Dehydration
Sunken fontanelle in infants
Absent tears
Sunken eyes
Skin tenting
Dry mucous membranes
Color
Cyanosis
Acrocyanosis (may be present if room temperature is cool)
Central cyanosis
Jaundice
Pallor
Breathing
Bradypnea/tachypnea
Stridor
Audible wheezing
Nasal flaring/grunting
Intercostal retractions
Level of Alertness
Awake and alert
Responds to verbal commands
Responds only to painful stimulation
Unresponsive

During the clinical exam, children should be allowed to remain in the position that they spontaneously assume for comfort. For children younger than 1 year, this is often in the arms of their primary caregiver. Illness may be marked by a patient's inability to find a position of comfort. Patients should not be forced to assume a different position because doing so could potentially compromise a tenuous airway.

> **!** *A child's level of reactivity and responsiveness is usually a reflection of the level of cerebral perfusion.*

An ill child may initially have increased irritability, but this may be followed by decreasing responsiveness, increasing flaccidity, and lethargy. This is observed in conditions such as hypoxia, uncompensated shock, and hypoglycemia. In most infants, alertness can be evaluated by observing the ability to fixate on objects, particularly a parent's face. The infant should turn toward sound and should follow an object horizontally, and starting at 1 month of age, should follow an object vertically as well. Older children should exhibit anxiety toward strangers and show clear recognition of parents.

III. RESPIRATORY SYSTEM AND AIRWAY

> !
>
> *Respiratory arrest is the most common cause of cardiopulmonary collapse in children.*
>
> !

Respiratory failure is particularly common in infants due to variable maturation in 3 areas:

- The central nervous system receptor and effector mechanisms for the respiratory drive
- Chest wall stability and respiratory muscular strength
- Conducting airways and the alveolar-capillary complex

The respiratory response to hypoxemia in neonates may be biphasic (ie, hyperpnea initially, followed by hypopnea and hypoventilation). This response occurs despite apparently normal central and peripheral chemoreceptors to oxygen and CO_2. The most common cause of cardiopulmonary collapse in children is respiratory arrest. This is potentially preventable by early recognition of loss of an adequate airway and pulmonary compromise.

A. Anatomic and Physiologic Considerations

The thorax is more cartilaginous in infants and young children and is, therefore, more compliant. In an infant, trying to increase negative intrathoracic pressure during respiratory distress is less effective in augmenting tidal volume because the chest retracts inward, reducing tidal ventilation and indirectly increasing the work of breathing. Soft-tissue retractions similarly reduce thoracic volume during vigorous respiratory efforts. In addition, the fact that an infant's ribs are aligned on a more horizontal plane decreases the inspiratory displacement of the thorax on the anteroposterior plane, further decreasing the efficiency of the bellows effect of the thorax.

The points of muscular insertion of the diaphragm on the thorax are more horizontal in the infant, resembling those of an adult with obstructive lung disease and a flattened diaphragm. Therefore, the lower thorax may be drawn inward during inspiration, causing reduced inspiratory volume. Immature intercostal muscles cannot assist active ventilation for several years after birth; thus, more dependency is placed upon diaphragmatic function and excursion. Compromise of diaphragmatic excursion by gastric distention, abdominal distension, surgery, and other factors may quickly evolve into compromised respiratory function.

Alveolar size and number increase substantially during childhood; lung compliance also increases. Tidal volume as a fraction of total lung capacity remains fairly constant through childhood at 6 to 7 mL/kg body weight. High intrinsic or externally supplied flow rates are required to deliver this tidal volume because children have a short inspiratory duration. Smaller anatomic conducting airways may produce high resistance if further narrowed by inflammation, edema, mucus, bronchospasm, bronchiolitis, and so forth. Such high peripheral airway resistance may also alter exhalation and induce dynamic closure of the airways and auto–positive end-expiratory pressure (auto-PEEP). Closing capacity in infants is within the functional residual capacity and, therefore, promotes airway closure during tidal breathing. These factors combine to produce less respiratory reserve in the pediatric patient. Consequently, children may decompensate rapidly, leading to cardiopulmonary arrest if there is no intervention.

The majority of deaths in children (especially those younger than 1 year) involve respiratory disorders resulting from infection, poisonings, trauma, submersion or suffocation, or sudden infant death syndrome.

B. Physical Examination

> !
>
> *Respiratory embarrassment is manifested by nasal flaring, tachypnea, grunting, and retractions.*
>
> !

Nasal flaring, tachypnea, grunting, and retractions are signs of increased work of breathing as the patient attempts to maintain adequate minute ventilation and oxygenation in response to pulmonary or airway compromise. Given the compliant nature of a child's chest wall, retractions can be quite profound, with evidence of subcostal, intercostal, and suprasternal retractions. Tachypnea is an important sign of illness in infants and young children, and bradypnea is an ominous precursor of impending respiratory arrest.

> !
>
> *Bradypnea is an ominous precursor of impending respiratory arrest.*
>
> !

Such extreme variations in respiratory rate have many etiologies, which are summarized in **Table 1-2.** It is important to remember that the normal respiratory rate of an infant or child is age dependent (see **Table 1-3**). As previously mentioned, a patient's position of comfort is usually the position that allows adequate gas exchange. For example, a child with upper airway obstruction (eg, epiglottitis) will usually attempt to sit forward, or tripod. Children should be allowed to choose their position of comfort; forcing a child into a different position may worsen respiratory distress and even precipitate respiratory arrest.

Table 1-2. Causes of Variations in Respiratory Rate

Tachypnea
Fever
Pain and anxiety
Hypovolemia
Respiratory disease
Metabolic acidosis
Heart failure
Adverse drug effect
Hyperviscosity syndromes

Bradypnea
Hypothermia
Central nervous system injury
Drug-induced depression
Neuromuscular disease
Severe shock
Metabolic disorders

Table 1-3. Normal Respiratory Rates in Children

Age	Respiratory Rate (breaths/minute)
Newborn - 1 year	30 - 60
1 - 3 years	25 - 40
3 - 12 years	20 - 30
> 12 years	12 - 20

The shape and movement of the chest during respiration will alert the observer to underlying respiratory problems. A rib-cage deformity, such as pectus excavatum, pectus carinatum, or scoliosis, may suggest the presence of restrictive lung disease or pulmonary hypoplasia, or lead to abnormal respiratory mechanics. Asymmetry of chest rise is indicative of unequal air entry and serious underlying pathology (see **Table 1-4**). Auscultation of breathing sounds will reveal the adequacy and symmetry of air entry and allow any other sounds, such as wheezes, crackles, and rubs, to become evident. Auscultation may be difficult or easy, depending on the child's level of cooperation. Because children have thinner chest walls than adults, breath sounds are easily audible but less easily localized, and other transmitted sounds often interfere with accurate auscultation. When a child is agitated and crying, adequate auscultation may not be possible.

> **!** *Children in respiratory distress should be allowed to choose their position of comfort.*

Table 1-4. Causes of Asymmetrical Chest Movement

- Unilateral pneumothorax
- Unilateral pleural effusion
- Foreign body aspiration with hyperinflation
- Mucus plugging of mainstem bronchus
- Lobar atelectasis

> **!** *Cyanosis is a poor indicator of hypoxemia in infants and children.*

In general, cyanosis of the skin and nail beds, if present, is indicative of hypoxemia. In cool temperatures and ambient lighting, it is possible to observe cyanosis of the nail beds (acrocyanosis), which is due to peripheral vasoconstriction in response to the cold. However, cyanosis may be a late finding in the hypoxemic child. For clinical cyanosis to be evident, more than approximately 5 grams of hemoglobin (Hgb) per deciliter (dL) must be desaturated, and its presence depends on the hemoglobin concentration.

Because children have lower hemoglobin concentration than adults, the blood oxygen content must fall to very low levels before cyanosis is evident. The advent of pulse oximetry has enabled the noninvasive measurement of oxygen saturation to accurately determine the degree of hypoxemia. A common error is equating adequate oxygen saturations with adequate ventilation and respiratory stability. Oxygen saturation alone does not provide enough information about the adequacy of ventilation. Alveolar ventilation is primarily responsible for removal of carbon dioxide and is represented by minute ventilation, which is the product of the respiratory rate and tidal volume. Although alveolar ventilation is a determinant of oxygenation, a patient may maintain adequate oxygen saturation in the face of inadequate ventilation, especially if supplemental oxygen is provided. Therefore clinical assessment, including attention to chest movement, respiratory rate, and work of breathing, is crucial to determine adequacy of ventilation. A useful adjunct to the clinical examination is noninvasive measurement of Pa_{CO_2} with the aid of end tidal capnography and transcutaneous carbon dioxide monitoring.

C. Airway Evaluation

Case Study

A 15-month-old boy was brought into the emergency department with sudden-onset acute respiratory distress after a choking episode. The patient was noted to be wheezing on auscultation. A chest radiograph reveals hyperinflation of the right lung. The patient is taken to the operating room for bronchoscopy. A large peanut fragment is removed from the right main-stem bronchus.

- Why is this patient wheezing?

- What noninvasive monitoring might be useful in evaluating this patient?

Airway obstruction, aspiration, and apnea are also serious hazards to respiratory function. Thus, ensuring a patent airway is the important first step in caring for children with respiratory compromise. In the case study above, the patient aspirated a foreign body that resulted in airway obstruction and respiratory failure. Many times the same signs and symptoms could easily be misinterpreted as indicators of reactive airway disease. The nasal pathway is the primary route for normal breathing (obligate nasal breathing) in neonates and young infants. Total airway resistance and the potential for compromised breathing are significantly greater in infants with nasal congestion, increased secretions, or a nasogastric tube.

> **!** *Nasal flaring is a sensitive indicator of respiratory distress in infants. Simply suctioning the nasal passages can be an important intervention in establishing airway patency.*

The anatomy of the pediatric airway, especially in infants and young children, predisposes these patients to airway obstruction when they are positioned incorrectly or are unable to maintain adequate hypopharyngeal tone. Children in this age group have a large occiput, a relatively large tongue, a larger, floppy epiglottis, and an anteriorly placed larynx. These factors, combined with decreased hypopharyngeal tone, lead to the loss of airway patency in obtunded patients because they are unable to keep these soft tissue structures apart.

In young children, common causes of airway obstruction are congenital, infectious (viral croup, bacterial tracheitis, or, less commonly, epiglottitis), or related to the ingestion of a foreign body. Clinical examination may help identify the site of obstruction. Asthma is not the sole reason for wheezing and lower-airway obstruction. Airway obstruction above the thoracic inlet tends to cause stridor (inspiratory noise), whereas intrathoracic obstruction tends to cause wheezing (expiratory noise). For children who present with stridor or wheezing unresponsive to appropriate bronchodilator and steroid therapy, a diagnosis of foreign body aspiration must be entertained.

D. Respiratory Failure

Children in respiratory distress progressing to respiratory failure will exhibit increased work of breathing until they experience muscle fatigue or are no longer able to compensate. Causes of respiratory failure in children can usually be grouped by age. In premature neonates, respiratory failure results from apnea of prematurity or infant respiratory distress syndrome, in which atelectasis and impaired gas exchange occur as a result of surfactant deficiency and ineffective chest bellows. In term neonates, bacterial pneumonia, sepsis, meconium aspiration, and congenital airway abnormalities are most common. In infants and toddlers, lower-respiratory disease from pneumonia, bronchiolitis, asthma, foreign-body aspiration, and upper-airway obstruction related to infection are common. The causes of respiratory failure in older children are similar to those found in adults.

Noninvasive monitoring has become indispensable in the evaluation of patients in respiratory distress. With pulse oximetry and end-tidal capnography, oxygenation and ventilation can be objectively evaluated. Ancillary investigative tests, such as chest radiographs, arterial blood gas tests, and other studies summarized in **Table 1-5,** are useful in determining respiratory failure, elucidating its etiology, and monitoring therapy. These tools are not substitutes for a clinical exam. Ultimately the clinical assessment and judgment of the healthcare provider are the most valuable tools for recognizing a patient in impending respiratory failure. Once that possibility is recognized, preparation and interventions can be made to secure an airway, ensure adequate ventilation, and facilitate transfer to a pediatric intensive care unit (PICU).

Table 1-5. Ancillary Studies to Evaluate Respiratory Status

Study	Evaluation
Arterial Blood Gas (in Room Air)	Hypoxemia = low Pao_2 (<60 mm Hg [<8.0 kPa]) Hypercarbia = high $Paco_2$ (>45 mm Hg [>6.0 kPa]) Acidosis = pH <7.35 Adequate Pao_2 does not mean adequate oxygenation if the Hgb is low pH >7.35 and $Paco_2$ 35-45 mm Hg in a child with severe increased work of breathing is a sign of impending respiratory failure
Pulse Oximetry (SpO_2)	Noninvasive measure of oxyhemoglobin Monitor oxygenation in response to treatment
Hemoglobin (Hgb) Concentration	Determinant of Arterial Oxygen Content (Cao_2) = (Hgb x 1.34 x Sao_2) + Dissolved Oxygen (0.0031 x Pao_2) Oxygen Delivery (Do) = Cao_2 x Cardiac Output
Capnography	Measure exhaled CO_2 from nasal cannula, endotracheal tube (ETT), or tracheostomy tube Noninvasively monitor adequacy of ventilation Confirm placement of ETT Detect lower-airway obstruction with waveform Determine physiological dead space
Peak Expiratory Flow Rate	Generates maximum flow during forced exhalation Decreases with lower-airway obstruction (asthma) Monitor bronchodilator therapy Requires cooperation to perform, and therefore may be useful only in older children
Chest Radiograph	Airway obstruction Pneumothorax and/or pleural effusion Parenchymal lung disease Atelectasis Barotrauma

IV. CARDIOVASCULAR SYSTEM

A. Anatomic and Physiologic Considerations

The circulating blood volume is higher per kilogram in children than in adults, but the absolute volume remains lower in children due to their small body size. Consequently, children are less able to tolerate small amounts of blood loss, and blood replacement is indicated when 5% to 10% of their circulating volume has been lost. Because an infant's ability to increase stroke volume is limited, any augmentation of cardiac output depends on the patient's heart rate and diastolic filling time. Cardiac output per kilogram of weight in the newborn (greater than 200 mL/kg/min) is higher than that of adults, with the cardiac index at birth (4 L/min/m^2) gradually falling to adult normative values (2.5-3 L/min/m^2) in adolescence. This occurs because oxygen consumption is dependent on cardiac output, and oxygen consumption per kilogram of body weight is greater in infants than in adults. Familiarity with the normative ranges of heart rates is important because those ranges vary with age, as can be seen in **Table 1-6.** Severe tachycardia will decrease diastolic filling time, resulting in a rapid fall in stroke volume. Bradycardia will result in decreased cardiac output and therefore decreased oxygen delivery, and is most often an ominous sign of significant hypoxemia or acidosis. Other arrhythmias usually do not produce significant changes in cardiac output unless sustained supraventricular tachycardia occurs. Ventricular arrhythmias are uncommon, but when present, they may signify congenital heart disease, myocarditis, cardiomyopathy, electrolyte abnormalities, or asphyxia.

Table 1-6. Normal Heart Rates in Children

Age	Heart Rate (Beats/Minute)
Newborn	80 - 200
< 2 years	80 - 180
2 - 10 years	60 - 150
> 10 years	60 - 100

Myocardial maturation influences the heart's response to volume challenges intended to increase preload. In infants younger than 8 weeks, cardiac output may not be increased by a fluid bolus, but thereafter the response is similar to that of adults. The central venous pressure, however, does not necessarily reflect circulatory blood volume or left ventricular efficiency. Left and right heart function may be disparate, and each side may fail independently. Therefore, pulmonary artery catheters may occasionally be required to monitor left and right heart filling pressures.

Pulmonary vascular resistance falls quickly after birth, reaching normal adult levels by 8 weeks of life. However, the pulmonary vasculature may remain very reactive to hypoxia, hypercapnia, hypothermia, or acidosis, thereby increasing afterload to the right ventricle. Myocardial anatomy changes after birth so that the larger right ventricle decreases in mass and the left ventricle increases in size and mass. The neonatal myocardium exhibits a limited response to catecholamines due to immaturity of sympathetic nervous system innervation as well as a reduced number of β_1-receptors, both of which increases over the first several weeks of life. The physiologic effects of exogenous catecholamine administration, therefore, may be quite variable, and careful titration to the individual child's response is essential.

B. Physical Examination

The physical examination of the cardiovascular system should focus on assessing tissue perfusion as it relates to circulation and end-organ function. This includes evaluation of skin color, temperature, capillary refill, pulse character, heart rate and rhythm, and blood pressure.

> !
>
> *Tachycardia is one of the earliest signs of shock.*
>
> !

Cardiac output in children, especially infants, is dependent on the patient's heart rate. As with heart rate and respiratory rate, blood pressure varies with age. Systolic blood pressure in the 5th percentile for the patient's age (**Table 1-7**) is at the lower limit of the acceptable range; a blood pressure below that indicates hypotension.

Hypotension in children from 1 to 10 years old can be quickly determined using either of the following formulas:

- Systolic blood pressure (mm Hg) <70 + (Age in Years × 2)
- Mean arterial pressure (mm Hg) <50 + (Age in Years × 2)]

Table 1-7. Lower Limit of Systolic Blood Pressure by Age

Age	Systolic Blood Pressure (mm Hg)
Newborn	60
< 1 year	70
1 - 10 years	70 + (Age in years × 2)
> 10 years	90

The end-organ systems of special relevance are the brain and the kidneys because the body's homeostatic mechanisms give priority to preservation of perfusion to these tissues. Brain and kidney function are assessed by evaluating the patient's mental status and urine output. Deterioration of end-organ function is a precursor to circulatory arrest. In addition to the clinical exam, several ancillary studies, listed in **Table 1-8,** should be used to fully evaluate and monitor the critically ill child. For additional information, see **Appendix 2**.

Table 1-8. Ancillary Studies to Evaluate Cardiovascular System

Study	Evaluation
Blood Gas	May use both arterial and venous blood gases if necessary Detects acid-base imbalances
Serum Lactate	Forms as result of tissue hypoxia and anaerobic metabolism Reflects poor tissue perfusion Serves as a prognostic indicator to assess response to therapy
Total serum CO_2	Measures all forms of CO_2 (primarily bicarbonate) Measures severity of metabolic acidosis
Hemoglobin Concentration	Gauges arterial oxygen content and therefore oxygen delivery Monitors ongoing blood loss in hemorrhagic shock
Urinary Catheter	Continuously monitors urine output Children: 1-2 mL/kg/h Adolescents: 0.5-1 mL/kg/h
Continuous Arterial Pressure Monitoring	Provides ongoing evaluation of blood pressure Supplies information on systemic vascular resistance and cardiac output through waveform analysis Monitors fluid resuscitation and inotropic/vasopressor therapy Facilitates arterial blood gas sampling
Central Venous Pressure Monitoring	Assesses preload and guides fluid therapy Increases in obstructive forms of shock Measures central venous oxygen saturation (Svo_2) Evaluates cardiac output and oxygen delivery
Chest Radiograph	Assesses for congestive heart failure Cardiomegaly Pulmonary edema Pleural effusion
Echocardiography	Shows contractility Measures estimated ventricular pressures Displays chamber size and wall thickness Demonstrates congenital anomalies Shows pericardial effusion

C. Shock

Shock may be defined as a state of circulatory dysfunction that fails to provide sufficient oxygen and nutrients to meet the metabolic needs of vital organs and peripheral tissues. For example, when a patient with hemorrhage continues to lose blood, the body compensates by trying to maintain adequate perfusion pressure to essential organs. The heart rate increases in an attempt to maintain adequate cardiac output as venous return diminishes along with a compensatory increase in systemic vascular resistance. This results in preservation of a normal blood pressure during the early phase (compensated phase) of shock, with hypotension occurring when the circulatory compensatory mechanisms are overwhelmed by uncorrected, ongoing blood loss. When hypotension is present, the patient is in late-stage (decompensated) shock, which is accompanied by weak, thready pulses, markedly prolonged capillary refill time, mottled extremities, and obtunded sensorium. Timely recognition of the shock state and aggressive intervention are essential to obtaining an optimal outcome. As soon as the diagnosis of shock is considered, early cardiopulmonary monitoring, vascular access, and treatment must be implemented.

> **!** *Fluid resuscitation is the initial therapy for most forms of shock.*

Rapid restitution of circulating intravascular volume is critical if end-organ damage is to be avoided. Hepatomegaly can be a sign of fluid overload in the pediatric patient; however, it must be viewed with caution. Disease processes common to children (eg, asthma, respiratory syncytial virus, and pneumonitis) can cause lung hyperinflation and displacement of the liver. Other signs of volume overload should also be considered in the evaluation of these patients. If a child with an enlarged liver fails to respond to initial fluid administration, radiologic examination of the chest may help to evaluate heart size. Crackles may occur late in children who are developing congestive failure, and a gallop may be difficult to discern in infants owing to their rapid heart rate. Possible etiologies of shock are listed in **Table 1-9.**

Table 1-9. Possible Etiologies of Shock

Hypovolemic Shock

Fluid losses: gastrointestinal disorders (acute gastroenteritis, pancreatitis), renal dysfunction

Blood loss: hemorrhage resulting from trauma or coagulopathy

Capillary leak: burns, intestinal ischemia caused by volvulus, intussusception, or necrotizing enterocolitis

Distributive Shock

Neurogenic shock: head injury, spinal cord injury

Anaphylaxis

Drug toxicity

Adrenal insufficiency: congenial adrenal hyperplasia

continued next page…

Table 1-9. Possible Etiologies of Shock (Continued)

Cardiogenic Shock
Congenital heart lesions
Myocardial dysfunction (systolic or diastolic): ischemic heart disease (Kawasaki disease), cardiomyopathies
Dysrhythmia: supraventricular tachycardia
Metabolic disorders
Drug poisoning
Septic Shock
Bacterial
Viral
Fungal
Rickettsial
Parasitic
Obstructive Shock
Aortic stenosis, coarctation of the aorta or other left-heart obstructive lesion (children <6 months)
Unrecognized pneumothorax
Cardiac tamponade
Pulmonary embolism

1. Hypovolemic Shock

Case Study

A previously healthy 4-month-old girl presents to the emergency department with a 4-day history of vomiting, loose watery stools, and low-grade fever. She became lethargic 24 hours earlier and has refused to drink water or tea offered by her grandmother.

- What is the etiology of shock in this scenario?

- What is lethargy a sign of?

- What are other signs of shock that you might expect to find?

The most common cause of shock in the pediatric patient is acute hypovolemia resulting from increased fluid and electrolyte losses (gastrointestinal disorders) or blood loss resulting from severe trauma. A detailed medical history should be obtained from the patient's caregiver and/or referring institution. A history of increased fluid losses (vomiting and diarrhea), lethargy, and decreased urine output is found in infants with hypovolemic shock. Blood pressure is maintained longer in hypovolemic children than in adults, and, as previously stated, blood pressure is not a clear indicator of the status of perfusion. Capillary refill and temperature of extremities are much more reliable indicators of hypovolemia because they may become abnormal much earlier than blood pressure in the child with shock. The primary treatment of hypovolemic shock is appropriate intravascular fluid volume resuscitation (see **Chapter 7**).

2. Cardiogenic Shock

Case Study

A 3-month-old girl with a history of a ventricular septal defect is sent from the pediatrician's office to the radiology suite for a chest radiograph. She presented with a 1-week history of progressive tachypnea, diaphoresis, weight loss, and decreased urine output. Her mother indicates that she had run out of medication. Examination reveals that the child is grunting, tachypneic, and diaphoretic. She has a loud precordial murmur and an enlarged liver.

- What studies should you perform to confirm your diagnosis?

- What interventions are required?

- What clinical signs would indicate a response to therapy?

Congestive heart failure in children is most often due to underlying congenital heart anomalies and often precedes low cardiac output syndrome. This can often be the result of acute or chronic changes in the heart's preload, afterload, contractility, or rate and rhythm. Signs and symptoms vary depending on the type of lesion (see **Chapter 18**). Infants with ductal dependent lesions will typically present in profound shock and have a history of poor feeding, tachypnea, lethargy, cyanosis, thready or absent femoral pulses, and poor or absent urine output (obstructive shock). Patients with non–ductal dependent lesions can present with a history of tachycardia, gallop rhythm, heart murmur, tachypnea, hepatomegaly, and failure to thrive. These patients will often respond to diuresis with a loop diuretic and to inotropic support and/or afterload reduction rather than fluid resuscitation (see **Chapter 18**). Early transfer to a PICU for further monitoring, inotropic support, and a complete evaluation by a pediatric cardiologist is recommended. Other common etiologies of cardiogenic shock include hypoxic-ischemic episodes after acute life-threatening events, near drowning, or strangulation.

3. Distributive Shock

Case Study

A 4-year-old boy has been admitted to the ward with a diagnosis of uncomplicated pneumonia. Ten minutes after receiving the first dose of IV antibiotic, he starts complaining of tightness of his chest and not feeling well. Upon arrival to his bedside, he is unresponsive with labored breathing and audible wheezing. He appears flushed, has an urticarial rash, and swollen eyes. He is warm, tachycardic, and has bounding pulses. His blood pressure is 80/20 mm Hg.

- What is the etiology of shock in this scenario?

- What would be your immediate response?

Distributive shock occurs as a result of an abnormality of vasomotor tone. This has the effect of redistributing blood volume and flow to the periphery causing a relative hypovolemia. In essence, the intravascular space has increased in size without an increase in intravascular volume. Patients appear flushed and have warm extremities with bounding pulses. Patients are typically tachycardic with a wide pulse pressure and brisk capillary refill. In anaphylaxis, there is release of histamine from the mast cells and basophils in the lung and gastrointestinal tract. The signs of anaphylaxis include wheezing, respiratory distress, urticaria, vomiting, swelling of the face and tongue, and hypotension. Subcutaneous epinephrine is the treatment of choice, along with antihistamines and systemic corticosteroids. In neurogenic shock, there is a loss of sympathetic tone, which results in decreased peripheral vasomotor tone. There is also vasodilatation without a compensatory rise in heart rate, as opposed to tachycardia, which is found with other forms of shock. This condition is resistant to fluid resuscitation but is responsive to appropriate α-adrengeric agents.

4. Septic Shock

Case Study

A 5-year-old boy is brought into the PICU from a referring hospital where he presented 5 days ago with fever, swelling of the left knee, and redness. He was treated with ceftriaxone and acetaminophen. He became oliguric, tachycardiac, and hypothermic, and received 500 milliliters of normal saline prior to transfer. On arrival to the PICU he is found to be lethargic, hypothermic, hypotensive, and tachycardiac.

- What type of septic shock is this patient in?

- What other ancillary tests might be useful in determining end organ perfusion?

- After receiving 100 mL/kg of crystalloid IV fluids, what other studies might you want to do to guide your ongoing management?

> ! *Tachycardia is a normal response to any stress in infants and children.*

The pathopysiology of septic shock is complex and exhibits the features of hypovolemic, distributive and cardiogenic shock. It is characterized by changes in mental status, fever or hypothermia, and perfusion abnormalities such as vasodilatation (warm shock) or vasoconstriction (cold shock). The presentation of septic shock is dependent on the timing of presentation, the infectious agent and host response. Cold shock reflects a low cardiac output state with poor peripheral perfusion and high systemic vascular resistance. These patients will present with tachycardia, prolonged capillary refill, mottled skin and weak pulses. In warm shock there is low systemic vascular resistance and high cardiac output. The clinical presentation of warm shock is vasodilatation, tachycardia, bounding pulses, brisk capillary refill and widened pulse pressure.

The therapeutic goal in septic shock is to restore and maintain optimal organ perfusion. Restoration of the patient's mental status and urine output (1 mL/kg/h) is an acceptable goal. Children in shock are usually severely hypovolemic and will respond to aggressive fluid resuscitation (see **Chapter 7**). Maintaining an optimal hemoglobin concentration for the patient's age is desirable for patients in shock (minimum 10 g/dL). Vasoactive agents are indicated in fluid-refractory shock, and administration of corticosteroids should be considered in catecholamine-refractory shock. Infants with sepsis are often profoundly hypoglycemic on presentation, and glucose determinations should be performed on all infants with suspected sepsis.

> !
>
> *In cases of shock it is desirable to maintain an optimal hemoglobin concentration for the patient's age (minimum 10 g/dL).*

5. Obstructive Shock

Case Study

A 2-week-old girl arrives by ambulance to the emergency department from her home, where she was found to be apneic by her father. She was intubated at the scene. On arrival, her heart rate is 200/min and her blood pressure is 40/20 mm Hg in her right arm. She is pale and hypothermic with no palpable pulses in her lower extremities.

- What is the etiology of shock in this scenario?
- What other ancillary tests would you perform?
- What medication should you immediately administer?

Patients presenting with obstructive shock will exhibit a rapid and often precipitous deterioration of their hemodynamic status. In infants, congenital lesions that interfere with outflow from the left ventricle, such as coarctation of the aorta or interrupted aortic arch, are common causes of obstructive shock. These infants develop signs of shock when the ductus arteriosus closes, thus interfering with the delivery of cardiac output to the distal aorta. A history of poor feeding, lethargy, decreased or absent urine output, decreased or absent femoral pulses, and metabolic acidosis is frequent. Inotropic support and a prostaglandin infusion should be initiated rapidly to reopen the ductus arteriosus and restore perfusion to the distal aorta in infants and children with suspected left-heart lesions. Administration of this medication should not be delayed to await a confirmatory echocardiogram.

> !
>
> *Administration of a prostaglandin should not be delayed to await a confirmatory echocardiogram.*

V. NERVOUS SYSTEM

Case Study

A 3-month-old girl with history of colic is brought into the emergency department by her mother's boyfriend after the infant apparently fell from her crib to the floor. On physical examination, she is unresponsive to stimulation. She has multiple bruises to the head, chest, and abdomen. Eye examination reveals retinal hemorrhages. A head computed tomographic scan reveals a subdural blood collection on the left parietal area, and a chest radiograph shows rib fractures. The caregiver is interviewed.

- Are the clinical findings consistent with the history provided?

- How would you describe this child's neurological status?

This child is a victim of abuse and has sustained a closed head injury as a result of nonaccidental head trauma. The Glasgow Coma Scale (GCS) is frequently used to evaluate a child's neurological status and level of consciousness. The GCS is difficult to apply in children, even when it is adapted for age (see **Table 16-1**). When assessing the need for further intervention, careful attention should be paid to the patient's ability to maintain the airway, the pupillary responses, the motor score, and, in infants, the fontanelle status. The pupillary response is used to rapidly evaluate brainstem function, but abnormalities in pupillary response, such as miosis and mydriasis, may also be found in many toxidromes as a result of poisoning. Other pertinent physical signs that should be assessed include muscle tone, muscle strength and power, facial symmetry, ataxia, and any abnormal movements of extremities and facial musculature.

> **!** *Hyponatremia, hypoglycemia, and hypocalcemia should be considered in infants and children presenting with seizures or altered mental status.*

In infants, seizures may be characterized by decreased alertness (the infant does not regard parents or track an object across the visual field), autonomic changes (tachycardia, elevated blood pressure, and dilated pupils), apnea, and subcortical muscle activity (bicycling movements of the legs, swimming movements of the arms, sucking, or tongue thrusting). Tonic-clonic muscle motion may not occur during seizures in infants because neurons and their connections have not fully developed. Hyponatremia and hypoglycemia should be considered in infants and small children presenting with coma and/or seizures. Hypocalcemia will cause seizures in infants and is commonly associated with tetany.

Any young child with a depressed level of consciousness, seizures, and/or coma should be evaluated for the possibility of occult trauma (eg, child abuse, especially shaken baby syndrome), even if there are no outward signs of injury. Infectious, metabolic, or toxic etiologies should also be considered.

VI. SEPSIS

Fever always suggests the possibility of serious bacterial disease. In the neonate, infections usually involve the bloodstream, although respiratory distress, temperature instability (including hypothermia), and gastrointestinal signs are frequent clinical findings of sepsis. The neonatal population is especially vulnerable, and the following factors increase their risk of infection:

- Decreased polymorphonuclear white cell function and storage reservoir
- Poor ability for antibody synthesis
- Reduced delivery of phagocytes to inflammatory sites
- Passive maternal immunity is depleted by 2 to 5 months after birth, and levels of immunoglobulin comparable to adult levels are not reached until 4 to 7 years of age

External signs other than fever should be sought. An exanthema or rash is often seen, and its characteristics, color, and distribution pattern may be specific to a particular infection. Examples of such exanthemas would be petechiae or purpura suggestive of meningococcemia, vesicular lesions indicative of herpes simplex or coxsackie viral infections, or erythematous rash with evidence of peeling secondary to staphylococcal or streptococcal infections.

Due to their incompletely developed immune systems, children are treated with empiric antibiotic therapy more frequently than are adults. For the same reason, antibiotics are considered emergency drugs, particularly for febrile infants under 2 months of age. Under the age of 3 years, the risk of occult bacteremia is increased if temperature is >40°C (>104°F) or white blood cell count is <500 cells/mm^3 or >15000 cells/mm^3. Absolute neutrophil count <1,000 cells/mm^3 or significant bands of 25% to 30% are also markers of severe bacterial infection in children. In such situations, a full workup is recommended and should include blood culture, urine culture, and lumbar puncture, if clinically indicated. Definitions for sepsis and organ dysfunction in pediatric patients (**Table 8-1**) are discussed at length in **Chapter 8.**

The features unique to the care of infants and children, as discussed in this chapter, severely limit the margin for error in the treatment of critically ill or injured pediatric patients. Therefore, specialty consultation should be requested early.

Key Points

Assessment of the Critically Ill Child

- A question that should be asked and answered in every healthcare provider's mind is, "Does this child look sick?" If the answer is yes, it is likely that the child is critically ill.
- Irritability is an early sign of a change in the mental status of young children.
- Children should always be examined in the position that they spontaneously assume for comfort. Forcing a child into a different position may worsen respiratory distress and even precipitate respiratory arrest.
- Early signs of respiratory distress in children include tachypnea, grunting, and nasal flaring.
- Ensuring a patent airway is the most important initial step in treating a child with respiratory compromise. Chest movement does not ensure a patent airway.
- A child's perfusion status is best assessed initially by capillary refill and temperature of extremities. Hypotension is a late finding in shock. Timely recognition of the shock state and aggressive intervention are essential to obtaining an optimal outcome.
- Intracranial hemorrhage in the young infant can cause hemodynamically significant blood loss.
- Infants and young children presenting with seizures should be evaluated for electrolyte imbalances and hypoglycemia.
- Young infants face an increased risk of infection due to their immature immune systems. Empiric antibiotics are considered emergency drugs for febrile infants younger than 2 months.

Suggested Readings

1. Carcillo JA, Fields AI, et al. Clinical practice parameters for hemodynamic support of pediatric and neonatal patients in septic shock. *Crit Care Med.* 2002;30:1365-1378.

2. Epstein D, Wetzel RC. Cardiovascular physiology and shock. In: Nichols DG, Ungerleider RM, Spevak PJ, et al, eds. *Critical Heart Disease in Infants and Children.* 2nd ed. Philadelphia, PA: Mosby Elsevier; 2006:17-72.

3. Goldstein B, Giroir B, Randolph A; and International Consensus Conference on Pediatric Sepsis. Definitions for sepsis and organ dysfunction in pediatrics. *Pediatr Crit Care Med.* 2005;6:2-8.

4. Hazinski M. Children are different. In: Hazinski M, ed. *Manual of Pediatric Critical Care.* 1st ed. St Louis, MO: CV Mosby; 1999:1-13.

5. Smith L, Hernan L. Shock states. In: Fuhrman BP, Zimmerman JJ, eds. *Pediatric Critical Care.* 3rd ed. St Louis, MO: CV Mosby; 2006:394-410.

6. Thompson AE. Pediatric airway management. In: Fuhrman BP, Zimmerman JJ, eds. *Pediatric Critical Care.* 3rd ed. St Louis, MO: CV Mosby; 2006:485-509.

7. Wood EG, Lynch RE. Electrolyte management in pediatric critical illness. In: Fuhrman BP, Zimmerman JJ, eds. *Pediatric Critical Care.* 3rd ed. St Louis, MO: CV Mosby; 2006:939-957.

Chapter 2:

Airway Management

Objectives

- Recognize signs and symptoms of an unstable airway.
- Recognize signs and symptoms of respiratory failure.
- Identify anatomic and physiologic variables involved in the management of the pediatric airway.
- Describe how to open and maintain an airway manually and with the help of airway adjuncts.
- Explain how to support a patient with bag-mask ventilation.
- Describe the preparation for and the sequence of intubating pediatric patients.
- Recognize the potential for difficult intubation and discuss alternative methods of establishing a stable airway.

Case Study

You are called to the bedside of a 7-month-old boy with respiratory syncytial virus bronchiolitis who has developed worsening retractions and desaturations over the last hour. You make the decision to intubate the patient.

- What signs and symptoms indicate airway instability?

- What interventions may be attempted to maintain the airway prior to deciding to intubate?

- What steps must be taken to ensure that intubation is as safe as possible?

I. INTRODUCTION

Respiratory distress due to problems at all levels of the respiratory tract, from the nose to the lungs, is a frequent occurrence in children. Respiratory failure is a common component of critical illness in children. The majority of cardiopulmonary arrests in children are heralded by respiratory failure.

> !
>
> *The ability to recognize airway compromise and to establish and maintain a patent airway is essential.*
>
> !

Airway management is challenging due to the anatomic differences that exist between children and adults as well as among children of different ages. Recognition and interruption of the progression from respiratory compromise to respiratory failure is fundamental to pediatric airway management. The ability to recognize airway compromise and to establish and maintain a patent airway is essential.

II. ANATOMIC AND PHYSIOLOGIC CONSIDERATIONS

The airway of a child changes dramatically from birth to adulthood. In order to assess and manage airway emergencies it is necessary to understand certain anatomic and developmental aspects of a child's airway. Some key developmental differences among infants, children, and adults are summarized below:

> !
>
> *Clearing the nasal passages by suctioning can significantly improve an infant's respiratory condition.*
>
> !

- In children, the nose provides nearly half of the total airway resistance. The infant's nose is short, soft, and small with nearly circular nares. Infants under 2 months of age are obligate nasal breathers. Although the nares double in size from birth to 6 months, they can be easily occluded by edema, secretions, or external pressure. Clearing the nasal passages by suctioning can significantly improve an infant's respiratory condition.

- A child's tongue is large in relation to the oral cavity. This relative disproportion is increased in developmental disorders such as Pierre Robin sequence and severe micrognathism. A large tongue in a relatively small oral cavity increases the difficulty of visualizing the larynx during laryngoscopy. Backward displacement of the tongue into the posterior pharynx as a result of decreased muscle tone due to sleep, depressed level of consciousness from head injury, sedation, or other nervous system dysfunction can result in upper airway obstruction.

- The level of the larynx in the neck changes from C2 in neonates to C3 to C4 in children and ends up at C5 to C6 in adults. The epiglottis in infants is at the level of the first cervical vertebrae and overlaps the soft palate. The high position of the larynx, combined with a large tongue and a small mandible, contributes to an infant's susceptibility to airway obstruction.

- Due to the high position of the larynx in infants and small children, the angle between the base of the tongue and the glottic opening is more acute, which increases the difficulty of visualizing the vocal cords during laryngoscopy. Therefore, a straight laryngoscope blade, such as a Miller, may be superior for creating a straight plane from the mouth to the glottis.

■ An infant's epiglottis is long, soft, and omega (Ω) shaped, whereas an adult's epiglottis is shorter, more rigid, and flatter. A longer and softer epiglottis is more difficult to control during laryngoscopy.

- Using a straight laryngoscope blade, which lifts the epiglottis and exposes the vocal cords, can overcome this difficulty.

■ A pediatric larynx is funnel shaped, with the subglottic portion angled posterior to the supraglottic portion. Consequently the narrowest portion of the larynx is in the subglottic space. An adult's larynx is barrel shaped, with the narrowest portion at the level of the vocal cords.

> **!**
>
> *A pediatric larynx is funnel shaped; the narrowest portion of the larynx is the cricoid cartilage. An adult larynx is barrel shaped; the narrowest portion is the vocal cords.*
>
> **!**

■ The internal diameter of a pediatric trachea is approximately one-third that of an adult, resulting in higher airflow resistance. Resistance to airflow is a function of $1/r^4$, where r is the airway radius. A small decrease in airway diameter (2 × radius) due to edema or secretions causes a far greater increase in resistance in a child than in an adult.

■ The length of a newborn's trachea is approximately 5 centimeters, and the trachea of an 18-month-old infant is approximately 7 centimeters long. Given the short length of the trachea, both right main-stem bronchus intubation and accidental extubation are common.

■ The chest wall of infants is relatively weak and unstable.

- The use of abdominal muscles leads to a characteristic see-saw, or abdominal, breathing pattern.

- Intercostal, subcostal, and suprasternal retractions become prominent as airway obstruction or lung disease increases work of breathing.

- Fatigue of respiratory muscles may lead to decreased respiratory effort as respiratory failure progresses.

III. ASSESSING RESPIRATORY STATUS

In children, as in adults, assessment of airway patency and spontaneous respiratory effort is a crucial first step. The clinician must recognize signs of distress as well as look, listen, and feel for diminished or absent air movement.

A. General Principles of Airway Assessment

Observe the general appearance of the child with careful attention to

- Muscle tone and spontaneous and reactive movement
- Alertness/interaction with environment or caregiver
- Inconsolable crying or agitation
- Ability to speak or cry (phonation and crying require air movement)
- Injury to the airway or other conditions (eg, cervical spine fracture or facial burns) that will affect assessment and manipulation of the airway
- Signs of congenital malformations of the face, mouth, or tongue that might contribute to respiratory problems
- It is possible that ventilation may be adequate with minimal thoracic excursion but that respiratory muscle activity and even vigorous chest movement do not ensure that tidal volume is adequate
- Signs of airway obstruction due to decreased level of consciousness

Assess the child's respiratory rate based on the following facts:

- Normal respiratory rate varies with age (**Table 2-1**).

Table 2-1. Age-Normal Respiratory Rates

Age	Respiratory Rate (Breaths per Minute)
Newborn	30-60
6 months	25-40
1-3 years	20-30
6 years	18-25
10 years	15-20

- Respiratory rate is best assessed by observation: expose child's chest and watch the rise and fall of the chest and abdomen.
- A respiratory rate greater than 60 breaths per minute is abnormal in a child of any age.
- An abnormally slow rate may herald respiratory failure.

Consider work of breathing.

- Intercostal, subcostal, and suprasternal retractions increase with progressive respiratory distress. Decreasing respiratory rate and diminished retractions in a child with a history of distress may signal severe fatigue.
- Increased inspiratory effort often amplifies airway resistance, causing collapse of the compliant upper airway and producing stridor.

> **!** *A respiratory rate greater than 60 breaths per minute is abnormal in a child of any age.* **!**

- Nasal flaring is an effort to increase airway diameter and is often seen with hypoxemia.
- Grunting is an expiratory noise produced by an effort to prevent airway collapse by generating positive end-expiratory pressure (PEEP).

Auscultate over the mouth, nose, and neck as well as the central and peripheral chest. Listen for quality, pitch, right-to-left symmetry and magnitude of breath sounds.

- Obstruction or narrowing of the extrathoracic airway (nose, posterior pharynx, larynx, and subglottic space) causes high-pitched inspiratory noise (stridor) and retractions.
- Obstruction or narrowing of the intrathoracic airways results in signs and symptoms that occur predominantly during expiration. Wheezing (high-pitched expiratory sounds) is caused by expiratory obstruction.
- Incomplete obstruction (during which a limited amount of air can be inspired and expired from the lungs) due to pharyngeal soft-tissue collapse, a mass, or a foreign body in the airway may be associated with snoring, stridor, gurgling, or noisy breathing.
- Complete airway obstruction (during which no air can be inspired or expired from the lungs) is likely when respiratory effort is visible but breath sounds are absent.
- Crackles are end-inspiratory noises usually heard with parenchymal lung diseases such as pneumonia and bronchiolitis and are loudest in the peripheral lung fields.
- Asymmetry of breath sounds is an important clue. Breath sounds may be diminished or absent on one side in the presence of pneumothorax or pleural effusion or when a tracheal tube is placed in the opposite main bronchus.

Evaluate mental status.

- Agitation and irritability may indicate hypoxemia. Lethargy in the presence of acceptable oxygen saturation may reflect a very elevated carbon dioxide tension.
- Assess presence and strength of protective airway reflexes (ie, cough and gag). Use caution because overly aggressive stimulation of the posterior pharynx while assessing those reflexes may precipitate emesis and aspiration of gastric contents. Moreover, stimulation of the posterior pharynx may convert partial upper airway obstruction due to illnesses such as epiglottitis to complete airway obstruction.

> ! *Agitation and irritability may indicate hypoxemia.* !

If respiratory efforts are absent and an immediate remedy is not available, proceed to manual support and assisted ventilation while preparing to establish an artificial airway.

IV. MONITORING RESPIRATORY FUNCTION

A. Longitudinal Physical Assessment

Once a patient is found to be in respiratory distress, frequent, repeated assessments are necessary to look for improvements resulting from intervention or for continuing clinical deterioration that necessitates further action. Constant vigilance is required once a patient is intubated and placed on a mechanical ventilator. Auscultation and observation are important tools for monitoring respiratory function.

B. Arterial Blood Gas

Arterial blood gas measurement may be helpful when either the etiology or the degree of respiratory insufficiency is unknown. Careful consideration should be given, however, to the fact that arterial puncture is a painful procedure. The agitation induced by arterial puncture might worsen the respiratory distress of some children.

A systematic approach to arterial blood gas interpretation consists of

- Determining the degree of alveolar ventilation based on the $Pa{CO_2}$
- Assessing whether the patient's pH can be explained solely on the basis of $Pa{CO_2}$ or if a metabolic component exists
- Determining whether the ventilatory or metabolic event was primary or compensatory

- Assessing the effectiveness of correction of any hypoxemic state
- Arterial blood gas disorders are classified into 4 main categories: hypoventilation, alveolar hyperventilation, metabolic acidosis, and metabolic alkalosis.

1. Hypoventilation

Hypoventilation (respiratory acidosis) results in an elevation of PCO_2 which, causes the HCO_3^-:PCO_2 ratio to decrease and results in a decrease in pH. Carbon dioxide retention can be caused by hypoventilation or a ventilation-perfusion inequality. Increasing ventilation in most cases will correct respiratory acidosis. If the patient is unstable, manual bag-mask ventilation is indicated until the underlying problem can be addressed.

If respiratory acidosis persists (as seen in chronic ventilatory failure), the kidneys respond by conserving HCO_3^-. Renal compensation is typically not complete, and so the pH approaches but does not fully return to 7.4.

2. Alveolar Hyperventilation

Alveolar hyperventilation (respiratory alkalosis) results in a decreased PCO_2, which in turn elevates the pH. Bicarbonate and base excess remain in the normal range because the kidneys have not had time to establish adequate compensation. Pain and anxiety may cause acute hyperventilation and alkalosis in children. Hypoxemia may lead to increased minute ventilation and respiratory alkalosis.

3. Metabolic Acidosis

A primary decrease in bicarbonate in turn leads to a decreased pH. Bicarbonate can be lowered by accumulation of acids in the blood, as in uncontrolled diabetes mellitus, and production of lactic acid in the setting of tissue hypoxia. Respiratory compensation occurs by an increase in ventilation that lowers the PCO_2 and in turn raises pH.

Respiratory insufficiency in the presence of metabolic acidosis is concerning due to the degree acidosis that results when a patient is unable to increase ventilation.

4. Metabolic Alkalosis

An increase in HCO_3^- raises the HCO_3^-:PCO_2 ratio and thus the pH. Compensation occurs by hypoventilation and CO_2 retention. Metabolic alkalosis is seen in the child with pyloric stenosis who loses large amounts of stomach acid due to vomiting. The ability of the child to compensate for metabolic alkalosis by hypoventilation is limited by hypoxia.

For additional information, please see **Appendix 3.**

C. Pulse Oximetry

Pulse oximetry provides continuous, noninvasive measurement of arterial oxyhemoglobin saturation (Sao_2). Figure 2-1 shows the oxyhemoglobin saturation curve, which is a graph of oxyhemoglobin saturation versus partial pressure of oxygen (Pao_2). Under normal conditions, hemoglobin is 90% saturated with oxygen at a Pao_2 of about 60 mm Hg (8.0 kPa). Raising the Pao_2 above 60 mm Hg does not result in an appreciable increase in hemoglobin saturation. However, due to the sigmoidal shape of the oxyhemoglobin saturation curve, once the Pao_2 drops below 60 mm Hg, the saturation changes rapidly with small changes in Pao_2.

Figure 2-1. Oxyhemoglobin Saturation Curve

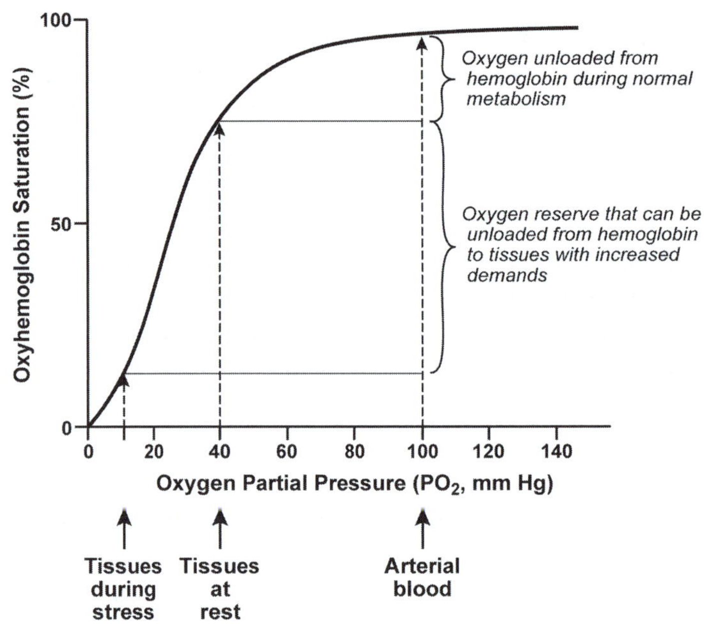

The oxyhemoglobin dissociation curve relates the partial pressure of oxygen (PO_2) to oxyhemoglobin saturation. Near-maximal saturation of hemoglobin occurs at a PO_2 of 60 mm Hg (8.0 kPa). PO_2 values above this point provide only a modest increase in oxyhemoglobin saturation. Note, however, that a rapid decrease in oxyhemoglobin saturation occurs when the PO_2 drops below 60 mm Hg (8.0 kPa). Reproduced with permission from Mayo Clinic.

The limitations to pulse oximetry that are relevant in managing critically ill patients include the following:

- Pulse oximetry requires pulsatile blood flow. In the presence of shock and poor perfusion, the accuracy and signal strength become unreliable.
- In carbon monoxide poisoning, most pulse oximeters will read falsely high for oxyhemoglobin saturation. The inaccuracy occurs because carboxyhemoglobin absorbs light at a similar wavelength as oxyhemoglobin. Blood gas measurement with co-oximetry is the only way to determine the true oxyhemoglobin and carboxyhemoglobin saturations.

> !
>
> *Normally, hemoglobin is 90% saturated with oxygen at a Pao2 of about 60 mm Hg (8.0 kPa). Raising the Pao2 above 60 mm Hg does not result in an appreciable increase in hemoglobin saturation.*

- Pulse oximetry is not accurate in methemoglobinemia.
- Oxygen saturation may be underestimated in patients with sickle cell disease and acute vasoocclusive crisis.
- Intravenous dyes and certain colors of nail polish falsely lower pulse oximetry readings.
- The accuracy of the pulse oximeter should be questioned when a patient's appearance and heart rate do not correlate with the pulse oximeter reading.
- It is always safer to question elevated saturations and accept decreased saturations as accurate until proven otherwise.

D. Exhaled Carbon Dioxide

End-tidal CO_2 monitoring can be used to estimate the arterial CO_2 tension. Quantitative continuous capnography can be performed via nasal cannula or with devices that attach to the tracheal tube. Qualitative (colorometric) devices are available that change color when exhaled CO_2 is present. These are generally used for confirmation of tracheal tube placement and are discussed later in this chapter.

In the presence of ventilation-perfusion mismatch, airway obstruction, or tracheal tube leak, end-tidal CO_2 values may not accurately reflect true arterial CO_2 levels.

V. AIRWAY MANAGEMENT

A. Oxygen-Delivery Systems

Oxygen should be administered immediately in virtually every setting where respiratory difficulty is suspected. Infants and children consume 2 to 3 times more oxygen per kilogram of body weight than adults under basal conditions and even more when they are ill or stressed. Several key points regarding administration of oxygen to children are as follows:

- When attempting to administer oxygen to an alert child it is important to balance the need to increase oxygen delivery against the potential effect of promoting agitation, thus increasing oxygen consumption.
- If a child is intolerant of one method of oxygen delivery (eg, nasal cannula), another method should be tried (eg, face tent). It is often helpful to have a parent hold the child and assist with placement of O_2 delivery devices.
- Children will often assume a position that maximizes airway patency and minimizes respiratory effort. They should be allowed to remain in their position of comfort.

- Oxygen administration will have limited effect in the presence of airway obstruction. In a somnolent or obtunded child the airway can be obstructed due to neck flexion, relaxation of the jaw, posterior displacement of the tongue against the pharynx, and collapse of the hypopharynx. Before using airway adjuncts, attempt to open the airway using manual methods. The airway should be cleared of secretions to optimize the patient's effort.

- In patients who are making respiratory efforts but are not moving an adequate amount of air, spontaneous respiratory efforts can be assisted with a bag-mask device. These patients can then be transitioned to noninvasive or invasive forms of ventilation.

> !
> *Oxygen should be administered when respiratory difficulty is suspected.*
> !

See **Appendix 4** for additional discussion on airway adjuncts.

1. Simple Oxygen Mask

The simple oxygen mask is a low-flow device that delivers oxygen with a flow rate of 6 to 10 liters per minute. The oxygen concentration delivered to the patient can reach a maximum of 60% due to entrainment of room air through the exhalation ports of the mask. It is important to maintain an oxygen flow rate of at least 6 liters per minute to sustain an optimal inspired oxygen concentration and prevent rebreathing of exhaled carbon dioxide.

2. Partial Rebreathing Mask

A partial rebreathing mask consists of a simple face mask with a reservoir bag. It provides oxygen concentrations of 50% to 60%. During inspiration the patient draws gas predominantly from the fresh oxygen inflow and the reservoir bag, so entrainment of room air through the exhalation ports is minimized. An oxygen flow rate of 10 to 12 liters per minute is usually required.

3. Non-rebreathing Mask

A non-rebreathing mask consists of a face mask and reservoir bag with a valve incorporated into one or both exhalation ports to prevent entrainment of room air during inspiration. Another valve between the reservoir bag and the mask prevents flow of exhaled gas into the reservoir. An inspired concentration of 95% can be achieved with an oxygen flow rate of 10 to 15 liters per minute and use of a well-sealed mask.

4. Face Tent

A face tent is a high-flow soft plastic bucket that children often tolerate better than a face mask. Even with a high oxygen flow rate, inspired oxygen concentrations over 40% cannot be reliably provided. A face tent permits access to the face without interrupting oxygen flow.

5. Nasal Cannula

A nasal cannula is a low-flow oxygen delivery system that is useful when low levels of supplemental oxygen are required. The net FIO_2 depends on the child's respiratory effort, size, and minute ventilation in comparison with the nasal cannula flow.

B. Maneuvers to Open and Maintain the Airway

The airway has oral, pharyngeal, and tracheal components. Maximal opening of the airway is obtained by aligning the oral, pharyngeal, and tracheal axes as shown in **Figure 2-2.** Children younger than 2 years have relatively large heads for their body size, which results in slight neck flexion when they are in the supine position. Children in this age group usually benefit from a small roll placed under the shoulders that allows the head to fall back into proper position. A thin towel or blanket is usually sufficient for this purpose. Care must be taken to avoid overextension of the neck, which will result in obstruction. In older children a small roll under the back of the head helps facilitate proper alignment of the axes.

Figure 2-2. Aligning the Oral, Pharyngeal, and Tracheal Axes

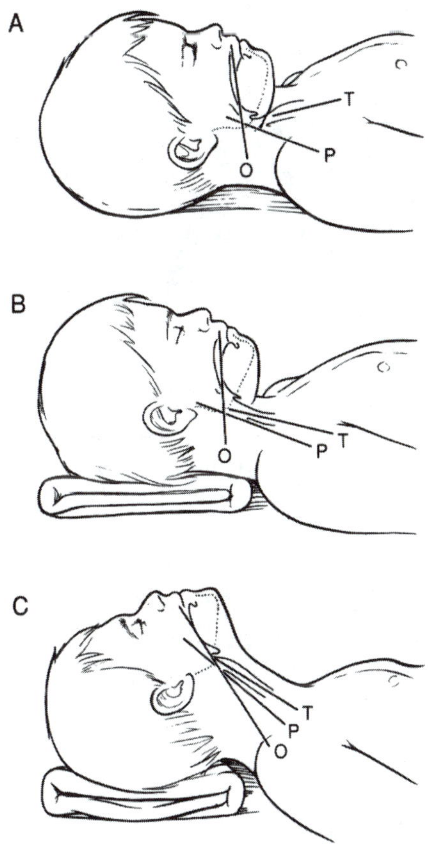

A, Maximal opening and visualization of the airway is obtained by aligning the oral (O), pharyngeal (P), and tracheal (T) axes. This is accomplished by placing a patient in the sniffing position. B, A folded sheet or towel placed under the occiput aligns the pharyngeal and tracheal axes. C, Extension of the neck into the sniffing position then results in approximate alignment of all 3 axes. Proper positioning places the external ear canal anterior to the shoulder. In children younger than 2 years, a folded towel or sheet is placed under the shoulder rather than under the occiput due to the relatively large forehead-to-occiput distance in this age group. Reproduced with permission of the American Heart Association ©2006.

Partial or complete airway obstruction caused by pharyngeal soft tissue collapse or posterior movement of the tongue can usually be relieved by manual maneuvers. These include positioning the patient to maximize airway patency and manipulating the jaw and head to open the airway. The first and simplest intervention is the jaw-thrust maneuver illustrated in **Figure 2-3.** The clinician's fingers are placed along the posterior rami of the mandible and the mandible is lifted upward or forward. The jaw-thrust maneuver can be performed safely in a patient with a suspected cervical spine injury because neck alignment is not altered. Often, a jaw thrust alone will reverse oxygen desaturation that occurs during deep sedation.

Figure 2-3. Jaw-Thrust Maneuver

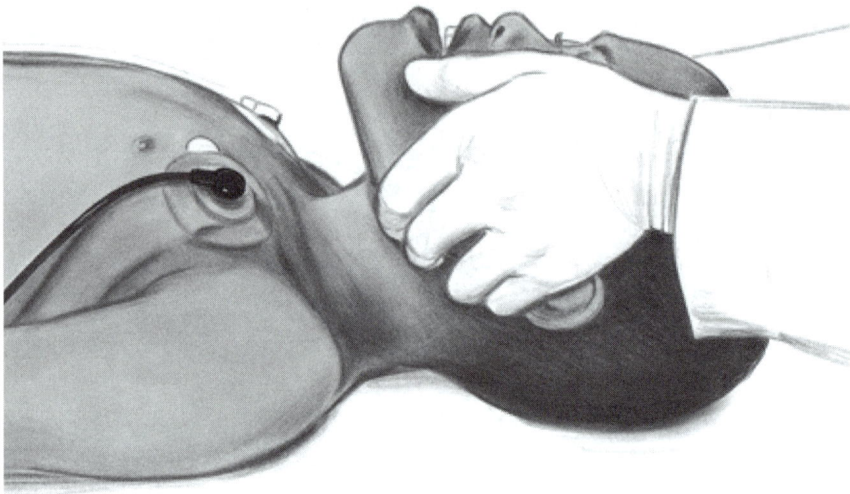

Place fingers on the posterior rami of both mandibles and lift in an anterior direction.
Reproduced with permission of the American Heart Association ©2006.

A complementary maneuver for opening an obstructed airway is the chin-lift maneuver. The clinician slightly hyperextends the head on the neck to place the patient in the sniffing position. In this position, the ear canal is just above or even with the top of the shoulder when viewed from the side.

Jaw-thrust and chin-lift maneuvers ease obstruction in spontaneously breathing patients but should also be used when supporting a patient with bag-mask ventilation in order to provide an unobstructed airway.

When a cervical spine injury is suspected, the patient's head should remain in the neutral position at all times, by active stabilization if necessary. Lateral rotation of the head must be avoided. The potential or actual presence of cervical spine injury should not stop or prevent efforts to maintain an unobstructed airway.

> **!**
>
> *Airway obstruction caused by pharyngeal soft tissue collapse or posterior movement of the tongue can usually be relieved by a jaw-thrust or chin-lift maneuver.*

C. Oropharyngeal and Nasopharyngeal Airways

An oropharyngeal (OP) airway consists of a flange, a short bite-block segment, and a curved body usually made of plastic and shaped to provide an air channel and a suction conduit through the mouth. The curved body of the oropharyngeal airway is designed to fit over the back of the tongue to hold it and the soft hypopharyngeal structures away from the posterior wall of the pharynx. The plastic flange should rest against the outer surface of the teeth while the distal end curves around the base of the tongue. If the oropharyngeal airway is too small, it may push the tongue back over the glottic opening; if it is too large, it may stimulate gagging and emesis.

An OP airway is used only in unconscious patients. In conscious or semiconscious patients, an oropharyngeal airway will stimulate gagging, vomiting, and possibly laryngospasm. Oropharyngeal airways can be used to maintain an open airway during bag-mask ventilation. The technique for inserting an OP airway is described in **Table 2-2** and illustrated in **Figure 2-4.**

Table 2-2. Insertion of an Oropharyngeal Airway

Select the proper size airway. As shown in **Figure 2-4,** the correct size extends from the corner of the mouth to the earlobe.

If the airway is too short, it won't hold the tongue out of the way.

If it is too long, it may obstruct breathing.

- Open the patient's mouth.
- To avoid obstructing the airway with the tongue, insert the airway upside down.
- Advance the airway gently until resistance is encountered. Turn the airway 180 degrees so that it comes to rest with the flange on the patient's teeth.

Note: An alternative method, preferable in small infants, is to press the tongue down and forward with a tongue depressor. The oral airway can then be passed (in its final alignment) into position over the tongue.

A nasopharyngeal (NP) airway is a soft rubber or plastic tube that provides a conduit for airflow between the nares and the pharynx. In addition, the NP airway pushes the tongue forward, which relieves airway obstruction. The diameter of a nasopharygeal airway should be the largest that will easily pass through the nostril into the nasopharynx. Its length should extend to the nasopharynx, but it should not be so long that it obstructs gas flow through the mouth or touches the epiglottis.

Nasopharyngeal airways are less likely to stimulate vomiting and may be used on patients who are responsive but need assistance in keeping the tongue from obstructing the airway. They are especially helpful in facial and airway deformities such as Pierre-Robin syndrome.

Relative contraindications to NP airways include coagulopathy, basilar skull fracture, and nasal infection or deformity. Unlike oral airways, they may be used in conscious patients.

The technique for placing an NP airway is described in **Table 2-3** and illustrated in **Figure 2-5.**

Figure 2-4. Oral Airway Placement

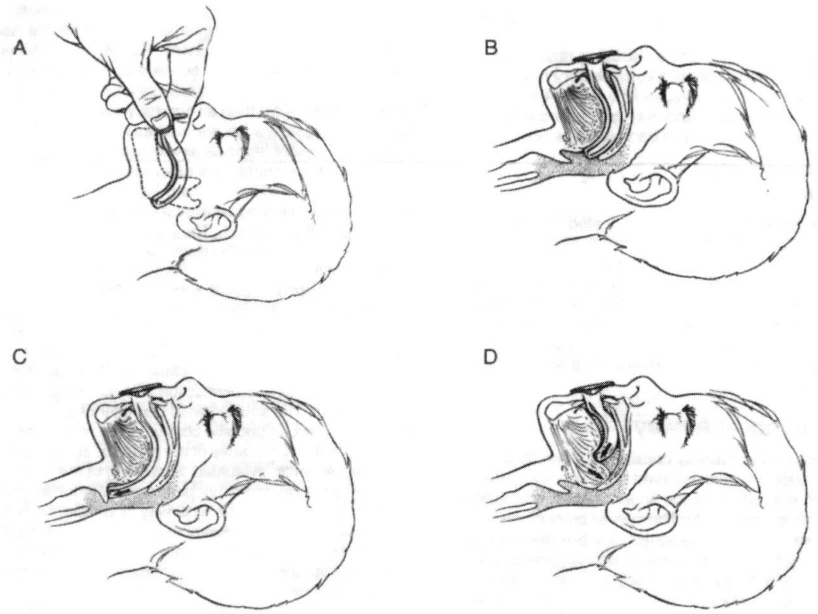

An airway of proper size will relieve obstruction caused by the tongue without damaging laryngeal structures. A, The appropriate size can be estimated by holding the airway next to the child's face. The tip of the airway should end just cephalad to the angle of the mandible. B, Example of an OP airway in correct position and its relationship to airway structures. C, If the OP airway is too big, its tip will hit the epiglottis, pushing it downward and obstructing the glottic opening. D, If the OP airway is too small, it will worsen obstruction by pushing the tongue backwards into the posterior pharynx. Reproduced with permission of the American Heart Association ©2006.

Table 2-3. Insertion of a Nasopharyngeal Airway

Choose an airway of the proper size. The length of the airway should be roughly the distance from the tip of the nose to the meatus of the ear.

Lubricate the nasopharyngeal airway with surgical lubricant.

If possible, vasoconstriction with phenylephrine nose drops (and topical anesthesia with lidocaine if the patient is awake) should precede any nasal instrumentation. However, in an acute situation, the lubricating qualities of lidocaine ointment may suffice.

The tip of the airway should be inserted perpendicularly to the face and not upward toward the cribriform plate. The bevel should point toward the base of the naris or toward the septum. If the airway cannot be inserted into one nostril, try the other.

It is helpful to listen by ear or stethoscope for air movement through the NP airway as it is placed. It is correctly positioned when airflow through the tube is present.

Once the airway is placed and secured, attention should be directed to maintaining its patency and position. An NP airway should be treated similarly to an endotracheal tube with regard to suctioning and patency. If airflow through the tube cannot be auscultated, the tube is either obstructed or malpositioned.

Note: If a commercial nasopharyngeal airway of the proper size is not available, an endotracheal tube of appropriate size can be used instead. Measure the distance from the tip of the patient's nose to the meatus of the ear and use that quantity to determine how much extra length should be cut from the tube prior to insertion.

Figure 2-5. Endotracheal Tube Used as a Nasopharyngeal Airway

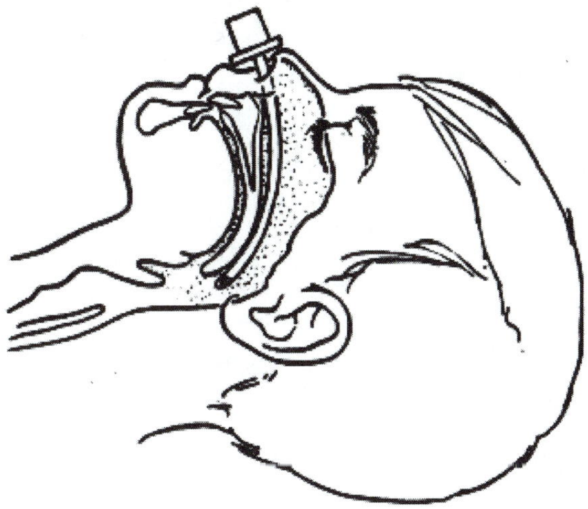

Example of an endotracheal tube used as a nasopharyngeal airway. The insertion technique is described in **Table 2-3.** Note that the 15-millimeter adapter must be inserted firmly and that the tube must be taped securely to prevent inadvertent advancement.

D. Bag-Mask Ventilation

Bag-mask ventilation is used to ventilate apneic patients and to assist patients with inadequate spontaneous ventilation. Bag-mask ventilation requires skill and practice and is challenging to perform effectively. However, if performed properly, it can be used to oxygenate and ventilate patients indefinitely, obviating the need to rush to tracheal intubation. Knowing how to provide adequate bag-mask ventilation is the most important airway skill that any healthcare provider can possess.

The 3 keys to providing adequate ventilation are to

- Maintain an open airway
- Establish a seal between the patient's face and the mask
- Deliver optimal minute ventilation from the resuscitation bag to distal lung units

Positioning the patient appropriately is an essential first step. Maintaining a jaw thrust by positioning the last 3 fingers of one hand under the bony part of the mandible will facilitate ventilation. Keep these fingers off the soft tissue below the mandible to avoid occluding the airway. It may be necessary to move the patient's head and neck gently through a variety of positions to determine the optimum position for airway patency and effective ventilation. A neutral sniffing position without hyperextension is appropriate for infants and toddlers.

The technique for bag-mask ventilation is illustrated in **Figure 2-6.** The hand position is called the E-C clamp technique. The thumb and forefinger form a C shape and exert downward pressure on the mask while the remaining fingers of the same hand, forming an E, lift the jaw and pull the face toward the mask. This should create a tight seal. Once the mask is correctly applied, the other hand is used to compress the bag with until the chest rises. It is better to lift the patient's face into the mask than to push the mask onto the patient's face.

Figure 2-6. Bag-Mask Ventilation

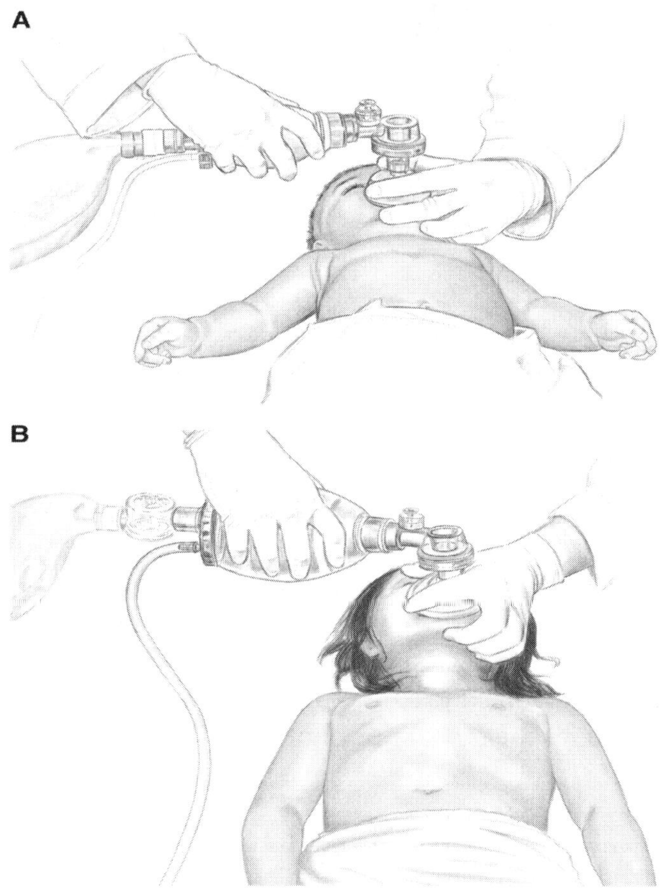

Note the E-C clamp technique as described in the text. Reproduced with permission of the American Heart Association ©2006.

Gentle cricoid pressure (**see Figure 2-7**) applied by another rescuer may reduce gastric inflation and decrease the risk of aspiration during bagging. Cricoid pressure should be used only in an unconscious victim. Excessive pressure on the cricoid cartilage should be avoided; only 1 finger is necessary in a young child or infant.

Figure 2-7. Cricoid Pressure (Sellick Maneuver)

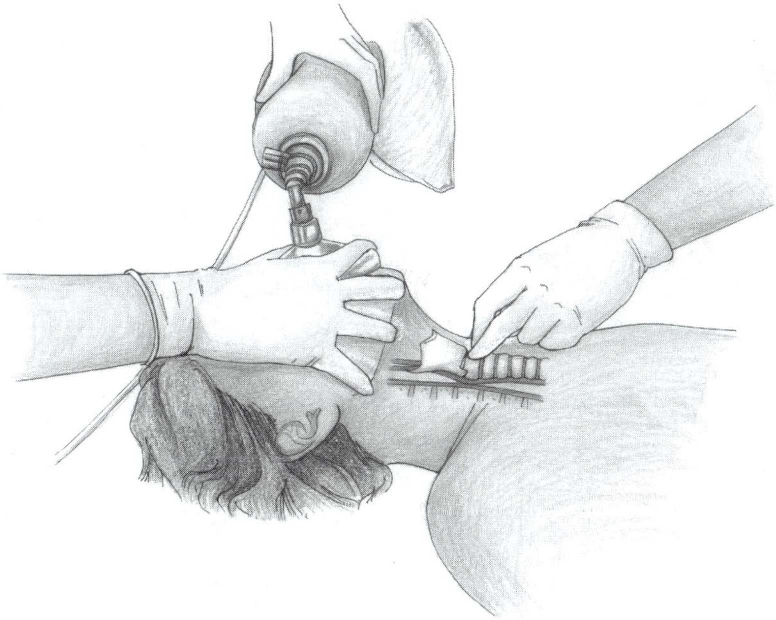

Gentle pressure on the cricoid cartilage by a second person may reduce gastric inflation and decrease the risk of aspiration during bagging. In an infant or child, cricoid pressure can also improve an intubator's view of the larynx. Reproduced from ICU web, copyright Kathy Mak 2004.

Ventilation provided by 2 rescuers (**Figure 2-8**) can be more effective when there is significant airway obstruction or poor lung compliance. In this technique, 1 rescuer uses both hands to open the airway by placing 3 fingers of each hand on both posterior rami of the patient's mandible and maintains a tight mask-to-face seal while the other rescuer compresses the ventilation bag. Again, the rescuer holding the face mask should concentrate on lifting the jaw and face into the mask in preference to pushing the mask onto the face.

The 2-rescuer technique may be essential in children with difficult airways (eg, epiglottitis or foreign body aspiration with complete obstruction). If a patient has any respiratory effort at all, ventilations should be timed with the patient's own inspiratory efforts. Allowing expiration to occur fully prior to providing another breath avoids hyperinflation with consequent hemodynamic and oxygenation problems. Use only the force and tidal volume necessary to make the chest rise. Excessive volumes may compromise cardiac output, distend the stomach, increase the risk of vomiting and aspiration, and add to the risk of barotrauma.

Figure 2-8. Two-person Bag-Mask Ventilation

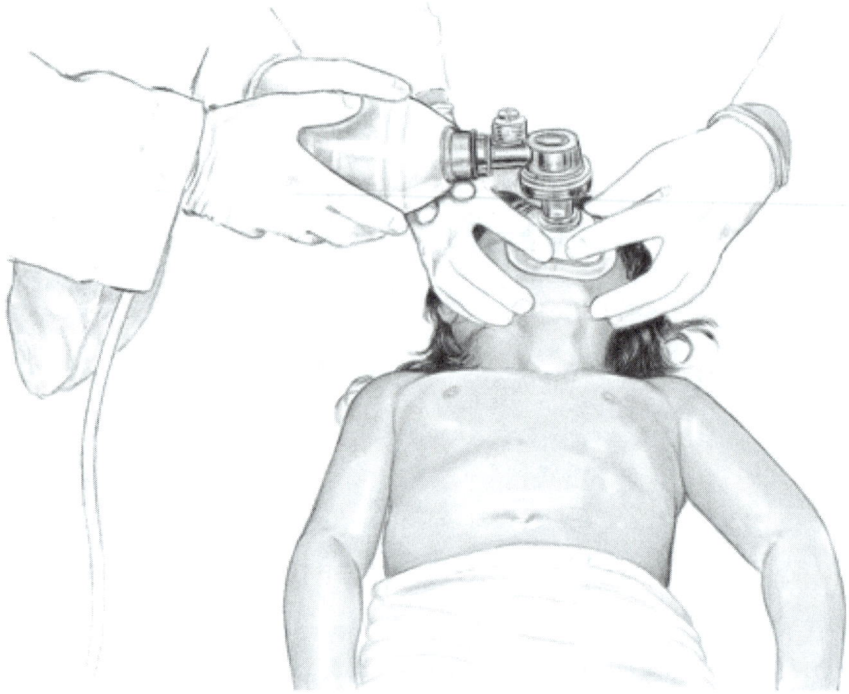

To maintain a tight seal, avoid pushing the mask onto the face but instead use both hands to lift the mandibular rami anteriorly into the mask. Reproduced with permission of the American Heart Association ©2006.

To assess the adequacy of bag-mask ventilation,

- Evaluate chest rise and presence of bilateral breath sounds
- Evaluate clinical response, including improved heart rate and return of good color
- Monitor oxygen saturation

E. Ventilation Bags

There are 2 types of ventilation bags: self-inflating and flow inflating. Ventilation bags used for resuscitation should be self-inflating and a suitable size for the child. Neonatal bags (250 mL) hold only enough volume to be used with neonates. Their volume and inspiratory pressure are inadequate for term newborns. Pediatric bags (450-500 mL) are adequate for full-term newborns, infants, and children.

Many self-inflating bags are equipped with pressure-limited pop-off valves set at 35 to 40 cm H_2O. In patients with significant pulmonary disease or anatomic obstruction of the airway, these valves may need to be inactivated in order to achieve adequate chest rise.

Flow-inflating bags require additional expertise.

F. Troubleshooting

When adequate chest rise does not occur:

- Reposition the head. Make sure the head and neck are not hyperextended and thus causing airway obstruction.
- Ensure that the mask is the appropriate size and that it is applied snugly on the patient's face.
- Make sure that you are lifting the child's jaw to the mask and not pushing the mask onto the child's face.
- Suction the airway if excessive secretions are noted.
- Place an oropharyngeal airway.
- Disable the pop-off feature of the ventilator bag.
- Use the Sellick maneuver to decrease abdominal distension.
- Assess the need for a nasogastric tube to decompress the stomach and protect against aspiration.
- Check for the presence of a foreign body.

When chest rise is appropriate, but oxygen saturation remains low:

- Check if the bag is connected to an appropriate oxygen source.
- Assess the need for higher pressures and the need to disable the pop-off valve.
- Consider using a positive end-expiratory pressure (PEEP) valve. Patients with lung disease might require additional pressure for improved oxygenation.
- In children with partial airway obstruction application of 5 to 10 cm H_2O of continuous positive airway pressure may maintain adequate airway patency.

VI. TRACHEAL INTUBATION

Tracheal intubation is required when less invasive methods of airway management prove inadequate. Many indications signal the need for intubation. The most common is respiratory failure. Respiratory failure is typically due to lower airway or parenchymal disease, such as bronchiolitis or pneumonia, and may result in failure of oxygenation, ventilation, or both. Upper airway obstruction due to foreign bodies, infectious processes, tracheomalacia and stenosis, or extrinsic compression all may require intubation. Another reason for intubation is to provide cardiovascular and neurologic support. Indications for tracheal intubation are summarized in **Table 2-4.** See **Appendix 5** for discussion of endotracheal intubation.

Table 2-4. Indications for Tracheal Intubation

Respiratory failure
Pa_{O_2} <60 mm Hg (8.0 kPa) with F_{IO_2} >0.6 (excludes cyanotic heart disease)
Pa_{CO_2} >55 mm Hg (7.3 kPa)
Excessive work of breathing
Upper airway obstruction
Hemodynamic instability (shock)
Loss or inadequacy of airway protective reflexes
Neuromuscular weakness
Therapeutic purposes
Severe metabolic acidosis
Head trauma (intracranial hypertension)
Need for deep sedation
Airway protection

A. Tracheal Tubes

Tracheal tubes (TTs) are sterile polyvinyl chloride tubes with a standard 15-millimeter adapter for attachment to a bag-mask device or ventilator tubing. They typically have centimeter markings on the side to document the depth of insertion as well as a vocal cord mark at the distal end to help approximate placement while intubating. Tubes are available in cuffed and uncuffed varieties. Historically, uncuffed tubes were recommended for children younger than 8 years because in that age group the trachea is narrowest at the cricoid ring. Uncuffed tubes allow a snug fit but avoid tracheal wall trauma from excessive cuff inflation. Currently, cuffed tubes are constructed with a low-pressure cuff designed to minimize trauma to the tracheal mucosa. Cuffed tracheal tubes are very helpful in patients with severe lung disease who may require high peak inspiratory pressure or PEEP. A cuffed tracheal tube should be inflated only the minimum amount necessary to eliminate any air leak around the tube. In many cases, there will be no air leak, even with the cuff deflated.

Whether a tracheal tube is cuffed or uncuffed, proper fit is essential. When inserted, the tube should fit snugly into the trachea but should pass smoothly, without the need for excessive force. There are several methods of determining proper tube size based upon a patient's age and size. A commonly used formula to calculate uncuffed tube size based on age is

$$\textbf{Tube Size (mm ID)} = \frac{\textbf{Age (Years)}}{4} + 4$$

Cuffed tubes should be downsized by 0.5 millimeters when using this formula. The depth of insertion can be estimated by multiplying the inner diameter (ID) of the tube by 3:

Depth of Insertion at Lip = ID of Selected Tube × 3

These formulas yield estimates, and adjustments may be needed for specific patients. In all cases, tubes a size above and a size below the estimated size should be available during intubation. Depth of insertion should be assessed by auscultation of breath sounds and with a chest radiograph obtained as soon as possible after intubation.

B. Laryngoscopes

The laryngoscope displaces the tongue and permits direct visualization of the larynx, vocal cords, and trachea. It consists of a handle (with battery) and a blade that has a light source at its tip. There are 2 types of blades, straight (eg, Miller, Robertshaw) and curved (eg, Macintosh), as shown in **Figure 2-9.** Each is used in a slightly different manner during intubation. Straight blades are typically used in infants and toddlers and are designed to lift the epiglottis out of the way, thus revealing the larynx and vocal cords. Curved blades are typically used in older children and adults, and are placed into the valleculla. Lifting the blade in the anterior direction lifts the epiglottis and reveals the vocal cords and related structures.

Figure 2-9. Laryngoscope Blades

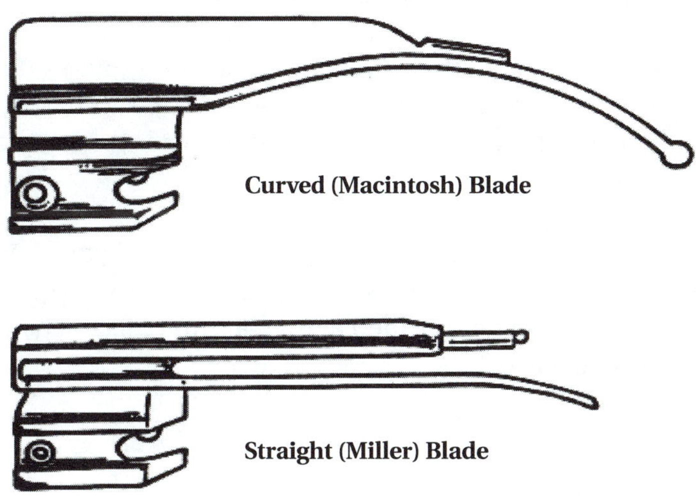

C. Sedation and Analgesia

Most patients require sedation prior to laryngoscopy and intubation. The goal is to depress the child's level of consciousness sufficiently to produce appropriate conditions for intubation. Those conditions include adequate sedation, analgesia, and amnesia plus blunting of the physiologic responses to airway manipulation, all with a minimum of hemodynamic compromise. Factors that play a role in the selection of sedating agents include, but are not limited to, the agent's rapidity of onset, the patient's hemodynamic status, the need to prevent increases in intraocular or intracranial pressure that may be caused by intubation, and whether the patient is in a fasting state. In many cases it is ideal to allow for the maintenance of spontaneous ventilatory drive during intubation. A wide variety of medications may be used for sedation, each with its own risks and benefits. In general, medications that act rapidly and are cleared quickly are ideal. Medications that clear quickly help to limit the duration of potential complications. However, the short duration of some agents can result in a patient's being intubated (which is painful and frightening) with inadequate sedation and analgesia. Thus it is important to continually reassess the child's level of consciousness during and after intubation and to give additional medication as appropriate. Providers should be familiar with the medications used at their institution because it is imperative to anticipate side effects that may occur and be prepared to address them. A brief overview of some of the medications commonly used in tracheal intubation is presented in **Table 2-5.**

D. Neuromuscular Blockade

Patients with inadequate relaxation despite adequate sedation may require neuromuscular blockade (or paralysis) as an adjunct to intubation. Therefore it is vitally important to understand the power and risks of pharmacologic paralysis. Once neuromuscular blockers have been administered to a patient, all spontaneous respiratory effort ceases. Moreover, in patients with partial airway obstruction, neuromuscular blockade may worsen pharyngeal collapse, potentially resulting in complete airway obstruction. It is thus imperative to be able to maintain patency of the airway with bag-mask ventilation prior to neuromuscular blockade. If adequate chest rise and oxygen saturations cannot be readily maintained with bag-mask ventilation, neuromuscular blockers should not be given until a clinician highly skilled in advanced airway management is present. For the same reason, it is advisable to use, whenever possible, a rapidly acting and quickly cleared neuromuscular blocker. Some frequently used neuromuscular blockers are shown in **Table 2-6.**

As with sedatives, it is necessary to be familiar with the pharmacology and side effects of neuromuscular blocking agents prior to using them. Succinylcholine, in particular, can cause hyperkalemia and malignant hyperthermia. Anyone who administers succinylcholine should be familiar with the management of those conditions.

Neuromuscular blockers provide no sedation or analgesia. Long-acting blockers, like vecuronium, often last longer than the short-acting sedative and analgesic medications given prior to intubation. Additional sedation should be provided at regular intervals to ensure that the patient does not awaken during neuroblockage.

Table 2-5. Medications Used to Facilitate Tracheal Intubation

Agent	Dosing	Onset and Duration	Benefits	Cautions
Fentanyl	1-2 μg/kg IV bolus every 2 minutes titrated to effect	Onset: Immediate Duration: 30-60 minutes	Rapid onset Short acting Reversible Relatively stable hemodynamic profile	Rigid chest syndrome Respiratory depression Lacks amnestic properties
Midazolam	0.05-0.1 mg/kg IV bolus every 5 minutes titrated to effect	Onset: 1-5 minutes Duration: 20-30 minutes	Rapid onset Short acting Provides amnesia Reversible	Lacks analgesic properties Respiratory depression Hypotension and bradycardia
Ketamine	1 mg/kg IV bolus every 5 minutes titrated to effect	Onset: 1-2 minutes Duration: 10-30 minutes	Rapid onset Airway-protective reflexes remain intact No hypotension or bradycardia	Increases airway secretions and laryngospasm (blunted with atropine) Elevates intracranial and ocular pressure Emergence reactions (blunted with benzodiazepines)
Etomidate	0.3 mg/kg IV bolus initially; 0.1 mg/kg bolus every 5 minutes thereafter titrated to effect	Onset: 10-20 seconds Duration: 4-10 minutes	Rapid onset Short acting Stable hemodynamic profile	Potential for adrenal inhibition May cause myoclonus Not recommended for children under 10 years
Thiopental	2-3 mg/kg IV bolus repeat as needed	Onset: 30-60 seconds Duration: 5-30 minutes	Ultra short-acting barbiturate Decreases intracranial pressure	Cardiovascular and respiratory depression Not FDA approved for children
Propofol	1-3 mg/kg IV bolus initially; 0.5-2 mg/kg bolus every 3-5 minutes thereafter titrated to effect	Onset: 30-60 seconds Duration: 5-10 minutes	Intravenous general anesthetic Rapid onset and recovery	Cardiovascular and respiratory depression Contraindicated in patients with egg allergy

Table 2-6. Frequently Used Neuromuscular Blockers

Agent	Dosing	Onset and Duration	Benefits	Cautions
Succinylcholine (depolarizing neuromuscular blockade)	1 mg/kg IV bolus	Onset: 30-60 seconds Duration: 4-6 minutes	Rapid onset Short duration	Causes muscle fasciculations (may be blunted with low dose nondepolarizing neuromuscular blocker) Potentiates hyperkalemia (contraindicated in head trauma, crush injury, burns, hyperkalemia) May induce neuroleptic malignant syndrome
Vecuronium (nondepolarizing neuromuscular blockade)	0.1 mg/kg IV bolus	Onset: 1-3 minutes Duration: 30-40 minutes	No fasciculations	Slower onset Longer duration of action
Rocuronium (nondepolarizing neuromuscular blockade)	0.6 –1 mg/kg IV bolus	Onset: 30-60 seconds Duration: 30-40 minutes		

E. Rapid Sequence Intubation

Rapid sequence intubation (RSI) is employed when there is increased concern about aspiration (eg, full stomach) and there is no suspicion of a difficult intubation. The goal of RSI is to obtain airway control with a tracheal tube as quickly as possible, thus minimizing aspiration risk. Preoxygenation by face mask is provided to increase the available oxygen in the lungs during the procedure. When all necessary intubation equipment and personnel are prepared, rapidly acting sedative, analgesic, and paralytic drugs are given simultaneously. Cricoid pressure is applied at the outset and maintained until the trachea is intubated and adequate confirmatory maneuvers are completed.

> **!** *Rapid sequence intubation is used only when all evidence indicates a normal airway. It should not be used if there is any concern that intubation will be difficult.* **!**

F. Other Intubation Equipment

Appropriate intubation supplies and equipment, as listed in **Table 2-7,** should be assembled at the bedside prior to beginning an intubation procedure. Cardiopulmonary monitoring and pulse oximetry should be used throughout the procedure. Suction equipment with a large-bore, rigid suction device (such as a Yankauer) should be present to suction the oropharynx of mucous, blood, and particulate matter. A flexible suction catheter to suction the tracheal tube is helpful as well.

Table 2-7. Intubation Supplies and Equipment

Intubation Supplies	Comments
Cardiopulmonary monitor and pulse oximeter	Continuous monitoring before, during, and after intubation
Suction devices	Yankauer and tracheal tube suction; test prior to starting
Stylet	Ensure appropriate size and ease of removal
Bag, face mask, and oxygen supply	Test size and function prior to starting
Tracheal tubes	A size above and a size below the anticipated size should be at the bedside
Laryngoscope	Ensure light is properly functioning; various sizes and types of blades should be at the bedside
End-tidal CO_2 detector	Turns yellow when carbon dioxide is detected
McGill forceps	For grasping and advancing the tracheal tube during nasotracheal intubation
Oxygenating stylet	May be used to insufflate oxygen and as a guide for tracheal tube placement
Tape or tube-securing device	Adhesive

A stylet should be used to add rigidity to the tracheal tube. To avoid airway trauma, ensure that the stylet does not protrude from the distal end of the tracheal tube. Also make sure the stylet can be removed easily from the tube once it is in position. Many successfully placed tracheal tubes have become dislodged in the process of removing tight stylets.

An end-tidal CO_2 detector should be attached to the TT after intubation to confirm proper placement in the trachea. Colorimetric end-tidal CO_2 devices change color from purple to yellow to confirm the presence of exhaled CO_2 and tracheal placement. The endotracheal tube should be secured with tape or a TT-securing device with attention to the depth; inadvertent displacement can compromise oxygenation and ventilation.

G. Intubation

Proper positioning is a key element of successful intubation. To visualize the glottis clearly, the oral, pharyngeal, and tracheal axes must be brought into alignment as described above and shown in **Figure 2-2.** Alignment of the 3 airway axes can be achieved with slight hyperextension of the head on the neck into the sniffing position, with the ear canal just above or even with the top of the shoulder when visualized from the side. Children younger than 2 years have relatively large heads for their body size, which results in slight neck flexion when they are in the supine position. Children in this age group usually benefit from a small roll (thin towel or blanket) placed under the shoulders, which allows the head to fall back into proper position but avoids hyperextension. In older children a small roll under the occiput helps facilitate proper alignment of the axes. In patients with suspected cervical spine injury, the head should remain in the neutral position at all times and the spine should be stabilized while intubating.

When possible, it is advantageous to preoxygenate patients to 100% oxygen saturation with bag-mask ventilation prior to attempting intubation. Each laryngoscopy and tracheal tube placement attempt should be limited to approximately 30 seconds. An assistant should monitor vital signs continuously. All attempts must be expedient, and failed attempts should be terminated prior to desaturation. After each unsuccessful attempt, the patient should again receive bag-mask ventilation to optimize oxygenation before the next attempt.

Figure 2-10. Insertion of Laryngoscope Blades

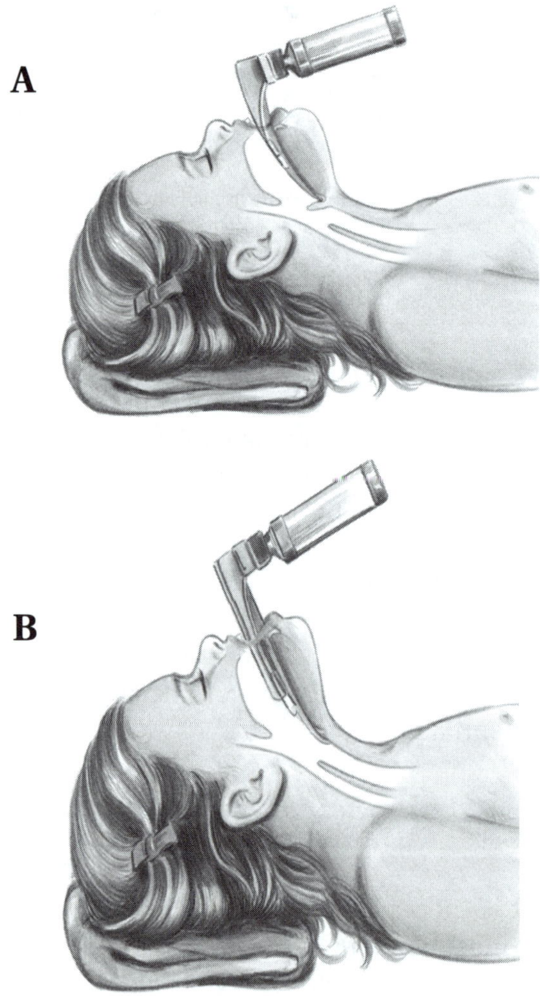

A, Insertion of a curved laryngoscope blade. B, Insertion of a straight laryngoscope blade. Insertion techniques are summarized in **Table 2-8**. Reproduced with permission of the American Heart Association 2006.

Not all intubation attempts will be successful, and anticipation of a difficult airway is a vital part of the preintubation assessment. A history of prior difficult intubation, obstructive sleep apnea, or frequent snoring should raise concern about the level of difficulty to be expected. Patients with facial abnormalities such as micrognathia, midface hypoplasia, small mouths, large tongues, and morbid obesity often are difficult to intubate. Limited mobility of the temporomandibular joint or the cervical spine as well as bleeding, masses, or foreign bodies in the upper airway all present challenges to tracheal intubation.

A backup plan should always be developed prior to intubation. Supplies should be available for multiple attempts, advanced intubation techniques, and cricothyrotomy. If a difficult intubation is anticipated and patient stability permits, it is advisable to have more experienced clinicians present prior to proceeding.

Orotracheal intubation is the most common and preferred method of intubation during emergency situations. The technique is summarized in **Table 2-8.**

Table 2-8. Technique for Orotracheal Intubation
Ensure that the patient is positioned correctly.
Hold the laryngoscope in your left hand and advance the blade along the right side of the mouth to the base of the tongue.
Sweep the blade to the midline, thus lifting the tongue out of the visual field and providing an area on the right side of the mouth where the tube can be advanced without losing direct visualization of the laryngeal structures. Taking an extra moment to ensure that the tongue is properly displaced will ensure optimal visualization and facilitate successful intubation.
When using a straight blade, position the distal end of the blade just below (posterior to) the epiglottis so it may be used to lift the epiglottis anteriorly. Often, a straight blade will initially enter the esophagus upon insertion. If the blade tip is in the esophagus, slowly backing out the blade will cause the larynx to fall into view as the blade leaves the esophageal inlet. When a curved blade is used, the end of the blade is placed into the vallecula above (anterior to) the epiglottis. The insertions of a straight blade and a curved blade are illustrated in **Figure 2-10.**

The anterior placement of the pediatric airway sometimes makes visualization of the epiglottis and larynx difficult. Slight pressure on the cricoid cartilage (Sellick maneuver) may move the larynx the airway posterior and improve visualization.

Once either a straight or a curved blade is properly positioned, the laryngoscope handle should be lifted anteriorly along an axis that is approximately 45° from the bed, providing a clearer view of the larynx. Do not lever the blade upwards, as this will result in trauma to the lips, gums, and teeth from the proximal end of the blade and the handle. Remember, even in an edentulous infant, teeth are developing right below the gum line.

Once the larynx is well visualized (**Figure 2-11**) make every effort not to take your eyes off the larynx. To facilitate continuous visualization of the larynx, an assistant should place all necessary equipment in the intubator's free hand. Advance the tube from the right corner of the mouth through the vocal cords. Do not advance the tube down the flange of the blade because doing so will obscure the larynx. A good rule of thumb is that if the operator does not see the tube go through the vocal cords, it has not gone through the vocal cords.

Figure 2-11. Visualization of the Larynx During Laryngoscopy

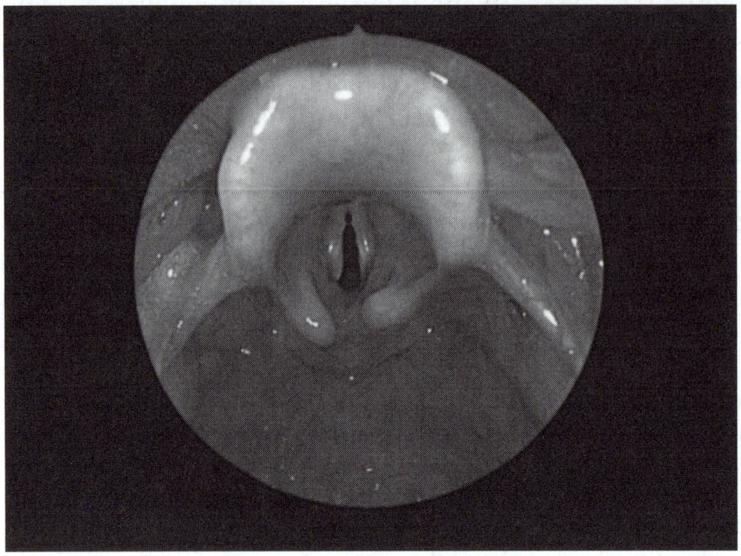

Image is courtesy of Sanjay Parikh, MD, The Children's Hospital at Montefiore Reproduced with permission.

The tip of the tracheal tube should be placed at the mid-tracheal level. Mid-tracheal placement is facilitated in uncuffed tubes by placing the distal black marker on the tube at the level of the cords. Cuffed tubes should be positioned with the cuff just below the vocal cords.

Once the tube has been inserted, confirm proper tracheal placement.

Correct placement is initially confirmed by seeing the tube pass through the vocal cords into the trachea. Look for symmetric chest rise and listen for equal breath sounds while delivering positive pressure breaths. If the tube is in the right mainstem bronchus, breath sounds will be more prominent over the right chest, signaling that the tube needs to be repositioned. Slowly pull the tube back while listening to the left chest. When breath sounds become audible on the left, the tube has entered the trachea. Obtain a chest radiograph to determine the actual position and guide further adjustment. Listen over the stomach; if the tube is in the trachea, breath sounds will be absent over the abdomen. Water vapor in the tracheal tube suggests but does not confirm tracheal placement. An end-tidal CO_2 detector may also be used to ensure proper placement. It is important to remember that during cardiac arrest or when cardiac output is very low, there is minimal to no blood flow to pulmonary capillaries and consequently very little to no CO_2 delivered to the lungs for exhalation. In such cases, CO_2 may not be detected despite proper tube placement, so other methods of confirmation are necessary. Because no single method is completely dependable in all situations, multiple methods of confirmation should always be used. If any question exists, perform laryngoscopy to obtain visual confirmation that the tracheal tube is passing through the vocal cords. A chest radiograph should be acquired as soon as possible to ensure proper position and to evaluate for complications such as pneumothorax.

The tracheal tube should be well secured to the patient's face to avoid unintentional extubation. This can be achieved with adhesive (eg, tincture of benzoin) and tape. Two pieces of tape can be partially ripped so that each resembles a pair of pants. The "waist" of the tape is placed on the patient's cheek, one leg is placed above the patient's upper lip, and the other is tightly wrapped around the tube. The other piece of tape is placed below the lower lip in the same manner. Commercially manufactured tube holders are also available.

Following intubation, monitoring by ECG, pulse oximetry, and end-tidal CO_2 should be continued. Once a patient is connected to a ventilator, an arterial blood gas study should be obtained as soon as possible.

H. Complications

The physiologic alterations that occur when positive pressure ventilation is initiated can lead to complications that can be anticipated and rapidly treated. As noted above, bag-mask ventilation delivers some of the volume from each positive pressure breath to the stomach, leading to distention (which may make it difficult to adequately ventilate the patient) and aspiration. To decrease the likelihood of aspiration, a naso- or orogastric tube should be placed to help decompress the stomach and remove stomach contents.

Stimulation of the airway results in activation of the vagus nerve. When a patient is intubated, this appears clinically as bradycardia. Atropine 0.01 to 0.02 mg/kg (maximum single dose 1 mg, minimum single dose 0.1 mg) can be administered to overcome this response. In patients who are bradycardic at baseline, or in whom there is concern for vagal-mediated bradycardia, atropine may be given prior to attempting intubation. Atropine is also used to decrease airway secretions in patients who receive ketamine for sedation.

Positive pressure ventilation has the potential to cause barotrauma to the alveoli, occasionally resulting in leakage of air into the pleural space (pneumothorax). As air accumulates in the pleural space, the lung becomes compressed, compromising oxygenation and ventilation. If the air leak is ongoing, the pressure in the pleural space rises, causing a tension pneumothorax. When a tension pneumothorax is present, the mediastinum shifts toward the uninvolved side, impairing venous return to the heart and compromising cardiac output. Signs of tension pneumothorax include deviation of the trachea away from the affected side, diminished breath sounds on the affected side, tachycardia, and falling blood pressure. Treatment should be emergent and should not be delayed while awaiting a chest radiograph. A tension pneumothorax can be decompressed by the sterile passage of an 18-gauge angiocatheter into the pleural space over the top of the third rib in the midclavicular line. A rush of air will be heard as the air under pressure escapes the pleural space. Definitive treatment is with a thoracostomy tube, which should be placed as soon as possible.

Another complication of positive pressure ventilation is decreased cardiac output. The increase in intrathoracic pressure induced by positive pressure ventilation impairs venous return to the right side of the heart, thus decreasing preload. In patients who are dehydrated and in those with compromised hemodynamic function, this impairment may produce clinically relevant decreases in cardiac output and hypotension. Fluid resuscitation will often restore preload and improve cardiac output. Practitioners should be ready to provide advanced cardiac care when hypotension is refractory to volume resuscitation.

I. Troubleshooting

Acute respiratory deterioration can occur in an intubated patient for a variety of reasons. A commonly used mnemonic to help assess the situation is DOPE: dislodgement of the tube, obstruction of the tube, pneumothorax, and equipment failure. View chest rise and auscultate the chest to ensure proper positioning of the tracheal tube. Asymmetric breath sounds may represent improper tube position or pneumothorax. When asymmetry is present, a chest radiograph can help diagnose the problem. Suction the tube to clear secretions from the lumen. If the patient is on a ventilator, check that it is functioning properly. In cases of uncertainty, it may be helpful to remove the patient from the ventilator and ventilate manually with 100% oxygen.

Respiratory deterioration may often be secondary to the patient's underlying condition. Adjustments to the ventilator and other respiratory therapies may be required to improve the child's respiratory status.

VII. FAILED INTUBATION

When respiratory failure occurs, tracheal intubation is the standard method of controlling the airway and supporting pulmonary function. Sometimes intubation is unachievable due to complete upper airway obstruction, anatomic airway abnormalities, severe facial trauma, or similar circumstances. It is important to have a backup plan in the event that a tracheal tube cannot be placed. First and foremost, bag-mask ventilation can be provided indefinitely as long as adequate oxygen saturations can be maintained. See **Appendix 4** for additional discussion of airway adjuncts.

A. Laryngeal Mask Airway

When it is impossible to intubate or manually mask ventilate a patient, a laryngeal mask airway is a useful adjunct that provides an open airway and permits gas exchange. A laryngeal mask airway consists of a tube with a cuffed, masklike projection at the distal end. When properly placed, it sits just above the glottic opening and seals off the esophagus from the trachea. Laryngeal mask airways now come in sizes appropriate for children.

The weight range appropriate for the size of a given laryngeal mask airway is printed on the mask itself. **Figure 2-12** shows the insertion technique. The laryngeal mask airway is held like a pencil with the distal opening facing away from the operator (so that it ends up facing anteriorly when placed). The balloon is placed against the hard palate, which is used as a guide as the laryngeal mask airway is slid into the airway. Once definite resistance is felt, the balloon is inflated and bag ventilation can be initiated. Assessment of air entry is the same as for intubated patients, with attention to symmetric lung inflation.

Figure 2-12. Insertion Technique for Laryngeal Mask Airway

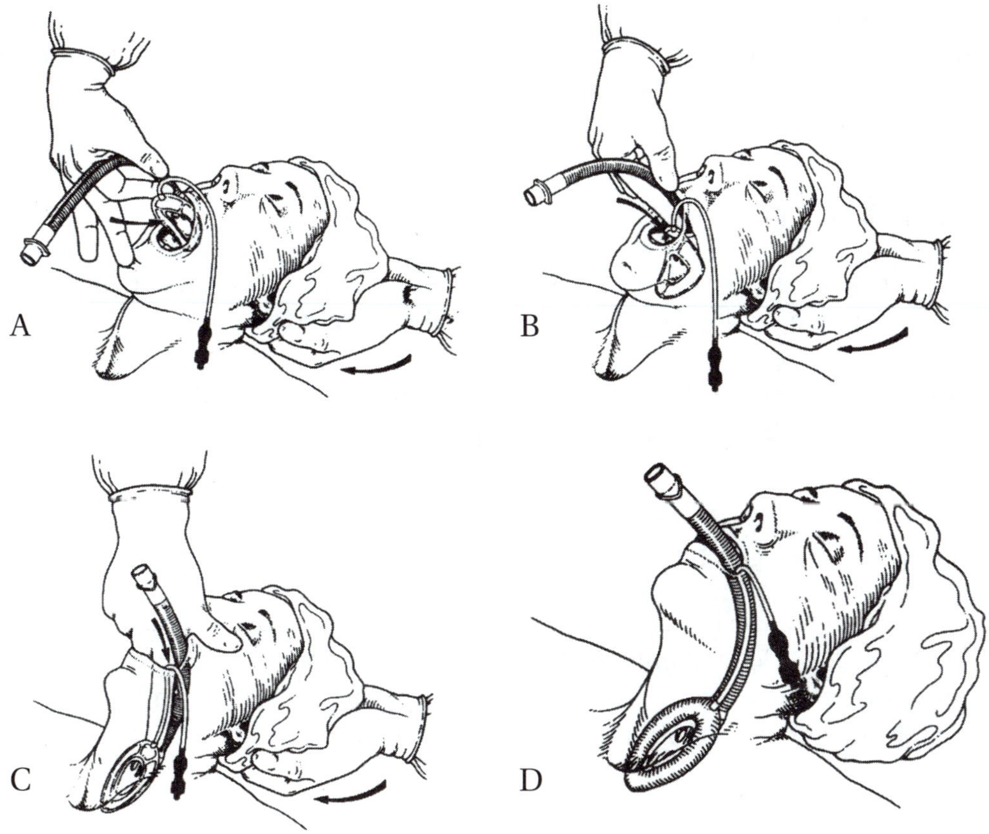

A, insert lubricated and deflated mask into the open mouth with the bowl facing anterior. B, hold the device like a pencil pressing against the palate and pharyngeal wall with the index finger. C, continue inserting the cuff behind the tongue into the hypopharynx until finite resistance is felt. D, without holding the divice, inflate cuff with enough air to obtain a seal. Attach manual ventilation device and assure chest movement. From Brain AIJ: *The Intavent Laryngeal Mask Instruction Manual.* Berkshire, UK, Brain Medical, 1992.

A special type of laryngeal mask airway, the intubating laryngeal mask airway, is commercially available for use in larger patients. An intubating laryngeal mask airway has a bar at the distal end that elevates the epiglottis and is wide enough to accommodate a special tracheal tube being passed through the lumen. Once in position, a tracheal tube is passed through the laryngeal mask airway. The epiglottis-elevating bar is forced up, lifting the epiglottis and allowing the tracheal tube to be passed into the trachea. The intubating laryngeal mask airway is then removed over the tracheal tube, which is left in position.

B. Esophageal-Tracheal Double-Lumen Airway Device

In children over 4 feet tall, it is possible to place an esophageal-tracheal double-lumen airway device. These tubes contain two lumens as well as proximal and distal balloons. They are placed blindly and almost always end up in the esophagus. Both balloons are then inflated to create a seal.

When properly positioned, the distal balloon obstructs the esophagus and the proximal balloon obstructs the distal pharynx. The proximal tube holes are above the distal balloon. Thus, air is forced out of the proximal tube down the trachea. If the tube happens to end up in the trachea, the distal tube may be used to ventilate the patient. A similar device, a laryngeal tube with only one lumen, is available in multiple sizes.

C. Intubating Stylets

When a patient's vocal cords are well visualized but the tracheal tube cannot be passed, it may be easier to pass an intubating stylet. These stylets are hollow and have a connector at the end that can be attached to an oxygen source or a bag-mask device. Once in place, they can be used to hand ventilate the patient. A tracheal tube can then be passed over the stylet into the trachea, and the stylet can be removed, leaving the tracheal tube in place.

D. Fiberoptic Intubation

Operators familiar with the use of intubating bronchoscopes can provide assistance with a difficult airway. The tracheal tube is loaded onto the bronchoscope, and the bronchoscope is placed into the trachea through the vocal cords under direct visualization. The TT is then slipped off the end of the bronchoscope and left in proper position within the trachea.

E. Cricothyrotomy

In extreme situations, cricothyrotomy may be performed. With the patient's neck hyperextended, the cricothyroid membrane is located by palpation between the thyroid cartilage and the cricoid cartilage. The area is sterilized, and an IV catheter (catheter over needle) is placed through the cartilage into the trachea. Proper completion of this step is confirmed by the patient's aspiration of air, after which the needle is withdrawn while advancing the catheter. The catheter can then be attached to a positive pressure device connected via the luer lock. A 5-milliliter syringe barrel (with the plunger removed) will accept a standard 15-millimeter adapter and manual ventilation can be carried out. Commercially available cricothyrotomy kits contain all the necessary supplies.

F. Planning for a Difficult or Failed Intubation

Whenever an airway proves difficult to intubate or even when difficulty is anticipated prior to intubation, backup personnel with expertise in the management of the pediatric airway should be summoned. Anesthesiologists, otolaryngologists, and pediatric intensivists are considered experts by training in maintaining difficult airways. An algorithm for dealing with difficult intubation is presented in **Appendix 6.**

Key Points

Airway Management

- Accurate assessment of work of breathing, airway patency, respiratory drive, and consciousness are crucial first steps in the management of children with breathing difficulty.
- Maintaining a patent airway with manual methods such as oropharyngeal airways and NP tubes is an important skill in airway management.
- All providers who care for ill children should be able to supply adequate oxygenation and ventilation with bag-mask ventilation.
- It is imperative that all necessary supplies and personnel be present prior to before intubation is attempted.
- Expertise with sedatives, analgesics, and neuromuscular blockers is a prerequisite for intubation.
- A backup plan should be developed before a potentially difficult intubation is attempted. The use of airway adjuncts such as a laryngeal mask airway and cricothyrotomy may be lifesaving when intubation cannot be achieved.

Suggested Readings

1. American Heart Association. Respiratory management resources and procedures. Pediatric Advanced Life Support. 2006.
2. American Society of Anesthesiology. Practice guidelines for the management of the difficult airway. *Anesthesiology.* 2003;98:1269-1277.
3. Thompson AE. Pediatric airway management. In: Fuhrman BP, Zimmerman JJ, eds. *Pediatric Critical Care.* St Louis, MO: Mosby; 2006:485.
4. deCaen A, Duff J, Covadia AH, et al. Airway Management. In: Nichols DG, ed. *Rogers' Textbook of Pediatric Intensive Care.* 4th ed. Philadelphia, PA: Lippincott Williams & Wilkins:208:303-322.

Chapter 3:

Cardiopulmonary/Cerebral Resuscitation

Objectives

- To rapidly identify the need for cardiopulmonary resuscitation and to provide excellent cardiopulmonary resuscitation.
- To rapidly identify the need for cardiopulmonary resuscitation
- To provide excellent mechanical and pharmacologic cardiopulmonary resuscitation
- To understand the physiology of cardiopulmonary resuscitation

Case Study

A 2-month-old infant is brought to the emergency department by a parent who reports that she was well until 1 hour ago. Since then, she has become progressively lethargic, and she is now unresponsive. Initial assessment reveals irregular, gasping respirations, no palpable pulse, and a heart rate of 250 beats/min on electrocardiogram. Bag-mask ventilation is initiated with good chest rise, and chest compressions are begun.

- What are the key aspects of the initial assessment of this infant?

- What is the most important next step?

- What is the likely diagnosis and what are the next management steps?

I. INTRODUCTION

Successful resuscitation of a child with a cardiac arrest depends upon effective cardiopulmonary resuscitation (CPR), which optimizes coronary perfusion pressure and cardiac output to critical organs, supporting vital organ viability. Clinicians responsible for resuscitating children from cardiac arrest need a solid understanding of the physiology of cardiac arrest, CPR, the pharmacology of medications used during and after resuscitation, and post-resuscitative care.

Pediatric cardiac arrests most often result from respiratory arrests: they result from lack of cellular substrate rather than from a primary cardiac event. Thus, the initial resuscitation of a child must emphasize restoration of respirations. Chest-compression-only resuscitation, while sometimes appropriate for adults, is inappropriate for children.

Although sudden death from cardiac causes is unusual in children, it is estimated that several thousand Americans under the age of 20 years die annually from sudden cardiac causes. In children younger than 1 year, sudden cardiac death is usually associated with complex congenital cardiac disease. After the first year, the most common causes of sudden cardiac death in the pediatric population include myocarditis, hypertrophic cardiomyopathy, coronary artery disease, congenital coronary artery anomalies, conduction system abnormalities, mitral valve prolapse, and aortic dissection.

Sudden infant death syndrome is the leading cause of out-of-hospital pediatric cardiac arrest, followed by trauma, airway obstruction, and near drowning. The survival rate following out-of-hospital cardiac arrest is approximately 12%, while only 4% survive neurologically intact. Survival rates following in-hospital cardiac arrest range from 14% to 44%, depending on circumstances. Future pediatric resuscitation research must focus not only on how to increase survival from cardiac arrest but also on how to ensure that the survivors remain neurologically intact.

II. PRIMARY RESPONSE

A. Leadership and Organization

The first step in any resuscitation is organizing the team and clearly identifying the team leader. The presence of one definitive leader is vital to the conduct of an efficient and effective resuscitation. Leaders must assign tasks to specific individuals rather than direct requests to the room at large. The team leader not only must determine which medications should be given and what other interventions must be performed (with appropriate input from other team members), but also must supervise the proper administration of chest compressions, direct unnecessary personnel away from the bedside, and ensure a calm, focused resuscitation environment. Ideally, the team leader should supervise all aspects of the resuscitation attempt and should not be involved in tasks, such as administering chest compressions. However, the team leader often possesses the most refined airway and vascular access skills; when this is the case, he or she must continue to oversee the resuscitation while intubating or placing vascular access devices.

B. Medical Assessment and Monitoring

The diagnosis of cardiopulmonary arrest is based on the absence of a palpable pulse in a major artery (carotid, femoral, brachial) in the presence of unconsciousness and apnea. When a child has physiologic monitors in place, they will often alert caregivers of an actual or impending cardiac arrest. The electrocardiogram (ECG) may indicate a non-perfusing rhythm, such as ventricular fibrillation or asystole; end-tidal carbon dioxide ($ETCO_2$) will fall precipitously when the lack of cardiac output results in decreased delivery of carbon dioxide to the lungs; and a pulse oximeter will lose its regular waveform in the absence of pulsatile blood flow. If physiologic monitors are not in place when a cardiac arrest is suspected, they should be placed immediately but without delaying resuscitation.

Attention must be paid in the early minutes of resuscitation to determine the cause of the arrest. Many children will not be successfully resuscitated unless the underlying problem is corrected. A focused physical exam should be conducted, and a brief history should be elicited if it is not already known. A cardiorespiratory monitor should be placed, and the ECG should be examined. Early in the course of an attempted resuscitation, a blood gas analysis should be performed, and key electrolytes (Na^+, K^+, Ca^{2+}) should be measured (ideally with point-of-care testing).

III. MECHANICS OF CARDIOPULMONARY RESUSCITATION

Management of the child with a cardiac arrest proceeds in accordance with the ABC algorithm (airway, breathing, circulation) (See **Appendix 7**); however, the patient with ventricular fibrillation (VF) or pulseless ventricular tachycardia (VT) should receive electrical defibrillation without delay. Airway access in patients with VF or pulseless VT should be obtained after defibrillation. Cardiopulmonary resuscitation should be conducted continuously until the shock can be delivered.

A. Airway

Although tracheal intubation is optimal for resuscitation, multiple attempts at intubation by unskilled individuals may seriously compromise future attempts. The child's airway can usually be managed effectively with bag-mask ventilation, using proper head positioning and jaw thrust, while awaiting the arrival of an individual with pediatric airway skills. The use of bag-mask devices, however, may result in a significant risk of gastric inflation followed by pulmonary aspiration. Abdominal distension can significantly compromise oxygenation and ventilation; therefore, the stomach should be vented with a nasogastric or orogastric tube when excessive gastric inflation occurs. Excessive inflation pressures should be avoided. Effective ventilation is best judged by visualizing chest excursions and listening to the quality of breath sounds.

Endotracheal intubation should be attempted as soon as appropriate personnel and equipment are available. It is essential to confirm appropriate placement of the endotracheal tube, ideally by measuring $ETCO_2$. A disposable colorimetric $ETCO_2$ is useful in verifying endotracheal tube placement in children when in-line capnography is not available. However, it is important to understand that $ETCO_2$ measurements are meaningful only when there is effective pulmonary circulation; a lack of color change may reflect either improper tube positioning or lack of effective chest compressions. In the very small infant, the amount of exhaled CO_2 may be too small to cause a convincing color change.

B. Breathing

In the inpatient environment, the equipment necessary to emergently ventilate a child should be readily available. In venues where pediatric cardiac arrests are uncommon, it is particularly important for the child's primary caregivers to know where appropriate equipment is kept because support staff may be unfamiliar with the equipment. An appropriately sized ambu bag should be used for ventilation; it is easy to overventilate small children if an adult bag is used. Similarly, if an infant bag is used for an older child, it will be difficult to achieve effective ventilation. If no chest movement occurs during bag-mask ventilation despite an apparently tight seal between the mask and the child's face, upper airway obstruction, whether anatomic or due to a foreign body, must be considered. Care providers should be familiar with the use of oral airways, which can dramatically improve ventilation in the child with a large tongue, a small jaw, or other anatomic variants.

While restoring effective ventilation to the child with cardiac arrest is critical, overventilation should be avoided. Overventilation is common during CPR and results in higher mean intrathoracic pressure with resultant decreased venous return, reduced cardiac output, and increased frequency of pneumothorax. In cardiopulmonary arrest, a lower-than-normal minute ventilation may be appropriate because cardiac output and delivery of CO_2 to the lungs are low. If there is no artificial airway in place, 2 breaths should be given after 15 chest compressions. Once an artificial airway is in place, ventilations should be given at a rate of 8 to 10 per minute without pausing between chest compressions (**Table 3-1**).

Table 3-1. Ventilation and Chest Compressions During Pediatric CPR

Ventilation Mode	Respirations	Chest Compressions	Notes
Bag-mask ventilation	2 respirations after each 15 chest compressions If 1 rescuer only, 2 respirations after each 30 compressions	100 per minute	Ventilate stomach to alleviate gastric inflation.
Endotracheal intubation	8-10 respirations per minute	100 per minute	Do not pause compressions during ventilation. Confirm appropriate positioning of the endotracheal tube.

C. Circulation

Ensuring effective chest compressions is one of the most important tasks of the team leader. During cardiac arrest, chest compressions provide the sole perfusion to a child's vital organs, yet providers frequently deliver chest compressions too slowly and without adequate force. Key steps to providing quality chest compressions include (1) ensuring an adequate rate (100 compressions per minute), (2) ensuring adequate chest wall depression (one-third to one-half of the anterior-posterior chest diameter, (3) releasing completely between compressions to allow full chest wall recoil, and (4) minimizing interruptions in chest compressions (**Table 3-2**).

Table 3-2. Keys to Generating Effective Cardiac Output During CPR

- Push hard.
- Push fast.
- Release completely.
- Do not interrupt compressions unnecessarily.

In small infants, circumferential chest compressions are preferred whenever the person providing compressions can comfortably encircle the chest with his or her hands. With the circumferential technique, the provider's thumbs depress the sternum, and the fingers support the infant's back and circumferentially squeeze the thorax. In larger infants, the sternum can be compressed using 2 fingers, and in children, either 1 or 2 hands should be used, depending on the size of the child and the rescuer. Whichever method is used, focused attention must remain on delivering effective compressions with minimal interruptions. In all cases other than circumferential CPR, a backboard must be used. Because it is tiring to deliver chest compressions properly, providers should rotate as frequently as necessary to ensure that compressions are not compromised by the provider's muscle fatigue. In larger children, providers may need to rotate as frequently as every 1 minute to ensure that compressions are delivered with adequate rate and force.

Optimal coronary perfusion pressure and cardiac output during CPR is consistently associated with improved chance for return of spontaneous circulation and with good short and long-term outcome. Ensuring rapid, strong, minimally interrupted chest compressions enhances cardiac output, while administration of vasoconstricting medications increases diastolic blood pressure and coronary perfusion pressure.

D. Mechanisms of Blood Flow

External chest compressions provide cardiac output through two mechanisms: the cardiac pump mechanism and the thoracic pump mechanism. In the cardiac pump mechanism of blood flow, blood is squeezed from the heart by compression of the heart between the sternum and the vertebral column, exiting the heart anterograde because of closure of the atrioventricular valves. Between compressions, ventricular pressure falls below atrial pressure, allowing the atrioventricular valves to open and the ventricles to fill. This sequence of events resembles the normal cardiac cycle.

With the thoracic pump mechanism of blood flow, the heart is a passive conduit for blood flow. The intrathoracic pressure is higher than the extrathoracic pressure during the compression phase of CPR, at which time blood flows out of the thorax, with venous valves preventing excessive retrograde blood flow. During the release phase of chest compressions, chest recoil results in negative intrathoracic pressure, drawing blood into the thorax. In adults, the thoracic pump mechanism likely dominates, but in infants, the smaller, more compliant chest wall allows for direct cardiac compression as well. Experimental and clinical data support both mechanisms of blood flow during CPR in human infants.

E. Vascular Access and Ongoing Monitoring

1. Vascular Access

A key to successful CPR is the early establishment of a route for administering medication. If an intravenous line cannot be established rapidly, the intraosseous or endotracheal route should be used.

> !
>
> *Move quickly to place an intraosseous needle if intravenous access is not immediately achievable.*
>
> !

a. Intravenous Access

For patients with impending cardiac arrest and no vascular access, a brief attempt should be made to insert a peripheral intravenous catheter. If access is not achieved quickly, an intraosseous needle should be placed. For young children in cardiac arrest without vascular access, an intraosseous needle should be placed without delay. In the older child with visible or easily palpable veins, it is appropriate to attempt peripheral intravenous catheterization before using an intraosseous needle. If neither a peripheral venous catheter nor an intraosseous needle is feasible, the most skilled practitioner should place a central venous catheter at the site with which he or she has the greatest comfort.

b. Intraosseous Access

Placing an intraosseous needle is not difficult but should be approached methodically and carefully. Ideally, a specialized intraosseous needle should be used (**See Appendix 8**). (These should be stocked in resuscitation carts in any venue where children are cared for.) If an intraosseous needle is unavailable, a standard 16- or 18-gauge needle or a bone marrow needle may be used, though their use may be more difficult. The needle should be inserted with a back-and-forth rotating motion at a 90-degree angle into the anterior surface of the tibia, 1 to 3 centimeters below the tibial tuberosity. When the needle passes through the cortex into the marrow, there is loss of resistance. In young infants, it is very easy to pass the needle completely through the bone; therefore, the minimum necessary pressure should be applied. When the needle is in the marrow cavity, it will stand upright without support. It loses the upright position if it has slipped into the subcutaneous tissue. Free flow of the drug or fluid infusion without significant subcutaneous infiltration should also be demonstrated. (A needle that has passed completely through the bone may stand upright without support but will be associated with subcutaneous infiltration.) The technique has a low complication rate, although possible complications include osteomyelitis, fat and bone-marrow embolism, and the most common complication, compartment syndrome. An intraosseous needle should be replaced by a definitive intravenous catheter as soon as practical.

All medications and fluids used during CPR, including whole blood, can be given by the intraosseous route. An intraosseous needle may also be used to obtain initial blood samples, although acid-base analysis will be inaccurate after administration of sodium bicarbonate via the intraosseous catheter. The intraosseous route of drug administration is preferred to the endotracheal route because medications will appear more rapidly in the central circulation. Intraosseous needles are appropriate for use in all children.

> **!**
>
> *Medications that can be administered endotracheally: Lidocaine Atropine Naloxone Epinephrine (LANE)*
>
> **!**

c. Administration of Endotracheal Medication

In the absence of other vascular access, medications including lidocaine, atropine, naloxone, and epinephrine (remember the mnemonic "LANE") can be given through an endotracheal tube. The use of ionized medications, such as sodium bicarbonate or calcium chloride, is not recommended by this route. Drugs should be administered with a maximum of 5 milliliters of volume in the infant and 10 milliliters of volume in the older child. Absorption into the systemic circulation may also be enhanced by deep intrapulmonary administration. This can be accomplished by passing a feeding tube through the endotracheal tube for the administration of medication.

2. Monitoring During Cardiopulmonary Resuscitation

A recurring, basic clinical examination is vital during cardiac arrest. The team leader should carefully evaluate the adequacy of chest expansion and of breath sounds and constantly reevaluate the adequacy of chest compressions. An indwelling arterial catheter, when available, is a valuable monitor in assessing arterial blood pressure. Specific attention should be paid to diastolic blood pressure because it relates directly to adequacy of coronary perfusion during CPR. In addition, arterial access allows for frequent blood sampling, particularly for measurement of arterial pH and blood gases. Pulse oximetry can be used during CPR to determine oxygen saturation and to suggest adequacy of cardiac output on the basis of a pulsatile waveform. The ECG can suggest metabolic imbalances and show electrical disturbances.

A quantitative $ETCO_2$ monitor is helpful to indicate the adequacy of chest compressions during CPR. The generation of exhaled carbon dioxide depends upon pulmonary blood flow; therefore, $ETCO_2$ rises with increasing cardiac output. In adults, achieving an $ETCO_2$ above 10 mm Hg is correlated with return of spontaneous circulation. If an $ETCO_2$ monitor reads less than 10 mm Hg, efforts should be taken to enhance the quality of chest compressions (push hard, push fast, release completely, optimize hand position).

Temperature should be monitored during and after CPR. When a patient's cardiac arrest is caused by hypothermia, resuscitation must be continued until the patient's core temperature has risen above 35°C (95°F). (Use of a glass bulb thermometer may be necessary in the severely hypothermic patient.) Repeated measurements of core body temperature should be made at several sites (rectum, bladder, esophagus, axilla, and tympanic membrane), if possible, to avoid misleading temperature readings from a single site that might be affected by alterations in regional blood flow during CPR.

IV. DEFIBRILLATION AND CARDIOVERSION

> !
>
> *Do not delay defibrillation to establish an artificial airway.*
>
> !

In the child with ventricular fibrillation or pulseless ventricular tachycardia, defibrillation should proceed without delay to establish either an artificial airway or vascular access. Defibrillation achieves simultaneous depolarization and sustained contraction of a critical mass of myocardium, which allows return of spontaneous, coordinated cardiac contractions, assuming the myocardium is well oxygenated and the acid-base status is relatively normal. Successful defibrillation becomes less likely as delay lengthens. If defibrillation is not successful after a single attempt, CPR should be performed for 2 minutes before subsequent attempts. Drug treatment may be required as an adjunct to defibrillation but cannot be solely relied on to terminate ventricular fibrillation. Automated external defibrillators may be used in children over 1 year of age. In children between 1 and 8 years of age, the use of an attenuated shock (using pediatric cables or by activation of a key or a switch, depending on the model of defibrillator) is preferable (See **Appendix 9**).

In the majority of adult cases, energy levels of 100 to 200 joules are successful when shocks are delivered with minimal delay. In children, the initial energy level should be 2 joules per kilogram, increasing to 4 joules per kilogram for subsequent attempts. The goal of defibrillation is to deliver electrical current to a critical mass of ventricular muscle while avoiding a higher-than-necessary current that could further damage the heart. The most reliable predictor of successful defibrillation is the duration of fibrillation prior to the first countershock. Acidosis and hypoxia decrease the success of defibrillation.

A. Practical Aspects of Pediatric Defibrillation

Paddle size and position should be selected to capture the largest mass of myocardium in the path of the current. The largest paddle size appropriate for the patient should be used because a larger size reduces the density of current flow, which in turn reduces myocardial damage. Generally, adult paddles should be used in children weighing more than 10 kilograms, and infant paddles should be used in children weighing less than 10 kilograms. Paddle force is important as well. If the entire paddle does not rest firmly on the chest wall, a current of high density will be delivered to a small contact point. Paddles should be positioned on the chest wall so that the bulk of myocardium lies directly between them. One paddle is placed to the right of the upper sternum below the clavicle, and the other is positioned just below and to the left of the left nipple. An alternative approach is to place one paddle anteriorly over the left precordium and the other paddle posteriorly between the scapulae.

> !
>
> *Adult defibrillator paddles should be used for children weighing more than 10 kg. The use of self-adherent pads is preferable when possible.*
>
> !

The interface between the paddle and the chest wall may be gel pads, electrode cream, or electrode paste. The electrode cream produces lower impedance than the paste. Electric current follows the path of least resistance, so care should be taken that the substance from one paddle does not touch that of the other paddle. This is especially important in infants, in whom the distance between paddles is short. If the gel is continuous between paddles, a short circuit is created, and an insufficient amount of current will cross the heart. Use of bare metal paddles increases the risk of arcing and worsens cutaneous burns from defibrillation. The use of self-adhesive pads is preferable when feasible.

Poorly applied defibrillator paddles may spark, which can result in a fire in an oxygen-enriched atmosphere. Therefore, any sources of free-flowing oxygen should be removed to a distance of at least 1 meter from the patient. Potentially hazardous oxygen sources include nasal cannula oxygen, blow-by oxygen, and nebulizers powered by oxygen. In contrast, oxygen in a closed circuit may remain on the patient. For example, it is not necessary to disconnect a ventilator from a patient's endotracheal tube. However, if a ventilator is disconnected, it should be turned off due to the large amount of oxygen flow that it may generate. Key aspects of pediatric defibrillation are summarized in **Table 3-3**.

Table 3-3. Key Aspects of Pediatric Defibrillation

- Do not delay defibrillation to establish an artificial airway.
- The initial energy level is 2 joules/kg; the subsequent energy level is 4 joules/kg.
- Use adult paddles for patients weighing more that 10 kilograms.
- If defibrillation is unsuccessful, perform 2 minutes of CPR before attempting defibrillation again.
- Remove sources of free-flowing oxygen to a distance of 1 meter from the patient. There is no need to disconnect an intubated patient from a ventilator prior to defibrillation.

B. Transcutaneous Cardiac Pacing

Transcutaneous cardiac pacing (TCP) may be considered in children whose primary problem is impulse formation or conduction with preserved myocardial function, such as patients with high-grade atrioventricular block and a slow ventricular escape rate. Transcutaneous pacing is not useful in patients with bradycardia resulting from lack of substrate delivery to the myocardium following prolonged shock or cardiac arrest. In those cases, pacing attempts usually result in electrical but not mechanical cardiac capture and delay or interfere with other resuscitative efforts (see **Appendix 10**).

To set up pacing, 1 electrode is placed anteriorly at the left sternal border and the other posteriorly just below the left scapula. Smaller electrodes are available for infants and children, but adult-size electrodes can be used in children over 15 kilograms. The ECG leads should be connected to the pacemaker, and an age-appropriate heart rate should be used. The stimulus output should be set at zero when the pacemaker is turned on, then increased gradually until electrical capture is seen on the monitor. After electrical capture is achieved, one must ascertain whether an effective arterial pulse is generated. If not, other resuscitative efforts should be employed.

The most serious complication of TCP is the induction of a ventricular arrhythmia. Fortunately, this is rare and may be prevented by pacing only in the demand mode. Mild skin irritation beneath the electrodes is common. Contraction of skeletal muscles can be minimized by using large electrodes, a pulse duration of 40 milliseconds, and the smallest stimulus required for capture.

V. MEDICATIONS USED DURING CARDIOPULMONARY RESUSCITATION

Among the medications that may be used during CPR are epinephrine, atropine, sodium bicarbonate, calcium, glucose, amiodarone, and lidocaine. Basic information about these medications is presented below and summarized in **Table 3-4**.

Table 3-4. Medications Used During Pediatric CPR

Medication	Dose	Notes
Epinephrine	0.1 mL/kg of 1:10,000 concentration	Routine use of high-dose epinephrine should be avoided.
Atropine	0.02 mg/kg	Minimum dose: 0.1 mg Maximum dose: 2 mg
Sodium bicarbonate	1 to 2 mEq/kg, repeated as necessary	Routine use is controversial. Specific indications: tricyclic antidepressant overdose, hyperkalemia, hypermagnesemia, and sodium channel blocker poisoning
Calcium	Calcium chloride: 20 mg/kg Calcium gluconate: 30-100 mg/kg	Routine use is controversial. Specific indications: ionized hypocalcemia, hyperkalemia, hypermagnesemia, and calcium channel blocker overdose
Glucose	D50: 1 mL/kg D25: 2 mL/kg D10: 5 mL/kg	Use only in the child with known or highly suspected hypoglycemia or in conjunction with insulin for the patient with hyperkalemia.
Amiodarone	5 mg/kg	Either amiodarone or lidocaine is acceptable therapy for the child with shock-resistant ventricular fibrillation or pulseless ventricular tachycardia.
Lidocaine	1 mg/kg	Either amiodarone or lidocaine is acceptable therapy for the child with shock-resistant ventricular fibrillation or pulseless ventricular tachycardia.

Abbreviations: D50, 50% dextrose; D25, 25% dextrose; D10, 10% dextrose.

A. Epinephrine

Epinephrine (adrenaline) is an endogenous catecholamine with potent α- and β-adrenergic receptor stimulating properties. Epinephrine is the first-line medication for the majority of cardiac arrests. Through its α-adrenergic effects, it causes extreme vasoconstriction, increasing systemic vascular resistance and diastolic blood pressure. During CPR this increase in aortic diastolic pressure is critical for maintaining coronary blood flow and enhancing the success of resuscitation. In patients with ventricular fibrillation, epinephrine may also increase the likelihood of successful defibrillation by increasing the vigor and intensity of ventricular fibrillation.

> **!** *Routine use of high-dose (1:1000) epinephrine should be avoided.* **!**

Doses of epinephrine that are higher than necessary may be deleterious, and routine use of high-dose epinephrine in in-hospital pediatric cardiac arrest should be avoided. Epinephrine may worsen myocardial ischemic injury secondary to increased oxygen demand and may result in post-resuscitative tachyarrhythmias, hypertension, and pulmonary edema. Prolonged peripheral vasoconstriction by excessive doses of epinephrine may delay or impair reperfusion of systemic organs, particularly the kidneys and organs of the gastrointestinal tract. In a randomized controlled trial comparing high-dose to standard-dose epinephrine use in children with in-hospital cardiac arrest refractory to an initial standard dose of epinephrine, those receiving high-dose epinephrine were less likely to survive to 24 hours. There was also a trend toward decreased survival to hospital discharge in patients who received high-dose epinephrine.

The dose of epinephrine is 10 µg/kg (0.1 mL/kg of 1:10,000 concentration). Use 100 µg/kg when given through an endotracheal tube.

B. Atropine

Atropine is indicated for the treatment of bradycardia, second- and third-degree heart block, and slow idioventricular rhythms. Atropine is particularly effective in clinical conditions associated with excessive parasympathetic tone. However, epinephrine remains the first-line medication for children with asystole or bradycardia associated with severe hypotension. Atropine blocks cholinergic stimulation of the muscarinic receptors of the heart, increasing the sinus rate and shortening atrioventricular node conduction time. Atropine has little effect on systemic vascular resistance, myocardial perfusion pressure, or contractility.

The recommended dose of atropine is 0.02 mg/kg, with a minimum dose of 0.1 milligram and a maximum dose of 2 milligrams. Doses smaller than 0.1 milligram, even in small infants, may result paradoxically in bradycardia due to a central vagal effect at a dose that is too low to provide anticholinergic effects on the heart. Atropine may be given by any method, including intravenous, intraosseous, endotracheal, intramuscular, and subcutaneous routes. Its onset of action occurs within 30 seconds, and its peak effect occurs between 1 to 2 minutes after an intravenous dose. The recommended adult dose is 0.5 milligram every 5 minutes until the desired heart rate is obtained, up to a maximum of 2 milligrams.

C. Vasopressin

Vasopressin is a long-acting endogenous hormone that causes vasoconstriction, increasing systemic vascular resistance and hence increasing diastolic blood pressure and coronary blood flow. Although there is very little information regarding the use of vasopressin in pediatric cardiac arrest, its use may be considered in children with refractory diastolic hypotension. Given the paucity of pediatric data, vasopressin is considered Class Indeterminate by the American Heart Association for use during pediatric cardiac arrest, although it is Class IIB for adults (40 U to replace the second or third dose of epinephrine, dose not repeated). For use in children, the dose would be 0.5 U/kg.

D. Sodium Bicarbonate

The routine use of sodium bicarbonate during CPR is controversial, and sodium bicarbonate remains American Heart Association Class Indeterminate. In specific situations, however, administration of sodium bicarbonate is specifically indicated. These include tricyclic antidepressant overdose, hyperkalemia, hypermagnesemia, and sodium channel blocker poisoning.

Severe acidosis itself has many potentially deleterious effects that should be considered. Acidosis may depress myocardial function, prolong diastolic depolarization, depress spontaneous cardiac activity, decrease the electrical threshold for ventricular fibrillation, and reduce the cardiac response to catecholamines. Acidosis also vasodilates systemic vessels and attenuates the vasoconstrictive response of peripheral vessels to catecholamines. In patients with a reactive pulmonary vascular bed, acidosis exacerbates pulmonary hypertension. Therefore, correction of even mild acidosis may be helpful in resuscitating patients with elevated pulmonary vascular resistance. Acidosis may also increase the threshold for myocardial stimulation in a patient with an artificial cardiac pacemaker.

Potentially adverse effects of bicarbonate administration include metabolic alkalosis, hypercapnia, hypernatremia, and hyperosmolality. Alkalosis causes a leftward shift of the oxyhemoglobin dissociation curve and so impairs release of oxygen from hemoglobin to tissues at a time when oxygen delivery may already be low. Alkalosis may also result in ionized hypocalcemia by increasing the protein binding of ionized calcium. The marked hypercapnic acidosis that occurs during CPR on the venous side of the circulation, including the coronary sinus, may be worsened by the administration of bicarbonate. Paradoxical worsening of intracellular acidosis after bicarbonate administration is possible due to the rapid entry of carbon dioxide into cells with a slow egress of hydrogen ions out of cells. The dose of sodium bicarbonate, when used, is 1 to 2 mEq/kg.

E. Calcium

The administration of calcium during CPR should be restricted to cases with a specific indication for calcium, including hypocalcemia, hyperkalemia, hypermagnesemia, and overdose of calcium channel blocker. Intracellular calcium overload occurs during cerebral ischemia by the influx of calcium through voltage-dependent and agonist-dependent calcium channels, and administration of unnecessary exogenous calcium may worsen ischemia-reperfusion injury. Calcium plays an important role in the process of cell death in many organs, possibly by activation of intracellular enzymes such as nitric oxide synthase and phospholipase A and C.

Although excess calcium may be deleterious, ionized hypocalcemia should be promptly identified and corrected. Given that severe ionized hypocalcemia may occur during prolonged arrest and is associated with critical illness, ionized calcium levels should be routinely checked during CPR. Ionized hypocalcemia also occurs after massive or rapid transfusion of blood products due to the presence of citrate and other calcium-binding preservatives in stored blood products. The calcium ion is essential to myocardial excitation-contraction coupling in increasing ventricular contractility and in enhancing ventricular automaticity during asystole. Ionized hypocalcemia is associated with decreased ventricular performance and peripheral blunting of the hemodynamic response to catecholamines.

The pediatric dose of calcium chloride for resuscitation is 20 mg/kg. The adult dose is 200 mg (2 mL of the 10% solution). Calcium gluconate is as effective as calcium chloride in raising ionized calcium concentration during CPR. Calcium gluconate is given at a dose of 30 to 100 mg/kg, with a maximum dose of 2 grams in pediatric patients. Calcium should be given slowly through a large-bore, free-flowing intravenous catheter, preferably a central venous catheter. When administered too rapidly, calcium may cause bradycardia, heart block, or ventricular standstill. Severe tissue necrosis occurs when calcium infiltrates into subcutaneous tissue.

F. Glucose

In a child with documented hypoglycemia, glucose should be administered without delay (1 mL/kg of 50% dextrose in the older child with central venous access, 2 mL/kg of 25% dextrose in the child without central venous access, or 5 mL/kg of 10% dextrose in an infant). However, glucose should not be routinely administered in the absence of documented or highly suspected hypoglycemia. Hyperglycemia may exacerbate ischemic neurologic injury due to an increased production of lactic acid in the brain by anaerobic metabolism. During ischemia under normoglycemic conditions, brain lactate concentration reaches a plateau. In a hyperglycemic milieu, however, brain lactate concentration continues to rise for the duration of the ischemic period. Clinical studies have shown a direct correlation between high initial postcardiac arrest serum glucose concentration and poor neurologic outcome, though the higher glucose concentration may be a marker rather than a cause of more severe brain injury.

Some groups of patients, including premature infants and debilitated patients with low endogenous glycogen stores, are prone to developing hypoglycemia during and after physiologic stress, such as surgery. Bedside monitoring of serum glucose is critical during and following a cardiac arrest and allows for intervention before the critical point of low substrate delivery has been reached.

G. Amiodarone

Amiodarone has now supplanted lidocaine as the first drug of choice for the medical management of shock-resistant ventricular tachycardia and fibrillation in adults. Compared to lidocaine, amiodarone results in a higher rate of survival to hospital admission in adults with shock-resistant out-of-hospital ventricular fibrillation, but there is limited data for or against its use in pediatric ventricular fibrillation or pulseless ventricular tachycardia. Nevertheless, amiodarone is used widely for serious pediatric arrhythmias in the non-resuscitation environment and appears to be effective and to have an acceptable short-term safety profile. This growing pediatric experience among experts and inference from adult studies led to the inclusion of amiodarone as a choice for treatment of ventricular tachycardia or pulseless ventricular tachycardia in the 2000 American Heart Association Pediatric Advanced Life Support guidelines. The pediatric dose of amiodarone is 5 mg/kg. This dose can be repeated if necessary to control the arrhythmia. Intravenous loading doses are followed by a continuous infusion of 10 to 20 mg/kg/day if there is a risk that arrhythmia will recur.

Hypotension is commonly reported with intravenous amiodarone administration and may limit the rate at which the drug can be given. The overall hemodynamic impact of amiodarone will depend on the balance of its effect on rate control, myocardial performance, and vasodilation. Owing to the potential for profound vasodilation in children, many recommend that it be given over 10 minutes, as detailed in the package insert. We recommend starting a slow IV push (at a rate that would deliver the whole dose over 2-3 minutes) until the arrhythmia is controlled and then a slower bolus (up to 10 minutes) for the remainder of the dose. An alternative dosing regimen that has been described is to give 1 mg/kg pushes every 5 minutes up to 5 mg/kg. The use of the small aliquot bolus technique may be particularly appropriate for infants from 6 to 12 months of age.

The use of amiodarone should be avoided in combination with other drugs that prolong the QT interval and in the setting of hypomagnesemia and other electrolyte abnormalities. Severe bradycardia and heart block have been described with amiodarone administration, especially in the postoperative period.

H. Lidocaine

Either lidocaine or amiodarone is an acceptable first-line antiarrhythmic medication for children with ventricular fibrillation or pulseless ventricular tachycardia. Lidocaine has no effect on atrioventricular nodal conduction time, so it is ineffective in the treatment of atrial or atrioventricular junctional arrhythmias. In healthy adults, no change in heart rate or blood pressure occurs with lidocaine administration. In patients with severe, typically acute cardiac disease, there may be a decrease in ventricular function when a lidocaine bolus is administered intravenously.

The pediatric dose of 1 mg/kg of lidocaine may be given IV push, followed by a constant intravenous infusion at a rate of 25 to 50 µg/kg/minute. If the arrhythmia recurs, a second intravenous bolus at the same dose can be given.

Toxic effects of lidocaine occur when the serum concentration exceeds 7 to 8 µg/mL and include seizures, psychosis, drowsiness, paresthesias, disorientation, agitation, tinnitus, muscle spasms, and respiratory arrest. The treatment of choice for lidocaine-induced seizures is a benzodiazepine such as midazolam or lorazepam, or a barbiturate such as phenobarbital, which also increases the hepatic metabolism of lidocaine.

VI. SPECIFIC SITUATIONS REQUIRING CARDIOPULMONARY RESUSCITATION

A. Bradycardia

The most common cause of bradycardia in children is hypoxemia. Therefore, early resuscitative efforts should focus on adequacy of respiratory support. If symptomatic bradycardia persists, it should be treated with epinephrine (10 µg/kg) or atropine (epinephrine is the first-line therapy if the child is severely hypotensive). The adequacy of perfusion determines when to initiate chest compressions in a child with bradycardia. Cardiac pacing for bradycardia should be considered when the bradycardia results from a failure of impulse generation rather than from a lack of substrate delivery (see "Transcutaneous Cardiac Pacing," above).

B. Asystole

The management of asystole proceeds along the same algorithm as symptomatic bradycardia. However, the ECG should be closely examined to ensure that what appears to be asystole is not, in fact, fine ventricular fibrillation.

C. Pulseless Ventricular Tachycardia

Case Study

A previously well teenager is admitted for observation following a syncopal episode. While watching TV, he collapses. Chest compressions are started and bag-mask ventilation is initiated, and when a cardiac monitor is placed, it shows ventricular tachycardia. The patient is unresponsive without a palpable pulse. The defibrillator is brought into the room, but the anesthesia resident asks everyone to hold on so she can get the patient intubated.

- What is the most appropriate immediate action at this point?
- If a single attempt at cardioversion is unsuccessful, what is the next immediate action?
- What medications should be considered if the patient remains in pulseless ventricular tachycardia?

Asynchronous cardioversion (defibrillation) (2 J/kg) is the primary treatment for unstable ventricular tachycardia. Cardioversion should not be delayed to establish an airway or vascular access. In the patient who does not respond to cardioversion, 10 µg/kg (0.1 mL/kg dose of 1:10,000) epinephrine should be administered and circulated with 2 minutes of CPR prior to reattempting cardioversion with 4 J/kg. In persistent pulseless ventricular tachycardia, epinephrine can be administered every 5 minutes. Amiodarone (5 mg/kg) or lidocaine (1 mg/kg) should be administered to children with persistent ventricular tachycardia refractory to epinephrine and cardioversion. Ventricular tachycardia with pulse present and poor perfusion should have synchronized cardioversion attempted with 0.5 to 1 J/kg.

D. Ventricular Fibrillation

Ventricular fibrillation is managed in the same way as pulseless ventricular tachycardia, except that asynchronous cardioversion (defibrillation) should be used.

E. Supraventricular Tachycardia

Supraventricular tachycardia (SVT) is a common arrhythmia in infants and children that may be associated with severe circulatory compromise or even cardiac arrest. Therapy for this arrhythmia should be based on the child's hemodynamic status. In the child with hemodynamically unstable

SVT, immediate cardioversion with 0.5 J/kg should be performed, increasing to 1 J/kg if 0.5 J/kg is ineffective. Adenosine may also be considered first-line therapy, although intravenous access is required. In the unstable patient, cardioversion should not be delayed by attempts to achieve vascular access.

The underlying mechanism of SVT in children is usually a reentry circuit involving the atrioventricular node. Adenosine causes a temporary block in the atrioventricular node and interrupts this reentry circuit. The initial dose is 0.1 mg/kg given as a rapid IV bolus. Central venous administration is preferable because the drug is rapidly metabolized by red blood cell adenosine deaminase and so has a half-life of only 10 seconds. When the drug is given peripherally, the catheter should be immediately and rapidly flushed with 10 milliliters of saline. If SVT persists, successive doses of 0.2 and 0.4 mg/kg should be used. In neonates, a smaller initial dose of 0.05 mg/kg is given and increased by 0.05 mg/kg/dose up to a maximum dose of 0.25 mg/kg until termination of the arrhythmia. The use of amiodarone or procainamide for hemodynamically unstable SVT refractory to adenosine and cardioversion should be considered.

F. Pulseless Electrical Activity

Case Study

A 6-year-old girl with necrotizing pneumonia and septic shock is being managed with positive-pressure ventilation and dopamine at 10 µg/kg/min, with acceptable blood pressure and a pulse oximeter reading in the mid-90s. Acutely, her pulse oximetry reading falls to 70% and then loses its waveform, and the waveform on her arterial catheter becomes flat.

- What is the most important immediate step?
- Assessment of airway and breathing reveals no breath sounds on the right. What is the most important next immediate step?
- A needle is inserted in the second intercostal space in the mid-clavicular line with prompt return of spontaneous circulation.

Pulseless electrical activity (PEA) is defined as organized ECG activity, excluding ventricular tachycardia and fibrillation, without clinical evidence of a palpable pulse or myocardial contractions. The most common causes of PEA can be remembered as the 4 Hs (hypovolemia, hypothermia, hypoxemia, hyperkalemia [or other metabolic disorder]) and the 4 Ts (tension pneumothorax, thromboembolism [pulmonary or coronary], tamponade, toxins), as summarized in **Table 3-5**. All of these causes of PEA are potentially reversible; therefore, prompt efforts should be made to identify and correct them. While such efforts are under way, epinephrine (10 µg/kg) may be administered every 5 minutes. When the cause of PEA is unknown and the patient does not respond to medications, consideration should be given to administering a fluid bolus and inserting catheters into the pleural spaces to rule out pneumothorax and into the pericardial space to rule out cardiac tamponade.

Table 3-5. Causes of Pulseless Electrical Activity

The 6Hs	The 5Ts
• Hypovolemia	• Tension pneumothorax
• Hypothermia	• Thromboembolism (pulmonary or coronary)
• Hypoxemia	• Tamponade
• Hyperkalemia (or other metabolic disorder)	• Toxins
• Hypoglycemia	• Trauma (hypovolemia)
• Hydrogen ion (acidosis)	

G. Hyperkalemia

A child with a hyperkalemic cardiac arrest may be identified by history, the progression of ECG changes leading up to the arrest, or initial lab results. A high index of suspicion must be maintained for hyperkalemia as a cause of cardiac arrest because it requires specific therapy. Along with the usual resuscitation algorithms, immediate therapy to antagonize the effects of elevated serum potassium is necessary (**Table 3-6**). The serum potassium concentration must be monitored frequently during this treatment, preferably by point-of-care testing modalities. Given that several of these therapies shift potassium intracellularly, therapy to remove potassium from the body (furosemide, hemodialysis) may also be indicated.

Table 3-6. Treatment of Hyperkalemia

Therapy	Dose	Mechanism of Action
Sodium bicarbonate	1 mEq/kg (more if patient has a substantial acidosis)	Enhances potassium/hydrogen exchange at cell membranes, driving potassium into the intracellular space
Calcium	Calcium gluconate (10%) 100 mg/kg Calcium chloride (10%) 20 mg/kg	Antagonizes the membrane actions of potassium, lessening the chance of arrhythmias
Insulin and glucose	Insulin 0.1 U/kg	Stimulates potassium entry into cells
	2 mL/kg of 25% dextrose	Prevents hypoglycemia from insulin administration
		Dextrose should be given prior to or concomitantly with insulin.

H. Anaphylaxis

Anaphylaxis is an unusual, but potentially reversible, cause of cardiac arrest. Manifestations of anaphylaxis include skin reaction (usually flushing, paleness, or urticaria), airway edema with possible airway obstruction, bronchospasm, and cardiovascular collapse.

Resuscitation of the child with anaphylaxis rests on reversing airway obstruction and restoring intravascular volume and vascular tone. In the patient with cardiac arrest, standard-dose epinephrine should be administered intravenously. In the child with impending cardiac arrest, 0.01 mL/kg of subcutaneous epinephrine (1:1000 concentration) may be preferred. Patients with anaphylactic shock have profound intravascular depletion that requires rapidly administered, high-volume fluid resuscitation. In addition to the usual resuscitation medications, treatment should include an antihistamine and a corticosteroid, such as diphenhydramine at a dose of 1 mg/kg and methylprednisolone at 2 mg/kg. Inhaled bronchodilators, such as albuterol, may help reverse bronchospasm, and inhaled racemic epinephrine may relieve airway edema. If severe airway obstruction occurs, endotracheal intubation or even cricothyrotomy may become difficult or impossible. Therefore, the airway should be secured early by a skilled practitioner.

VII. Post-resuscitation Management

Medical management of the child resuscitated from cardiac arrest should aim to match oxygen and substrate delivery to meet metabolic tissue demand and to minimize reperfusion injury and support cellular recovery. A complete reevaluation of the patient is necessary after resuscitation.

A. Ventilation

Both hypoventilation and hyperventilation should be avoided. Hyperventilation may decrease venous return by increasing mean intrathoracic pressure. Further, abnormally low $Paco_2$ causes cerebral vasoconstriction and may impair cerebral perfusion. Similarly, in the patient for whom cerebral edema is a concern, care should be taken to avoid hypoventilation with resultant cerebral vasodilation. Brief hyperventilation may be appropriate in the child with signs of cerebral herniation.

B. Temperature Management

Fever exacerbates neurologic injury following resuscitation from cardiac arrest; therefore, great care should be taken to prevent fever in these children. The use of a servo-controlled temperature regulating blanket is recommended. Induction of hypothermia (32°C-34°C [89.6°F-93.2°F]) should be considered for 12 to 24 hours in children who remain comatose following resuscitation. This may be achieved using cooling blankets and ice packs around the head and torso. A rectal temperature probe should be placed for continuous temperature monitoring.

C. Inotropes and Vasoactive Medications

Many children will require hemodynamic support following resuscitation. The choice of vasoactive agent should be based on physical exam and other available monitoring data. Some children may have an ongoing need for vasoconstrictors, whereas for others inotropy with vasodilation may be more appropriate. Intense vasoconstriction during cardiac arrest and CPR may improve coronary perfusion pressure and probability of return of spontaneous circulation, but the same intense vasoconstriction during the post-arrest resuscitative phase may increase left ventricular afterload and worsen myocardial ischemia and dysfunction.

D. Glucose Control

Both hyperglycemia and hypoglycemia should be avoided in the post-resuscitation phase. The choice of dextrose content for fluids administered in this phase should be determined by frequent monitoring of blood glucose levels.

VIII. ETHICAL ISSUES

A. Who Should Be Resuscitated?

In children with a progressive, terminal condition, performing CPR may prolong the dying process and deny family members a peaceful death for their child. For children with terminal conditions, caregivers should initiate a discussion of do-not-attempt-resuscitation (DNAR) orders well before a cardiac arrest becomes imminent. In the absence of a documented DNAR order or verbal parental request, the medical staff is obligated to perform CPR in the event of cardiac arrest. Slow codes, in which interventions are performed, but not promptly, are inappropriate. It is appropriate to consider a child's underlying condition when determining the appropriate duration of a resuscitation attempt. In the child with multisystem organ failure and incurable cancer, a 10-minute resuscitation attempt may be appropriate, whereas in cases of cold-water drowning, drug toxicity, or severe electrolyte disturbance, it may be appropriate to continue resuscitation efforts for 1 hour or more.

B. Family Presence During Resuscitation

Data suggest that parents who choose to remain in the room during an attempted resuscitation are not psychologically harmed by witnessing CPR. Parents who are present during a failed resuscitation may benefit from knowing that extreme measures were taken in the attempt to save their child's life and that they were with their child when he or she died. However, an appropriate staff person (physician, nurse, social worker) should be assigned sole responsibility for providing support to parents present during CPR. Family presence should be an option rather than an expectation.

C. Termination of Efforts

When excellent CPR is provided, children may have intact neurologic survival even after as much as 1 hour of CPR. However, if a child remains pulseless after 30 minutes of CPR with an established airway and appropriate medical and other therapeutic interventions, consideration should be given to terminating resuscitation efforts. If a child is profoundly hypothermic, resuscitation should not be terminated until after rewarming has occurred. If emergency extracorporeal membrane oxygenation is immediately available, it may be appropriate to continue CPR for 1 hour or more while extracorporeal membrane oxygenation is being established.

Key Points

Cardiopulmonary/Cerebral Resuscitation

- The presence of one definitive leader is vital to the conduct of an efficient and effective resuscitation.
- If an intravenous line cannot be established rapidly, medications should be administered via the intraosseous or endotracheal route.
- To ensure high-quality CPR, providers should push hard at a rate at 100 compressions per minute, ensuring proper positioning and full release, and rotating providers frequently.
- While rapid ventilation may be necessary immediately following a hypercarbia-induced cardiac arrest, ongoing hyperventilation or hyperventilation in the child with primary cardiac arrest is probably deleterious.
- Avoid routine use of high-dose (1:1000) epinephrine.
- In the child with ventricular fibrillation or pulseless ventricular tachycardia, defibrillation should proceed without delay to establish either an artificial airway or vascular access.
- If a manual defibrillator is not available, the use of an automated external defibrillator is acceptable in children older than 1 year, preferably with the use of pediatric cables or adaptors in children younger than 8 years.
- To optimize post-resuscitation management, avoid hyper- and hypotension, hyper- and hypoglycemia, and hyponatremia. Consider the use of induced hypothermia for 12 to 24 hours in patients who remain comatose following resuscitation.

Suggested Readings

1. American Heart Association. 2005 American Heart Association guidelines for cardiopulmonary resuscitation and emergency cardiovascular care. *Circulation.* 2005;112(suppl 4):S1-S203.

2. Donoghue AJ, Nadkarni V, Berg RA, Osmond MH, Wells G, Nesbitt L, Stiell IG. Out-of-hospital pediatric cardiac arrest: an epidemiologic review and assessment of current knowledge. *Ann Emerg Med.* 2005;46(6):512-522.

3. Perondi MB, Reis AG, Paiva EF, Nadkarni VM, Berg RA. A comparison of high-dose and standard-dose epinephrine in children with cardiac arrest. *NEJM.* 2004;350(17):1722-1730.

Chapter 4:

Diagnosis and Management of the Child With Acute Upper Airway Disease

Objectives

- Explain the anatomic and developmental differences that make infants and children prone to disorders of the upper airway.
- Describe how to assess children with upper airway disorders.
- Summarize diagnosis and treatment of children with upper airway disorders.
- Identify common disorders of the upper airway.

Case Study

You are called to the bedside of a 6-month-old boy who has developed a barky cough and is having difficulty breathing. When you approach the patient you see deep subcostal retractions and upon auscultation over the trachea you hear high-pitched inspiratory noise.

- What immediate actions should you take?

- What problems are in your differential diagnosis?

- What does the high pitched noise signify?

I. INTRODUCTION

Problems related to the upper airway occur frequently in infants and children. Upper airway problems range from benign and self-limiting, such as most cases of viral croup, to immediately life threatening, as in cases of acute upper airway obstruction due to foreign body aspiration. Management strategies for upper airway–related disorders range from calm reassurance to urgent life-saving intervention. Knowledge of the etiologies of upper airway diseases in children, how to assess their severity, and approaches to treatment is important for treating hospitalized children.

II. ANATOMIC DIFFERENCES BETWEEN CHILDREN AND ADULTS

A. Airway

The airway of a child changes continuously from birth until approximately 8 years of age, when it becomes anatomically similar to an adult's airway. In addition to airway disorders related to small size and normal anatomic development, congenital abnormalities occur that affect the airway. Pediatric patients are more susceptible to several illnesses, one being viral croup, that are not so problematic for adults because they have larger airways. After children reach age 8, their upper airway problems become similar to those found in adults.

Chapter 2 on airway management describes many of the developmental differences that exist between newborn, infant, pediatric, and adult airways and the impact of those differences on airway management. **Table 4-1** highlights some differences between the infant and adult airways.

Table 4-1. Anatomic Differences between Infant, Pediatric, and Adult Airways

	Newborn	Pediatric (at Age 1 Year)	Adult
Air entry	Obligate nasal breather	Mouth and nose	Mouth and nose
Tracheal diameter	4 mm	5-6 mm	18 mm
Laryngeal shape	Funnel	Funnel	Barrel
Narrowest portion	Cricoid	Cricoid	Laryngeal inlet
Epiglottis	Long, soft, (omega) shaped	Long, soft, (omega) shaped	Short, firm

continued next page...

Table 4-1. Anatomic Differences between Infant, Pediatric, and Adult Airways (Cont)

	Newborn	Pediatric (at Age 1 Year)	Adult
Laryngeal inlet	C1	C3-C4	C5-C6
Proportion of tongue to jaw	Tongue relatively large in proportion to oral cavity (jaw space)	Proportion of tongue to jaw space changes continually up to approximately 8 years of age	Tongue easy to displace into jaw
Position of larynx on laryngoscopy	Anterior, cephalad	Transition between infant and adult position	More posterior, caudad
Trachea	Soft cartilage	Firmer but still collapsible cartilage	Firm, more rigid tracheal cartilage

At birth, and for some time afterward, infants are obligate nasal breathers. This makes them prone to distress from congenital and acquired nasal obstruction. Congenital causes of nasal obstruction include unilateral and bilateral choanal stenosis. Acquired causes of nasal obstruction include mucous plugging and edema from upper respiratory tract infections due to respiratory syncytial virus (RSV) or other viruses. Suctioning to clear the nasal passages of infants can result in substantial improvement in respiratory status. As a child ages, oral breathing becomes possible, but there continues to be a preference for the nose.

A small chin is developmentally appropriate at birth in that it facilitates both vaginal delivery and breast-feeding. Anatomically, a small chin is manifested by short mandibular rami and short distance from chin to hyoid cartilage. A small chin contributes to a smaller jaw space and is one reason that the tongue is relatively large for the size of the oral cavity around birth. A relatively large tongue-to-mouth ratio facilitates obligate nasal breathing, which, in turn, permits a child to feed without aspirating. The ratio of tongue size to oral cavity size decreases as a child grows. A large tongue in a relatively small mouth, though anatomically normal, makes infants with a decreased level of consciousness more prone to develop upper airway obstruction from the tongue falling back into the pharynx.

In the Pierre Robin sequence (micrognathia, relative macroglossia, cleft palate) there is such severe disproportion in size between the tongue and mouth that the tongue may be pressed back into the pharynx, obstructing all air movement. A small submental space in infants results in less space into which the tongue can be displaced during laryngoscopy and adds difficulty to intubation. Airway visualization by laryngoscopy is always more difficult in patients with disorders in which micrognathia, macroglossia, or both are present.

The airway diameter of newborns, infants, and children increases with growth until the mid-teens, when it reaches adult caliber. The narrower airway diameter of infants and children results in increased resistance to airflow. Resistance to airflow is described mathematically by the Hagen-Poiseuille equation:

$$R = 8\eta l/\pi r^4$$

In this equation, R is resistance, η is the viscosity of the gas, l is the length of a tube that air flows through, and r is the radius of the airway. From the equation, it is seen that resistance goes up exponentially to the fourth power as airway diameter (2 times the radius) decreases. Therefore, even though the absolute volume of gas that flows is less, resistance to airflow is greater in infants and children. In a small airway, very small decreases in airway caliber will result in significant increases in airflow resistance.

Figure 4-1 illustrates the relative increase in resistance when 1 millimeter of circumferential airway edema occurs in an infant airway that is 4 millimeters in diameter compared to the increase in resistance that occurs when the same amount of circumferential edema occurs in the 8-millimeter-diameter airway of an older child or teen. Airways with 1 millimeter of circumferential edema are on the right. Remembering that 1 millimeter of circumferential edema results in a 2-millimeter decrease in diameter and using Posiseulle's law, it is seen that the $1/r^4$ relationship of airway radius to resistance results in a 16-fold increase in airway resistance in the 4-millimeter airway compared to a 3-fold increase in resistance in the 8-millimeter airway.

Figure 4-1. Age-dependent Effects of Reduction in Airway Caliber on Airway Resistance

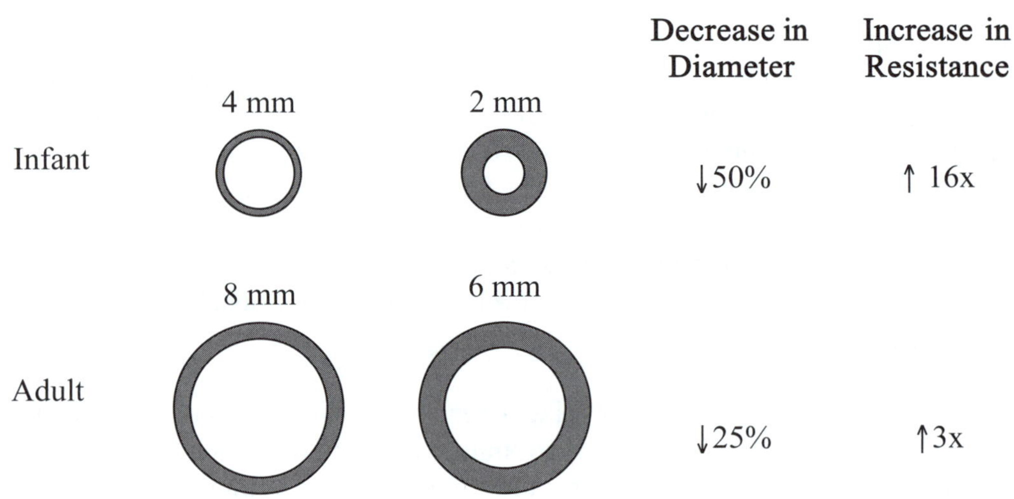

Until a child reaches approximately 8 years of age, the narrowest portion of the airway is in the subglottic space. The infant and pediatric larynxes have a funnel shape rather than the barrel shape of an adult larynx. Thus, the adult airway is narrowest at the vocal cords, or laryngeal inlet, whereas the infant and pediatric airways continue to narrow below the vocal cords to their narrowest portion at the level of the cricoid cartilage. The narrowest portion of the upper airway being located in the subglottic space creates a susceptibility to significant airflow compromise in an infant in response to even small amounts of tissue edema caused by infectious and noninfectious reasons. As the airway diameter increases with growth, the increases in resistance related to airway edema become less significant. Thus, it is extremely unusual, barring other anatomic abnormalities, for adults to have significant distress from viral laryngotracheobronchitis (croup) even though they may be infected with the same virus.

Although passing an endotracheal tube through the vocal cords always places a patient at risk for vocal cord injury, a narrow subglottic space makes infants and children susceptible to subglottic injury as well. Inappropriately large endotracheal tubes, repeat intubations, excessive movement, and thrashing while tracheally intubated all may contribute to subglottic injury and edema that may develop into scar tissue leading to subglottic stenosis.

B. Epiglottis

The epiglottis of infants and young children differs in shape and consistency from an adult epiglottis. The epiglottis of infants and children is longer, softer, and assumes an omega-like shape (Ω). The adult epiglottis, in contrast, is shorter, firmer, and squarer. The characteristics of the infant larynx create a need for the epiglottis to be actively displaced from the glottic opening during laryngoscopy for tracheal intubation. The shape of an infant's epiglottis, when exaggerated, contributes to laryngomalacia. In laryngomalacia, an infant shows signs of inspiratory upper airway obstruction that are due to the collapse of the epiglottis and laryngeal components over the laryngeal inlet on inspiration.

C. Larynx

The larynx of infants and young children is anterior and cephalad compared with the larynx of an adult. The impact of this relationship on airway visualization during intubation is discussed in the chapter on airway management.

D. Trachea

During infancy, tracheal cartilage is soft and collapsible. The cartilaginous tracheal rings become more rigid with growth. One result of a child's trachea having a less rigid skeleton than that found in adults is that the walls of the extrathoracic trachea can collapse inward when an infant creates significant negative inspiratory force by inhaling against an obstructed upper airway. **Figure 4-2** illustrates this point.

Figure 4-2. Extrathoracic Tracheal Collapse With Forceful Inspiration Against a Subglottic Obstruction

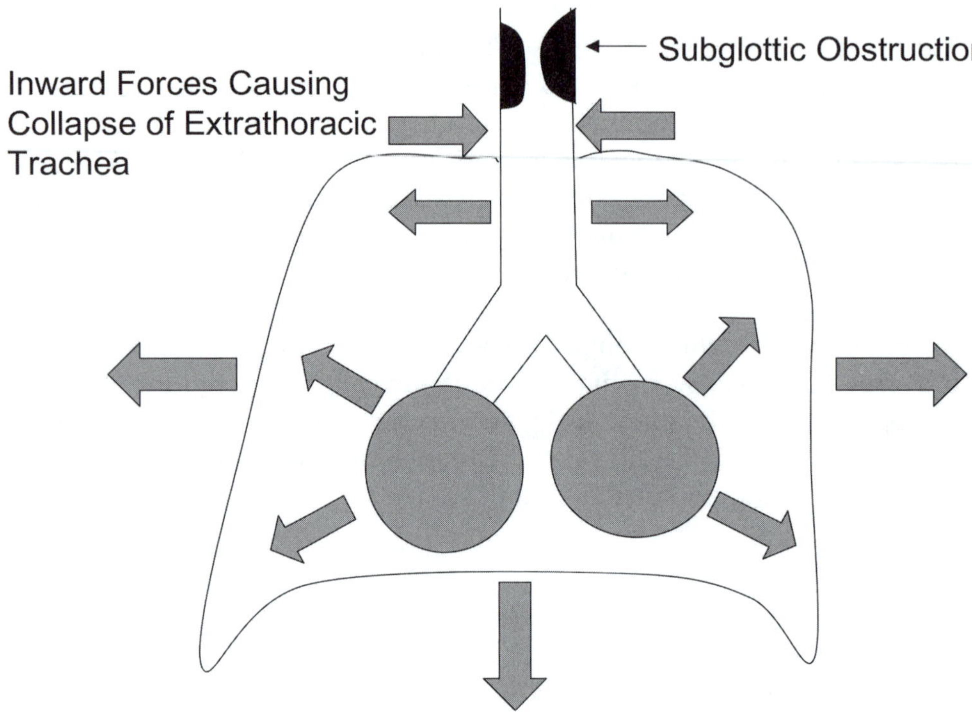

The extrathoracic and intrathoracic portions of the trachea react differently to forces generated by breathing. The portion of the trachea from the subglottic space to the thoracic inlet is extrathoracic. The trachea from the thoracic inlet to the carina is intrathoracic. The intrathoracic section of the trachea sits within the chest, surrounded by lung and pleura, and is thus subject to the forces generated within the chest during inspiration and expiration. The pleural pressure is negative during quiet inspiration and very negative when there is increased airway resistance due to partial or complete airway obstruction. This negative inspiratory force is generated by the downward movement of the diaphragm during quiet breathing and is augmented by the accessory muscles of inspiration (external intercostals, scalenes, and sternocleidomastoids) during periods of distress. The negative pleural pressure creates a pressure gradient from the alveoli (where it is most negative) to the mouth (where it is approximately zero). The pressure gradient drives airflow into the lungs. When the diaphragm contracts (and in distress, the accessory muscles of respiration as well), the negative intrathoracic pressure is transmitted to the outside of the trachea to serve as a distending force that keeps the intrathoracic airways open.

Intrapleural pressure becomes very positive during forced expiration, as occurs in diseases such as asthma. When the intrapleural pressure becomes positive, the airway pressure gradient becomes very positive in the alveoli and decreases as it moves toward the mouth, where it is zero. A gradient is necessary for air movement to occur. As the pressure gradient decreases toward the mouth, there may come a point, known as the equal pressure point, where the pressure in the airways becomes equal to the intrapleural pressure. At any point closer to the mouth than the equal pressure point, the sum of forces favors closure of the airways.

Thus, the intrathoracic airways, including the intrathoracic trachea, will remain open when inspiratory effort is increased but are prone to closure when expiratory forces are increased. The extrathoracic trachea behaves in a manner opposite to the intrathoracic trachea. In the extrathoracic trachea there is no tethering of the outer trachea to the lung and pleura that creates a distending force to counterbalance the negative intratracheal pressure that occurs during inspiration. During quiet breathing, and when the tracheal cartilage is formed normally, there is no significant tracheal collapse during inspiration. However, when a patient breathes against a partial upper airway obstruction, as occurs in laryngomalacia or viral croup, the tracheal walls can partially collapse, thus further increasing airway resistance. Collapse of the extrathoracic trachea during inspiration and of the intrathoracic trachea during expiration is much worse in the presence of poor cartilaginous ring development, as is seen in tracheomalacia.

The extrathoracic trachea is not subject to collapse during forced exhalation. These differences between the intrathoracic and extrathoracic airways provide the basis for understanding why problems of the nose, pharynx, larynx, and subglottic trachea have their greatest impact on inspiration, whereas problems of the lower (intrathoracic) airways tend to have greater impact upon exhalation. A tendency for the subglottic, but extrathoracic, trachea to narrow or close when there is very negative intrapleural pressure also explains why patients with upper airway obstruction do worse when they are agitated. See **Figure 4-2.**

!

Changes in Pediatric Airway with Partial Obstruction

Airflow restriction is related to where the obstruction is located.

- *Extrathoracic Obstruction →*
  Inspiratory Airway Collapse → Stridor
- *Intrathoracic Obstruction →*
  Expiratory Airway Collapse →
  Wheezing on Expiration

In severe cases (eg, laryngotracheobronchitis), both may be present.

!

III. DISORDERS THAT AFFECT CHILDREN'S AIRWAYS

Table 4-2 lists some of the disorders that affect the pediatric airway and may present as partial or complete obstruction of the upper airway. The causes are organized by category and discussed below, along with specific approaches to management. General approaches to management are discussed in greater detail in a later section.

Table 4-2. Causes of Disorders That Affect the Pediatric Airway

Causes
Anatomic Disorders
Altered level of consciousness (airway muscle laxity)
Tonsillar hypertrophy
Subglottic stenosis (acquired or congenital)
Macroglossia
Micrognathia
Vocal cord paralysis
Choanal stenosis
Pierre Robin sequence
External or Internal Compression Disorders
Tumor
Hemangioma
Hematoma
Cyst
Papilloma
Vascular rings and slings
Infectious Disorders
Laryngotracheobronchitis (croup)
Epiglottitis (supraglottitis)
Bacterial tracheitis
Retropharyngeal (Parapharyngeal) abscess
Peritonsillar abscess
Infectious mononucleosis
Miscellaneous Disorders
Airway Trauma
Postextubation airway obstruction
Angioedema
Spasmodic croup
Foreign body aspiration
Airway trauma
Thermal and chemical burns

A. Anatomic Disorders

1. Altered Level of Consciousness

Altered level of consciousness (LOC) is frequently responsible for upper airway obstruction in patients of all ages. For the developmental reasons discussed previously, younger patients are more prone to upper airway obstruction related to a decreased level of consciousness. For example, the decreased level of consciousness that accompanies the postictal state after a seizure, especially when barbiturates or benzodiazepines have been administered, can lead to upper airway obstruction. Many decreases in oxygen saturation that occur during procedural sedation are related to upper airway obstruction. A child injured in an automobile or bicycle collision and who has decreased LOC is likely to have a partially obstructed airway and may benefit significantly from maneuvers that open and maintain airway patency while protecting the neck's spinal alignment. See **Chapter 2.**

2. Tonsillar-Adenoidal Hypertrophy

Tonsillar-adenoidal hypertrophy by itself and combined with obesity is responsible for obstructive sleep apnea and even for acute upper airway obstruction. Though obstructive sleep apnea is mostly a chronic problem, there are situations in which such patients develop acute upper airway obstruction. Positive pressure ventilation by continuous positive airway pressure (CPAP) or bilevel positive airway pressure (BiPAP) is often helpful. In an acute emergency, a nasopharyngeal airway may be helpful. Tonsillectomy and adenoidectomy along with weight loss are the definitive treatments. Patients may continue to require positive airway pressure for some time after tonsillectomy and adenoidectomy. In acute situations, corticosteroids may be helpful in reducing tonsillar tissue size, especially when the cause is mononucleosis.

3. Subglottic Stenosis

Subglottic stenosis (SGS) can be congenital or acquired. Acquired SGS is frequently seen in the neonatal intensive care unit (NICU) in infants with a history of prematurity and intubation. Sometimes an acute intercurrent viral respiratory infection, especially RSV, can cause SGS to change rapidly from a chronic compensated problem to uncompensated respiratory distress. Racemic epinephrine, dexamethasone, and heliox are all useful interventions for ameliorating a severe event, but ultimately a patient with severe SGS requires airway endoscopy for definitive diagnosis and, potentially, laryngotracheal reconstruction.

4. Macroglossia and Micrognathia

Macroglossia (a large tongue) or micrognathia (small chin and jaw), or both, are components of several congenital craniofacial anomalies. The roles of macroglossia and micrognathia in upper airway obstruction were discussed above. Severe macroglossia and micrognathia can result in critical airway issues in the perinatal period. After the perinatal period, these issues become relevant when a patient either requires procedural sedation or anesthesia with tracheal intubation.

5. Vocal Cord Paralysis

Vocal cord paralysis can be either unilateral or bilateral. Unilateral vocal cord paralysis is manifested by weak cry and occasional stridor, and is usually well tolerated. The etiology of unilateral vocal cord paralysis is often idiopathic, but the condition is occasionally associated with injury to the recurrent laryngeal nerve during thoracic surgery. Bilateral vocal cord paralysis manifests as severe stridor and severe respiratory distress, though often with a normal cry. Bilateral vocal cord paralysis is often associated with central nervous system injury or disease. Children with bilateral vocal cord paralysis often require urgent airway management.

6. Choanal Stenosis and Choanal Atresia

Choanal stenosis and choanal atresia may be unilateral or bilateral. Given that infants are obligate nasal breathers, most children with choanal stenosis develop some degree of distress and poor feeding. Bilateral choanal stenosis almost always produces symptoms during the neonatal period. Diagnosis is confirmed by attempting to pass a soft catheter through the nose. Evaluation of the nose and nasopharynx by computed tomographic (CT) scanning is helpful in confirming the diagnosis and determining the extent of obstruction. Associated anomalies are common and occur in 20% to 50% of infants with choanal atresia. The syndrome of anomalies, known as the CHARGE association, includes **c**oloboma and other ophthalmologic anomalies, **h**eart disease, choanal **a**tresia, growth **r**etardation, **g**enital hypoplasia, and **e**ar anomalies. Choanal stenosis and choanal atresia are treated surgically.

Unilateral choanal stenosis may make it difficult or impossible to pass a nasogastric (NG) tube through the stenotic naris. If the NG tube is instead passed through the unobstructed nostril, an infant will become distressed due to occlusion of the one patent nare.

7. Pierre Robin Sequence

Pierre Robin sequence is an example of a congenital syndrome in which upper airway obstruction often occur and can be life-threatening. The primary defect is poor mandibular growth in utero that results in micrognathia, cleft palate, and glossoptosis (posterior displacement or retraction of the tongue). In Pierre Robin the oral cavity is too small for the tongue, which is usually a normal size. As a result of the mismatch between tongue and jaw sizes, affected infants are very prone to airway obstruction from posterior movement of the tongue against the retropharyngeal wall. Approaches to management include prone positioning to allow the tongue to move anteriorly and away from the pharynx. The placement of a nasopharyngeal (NP) tube made from an appropriately sized endotracheal tube can be life saving. The general technique for using NP tubes is presented in **Chapter 2,** but the approach presented in **Figure 4-3** focuses on differences specific to Pierre Robin sequence.

When air movement through the NP tube is heard and felt, the tube is in appropriate position; the patient will also be less distressed. The tube should be secured at this position with tape and adhesive in much the same way as an endotracheal tube. Though it does not pass through the vocal cords and into the trachea, the NP tube is nonetheless a lifeline through which the patient can move air. The tube should be suctioned as necessary to maintain patency. Should a patient with an NP tube for Pierre Robin develop distress, attention should be paid to suctioning and, if necessary, repositioning the tube until air movement is again heard. The tube has a dual purpose in that it not only serves as a conduit for air movement but also pushes the tongue slightly forward off the retropharyngeal wall, thus relieving that level of obstruction.

An additional life-saving maneuver that has been described for severe cases of obstruction in Pierre Robin sequence is to pull the tongue forward manually using a towel clamp or similar instrument. Passing a needle with size 0 silk through the tip of the tongue and pulling it forward and out of the mouth may serve a similar purpose. Definitive management for severe cases of Pierre Robin is surgical, occasionally with a need for tracheostomy.

Figure 4-3. Placement of Nasopharyngeal Tube for Airway Obstruction due to Pierre Robin Sequence

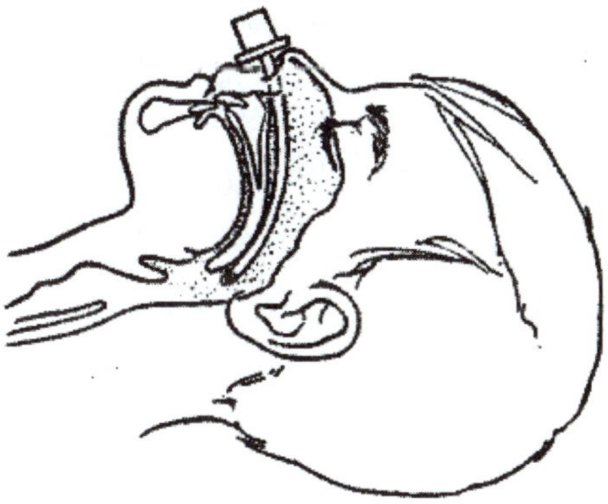

1. Use an uncuffed tracheal tube that fits in a nostril.
2. Match the length of the tube approximately to the distance between the naris and the tragus.
3. Lubricate the tube with surgical lubricant.
4. Insert the tube and advance it while listening for air movement.
5. Secure the tube carefully with tape and adhesive.
6. Suction frequently to maintain patency.
7. If air movement through the tube cannot be heard, reposition the tube until airflow is audible.

B. External or Internal Compression Disorders

External or internal compression of the airway can also result in upper airway obstruction. Tumors, hemangiomas, hematomas, cysts, papilloma, and vascular rings and slings can all present with signs and symptoms of upper airway obstruction. Often CPAP and BiPAP can temporarily reduce the degree of airway obstruction and improve airflow. When CPAP or BiPAP is started, it is helpful to auscultate for breath sounds over the lung fields while titrating pressures in order to find a pressure that results in opening of the airway. Positioning a patient with an anterior mediastinal mass upright, prone, or even on the side can take the pressure of anterior masses off the trachea and relieve obstruction.

C. Infectious Causes of Upper Airway Obstruction

Infectious causes of upper airway obstruction are very common and bring patients of all ages to medical attention. One significant change over the past 20 years is that epiglottitis has become very rare due to widespread use of the *Haemophilus influenzae* type B vaccine. Twenty years ago, almost every pediatric resident saw several children with epiglottitis per year arrive at the hospital. In the current era it is difficult to find a younger pediatric healthcare provider who has ever seen a case of epiglottitis. It is, however, such a fulminant and life-threatening infection that knowledge of its diagnosis and management remains important. Moreover, the evaluation and care of the patient with epiglottitis often serves as a paradigm of how to approach all problems that can result in severe upper airway obstruction.

Table 4-3 compares four of the most common infectious causes of upper airway obstruction.

Table 4-3. Common Infectious Causes of Upper Airway Obstruction

	Croup	Epiglottitis	Bacterial Tracheitis	Retropharyngeal Abscess
Onset	Gradual, viral prodrome, 1-7 days	Rapid onset, 6-12 hours	Viral prodrome followed by rapid deterioration	Viral prodrome followed by rapid deterioration
Typical Age at Onset	6 months–4 years	2-8 years	6 months–8 years	<5 years
Seasonal Occurrence	Late fall–winter	Throughout the year	Fall-winter	Throughout the year
Causative Agents	Parainfluenza, Respiratory Syncytial Virus, Influenza A	*H influenzae* type B (classically), *S pneumoniae,* GABHS	*S aureus* (classically), GABHS, *S pneumoniae*	Anaerobic bacteria, GABHS, *S aureus*
Pathology	Subglottic edema	Inflammatory edema of supraglottis	Thick, mucopurulent, membranous tracheal secretions	Abscess formation in deep cervical fascia
Fever	Low grade	High	High	High
Cough	Barking or seal-like	None	Usually absent	Usually absent
Sore Throat	None	Severe	None	Severe

continued next page...

Table 4-3. Common Infectious Causes of Upper Airway Obstruction (Continued)

	Croup	Epiglottitis	Bacterial Tracheitis	Retropharyngeal Abscess
Drooling	None	Frequent	None	Frequent
Posture	Any	Sitting forward, mouth open, neck extended (tripod position)	Any	Sitting forward, mouth open, neck extended (tripod position)
Voice	Normal or hoarse	Muffled	Normal or hoarse	Muffled
Appearance	Nontoxic	Toxic	Toxic	Toxic

Abbreviations: GABHS, group A β-hemolytic streptococcus; *H influenzae, Haemophilus influenzae; S aureus, Staphylococcus aureus; S pneumoniae, Streptococcus pneumoniae.*

1. Viral Laryngotracheobronchitis (Croup)

Viral laryngotracheobronchitis (croup) is the most common infectious cause of upper airway obstruction in children, primarily affecting children aged 6 months to 4 years, with a peak incidence between 1 and 2 years of age. Cases of croup can be seen throughout the year, with a peak incidence during early fall and winter. Croup is most commonly caused by parainfluenza virus type 1, though parainfluenza virus types 2 and 3, *H influenzae* types A and B, respiratory syncytial virus, adenovirus, and *Mycoplasma pneumoniae* may all cause croup as well. Most children with croup are managed as outpatients, but some do require hospitalization, and a small percentage of hospitalized children require tracheal intubation and mechanical ventilation. Children with croup usually present after several days of prodromal viral-like symptoms (cough, coryza, rhinorrhea, low-grade fever) with progressively worsening hoarseness and eventually develop a classic seal-like, barky cough and stridor. Stridor is classically inspiratory but may be biphasic as well, indicating airway edema that extends beyond the subglottic space into the intrathoracic trachea and bronchi. Radiographs of the airway (**Figure 4-4**) may demonstrate a classic steeple sign (narrowing of the subglottic trachea coming to a point at the level of the vocal cords). Lateral neck films in croup may show dilatation of the airway above the level of the vocal cords.

Figure 4-4. Laryngotracheobronchitis (Croup)

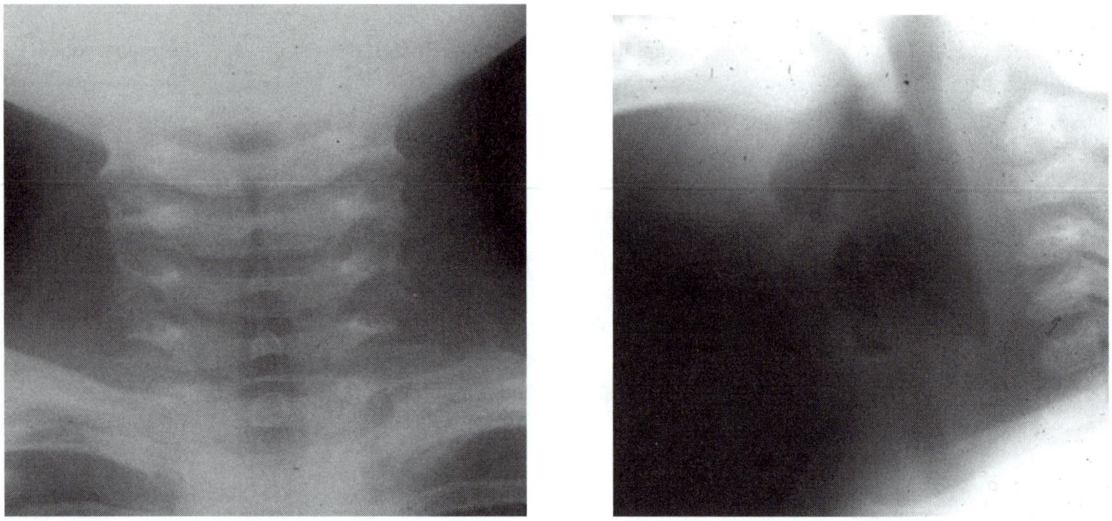

A B

A, Anteroposterior radiograph of the airway demonstrating narrowing of the airway in a steeple-like manner that is characteristic of viral laryngotracheobronchitis. B, A lateral neck radiograph of a patient with viral croup shows a sharp epiglottis, characteristic dilatation of the airspace above the level of the vocal cords, and narrowing of the subglottic air column. Radiographs courtesy of Terry Levin, MD, the Children's Hospital at Montefiore.

Croup is generally self-limiting and requires only supportive care with cool mist and IV fluids if a patient is unable to drink without difficulty. Nebulized racemic epinephrine rapidly reduces airway edema and improves symptoms. The reduction in edema is limited by the lifetime of the drug, however, and symptoms usually return within 2 hours. Corticosteroids have been shown to bring about significant improvement and are prescribed routinely. Heliox may be helpful, as described later in this chapter. Nasal CPAP and BiPAP have been used with some success and may hold off tracheal intubation. In the event that intubation is required, a smaller than normal tube size should be used, and the patient should remain intubated until an air leak develops around the tube. The treatment of croup is summarized in **Table 4-4.**

Table 4-4. Treatment of Croup

1. Minimize situations that may cause distress in the child, such as separation from parents and unnecessary examination and procedures.
2. Provide blow-by oxygen if desaturation or cyanosis is present.
3. Give oral, intramuscular, or intravenous dexamethasone, 0.6 mg/kg.
4. Administer nebulized racemic epinephrine, 2.25%, 0.5 mL in 2.5 mL saline.
5. If the response is good, observe the patient for 2 hours.
6. If the response is poor or if stridor rapidly recurs, admit the patient to the ICU for observation.
5. Consider heliox 60:40 or 70:30.
6. Consider nasal CPAP or BiPAP.
7. If intubation required, use a tube that is smaller than normal for age.

2. Epiglottitis (Supraglottitis, Panglottitis)

Epiglottitis (supraglottitis, panglottitis) is a true emergency. Though epiglottitis is rare due to widespread use of the *H influenzae* type B vaccine, having knowledge of this life-threatening infection is still very important. The name implies involvement of only the epiglottis, but because all of the supraglottic structures can be involved, the label "supraglottitis" or "panglottitis" is more correct. Historically, epiglottitis was most commonly caused by *H influenzae* type B (Hib) and was associated with bacteremia and severe toxicity. However, in the present era of widespread Hib vaccination, *Streptococcus pneumoniae*, group A β-hemolytic streptococci (GABHS), and *Staphylococcus aureus* are more common causes.

Children with supraglottitis usually present with rapidly progressive signs and symptoms, including high fever, irritability, drooling, dysphagia, dyspnea, and dysphonia. These children appear toxic and prefer to rest in the tripod position. Stridor occurs late in the course and is usually soft in comparison to the loud stridor that occurs with croup. When suspicion of epiglottitis is relatively low but not eliminated entirely, a lateral neck radiograph can be obtained. If epiglottitis is present, on lateral view, the epiglottis appears rounded, large, and thumb shaped in comparison to a normal epiglottis, which is sharp (**Figure 4-5**).

Figure 4-5. Lateral Neck Radiographs of a Healthy Patient and a Patient With Epiglottitis

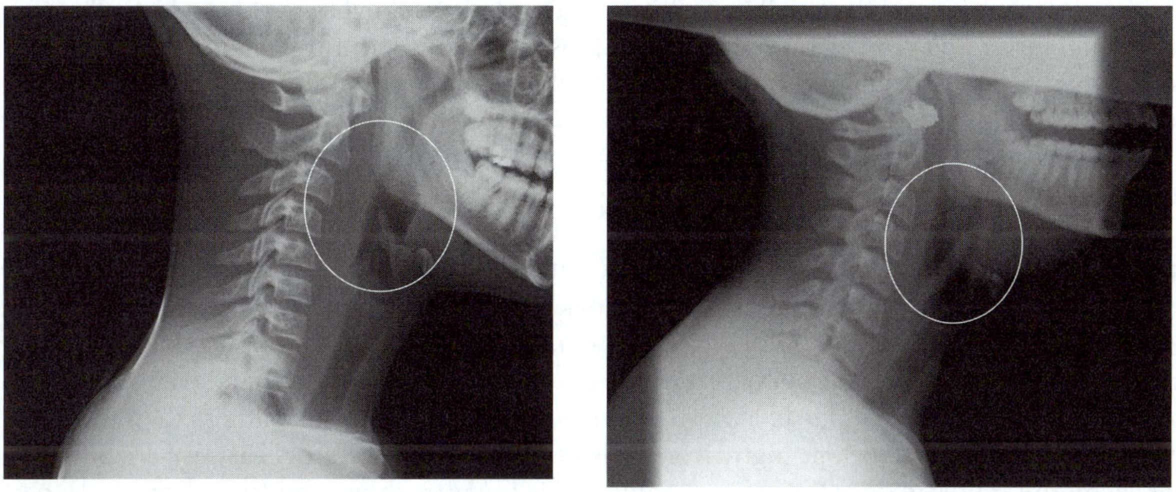

A B

A, The radiograph from a healthy patient shows a sharply defined epiglottis (circled). B, The radiograph from a patient with epiglottitis demonstrates an edematous, less clearly defined, thumb-like epiglottis (circled). The radiograph also shows edema of the aryepiglottic folds and other supraglottic tissues consistent with supraglottitis.
Radiographs courtesy of Terry Levin, MD, the Children's Hospital at Montefiore.

Even if the likelihood of epiglottitis is low, a healthcare provider trained in airway support and bag-mask ventilation must accompany a child sent to the radiology department for lateral neck radiographs. If epiglottitis is suspected based on history and physical exam, the patient should not go to radiology but should instead be brought to the operating room accompanied by a physician skilled in airway management and all necessary airway support equipment. The management of suspected epiglottitis is summarized in **Table 4-5.**

Table 4-5. Management of Suspected Epiglottitis

Low suspicion of epiglottitis → Send patient to radiology for lateral neck radiographs
High suspicion of epiglottitis → Send patient to operating room for direct examination under anesthesia and intubation
Whether suspicion is low or high, the patient should be
Accompanied by a physician skilled in airway management
Kept in a comfortable position
Transported with a bag-mask ventilator, with a mask of appropriate size and, if possible, a PEEP valve

All noxious interventions, such as IV insertion, blood work, and examination of the pharynx, should be deferred until the child is asleep in the operating room and the airway has been secured by tracheal intubation. The child should be permitted to remain in a position of comfort during the trip to the OR and even during mask induction of anesthesia. Once the child is anesthetized but still spontaneously breathing, the larynx is visualized by direct laryngoscopy, and if epiglottitis is found, the child should be tracheally intubated. Following intubation, cultures should be obtained of the epiglottis, tracheal secretions, and blood. An IV is then inserted, and broad-spectrum antibiotics effective against β-lactamase-producing organisms should be administered. Antibiotic choices include second- and third-generation cephalosporins such as cefuroxime or ceftriaxone or, alternatively, ampicillin-sulbactam. The endotracheal tube should be well secured, and the patient should then be brought to the intensive care unit. Improvement is usually rapid once antibiotics are started. The patient can be extubated when an audible air leak develops around the tracheal tube.

3. Bacterial Tracheitis

Bacterial tracheitis is a relatively uncommon but potentially life-threatening cause of upper airway obstruction in children. In bacterial tracheitis, thick mucopurulent membranous secretions obstruct the airway and cannot be cleared by cough. Hence, tracheal intubation is usually required. Children typically present with a viral prodrome of several days' duration that develops into a croup-like illness with low-grade fever, cough, and stridor. This croup-like illness then worsens rapidly, and the patient develops high fever, signs of increasing respiratory distress, inability to clear secretions, and a toxic appearance. Radiographic imaging shows a croup-associated steeple sign. The similarity of the prodromes of croup and bacterial tracheitis has led to an impression that bacterial tracheitis is a bacterial superinfection of viral croup. Bacterial tracheitis affects children aged 6 months to 8 years, with a peak incidence during the fall and winter.

Children who present with bacterial tracheitis to an emergency department may be indistinguishable from patients with epiglottitis and therefore should be managed according to a suspected epiglottitis protocol as described above. In other words, these children should be brought to an operating room where an otolaryngologist can examine the airway under anesthesia and establish the diagnosis. Direct inspection of the airway usually reveals subglottic edema with ulcerations, erythema, and pseudomembrane formation in the trachea. Historically, S aureus is the most common causative agent but *S pneumoniae*, GABHS, and viruses have also been identified. On occasion, a patient who has been in an intensive care unit with croup-like symptoms will acutely worsen and require tracheal intubation. At the time of intubation, copious thick secretions come up through the tracheal tube, lending support to a diagnosis of bacterial tracheitis.

Pulmonary and tracheal toilet, tracheal intubation, and broad-spectrum antibiotics directed against *Staphylococcus* and *Streptococcus* species are the basics of treatment. A second-generation cephalosporin such as cefuroxime is a reasonable choice of antibiotic. Extubation may be attempted following clinical improvement and development of an air leak around the tracheal tube. This may take 3 to 5 days.

4. Retropharyngeal Abscess

Retropharyngeal abscess (also known as parapharyngeal abscess) is an infection of the soft tissues of the posterior pharyngeal wall. The retropharyngeal space consists of a loose network of connective tissue and lymph nodes that drain the nasopharynx, paranasal sinuses, middle ear, teeth, and facial bones. Infection and abscess formation in this area usually result from lymphatic spread of infection or direct spread from the nasopharynx, paranasal sinuses, or middle ear. These lymph nodes atrophy during early childhood, thus decreasing the risk of disease in older children and adolescents. For this reason, direct trauma to the posterior pharynx from a pencil or stick in the mouth and ingestion of foreign bodies account for the majority of cases in older children and adolescents. Most cases occur in children less than 5 years of age, thereby overlapping the most common ages for epiglottitis and bacterial tracheitis.

Children with retropharyngeal abscesses have a nonspecific collection of symptoms that eventually coalesce as high fever, sore throat, and stiff neck. Symptoms are similar to epiglottitis, and physical exam may reveal a bulging unilateral neck mass. The neck stiffness may mimic the neck stiffness seen in meningitis. Diagnosis may be confirmed by the presence of an increased prevertebral soft tissue space on lateral neck radiograph (**Figure 4-6**). In addition to an abnormally wide prevertebral soft tissue space, a lateral neck radiograph may also show the presence of gas or air fluid levels in the retropharyngeal space as well as loss of the normal cervical lordosis. Blood cultures are usually negative, but abscess cultures often yield anaerobic organisms such as *Prevotella, Porphyromonas, Fusobacterium,* and *Peptostreptococcus.* Additionally, *S aureus,* GABHS, and *H influenzae* may be identified.

Figure 4-6. Retropharyngeal Abscess

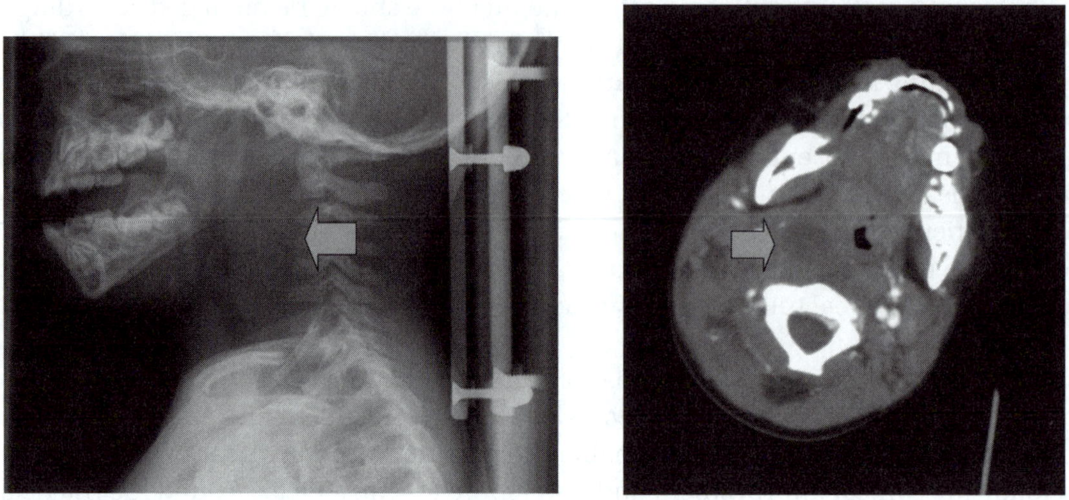

A   B

A, The arrow on the radiograph points to a widened distance between the air column and the anterior aspect of the spinal column (prevertebral space). B, The arrow on the CT image points to a retropharyngeal abscess. Radiographs courtesy of Terry Levin, MD, the Children's Hospital at Montefiore.

Management of retropharyngeal abscess includes broad-spectrum antibiotics that have anaerobic coverage and close observation. Abscess drainage is recommended for cases refractory to antibiotics. Complications are rare with early recognition and appropriate antibiotic treatment. Serious complications include rupture of the abscess into the posterior pharynx (resulting in aspiration of infectious material), lateral spread of infection, and dissection into the posterior mediastinum through fascial planes. Deaths have been reported.

5. Peritonsillar Abscess (Quinsy)

Peritonsillar abscess (quinsy) is the most common deep-space infection of the head and neck tissues in children. A peritonsillar abscess (PTA) results from direct contiguous spread of infection from the tonsils. Older children and adolescents are most commonly affected without seasonal preference. Children with PTA have sore throat, neck pain, pain with swallowing or dysphagia, and fever. Physical exam reveals enlargement of the cervical lymph nodes, uvular deviation, and muffled (hot potato) voice. Treatment options include broad-spectrum antibiotics, needle aspiration with opening of the abscess, incision and drainage, and tonsillectomy. Complications include extension of the infection, rarely acute upper airway obstruction, and rupture of the abscess with aspiration of purulent material.

6. Infectious Mononucleosis

Infectious mononucleosis may lead to acute upper airway obstruction due to enlargement of tonsils and adenoids. Fortunately, this complication, which tends to occur in younger children, is rare. Oral or parenteral corticosteroids may be helpful. Tracheal intubation or non-invasive positive pressure ventilation by CPAP or BiPAP may be required.

7. Miscellaneous Disorders

a. Airway Trauma

Traumatic injury to the upper airway may be caused by foreign bodies, thermal or chemical injury, or direct blunt or penetrating trauma. Foreign body aspiration is a leading cause of accidental death and severe neurologic impairment in young children. Infants are at significant risk of foreign body aspiration due to their tendency to put any and all objects into their mouths. Many aspirated foreign bodies pass through the vocal cords and lodge in the distal airways. Any foreign body that lodges in the larynx is immediately life-threatening. A high index of suspicion is always necessary in that an actual aspiration event is frequently not identified. Children with a history of choking and respiratory distress should undergo immediate rigid bronchoscopy for diagnosis and treatment.

Life-threatening airway obstruction may develop as a result of inhalation injury, laryngeal burns, or caustic ingestions. Any child with a scald injury to the face or neck should be evaluated by bronchoscopy for potential inhalational injury. Inhalation injury should be suspected in children with evidence of soot in sputum or vomitus, singed nasal hairs, facial burns, lip burns, wheezing, stridor, or extensive surface burns. Early endoscopic evaluation is helpful for determining the presence and extent of airway injury. Management of the airway includes early tracheal intubation because airway burns tend to worsen with edema for several days before they begin to resolve.

Blunt injury to the neck can cause edema and hematoma formation that can result in acute upper airway obstruction. Penetrating injury is less common in children. Imaging and surgical consultation are necessary.

b. Postextubation airway obstruction

Patients who are extubated sometimes develop signs and symptoms of airway obstruction. Referred to as postextubation croup, this is may be related to several factors including the size of the tracheal tube in relation to the airway; the duration of intubation; global body edema; and the amount of thrashing the patient did while intubated. Postextubation croup is often self limited and resolves over 12 – 24 hours but may also require interventions as described later in this chapter. On occasion, reintubation is necessary. Assessment and treatment is similar to viral croup. Dexamethasone may be administered both as treatment and as preextubation prophylaxis if there is suspicion that postextubation airway obstruction will occur. Repetitive bouts of postextubation airway obstruction requiring reintubation and even prolonged stridor after extubation are indications for bronchoscopy.

c. Angioedema

Angioedema is an immunologically mediated acute edema that may result in acute upper airway obstruction. The edema may affect the larynx; tissues of the head, neck, face, and lips; tongue; and pharynx. Angioedema most often occurs after ingestion of food or medication, upper respiratory infection, or insect sting. Intravenous corticosteroids, antihistamines, and subcutaneous epinephrine usually will bring about rapid improvement in symptoms. In the event that those medical interventions do not result in improvement or that they are not working rapidly enough, the airway should be secured in a child who demonstrates progressive signs and symptoms of acute upper airway obstruction.

d. Spasmodic Croup

Spasmodic croup is probably an allergic disease not caused by infection. In spasmodic croup, an infant typically wakes with sudden onset of respiratory distress, inspiratory stridor, and a loud, croupy cough. There may be a mild intercurrent upper respiratory illness. The episodes may recur on successive nights. There is often a history of asthma or allergies in the family. By the time the patient reaches the hospital, symptoms have usually resolved. The family often reports that when they brought the child into the cool night air to get in a car, wait for a cab, or wait for an ambulance the symptoms abated. Dysphagia, drooling, high fever, and a toxic appearance are all absent in spasmodic croup.

IV. PHYSICAL FINDINGS AND ASSESSMENT

A. History

A brief history and careful physical exam will provide much of the information necessary to obtain a diagnosis. In the face of severe distress and impending upper airway obstruction the gathering of history must be abbreviated, and emergent intervention takes precedence.

The duration of symptoms and their rapidity of onset is a key area on which to focus. Children with viral croup often have symptoms of upper respiratory infection for one or more days prior to the onset of stridor. Airway obstruction due to foreign body aspiration has an almost instantaneous onset. Epiglottitis has an acute onset, with fever and distress appearing without prodrome. Retropharyngeal and parapharyngeal abscesses typically cause upper airway obstruction after several days of sore throat and related symptoms. A period of intubation in the NICU may precede a presentation of subglottic stenosis.

Additional points to cover in a history include whether distress is stable or worsening, whether symptoms are intermittent or persistent, whether positional changes affect symptoms, presence or absence of fever, history of trauma or exposure to allergen, smoke, chemical vapors or steam, changes invoice quality, report of choking episode or possible foreign body aspiration.

B. Observation and Appearance

The degree of distress and severity of airway obstruction can often be ascertained by observation. Audible stridor indicates turbulent airflow through narrowed passages, but airflow is nonetheless present. Infants and young children with partial upper airway problems may appear calm, whereas older children and adults with partial airway obstruction will be agitated and extremely fearful. Some children, especially those with chronic airway obstruction, appear surprisingly at ease considering the difficulty they have breathing. Observe for accessory muscle use. Children who have been breathing against partially obstructed airways for several years often develop visible hypertrophy of accessory muscles of inspiration.

> !
>
> *Children with acute airway-related processes often adopt a position of comfort to maximize airway patency and airflow. It is important to try to maintain this positioning.*
>
> !

Children with acute airway-related processes often adopt a position of comfort in order to maximize airway patency and airflow. It is important to appreciate this positioning and attempt to maintain it. For example, a child who seems most comfortable in a caregiver's arms should not be removed from that position. The most comfortable position is usually upright, and a patient may vigorously resist being moved out of this position. Moving children out of their position of comfort may induce unnecessary fear and worsen the degree of airway obstruction. As discussed above, increasing respiratory effort against an upper airway obstruction will result in tracheal collapse and worsening of obstruction. Thus, it is crucial to maintain a patient with signs and symptoms of upper airway obstruction in as calm a state as possible. (Note that sedating a child with partial upper airway obstruction who is about to be intubated or positioning a patient to facilitate laryngoscopy may also result in complete airway obstruction.)

A tripod position, in which a child sits upright and leans forward on outstretched arms, is a sign of upper airway obstruction. By leaning forward, the patient tries to relieve upper airway obstruction by using gravity to move enlarged tonsils, redundant pharyngeal tissue, or an edematous epiglottis forward and away from the airway, thus opening an air passage. A component of the tripod posture is forward jutting of the jaw, which is an attempt by the patient to perform a jaw-thrust maneuver that will move pharyngeal contents anteriorly.

> !
>
> *Sedating a child with partial upper airway obstruction who is about to be intubated or positioning a patient to facilitate laryngoscopy may result in complete airway obstruction.*
>
> !

In laryngomalacia, the epiglottis is long and soft and closes in over the laryngeal inlet with inspiration. Given that the epiglottis is an anterior component of the larynx, placing an infant in a prone position permits gravity to move the epiglottis out of the way of the airway. Frequently an infant with laryngomalacia breathes more easily when placed in a prone position rather than a supine position.

A listless appearance may indicate fatigue and signify impending respiratory or cardiac arrest. Observe for cyanosis. Listen for the quality of cough or voice.

C. Physical Examination

The physical exam should focus on the quantity and quality of airflow. Inspiration and expiration are normally quiet. Noise, accessory muscle use, and an appearance of unease indicate the presence of a pathologic situation. Inspiratory noise that emanates from the nose or pharynx is called stertor. Partial nasal obstruction, tonsillar-adenoidal hypertrophy (infectious and noninfectious), peritonsillar abscesses, and parapharyngeal abscesses may all cause this sound. Noise cannot occur without air movement. The absence or disappearance of respiratory noise may indicate that partial upper airway obstruction has converted to complete upper airway obstruction.

> !
>
> *The absence or disappearance of respiratory noise may indicate that partial upper airway obstruction has converted to complete upper airway obstruction.*
>
> !

1. Inspiratory and Expiratory Noises

Inspiratory noise is characteristic of airway disorders from the nose to the subglottic, but extrathoracic, space. The presence of an expiratory component indicates that the process extends to the airways of the chest as well. For example, viral laryngotracheobronchitis may affect the airway from the level of the subglottic space (extrathoracic) to the bronchi (intrathoracic). The edema and mucous accumulation associated with severe croup may thus cause both inspiratory stridor from involvement of the extrathoracic airway and an expiratory component from involvement of the intrathoracic airways. Laryngomalacia involving the epiglottis, arytenoid cartilages, and laryngeal structures is extrathoracic and causes inspiratory noise. Tracheomalacia, in which the tracheal tissue is prone to collapse, may involve both the intrathoracic and the extrathoracic trachea. The extrathoracic trachea is prone to collapse with inspiration, whereas involved intrathoracic areas are prone to collapse with expiration, thus accounting for a characteristic biphasic stridor seen in severe tracheomalacia.

Stridor is a raspy, higher-pitched noise that is caused by air moving through narrowed passages of the supraglottic, glottic, and subglottic spaces. Stridor occurs most commonly with inspiration but may occur during expiration as well. It is most often associated with viral croup, subglottic stenosis, epiglottitis, and postextubation airway edema. Stridor may be present at rest or mainly during agitation. When airway edema is treated with nebulized racemic epinephrine, stridor may disappear and then return when the medication wears off.

Children and infants who are large enough to move sufficient amounts of air often manifest a characteristic barky or seal-like cough with viral croup. Sufficient airflow is required for a cough to be present, and thus absence of cough is not necessarily reassuring. Small infants with viral croup may not manifest a classical croupy cough.

Peritonsillar abscess is associated with a “hot potato voice,” which occurs due to pain and edema in the peritonsillar tissues that make it very difficult to enunciate clearly.

Noisy stertorous sounds are usually associated with obstruction in the nose or retropharynx. In patients who can open their mouths, it may be possible to see obstructing tonsillar tissue or an exudative pharyngitis associated with infectious mononucleosis. It is unwise to persist at trying to open the mouth of a child who resists doing so. A tongue blade should not be used to examine the pharynx of a child with suspected epiglottitis due to the risk of converting a partial upper airway obstruction into a complete obstruction.

Auscultation over the nares can determine the presence or absence of airflow. High-pitched sounds over the throat indicate narrowing of the air passage. During auscultation of the chest, careful attention should be paid to whether adventitious sounds are inspiratory, expiratory, or both, and to which component is louder. Sounds related to the trachea and bronchi will be louder centrally, whereas small, distal airway-related sounds will be more prominent in the peripheral chest.

2. Fever

The presence of fever depends on the etiology of the airway problem. Congenital and acquired disorders, such as laryngomalacia and subglottic stenosis, are not associated with fever. Viral laryngotracheobronchitis is infectious in etiology, and a low-grade fever may be present. High fevers are usually associated with bacterial infections of the airway, such as parapharyngeal abscess, epiglottitis, and bacterial tracheitis.

D. Measurements and Imaging

Pulse oximetry is neither threatening nor painful and is useful in assessing a patient with acute upper airway disease. Acceptable oxygen saturation indicates that even in the presence of clinically visible distress, gas exchange is sufficient to provide an adequate amount of oxygen to the bloodstream. A drop in oxygen saturation may suggest a worsening of obstruction or the development of muscle fatigue and impending respiratory arrest.

Upper airway diseases do not usually affect the regions of the lungs responsible for gas exchange, but if airway obstruction limits gas flow to the extent that inadequate oxygen reaches the alveoli, the patient will develop desaturation. A second mechanism of desaturation is ventilation-perfusion mismatch from atelectasis that develops when unrelieved inspiratory effort against an obstruction leads to respiratory muscle fatigue. The work of breathing and the oxygen consumption necessary to support the diaphragm and accessory muscles of inspiration can be tremendous when a patient breathes against a partially obstructed airway. The inability to meet the diaphragm's demand for oxygen in the face of inadequate gas flow ultimately results in anaerobic metabolism and lactic acidosis.

Although an arterial blood gas analysis can yield important and valuable information about a patient with upper airway disease, its utility is offset by the discomfort and difficulty of obtaining an arterial blood sample compounded by the agitation that drawing it induces. One of the prime directives of managing a patient with upper airway obstruction is to limit noxious stimuli, and ABG measurement in the absence of an indwelling arterial line is noxious.

> !
>
> *Although an arterial blood gas analysis can yield important and valuable information about a patient with upper airway disease, its utility is offset by the discomfort and difficulty of obtaining an arterial blood sample compounded by the agitation that drawing it induces.*
>
> !

Side stream end tidal CO_2 sampled via nasal cannula can be helpful in assessing ventilation adequacy in a patient with upper airway obstruction. However, the necessary devices are not that widely available, and more important, children with upper airway obstruction are very resistant to the placement of anything on their faces.

Radiographic imaging, when safe for a patient with a compromised airway, can yield helpful information. Anteroposterior and lateral neck views with filtering in place to gain increased soft tissue resolution may potentially show:

- Narrowing in the subglottic space consistent with viral croup (steeple sign) (**Figure 4-4**)
- Radio-opaque foreign bodies
- Enlarged, edematous epiglottis (thumb-print sign) consistent with epiglottitis (**Figure 4-5**)
- Hypertrophied adenoidal and tonsillar tissue
- Abnormally wide retropharyngeal or prevertebral tissues consistent with mass or with retropharyngeal or parapharyngeal abscess (**Figure 4-6**)

For comparison, films of a patient with normal airway anatomy are shown in **Figure 4-7.** Plain view radiographs of the chest can show a deviated or narrowed tracheal air column, compressed or narrowed bronchi, or the presence of atelectasis or pneumonia. More advanced imaging of the airways by techniques such as fluoroscopy and CT scanning with 3D reconstruction can also yield important information. The stability of the patient and the maintenance of the airway must be given top priority in planning all radiographic imaging.

Figure 4-7. Normal Airway

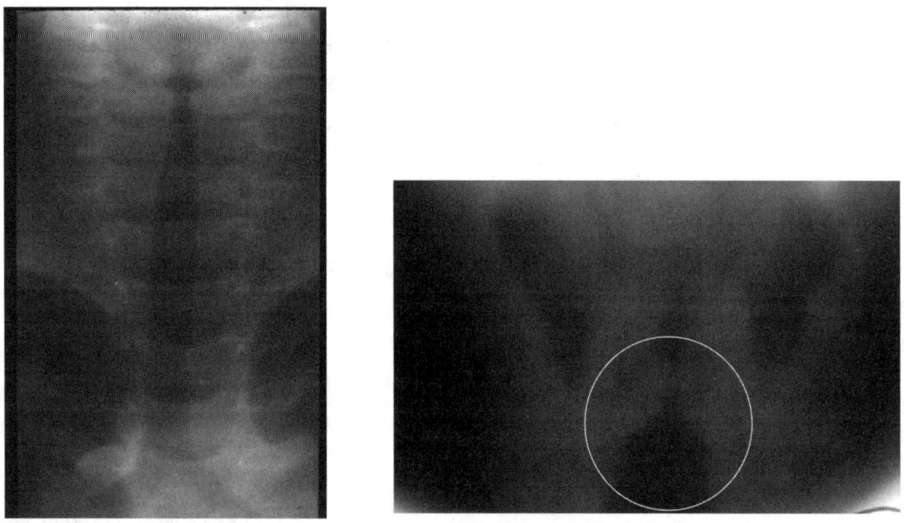

A B

A, An anteroposterior radiograph of a normal tracheal airway shows a widely patent air column with some narrowing at the level of the vocal cords. B, An airway tomogram demonstrates a widely patent tracheal air column coming to the level of the vocal cords (circled), showing the typical “shoulders” seen in a normal airway.
Radiographs courtesy of Terry Levin, MD, the Children’s Hospital at Montefiore.

> !
>
> *For very distressed patients of all ages with upper airway problems, the safest and most effective approach to diagnosis begins with monitored transfer to an operating room or intensive care unit.*
>
> !

For very distressed patients of all ages with upper airway problems, the safest and most effective approach to diagnosis begins with monitored transfer to an operating room or intensive care unit. In an OR or ICU, personnel skilled in medical and surgical airway management can together perform a careful examination of the airway by means of laryngoscopy or bronchoscopy. This multidisciplinary approach should be carefully defined and made a standard operating procedure in any facility that cares for children.

Scoring scales have been developed to assist in assessing the degree of respiratory compromise. One such assessment scale, the Westley croup score, provides a structured means for evaluating clinical change, either worsening or improving, and permits interobserver consistency. The scoring rubric (**Table 4-6**) is based on the presence and extent of inspiratory stridor, retractions, air entry, and cyanosis, and on the patient's mental status. A Westley croup score lower than 3 suggests mild disease, a score of 3 to 6 indicates moderate disease, and a score higher than 6 represents severe disease.

Table 4-6. Westley Croup Score

	(Points)					
Finding	**0**	**1**	**2**	**3**	**4**	**5**
Stridor	None	With agitation	At rest			
Retractions	None	Mild	Moderate	Severe		
Air Entry	Normal	Mild decrease	Marked decrease			
Cyanosis	None				With agitation	At rest
Level of Consciousness	Normal					Depressed

<3 points: mild disease

3-6 points: moderate disease

>6 points: severe disease

V. MANAGEMENT OF ACUTE UPPER AIRWAY DISEASE

Patients of all ages with upper airway obstruction will be very frightened and very uncomfortable. Painful or otherwise noxious interventions should be proportional to the level of distress and severity of clinical state. For example, an infant with mild-to-moderate viral croup who is able to drink and is comfortable in his caregiver's arms with blow-by humidified oxygen does not usually need arterial blood gas analysis, extensive blood tests, or even an IV. In upper airway disorders, probably more than in any other medical disorder, increased anxiety and agitation may worsen a patient's clinical condition. Interventions should be carried out in progressive steps from least to most invasive. In general, it is best to do the least, keeping in mind that in some circumstances definitive action may be required and cannot be delayed.

> **!** *Attempt to accomplish any interventions with patients in their position of comfort.*

As mentioned earlier, children who are awake will attempt to find and maintain a position of comfort that maximizes their ability to maintain their own airway. Allow this, and attempt to accomplish any interventions while patients are in their preferred position. When epiglottitis was more prevalent, affected infants and children were often seen in their caregivers' arms with their chins up and jutted forward in a spontaneous jaw-thrust position, all in an effort to maintain a patent airway in the presence of a swollen epiglottis. One general approach to treatment of such patients was to keep them in their caregivers' arms until they were brought to the operating room for mask induction and intubation.

When a patient is not awake or has an altered sensorium, attempt to find a position that maximizes airflow and minimizes obstruction. An infant with disorders of the chin and tongue, such as Pierre Robin sequence, may have a completely obstructed airway when lying supine but may be able to breathe easily when placed prone. In a spontaneously breathing patient, attempting to align the oral, pharyngeal, and tracheal axes, as is done to facilitate tracheal intubation, may maximize the airway. As described in **Chapter 2,** the airway axes can be lined up by placing a small roll under the shoulders of an infant or under the occiput of an older child, followed by careful neck flexion to place the patient in the sniffing position. Monitoring changes in airflow through the nose and mouth or watching oxygen saturation can help in assessing the utility of such maneuvers. Patients with severe tonsillar-adenoidal hypertrophy are usually able to move air more easily in an upright position.

Partial upper airway obstruction due to backward movement of the tongue and reduced hypopharyngeal tone occurs frequently in children with a decreased level of consciousness. It may be seen, for example, in a child involved in a bicycle or automobile collision who has sustained a closed head injury, a child recovering from surgical anesthesia, or a patient undergoing procedural sedation with opiates, benzodiazepines, or anesthetic agents such as propofol. In all these situations, the most likely cause of oxygen desaturation is upper airway obstruction. In a procedural sedation, administration of supplemental oxygen will delay desaturation by replacing the functional residual capacity of the patient with oxygen, but oxygen by itself will not be effective in the presence of airway obstruction. When sedation-induced airway obstruction occurs, opening the airway by means of chin lift, jaw thrust, or a combination of both will be more effective than supplemental oxygen in reversing oxygen desaturation. After the airway is opened, oxygen saturation will usually rise quickly provided the patient is not apneic.

> !
> *In sedation-induced airway obstruction, opening the airway by means of chin lift, jaw thrust, or a combination of both will be more effective than supplemental oxygen in reversing oxygen desaturation.*
> !

Maintaining airway patency by means of chin-lift and jaw-thrust maneuvers is a skill that all healthcare workers involved with seriously ill children should possess. These maneuvers are discussed in detail in **Chapter 2** on airway management.

A. Medical Interventions

1. Heliox

Helium-oxygen mixtures known as heliox are extremely useful when any form of obstruction limits airflow. Heliox comes in 60:40, 70:30, and 80:20 helium:oxygen mixtures. It can be administered by nonrebreathing facemask or by nasal cannulae. A significant improvement in comfort is often seen upon initiation of heliox therapy. The oxygen concentration in heliox is not high, and with an 80:20 mixture it is actually below the oxygen concentration of room air. Thus, heliox alone may not be adequate if a patient has a significant oxygen requirement due to parenchymal lung disease.

Heliox is effective because it is less dense than either oxygen or air. When airways become narrowed by edema, compression, or anatomic abnormality, the gas flow becomes turbulent due to abrupt changes in velocity. In croup, airflow becomes turbulent due to constriction in the subglottic space.

Heliox is a very leaky gas owing to the same properties that make it work for airway problems. For this reason, it is helpful to use a tight-fitting facemask and to minimize, when possible, connections that may decrease the amount of heliox that reaches a patient's airway.

2. Racemic Epinephrine

Racemic epinephrine (2.25% by nebulizer) is frequently used as a topical vasoconstrictor in the management of stridor due to viral laryngotracheobronchitis (croup). Racemic epinephrine is usually effective in postextubation croup as well. For children younger than 4 years the dose is 0.05 mL/kg mixed with 4.5 milliliters normal saline and administered by nebulizer every 2 to 4 hours. For children 4 years and older the dose is 0.5 milliliters mixed with 4.5 milliliters normal saline administered every 2 to 3 hours. The maximum dose is 0.5 mL every 1 to 2 hours. Onset of action can be expected in about 1 to 5 minutes, and the effect may last 1 to 3 hours. Although

Racemic epinephrine 2.25% administered by nebulizer
<4 years old: 0.05 mL/kg mixed with 4.5 mL normal saline every 2-4 hours
≥4 years old: 0.5 mL mixed with 4.5 mL normal saline every 2-4 hours
Maximum dose: 0.5 mL every 1-2 hours
Onset of action: 1-5 minutes
Duration of action: 1-3 hours
Possible rebound: 2-3 hours

racemic epinephrine is usually prescribed for croup, it is conceivable to attempt its use for almost any upper airway disorder in which tissue edema may be contributing factor. Rebound may occur in 2 to 3 hours and is cited as a reason for the hospital admission of children who receive racemic epinephrine in the emergency department. The subglottic narrowing of viral croup is of longer duration than the half-life of racemic epinephrine.

There is little information about the use of continuously nebulized racemic epinephrine, but if a patient with a complicated airway is showing some clinical response and the alternative is intubation, continuous nebulizer treatments may be of some help.

3. Dexamethasone

Dexamethasone administered orally or parenterally, by IM or IV routes, has been shown to be effective in viral laryngotracheobronchitis. The published dose is 0.6 mg/kg given once. For postextubation airway edema the dosing is 0.5-2 mg/kg/day IM or IV divided every 6 hours. When used to prevent postextubation croup, dexamethasone is started 24 hours prior to extubation and continued for 4 to 6 doses after extubation.

Dexamethasone
Viral croup → 0.6 mg/kg (PO, IM, IV) once
Postexubation stridor → 0.5-2 mg/kg/day IM or IV divided every 6 hours; start 24 hours prior to extubation and continue for 4-6 doses after extubation.

4. Noninvasive Positive-Pressure Ventilation

Noninvasive positive-pressure ventilation (NPPV) by either continuous positive airway pressure (CPAP) or bilevel positive airway pressure (BiPAP) may be useful in cases of upper airway obstruction due to viral croup or subglottic stenosis. The addition of positive pressure to the airways can decrease the amount of extrathoracic tracheal collapse that occurs when a patient attempts to inhale against a partial obstruction. Patients with upper airway obstruction due to tonsillar-adenoidal hypertrophy can experience significant relief from obstruction through the use of NPPV. Although NPPV may be beneficial, it may also force secretions down into the trachea and inhibit their clearance.

In cases of severe inspiratory difficulty, complete airway obstruction, or respiratory arrest, it is usually possible to support a patient by means of bag-mask ventilation. There should be no hesitation to attempt to supply such support. Due to the airway obstruction effective ventilation may be difficult to provide, and careful attention should be paid to airway maneuvers to maximize patency as well as to mask seal. It may be more effective to perform 2-person bag-mask ventilation (see **Chapter 2**) so that one person can concentrate on mask seal and airway patency and the other person can bag forcefully. The addition of a PEEP valve to the bag-mask ventilator provides a means to prevent end-exhalation airway collapse and may facilitate ventilation.

If foreign body aspiration is suspected and the patient is in respiratory failure and has not responded to basic life support interventions such as abdominal and chest-thrust maneuvers, direct laryngoscopy with removal of a visualized foreign object by Magill forceps should be considered.

Key Points

Diagnosis and Management of the Child With Acute Upper Airway Disease

- Airway maneuvers such as jaw thrust and chin lift can reverse hypoxemia due to upper airway obstruction caused by decreased levels of consciousness.
- A nasopharyngeal tube can be life saving in patients with severe airway obstruction due to Pierre Robin sequence.
- Children should be allowed to remain in their position of comfort for as long as possible.
- A multidisciplinary team with expertise in medical and surgical airway management should be assembled for cases of suspected epiglottitis and other severe cases of upper airway obstruction.
- Direct examination of the airway in the operating room by skilled anesthesiologists and otolaryngologists is the correct way to diagnose severe upper airway obstruction. Radiographic examination should be reserved for children who are relatively stable and whose diagnosis is in question.
- Bag-mask ventilation can provide lifesaving oxygenation and ventilation even in cases of complete airway obstruction due to epiglottitis.
- Heliox is useful in all varieties of upper airway obstruction.

Suggested Readings

1. Backofen JE, Rogers MC. Upper airway disease. In: Rogers MC, ed. *Textbook of Pediatric Intensive Care.* 2nd ed. Baltimore, MD: Williams & Wilkens; 1992:231-257.

2. Cherry JD. Croup. *N Engl J Med.* 2008;358:384-391.

3. Cote CJ, Todres ID, Ryan JF, Goudsouzian NG. *A Practice of Anesthesia for Infants and Children.* 3rd ed. Philadelphia, PA: Saunders; 2001.

4. McBride TP, Davis HW, Reilly JS. Otolaryngology. In: Zitelli BJ, Davis HW, eds. *Atlas of Pediatric Physical Diagnosis.* 3rd ed. St Louis, MO: Mosby; 1997:683-728.

5. Westley CR, Ross EK, Brooks JG. Nebulized racemic epinephrine by IPPB for the treatment of croup. *Am J Dis Child.* 1978;132:484-487.

6. Wheeler DS. The pediatric airway. In: Conway EE, Relvas MS, eds. *Pediatric Multiprofessional Critical Care Review.* Chicago, IL: Society of Critical Care Medicine; 2006:37-51.

7. deCaen A, Duff J, Couvadia AH, et al. Airway Management. In: Nochols DG, ed. *Rogers' Textbook of Pediatric Intensive Care.* 4th ed. Philadelphia, PA: Lippincott Williams & Wilkins; 2008:303-322.

Chapter 5:

Diagnosis and Management of the Child With Acute Lower Airway Disease

Objectives

- Summarize the pathophysiology of acute lower airway disease.
- Identify respiratory failure accompanied with or without respiratory distress.
- Initiate appropriate diagnostic and therapeutic interventions for the various causes of acute lower airway disease.

Case Study

A 5-year-old girl with a history of asthma since age 2 is brought to the emergency department due to worsening tachypnea and wheezing despite frequent albuterol inhalation treatments at home. Her vital signs are heart rate 135/min, respiratory rate 40/min, and pulse oximetry 89% on room air. She appears anxious. On auscultation she has bilateral inspiratory and expiratory wheezes with intercostal retractions.

- What is the diagnosis?

- What pharmacologic treatment should be initiated?

- What tests would be useful to evaluate the severity of the patient's condition?

I. INTRODUCTION

Respiratory failure is the inability of the pulmonary system to meet the metabolic needs of the body. The pulmonary system is involved in 2 crucial metabolic roles: elimination of CO_2 and blood oxygenation. There are 3 forms of respiratory failure: hypoxemic, hypercapnic, and mixed.

Hypoxemic respiratory failure is defined by a room air Pao_2 of ≤60 mm Hg (≤8.0 kPa). It may be caused by

- Ventilation/perfusion mismatch
- Decreased diffusion of oxygen across the alveolocapillary membrane
- Alveolar hypoventilation
- High altitude with low inspired oxygen tension

> **!** *Signs of respiratory failure include tachypnea, tachycardia, nasal flaring, retractions, and abnormal airway sounds, such as wheezing and grunting.*

Hypercapnic respiratory failure is defined by $Paco_2$ of ≥50 mm Hg (>6.7kPa) with an accompanying acidosis (pH <7.35). It may be caused by

- Decreased tidal volume
- Decreased respiratory rate
- Increased physiologic dead space
- Increased CO_2 production, which rarely produces significant hypercapnia

In both types of respiratory failure, hypoxemia is present to some degree. The diagnosis of respiratory failure by arterial blood gas analysis may not be readily available to the clinician at the time of the first encounter with the ill child. The clinician would need to rely on the clinical indicators of respiratory failure (**Table 5-1**).

Table 5-1. Clinical Indicators of Respiratory Failure

Clinical Indicators of Respiratory Failure
Marked tachypnea (respiratory rate >60 breaths/min abnormal at any age)
Bradypnea and/or apnea
Cyanosis
Worsening oxygen saturations despite intervention
Tachycardia or bradycardia
Poor or absent distal air movement
Lethargy, stupor, and coma

A. Management of Respiratory Failure

The initial goal of the management of respiratory failure is the restoration and stabilization of ventilation and oxygenation. The intervention should focus on a rapid assessment of the type and severity of respiratory compromise rather than on the precise etiology. An action plan with direct management should follow, emphasizing the need for frequent reassessment of the response to treatment and the planning of further interventions as needed.

> !
>
> *Provide 100% oxygen, and monitor oxygen saturation continuously with a pulse oximeter.*
>
> !

The most vital aspect of management is securing the patient's airway. While attempting to establish an airway, it may be necessary to assist ventilation with a bag-mask device (see **Chapter 2**). Oxygen saturation, end tidal CO_2, and cardiovascular monitoring should be implemented.

II. CAUSES OF ACUTE RESPIRATORY FAILURE

Acute respiratory failure develops in a variety of clinical settings. Respiratory failure in children typically results from diseases affecting the upper airway, lower airway, and lung parenchyma. Most of the time these entities produce respiratory distress. Diseases affecting other organ systems, including the cardiovascular and central nervous systems, may result in acute respiratory failure without respiratory distress.

A. Asthma

1. Pathophysiology of Asthma

Asthma is a highly prevalent, chronic inflammatory disease of the lower airway that is characterized by a reversible airway obstruction due to bronchial smooth muscle contraction, increased mucus production, and airway edema. There are various entities that can trigger asthma attacks; these include inhaled irritants, cigarette smoke, exercise, allergen exposure, respiratory viral infections, and psychological stress. The obstruction and increased airway resistance due to bronchoconstriction and airway edema diminish airflow (expiration greater than inspiration), interrupts pulmonary mechanics, and causes air trapping, hyperinflation, and ventilation-perfusion mismatch. Expiration becomes an active process, requiring accessory muscle use. Increased work of breathing, respiratory muscle fatigue, and hypoxia will ensue if asthma is left untreated and will lead to respiratory failure.

2. Clinical Findings and Diagnosis of Asthma

Children with severe acute asthma usually present with tachypnea, hyperpnea, retractions, and nasal flaring. These patients appear anxious; they may prefer a tripod sitting position, remain undistracted from just breathing, and be unable to speak in full sentences. The disease severity correlates poorly with the degree of wheezing.

> !
>
> *A silent chest with very limited airflow is a worrisome finding in children with asthma.*
>
> !

A chest radiograph is indicated in patients with severe disease in order to rule out air space disease, atelectasis, or the presence of pneumothorax. The typical blood gas in an asthmatic patient in the early stage of an acute asthmatic exacerbation shows mild hypoxemia and hypocapnia ($Paco_2$ <35 mm Hg [4.7 kPa]) due to hyperventilation. Normalization of the $Paco_2$ in a patient with worsening airway obstruction should be interpreted as a sign of respiratory muscle fatigue and impending respiratory failure.
The decision to intubate should be based on the overall clinical status.

3. Management of Asthma

Patients with acute moderate to severe asthma may benefit from the following interventions in addition to the general management already discussed:

- Administer nebulized albuterol or levalbuterol and reassess frequently. Albuterol is recommended at a dose of 0.05 to 0.15 mg/kg every 20 minutes for 3 doses. Continuous albuterol should be considered in patients falling to respond to the initial treatment. The recommended dose for continuous albuterol is 0.15 to 0.45 mg/kg every hour, with a maximum dose of 20 mg per hour. The recommended Levalbuterol dose is 0.075 mg/kg, (minimum dose of 1.25 mg) every 20 minutes for 3 doses followed by 0.075 to 0.15 mg/kg (not to exceed 5 mg) every 1 to 4 hours as needed. It is important to monitor serum potassium levels in patients undergoing continuous albuterol or levalbuterol therapy due to intracellular potassium shifts with resulting hypokalemia.

- Administer 250 micrograms of nebulized ipratropium bromide every 20 minutes during the first hour, followed by 250 to 500 micrograms every 6 hrs. This can be used simultaneously with albuterol.

- Administer methylprednisolone intravenously at a dose of 1 mg/kg every 6 hours or an equivalent IV corticosteroid. The duration of therapy is dictated by the clinical response. Consider gradually tapering the corticosteroids in patients requiring more than 5 to 7 days of therapy. Consider gastric prophylaxis with a histamine 2 (H_2) blocker.

- Administer terbutaline intravenously in patients who fail to improve or show deterioration with the above treatments. The recommended starting loading dose is 10 µg/kg over 10 minutes, followed by a continuous infusion of 0.1 to 1 µg/kg per minute. It is rare that a dose higher than 4 µg/kg per minute is needed.

■ Consider administering magnesium sulfate intravenously at a dose of 25 to 40 mg/kg over 30 minutes. Monitor for signs of hypermagnesemia, such as hypotension, nausea, and flushing. Serious toxicity involving cardiac arrhythmias, muscle weakness, areflexia, and respiratory depression may occur at higher doses.

The indications for endotracheal intubation include cardiac or respiratory arrest, profound hypoxemia, and respiratory failure. Older patients may benefit from a trial of noninvasive bilevel positive airway pressure (BiPAP) ventilation in an attempt to improve oxygenation and respiratory muscle fatigue (see **Chapter 6**).

The use of helium-oxygen mixtures (heliox) in concentrations of 80:20 (80% helium to 20% oxygen) and 70:30 (70% helium to 30% oxygen) are recommended as an adjuvant treatment in severe asthma. Due to its low density, heliox can potentially improve work of breathing by facilitating laminar gas flow in areas of high airway resistance and help in the delivery of albuterol. The use of heliox is recommended in non-hypoxemic patients who fail to respond to conventional treatments.

B. Bronchiolitis

Case Study

A previously healthy 1-month-old boy, born at 34 weeks gestation, is brought to the emergency department by his mother. She reports that about 1 week ago the infant developed a runny nose and some cough. His symptoms have not improved despite her giving him nebulized albuterol treatments every 6 hours as prescribed. During the last 12 hours he has been grunting, flaring, and retracting. He appears less active and has been feeding poorly. The mother is concerned because the infant stops breathing intermittently.

– What is the possible diagnosis?

– What pharmacologic treatment should be initiated?

– What tests would be useful to evaluate the severity of his condition?

1. Pathophysiology of Bronchiolitis

> **!** *The diagnosis of bronchiolitis needs to be considered in neonates presenting with apnea after hospital discharge.*

Bronchiolitis is a lower-airway-obstructive disease characterized by the presence of cough, wheezing, and copious secretions. It affects mostly infants and young children. It is the most frequent cause of apnea after hospital discharge in patients younger than 2 months of age. Respiratory syncytial virus (RSV) and human metapneumovirus (hMPV) are the most common causes and tend to occur in epidemics during winter and spring. Bronchiolitis may also occur with other viruses, including adenovirus, influenza, parainfluenza, or rhinovirus. The majority of infants and young children infected with these viruses develop a prodrome that includes low-grade fever, rhinorrhea, and poor feeding followed by cough and wheezing.

Preterm infants, infants with cyanotic congenital heart disease, infants with bronchopulmonary dysplasia (BPD), and children with immune deficiency or immune suppression are more susceptible to bronchiolitis. They have a tendency to develop a more severe illness with hypoxia, respiratory failure (ventilation-perfusion mismatch), and hypoventilation (respiratory muscle fatigue) requiring intubation and mechanical ventilation.

2. Diagnosis of Bronchiolitis

Rapid diagnostic assays are available for RSV but not for hMPV. Premature infants with a history of apnea of prematurity and BPD and infants younger than 3 months have an increased risk of bronchiolitis-associated apnea.

3. Management of Bronchiolitis

In addition to general management, patients with bronchiolitis may benefit from the following interventions:

- Frequent, gentle oral and nasal suctioning or in intubated patients, endotracheal tube suctioning
- Nebulized albuterol (see dosage in the section on asthma, above), followed by reassessment of the patient; repeated doses given only in patients with documented improvement
- Racemic epinephrine (2.25% solution: 0.05 mL/kg/dose diluted in 3 mL of saline via nebulizer); discontinued if no improvement is observed
- For children with severe respiratory distress, impending respiratory failure, or apnea, admission to a pediatric ICU for close observation and cardiopulmonary monitoring

Smaller endotracheal tubes are recommended for infants with history of prematurity and previous endotracheal intubation or for infants with subglottic stenosis.

C. Neoplastic Airway Obstruction

Case Study

A previously healthy 10-year-old girl is evaluated in the emergency department for gradual new-onset wheezing, increased work of breathing, and increased dyspnea in a supine position. Her mother also reports fever of 39°C (102.2°F), weight loss, and night sweats. The child prefers the sitting position and looks anxious. On exam, her vital signs are found to be respiratory rate

25/min, heart rate 120/min, and blood pressure 130/75 mm Hg; she has inspiratory and expiratory wheezes on auscultation with decreased breath sounds in the right upper chest. Despite your recommendation, the nurse places the patient in a flat supine position. The patient becomes more anxious, her oxygen saturations drops, and the engorgement of her neck veins increases.

- What is the most likely diagnosis?
- What treatment should be initiated?
- What tests would be useful to evaluate the severity of the patient's condition?

1. Pathophysiology of Neoplastic Airway Obstruction

Lymphoid malignancies (Hodgkin and non-Hodgkin lymphoma) and leukemic malignancies (acute lymphocytic leukemia) in children may present with an anterior or middle mediastinal mass. Tumor masses in this location produce superior vena cava (SVC) obstruction and compression of other mediastinal structures, such as the trachea, mainstem bronchus, pulmonary vessels, and aorta. Progressive venous congestion and airway compression will lead to the usual symptoms found in SVC: facial engorgement, headache, plethora, cyanotic facies, cough, dyspnea, orthopnea, hoarseness, and dysphagia.

2. Diagnosis of Neoplastic Airway Obstruction

Posterior, anterior, and lateral chest radiographs will show a widening of the mediastinum with tracheal deviation or compression.

3. Management of Neoplastic Airway Obstruction

In addition to general management, the following interventions may benefit the patient with neoplastic airway obstruction:

- The patient should be allowed to adopt a position of comfort. Avoid painful interventions that could potentially end in sudden airway collapse.
- Continuous positive airway pressure (CPAP) or BiPAP may be helpful in maintaining an open airway. Provide humidified oxygen.
- An experienced anesthesiologist and an ear, nose, and throat surgeon should be available in the event that endotracheal intubation is necessary. The patient's airway is best secured by having the patient breathe spontaneously.
- In the patient with SVC syndrome, it is important to secure IV access in the lower extremities.

> **!** *Sedation and airway instrumentation of children with neoplastic airway obstruction should be done by experienced anesthesiologists or intensivists. The use of sedatives and muscle relaxants can precipitate a total airway collapse.*

In some patients it is impossible to obtain a tissue sample before empiric emergency therapy is established. Chemotherapy, including steroids and or radiation therapy, may have to be delivered in consultation with a pediatric oncologist before the correct diagnosis is established. Studies for definitive diagnosis should be obtained as soon as the patient's clinical status allows it.

D. Cystic Fibrosis

Case Study

A 17-year-old girl with cystic fibrosis comes to the emergency department with a 1-week history of increased cough, wheezing, and change in the quantity and quality of her sputum. She has had chest pain and increased work of breathing since this morning. Her current O_2 saturations of 89% are considerably lower than her baseline.

– What is the most likely diagnosis?

– What treatment should be initiated?

– What tests would be useful to evaluate the severity of the patient's condition?

1. Pathophysiology of Cystic Fibrosis

Cystic fibrosis (CF) is an autosomal recessive disorder involving a mutation on the long arm of chromosome 7 that causes abnormal chloride and sodium ion transport across epithelial surfaces, resulting in viscid secretions that lead to blockage of airways. The lower airway is normal at birth but over time will develop obstructive pulmonary disease as a result of recurrent airway inflammation, chronic viscid mucus production, and recurrent infections. Children usually present with recurrent coughing and wheezing, bronchiolitis, asthma, and pneumonia. They eventually develop hyperinflation with chronic diffuse bronchiectasis. Pneumothorax occurs in about 10% of the patients and can be a common cause of chest pain and respiratory failure.

2. Diagnosis of Cystic Fibrosis

Patients with CF tend to have upper airway involvement with pansinusitis and nasal polyps. Bacteria responsible for exacerbations early in the disease process may include *Staphylococcus aureus, Haemophilus influenzae,* and *Klebsiella* species. *Pseudomonas aeruginosa* (mucoid strain), *Aspergillus fumigatus, Burkholderia cepacia,* and *Stenotrophomonas maltophilia* become the predominant responsible organisms later in the process. Sweat testing should be considered in patients with

- History of meconium ileus with prolonged jaundice in the neonatal period
- Rectal prolapse, chronic diarrhea with steatorrhea

- Nasal polyps and pansinusitis
- Chronic coughing and wheezing
- Documented *Staphylococcus aureus* pneumonia or documented pseudomonas in sputum culture
- Failure to thrive
- Digital clubbing
- Family history of CF

3. Management of Cystic Fibrosis

Respiratory failure is relatively uncommon in children with CF. It may, however, occur in undiagnosed children presenting with viral or bacterial pneumonia, in patients with advanced CF presenting with pneumonia or an acute pneumothorax, or in terminally ill CF patients presenting with right heart failure.

The patient with cystic fibrosis may benefit from

- Physical therapy and postural drainage
- Inhalation therapy with bronchodilators (see dosage in the section on asthma, above), mucolytic agents (acetylcysteine 3-5 mL of 20% solution via nebulizer 3 times a day), recombinant human DNase, and vasoconstrictors

Antibiotic treatment may vary from a short course of 1 antibiotic for uncomplicated cases to a continuous course of multiple antibiotics in complicated cases. Treatment should be initially directed against Pseudomonas species. Recommended therapy includes cefepime 150 mg/kg daily or ceftazidime 150 mg/kg daily in combination with tobramycin 7.5 mg/kg daily. Vancomycin 45 mg/kg daily should be considered in patients with suspected staphylococcus infections.

E. Pneumonia

1. Pathophysiology of Pneumonia

Pneumonia is an inflammation of the lung parenchyma characterized by a reduction in total lung capacity that is associated with a decrease in compliance. Expiratory flow rates are usually preserved, and major obstructive defects are rare. Progressive alveolar involvement and deterioration of gas exchange lead to respiratory distress and failure.

2. Diagnosis of Pneumonia

The diagnosis of parenchymal lung disease is somewhat challenging. Auscultative findings may be completely normal unless significant consolidation or small airway disease (fine crackles late in inspiration) exist. A chest radiograph is critical in both the diagnosis and the management of pneumonia. (See **Chapter 8** for further information.)

3. Management of Pneumonia

Noninvasive positive pressure ventilation with CPAP or BiPAP should be utilized in hypoxic children despite higher oxygen concentrations.

Consider adding a positive end-expiratory pressure (PEEP) valve to the bag-valve mask prior to intubating. Positive end-expiratory pressure will improve oxygenation and recruit collapsed alveoli.

> **!** *Cuffed endotracheal tubes should be used in patients with parenchymal lung disease when possible.* **!**

F. Acute Respiratory Distress Syndrome

1. Pathophysiology of Acute Respiratory Distress Syndrome

Acute respiratory distress syndrome (ARDS) is characterized by acute onset, diffuse bilateral alveolar opacities and pleural effusion in chest radiography, and no evidence of increase in left atrial pressure. The following 3 phases in the pathogenesis of ARDS have been described as: acute phase, subacute phase (fibroproliferative phase) and chronic phase (fibrosis).

The acute phase (several hours up to 5 days) of ARDS is characterized by an influx of protein-rich fluid into the airspace due to disruption of the alveolocapillary membrane secondary to injury to the vascular endothelium and the alveolar epithelium. The damage to the alveolar epithelium contributes to alveolar flooding and impedes edema fluid removal by disrupting the normal membrane fluid transport. There is also injury to type 2 alveolar cells, impeding surfactant production and differentiation to type 1 cells for alveolar repair. The inflammatory cascade is activated with the release of proinflammatory cytokines that amplify the inflamatory response. Edematous dependent regions of the lung collapse, leading to atelectasis and reduction in lung compliance. Hypoxemia results from intrapulmonary shunting with ventilation/perfusion mismatch.

The subacute phase of ARDS usually occurs 5 to 10 days after the onset and is characterized by the appearance in the alveolar space of fibroblasts and procollagen III peptides, resulting in progressive pulmonary fibrosis leading to CO_2 retention and changes in lung compliance.

2. Diagnosis of Acute Respiratory Distress Syndrome

In 1994, the American-European Consensus Conference proposed a new definition recognizing that the severity of lung injury can vary. Children with less severe hypoxia (PaO_2/FIO_2 ≥200 and ≤300) were considered to have acute lung injury (ALI), and children with more severe hypoxemia (PaO_2/FIO_2 ≤ 200) were considered to have ARDS. This difference has helped in the standardization of clinical research trials.

Some of the insults leading to ARDS include pneumonia, lung contusion, aspiration pneumonitis, hydrocarbon ingestion, smoke inhalation, multiple emergent transfusions, near drowning, and sepsis.

3. Management of Acute Respiratory Distress Syndrome

Patients with ARDS may benefit from the following:

> !
>
> *Mechanical ventilation is provided using a lung-protective strategy.*
>
> !

Noninvasive positive pressure ventilation with BiPAP or CPAP should be used to improve oxygenation and minimize iatrogenic oxygen toxicity.

Endotracheal intubation with a cuffed endotracheal tube should be performed in patients unable to tolerate noninvasive positive pressure ventilation or in patients that deteriorate rapidly despite its use. It is important to monitor and maintain the cuff inflation pressure at a level lower than 20 cm H_2O.

Patients should be ventilated with a lung-protective strategy (see **Chapter 6**). Permissive hypercapnia should be considered part of a lung-protective strategy in patients with severe lung disease requiring high ventilator pressures. Permissive hypercapnia is contraindicated in children with intracranial hypertension and sickle cell disease.

G. Pulmonary Edema

1. Pathophysiology of Pulmonary Edema

There are 2 types of pulmonary edema, high-pressure pulmonary edema and permeability pulmonary edema. High-pressure pulmonary edema is frequently cardiac in origin, whereas permeability pulmonary edema is typically caused by a disruption of the alveolocapillary membrane (see the section on the pathophysiology of acute respiratory distress syndrome above). The increase in capillary pressure associated with high-pressure pulmonary edema might be caused by conditions causing obstruction of blood flow through blood vessels (pulmonary venous obstruction) or through the heart (mitral valve stenosis) or by impaired left ventricular function. As the left ventricular pressure rises, a concomitant rise in left atrial pressure (hydrostatic pressure) is transmitted to the microvasculature, thereby increasing the rate of fluid flux into the interstitial space. This net flow overwhelms the lymphatic system's ability to clear the fluid. Edema fluid can break through the tight walls of the alveolar epithelium and cause flooding in the alveolar air space, producing hypoxemia. Peribronchial edema leads to small airway closing, decreasing pulmonary compliance, and increasing work of breathing. Increased hydrostatic pressure is the primary mechanism by which interstitial and alveolar flooding occurs.

2. Diagnosis of Pulmonary Edema

Patients with low plasma protein are more likely to develop pulmonary edema at lower levels of atrial pressure. Children might present with only mild dyspnea and failure to thrive. With worsening symptoms, chest radiography will show cephalization of fluid, pulmonary congestion, and clearly evident Kerley B lines.

3. Management of Pulmonary Edema

Patients with high-pressure pulmonary edema may benefit from:

- A timely cardiology consultation
- Bed rest in a semi-sitting position, with the head of the bed at 30 to 45 degrees
- Reduction of pulmonary venous return (preload) and systemic vascular resistance (afterload)
- Furosemide (1-2 mg/kg per day in divided doses every 6-12 hours) to reduce extracellular volume and decrease systemic venous return by lowering atrial filling pressure and improving cardiac function. The acute relief in pulmonary congestion is probably related to its furosemide's almost immediate venodilatory effect. It also promotes transcapillary refill from the interstitial space.
- Morphine (0.1-0.2 mg/kg/dose) to reduce preload by increasing venous capacitance. Morphine decreases venous return and reduces total peripheral resistance.
- Reduction of myocardial metabolic demand by treating hyperthermia, improving the work of breathing through the provision of oxygen (100% fraction of inspired oxygen [FIO_2]), and attempting noninvasive positive pressure ventilation. Endotracheal intubation should be considered in patients with persistent hypoxemia and respiratory failure despite maximum noninvasive supplementary oxygen support and in patients with hemodynamic compromise.

The cardiovascular collapse noted in some patients after endotracheal intubation and bagging may be the result of a further decrease in venous return with positive pressure ventilation.

Additionally, measures designed to minimize the increase in intrathoracic pressure, such as decreasing inspiratory time, decreasing tidal volume, and minimizing the amount of PEEP, need to be considered. Cardiopulmonary resuscitation (CPR) may be necessary, and clinicians must always be prepared for this possibility.

Key Points

Diagnosis and Management of the Child With Acute Lower Airway Disease

- Any intervention should focus on a rapid assessment on the type and severity of respiratory compromise rather than the precise etiology.
- Frequent reassessment of the response to treatment is vital for good outcome.
- Respiratory failure can exist with or without respiratory distress.
- In patients with asthma, the degree of wheezing is unrelated to the severity of the disease. A silent chest with very limited airflow is a worrisome finding.
- Chest radiography should be repeated between 6 and 24 hours after the initiation of therapy to ensure there is no progression of disease or unsuspected pathology.
- Cuffed endotracheal tubes should be used with patients when a significant change in compliance is anticipated.

Suggested Readings

1. Fraser RS. Histology and gross anatomy of the respiratory tract. In: Martin JG, Hamid Q, Shannon J, eds. *Physiologic Basis of Respiratory Disease.* Ontario, BC, Canada: Decker; 2005:1-14.

2. Mercier J, Dauger S, Durand P, et al. Acute respiratory syndrome in children. In: Fuhrman BP, Zimmerman JJ, eds. *Pediatric Critical Care.* 3rd ed. Philadelphia, PA: Mosby; 2006:731-743.

3. Ralston M, Hazinski MF, Zaritsky AL. Recognition of respiratory distress and failure. In: Ralston M, Hazinski MF, Zaritsky AL, eds. *Pediatric Advance Life Support.* Wheeling, IL: World Point; 2006:33-43.

4. Ralston M, Hazinski MF, Zaritsky AL. Management of respiratory distress and failure. In: Ralston M, Hazinski MF, Zaritsky AL, eds. *Pediatric Advance Life Support.* Wheeling, IL: World Point; 2006:45-59.

5. Rotta A. Asthma. In: Fuhrman BP, Zimmerman JJ, eds. *Pediatric Critical Care.* 3rd ed. Philadelphia, PA: Mosby; 2006:588-607.

6. Scharf S. Mechanical cardiopulmonary interactions in critical care. In: Dantzker DR, Scharf SM, eds. *Cardiopulmonary Critical Care.* 3rd ed. Philadelphia, PA: Saunders; 1998:75-91.

7. Switzer ND, Rajagopal A. Oncologic emergencies: pulmonary embolus, superior vena cava syndrome, cardiac tamponade, and respiratory emergencies. In: Shaw AD, Riedel BJ, Burton AW, eds. *Acute Care of the Cancer Patient.* Boca Raton, FL: Taylor and Francis Group; 2005:505-517.

Chapter 6:

MECHANICAL VENTILATION

Objectives

- Identify the indications, advantages, and disadvantages of noninvasive positive-pressure ventilation (NPPV).
- Describe the distinguishing characteristics of the different mechanical ventilators and their modes.
- Select ventilator settings for the initiation of mechanical ventilation.
- Explain the relationship between parameters of mechanical ventilation and modifications needed to avoid its harmful effects.
- List modalities for monitoring patients who are receiving mechanical ventilation, and state each modality's limitations.
- Briefly discuss approaches to weaning a patient from mechanical ventilation.
- Describe newer approaches to mechanical ventilation in patients with acute respiratory insufficiency and acute respiratory distress syndrome (ARDS).

Case Study

A 6-year-old male underwent thoracotomy and drainage of a pleural abscess 2 days ago. A left thoracostomy tube was left in place. The operative course was uneventful, and he was extubated on postoperative day 1 without difficulty. This morning, he is noted to have increased work of breathing and saturations of 92% on 5 L oxygen via facemask. A chest radiograph shows complete atelectasis of the left lung. He is started on bilevel positive airway pressure (BiPAP) with the following settings: peak inspiratory pressure (Ppeak) 12 cm H_2O, positive end-expiratory pressure (PEEP) 6 cm H_2O, fraction of inspired oxygen (F_{IO_2}) 50% with a backup rate of 20. A repeat chest radiograph 8 hours later shows near-complete reexpansion of the left lung.

- What was the most likely reason for the radiographic findings prior to the initiation of BiPAP?

- What are the advantages and disadvantages of BiPAP therapy in this setting?

- If the repeat chest radiograph did not show any improvement, what steps might have been taken to promote reexpansion of the lung?

I. INTRODUCTION

The recognition of and response to respiratory failure continues to be a top priority in the management of critically ill children. The anatomic considerations unique to the respiratory tracts of infants and children and the inherent lack of respiratory reserve during times of stress pose special challenges to the caretaker confronted with this urgent situation. Regardless, the goal is always the same: to restore and maintain adequate oxygenation and ventilation while optimizing patient comfort and avoiding further injury. Failure to accomplish this goal can lead to devastating consequences, including cardiopulmonary arrest and death.

This chapter briefly outlines the general approach to the management of the child requiring mechanical ventilation, with a focus on the use of mechanical ventilation in specific clinical settings in the child with normal lungs or mild respiratory disease. We both review conventional ventilation techniques and introduce more recent advances in respiratory support.

It is important to keep in mind that consultation with a specialist in the management of pediatric critical respiratory illness is essential when the patient is a child with more severe lung disease who requires ongoing care.

II. NONINVASIVE POSITIVE-PRESSURE VENTILATION

Noninvasive positive-pressure ventilation (NPPV) can augment oxygenation and ventilation without insertion of an artificial airway into the trachea. One form of NPPV, bilevel positive airway pressure (BiPAP), augments ventilation by delivering pressurized air through a facial or nasal mask or a mouthpiece. Both the nasal mask and the facemask must be tight fitting to avoid leakage of pressure. A helmet-like apparatus may improve patient tolerance.

The delivery of positive inspiratory pressure has been found helpful in patients with chronic obstructive lung disease, neuromuscular disorders, obstructive sleep apnea, cystic fibrosis, upper-airway obstruction, and thoracic dysplasia. It has also been used as a means to avoid intubation in patients with mild to moderate acute respiratory insufficiency. Noninvasive positive-pressure ventilation can significantly improve respiratory rate, heart rate, work of breathing, and dyspnea score in the acute setting, and it has been especially useful in previously healthy children with respiratory embarrassment due to muscle deconditioning following prolonged intubation.

Noninvasive positive-pressure ventilation is contraindicated in the following situations:

- Patients experiencing rapidly progressive respiratory failure
- Patients with hemodynamic instability
- Patients at significant risk of aspiration
- Patients who are unable to clear copious oropharyngeal secretions

The use of this form of respiratory support requires the patient's cooperation, including a willingness to tolerate little or no sedation. Initial settings for NPPV are presented in **Table 6-1**.

Table 6-1. Initial Settings for Noninvasive Positive-Pressure Ventilation

Age	Initial Setting
Infants <12 months	Nasal CPAP should be attempted first. If CPAP does not provide adequate support, tracheal intubation is indicated.
Infants 1-2 years	Ppeak: 8 cm H_2O; PEEP: 4 cm H_2O; F_{IO_2}: 1.0; ± backup rate appropriate for age and disease
Children >2 years	Ppeak: 10 cm H_2O; PEEP: 5 cm H_2O; F_{IO_2}: 1.0; ± backup rate: appropriate for age and disease

Note: Maximum settings are patient and age dependent, and effective delivery relies at least in part on the adequacy of the seal rather than the settings. If a Ppeak >18-20 cm H_2O and PEEP >12-15 cm H_2O can be tolerated by the patient but does not decrease work of breathing or improve oxygenation sufficiently, or if respiratory insufficiency is not improved, tracheal intubation is indicated.

Machines designed to deliver noninvasive positive-pressure ventilation offer a variety of modes:

1. **Spontaneous:** The patient triggers the inspiratory and expiratory pressure cycles and the rate and depth of breathing.
2. **Spontaneous/timed:** Similar to the spontaneous mode, but in addition machine breaths are delivered at a set frequency for patients that may be intermittently apneic.
3. **Timed positive pressure:** Breaths are delivered at a set frequency, but the patient can still breathe spontaneously.
4. **Continuous positive airway pressure (CPAP):** A baseline system pressure is provided (usually 4-8 cm H_2O for children), but respiratory drive and effort must be maintained by the patient.

Selection of the appropriate setting is based on the nature and severity of the patient's respiratory insufficiency. A word of caution: machines are often insufficiently sensitive to the respiratory efforts of small patients. Careful observation is required to prevent counterproductive or poorly timed mechanical breaths, that is, dyssynchrony.

The advantages of NPPV include decreased laryngeal trauma, decreased risk of ventilator-associated pneumonia (VAP) and tracheitis, and decreased need for sedation and analgesia. In addition, if a nasal mask is utilized, the patient can communicate verbally, cough and cooperate with pulmonary toilet, and take sips of clear liquids.

The disadvantages of NPPV in children include the breakdown of the skin over the nasal bridge and an increased risk of aspiration due to gastric distension. Masks may not fit tightly and may not provide effective ventilation, particularly in small patients. Restriction of activity is often needed to maintain optimal mask placement. Tracheal suctioning requires mask removal, which can lead to respiratory decompensation.

> !
>
> *Children on NPPV require close observation in a monitored pediatric intensive or intermediate care setting.*
>
> !

A. Continuous Positive Airway Pressure

Continuous positive airway pressure (CPAP) allows spontaneous breathing from a fresh gas source at an elevated baseline system pressure (higher than atmospheric pressure), thus preventing collapse of distal small airways and alveoli. It can be delivered via nasal cannula, mask, or tracheostomy or endotracheal tubes. Continuous positive airway pressure is not a true mode of mechanical ventilation because no additional positive pressure is applied above end-expiratory airway pressure during inspiration. Patient inspiration is initiated from the elevated baseline system pressure, and airway pressure returns to that level at the end of expiration. Therefore, CPAP allows application of positive end-expiratory pressure in a spontaneously breathing patient. The respiratory rate and tidal volume (V_T) are totally dependent on the patient's inspiratory effort because the patient inspires against the resistance of the endotracheal tube (ETT). For this reason, CPAP has been utilized in many PICUs as a means of assessing readiness for extubation. Continuous positive airway pressure can be delivered to infants younger than 1 year of age via nasal cannula and has been especially helpful in the treatment of apnea related to prematurity and apnea associated with viral respiratory infections.

III. MECHANICAL VENTILATORY SUPPORT

Indications for endotracheal intubation are addressed in **Chapter 2**. When hypoxic or hypercapnic respiratory failure cannot be treated by other means, the generally accepted indications for initiating mechanical ventilatory support listed in **Table 6-2** may apply.

Table 6-2. Indications for Mechanical Ventilatory Support

Ventilation abnormalities	Respiratory muscle dysfunction • Respiratory muscle fatigue • Chest wall abnormalities • Neuromuscular disease Decreased ventilatory drive Increased airway resistance and/or obstruction
Oxygenation abnormalities	Refractory hypoxemia Need for PEEP, as in pulmonary edema or pulmonary hemorrhage Excessive work of breathing

Mechanical ventilation is also indicated for the following purposes:

- To permit sedation and/or neuromuscular blockade
- To decrease systemic or myocardial oxygen consumption
- To allow hyperventilation as a temporizing measure to reduce intracranial pressure
- To facilitate alveolar recruitment and prevent and/or treat atelectasis
- To improve oxygen delivery in conditions associated with inadequate oxygen supply or increased oxygen demand (shock, sepsis, cardiopulmonary arrest)
- To protect the airway from aspiration in patients with loss of innate airway protective reflex function

A. Ventilator Variables

1. Phase Variables

Mechanical ventilators and their modes can be distinguished by the phase variables—trigger, limit, and cycle—that govern the characteristics of the inspiratory phase of each breath. The trigger variable regulates the start of each breath. The limit variable sustains inspiration. The cycling variable controls the termination of inspiration.

Early positive-pressure ventilators had no mechanism to detect patient effort; this resulted in asynchrony and poor tolerance by some patients. Engineers developed triggering mechanisms that detected decreases in the pressure within the ventilator circuit associated with the patient's respiratory effort. Newer ventilators can detect changes in flow as the patient inhales by providing a continuous stream of gas through the ventilator circuit and continually monitoring the returning flow.

2. Volume and Pressure

Common ventilator modes are limited by either volume or pressure. Guaranteeing V_T with volume-limited ventilation is generally preferred over pressure-limited ventilation. In the past, infants were ventilated primarily with pressure-limited modes due to limitations in flow delivery and imprecise tidal-volume measurement in older generation ventilators. With newer machines, nearly all patients, including premature infants, can be managed using a volume-control mode, although the prevailing culture has been slow to change.

3. Time Cycling, Flow Cycling, and Other Variables

> !
>
> *In children, guaranteeing V_T with volume-limited ventilation is generally preferred over pressure-limited ventilation.*
>
> !

Ventilator modes are typically time cycled; in other words, inspiration is terminated after a specified time. Flow cycling, an engineering advancement, is used in specialized modes of ventilation, such as pressure support.

Numerous other variables distinguish the newer ventilators and their unique modes of ventilation. Such features as gas source, valve response times, variable flows, and monitors can provide important tools for managing the difficult-to-ventilate patient.

IV. MODES OF MECHANICAL VENTILATION

Once the decision to initiate mechanical ventilation has been made, the form of ventilatory support that best satisfies the patient's needs must be determined. The choice of ventilator mode depends on how much of the function of gas exchange can be contributed by the patient and how much must be done by the machine. A trial of NPPV may be considered in some circumstances (see Section II of this chapter). Frequently used modes of ventilation include controlled mechanical ventilation (CMV), assist-control ventilation (AC ventilation), synchronized intermittent mandatory ventilation (SIMV), and pressure-support ventilation (PSV). These modes are achieved by using various combinations of the phase variables described above. They may be combined with the application of PEEP. Airway pressure and flow tracings of CPAP and 2 widely used modes of mechanical ventilation are illustrated in **Figure 6-1**. Each has advantages and disadvantages, as summarized in **Table 6-3**. In choosing a mode of ventilation, it is important to consider that 3 specific goals are (1) to provide adequate ventilation and oxygenation, (2) to reduce the work of breathing, and (3) to ensure patient comfort and synchrony with the ventilator.

Figure 6-1. Airway Pressure and Flow Tracings of CPAP and 2 Modes of Mechanical Ventilation

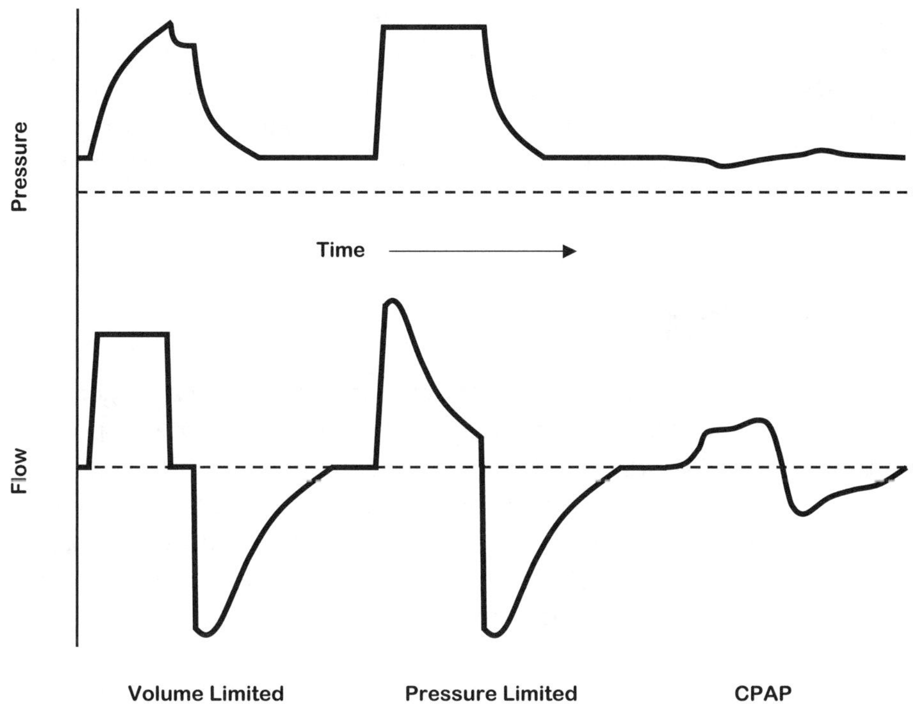

Table 6-3. Potential Advantages and Disadvantages of Selected Modes of Mechanical Ventilation

Mode	Advantages	Disadvantages
Controlled mechanical ventilation (CMV)	Rests muscles of respiration	Requires use of sedation/neuromuscular blockade; potential adverse hemodynamic effects
Assist-control (AC) ventilation	Patient can increase ventilatory support; reduced work of breathing compared to spontaneous breathing	Potential adverse hemodynamic effects; delivery of a full breath with each patient effort may lead to inappropriate hyperventilation, breath stacking, and inadvertent positive end-expiratory pressure (PEEP)
AC volume-control ventilation	Guarantees delivery of set tidal volume (unless peak pressure limit is exceeded)	May lead to excessive inspiratory pressures
AC pressure-control ventilation	Allows limitation of peak inspiratory pressures	Potential hyper- or hypoventilation with lung resistance/compliance changes
Synchronized intermittent mandatory ventilation (SIMV)	Less interference with normal cardiovascular function	Increased work of breathing compared to AC ventilation; added patient-ventilator synchrony
Pressure support ventilation (PSV)	Patient comfort; improved patient-ventilator interaction; decreased work of breathing	Apnea alarm is only backup; variable patient tolerance

A. Controlled Mechanical Ventilation

Controlled mechanical ventilation (CMV) delivers ventilator breaths at a preset rate. Each breath is time cycled and either volume limited or pressure limited. A preset V_T, as in volume-control ventilation, or a preset applied pressure and time, as in pressure-control ventilation, is delivered at a preset rate. Early ventilators had no triggering mechanisms to allow synchronization with patient respiratory effort and thus could be used effectively only in patients who were heavily sedated and pharmacologically paralyzed.

B. Assist-Control Ventilation

Assist-control (AC) ventilation is controlled mechanical ventilation with a triggering mechanism that allows synchronization with patient respiratory effort. A preset volume or pressure is delivered at a preset minimum rate. A full ventilator breath is also delivered with each spontaneous inspiratory effort; therefore, patients who are tachypneic due to their illness or agitation are likely to hyperventilate in this mode. The implementation of CMV in most contemporary ventilators is, in fact, AC ventilation. This mode of ventilation is commonly used when mechanical ventilation is initiated in patients with acute respiratory failure.

With proper use of AC ventilatory support, the work of breathing may be significantly decreased. However, if the ventilator and the patient are not in synchrony or if the ventilator flow rates are not matched with patient demand, this mode of support may actually lead to an increase in the work of breathing.

Decreasing the work of breathing may be important for clinical situations in which there is inadequate cardiac output. Resting the diaphragm and respiratory muscles allows redistribution of blood flow and better delivery of oxygen to vital organ systems.

!

In choosing a mode of ventilation, important goals to consider are:

(1) to provide adequate ventilation and oxygenation,

(2) to reduce the work of breathing, and

(3) to ensure patient comfort and synchrony with the ventilator.

!

C. Synchronized Intermittent Mandatory Ventilation

Synchronized intermittent mandatory ventilation (SIMV) delivers either volume-limited or pressure-limited breaths at a preset rate. Most frequently, SIMV is used with breaths in a volume-cycled mode. Unlike AC ventilation, no additional ventilator breaths are delivered above the preset rate. Spontaneous breathing above that rate is possible, but the V_T is limited to that which the patient can generate. The use of synchronization allows for enhanced patient-ventilator interaction by delivering the preset machine breaths in conjunction with the patient's inspiratory effort. When no effort is sensed, the ventilator delivers the preset V_T at an interval that depends on the set rate. Synchronized intermittent mandatory ventilation is often combined with PSV (see below) to augment the VT generated by the patient during spontaneous breathing. The level of pressure support should be selected to offset ETT resistance and is usually 5 to 10 cm H_2O.

One advantage of the SIMV mode is that it allows the patient to contribute to the minute ventilation requirement with spontaneous, negative-pressure breaths. The negative inspiratory pressure (relative to PEEP, not atmospheric pressure) leads to an increased venous return to the right side of the heart, which may improve cardiac output and cardiovascular function. Although this mode of ventilatory support may be more comfortable for some patients, SIMV is usually associated with more work of breathing than AC ventilation.

D. Pressure-Support Ventilation

Pressure-support ventilation (PSV) provides a preset level of inspiratory pressure with each breath. All breaths are flow cycled and pressure limited. This inspiratory assistance is generally selected to overcome the increased work of breathing imposed by the disease process, the ETT, the inspiratory valves, and other mechanical aspects of ventilatory support. The pressure support that is applied augments each patient-generated breath. With PSV, the patient controls the respiratory rate and exerts a strong influence on the duration of inspiration, inspiratory flow rate, and VT. The delivered VT is influenced by pulmonary compliance and resistance. Rapid changes in these parameters may alter the minute ventilation and work required of the patient. PSV can also be coupled with SIMV, primarily as a means to diminish work of breathing during spontaneous breaths.

The amount of pressure support set during mechanical ventilation is titrated to the patient's exhaled VT. Pressure support should be set to achieve adequate gas exchange and optimize patient comfort.

Pressure-support ventilation is a strictly spontaneous mode of ventilation, and when used alone it will not provide ventilation during periods of apnea. A backup, mandatory ventilation setting is therefore required and is standard on many ventilators. Potential benefits of PSV include improved comfort and tolerance for awake, spontaneously breathing patients and reduced work of breathing due to enhanced patient-ventilator interaction. Typically, as pressure support is increased in patients with lung disease, the patient's work of breathing and respiratory rate decrease, and VT increases. Alternatively, patients recovering from severe lung disease who were initially placed on high levels of pressure support can be effectively weaned from mechanical ventilation by gradually decreasing the pressure support, thus requiring progressively more work from deconditioned respiratory muscles. The presence of a bronchopleural fistula or an ET cuff leak may interfere with appropriate cycling in this mode because flow is accelerated to offset the pressure lost from escaping gas.

V. INITIAL VENTILATOR SETTINGS

When initiating ventilatory support, an FIO_2 of 1.0 is used to maximize the oxygen available during the transition to positive pressure ventilation and to compensate for any periods of respiratory or hemodynamic instability. Tidal volume levels are set between 8 and 10 mL/kg in patients with reasonably normal lung compliance. Higher VT levels are generally avoided to decrease the risk of trauma to the lungs. The choice of the initial respiratory rate in children is usually based on age and disease process and is subsequently titrated by measurement of pH and, to a lesser extent, $Paco_2$ in arterial blood. Guidelines for initiation of mechanical ventilation are listed in **Table 6-4.**

Table 6-4. Guidelines for Initiation of Mechanical Ventilation

1. Choose a ventilator mode with which you are familiar. The primary goals of ventilatory support are adequate oxygenation/ventilation, reduced work of breathing, synchrony between the patient and ventilator, and avoidance of high end-inspiration alveolar pressures.
2. The initial Fio_2 level should be 1.0.[a] The Fio_2 thereafter can be titrated downward to maintain a Spo_2 of 92% to 94%. In severe ARDS, $Spo_2 \geq 88\%$ may be acceptable, lowering the therapeutic goal in favor of minimizing ventilator-associated lung injury.
3. Initial VT should be set between 8 and 10 mL/kg and adjusted according to blood gas results. Patients with neuromuscular disease often require VT levels of 10 to 12 mL/kg to satisfy air hunger. In some patients with ARDS, a VT level of 5 to 8 mL/kg is recommended to avoid high inspiratory plateau pressures (>30 cm H_2O).
4. Choose a respiratory rate and minute ventilation appropriate for the particular clinical requirements. Rate is dependent upon age and disease process, generally 12 breaths/minute (adolescents) to 24 breaths/minute (neonates). Target pH primarily and $Paco_2$ secondarily.
5. Set the inspiratory time (TI) for each breath according to the patient's age and disease process. Neonates with normal lung function require TI of approximately 0.35-0.6 sec, whereas the TI for children older than 2 years is generally 0.85-1.0 second. In addition, the ratio of inspiratory to expiratory time (I:E ratio) should be set with the patient's specific needs in mind. Start with an I:E ratio of 1:2 in patients with healthy lungs. Patients with respiratory illnesses marked by difficulty with oxygenation (ARDS) may require a TI >1 and an I:E ratio >1:1, whereas patients with obstruction to outflow (as in asthma and bronchopulmonary dysplasia) will require ample expiratory time and I:E ratios of 1:3.5-4 to avoid auto-PEEP (see "Relationship of Inspiratory Time to Expiratory Time and Auto-PEEP," below). Keep in mind that the parameters for inspiration and exhalation are somewhat rate dependent.
6. Use PEEP to achieve and maintain optimal alveolar recruitment. In diffuse lung injury, PEEP will improve oxygenation and reduce the Fio_2 (see **Table 6-5**). If volume is held constant, PEEP increases mean airway pressure, but it may also increase peak inspiratory airway pressure, depending on the ventilator mode, and this may result in potentially undesirable consequences in ARDS. Set PEEP to 5 cm H_2O when initiating mechanical ventilation in children with healthy lungs. PEEP levels >15 cm H_2O are rarely necessary.
7. Set the trigger sensitivity to allow a minimal patient effort to initiate the inspiration. Beware of autocycling if the trigger setting is too sensitive.
8. When poor oxygenation, inadequate ventilation, or excessively high peak inspiratory pressures are thought to be related to patient intolerance of ventilator settings and cannot be corrected by ventilator adjustments, consider sedation, analgesia, and/or neuromuscular blockade.
9. Call a pediatric critical care consultant or other specialist in respiratory care for assistance.

Abbreviations: ARDS, acute respiratory distress syndrome; PEEP, positive end-expiratory pressure; Spo_2, peripheral oxyhemoglobin saturation; VT, tidal volume.

[a] The exception to this recommendation is the patient with congenital heart disease, whose condition will be exacerbated by oxygen-driven decreases in pulmonary vascular resistance.

!

As a general rule Fio_2, mean airway pressure, and PEEP affect the Pao_2, whereas respiratory rate, dead space (VD), and VT determine alveolar minute ventilation and $Paco_2$.

VI. CONTINUING CARE DURING MECHANICAL VENTILATION

After mechanical ventilation has been initiated, the parameters listed below should be assessed frequently to guide changes in the ventilator settings. Care should be taken when any change in ventilator settings is made because adjusting one parameter is likely to affect the others. This interdependency of parameters may cause a change that is beneficial in one respect but harmful in another. In complex patient-care situations, such as those discussed later in this chapter, a critical care consultation should be obtained.

A. Fraction of Inspired Oxygen

Inspired oxygen may be harmful to the lung parenchyma after prolonged exposure due to the production of toxic oxygen-derived radicals. Although the precise threshold for concern is not known, it is desirable to reduce the FIO_2 to 0.5 (50% oxygen) or below as soon as possible (ideally within the first 24 hours). However, except in the premature neonate, to whom oxygen toxicity may be equally damaging, hypoxemia is usually considered a greater risk to the patient than high FIO_2 levels.

The primary determinants of oxygenation during mechanical ventilation are FIO_2 and mean airway pressure ($P\overline{aw}$). In the patient with acute lung injury or acute respiratory distress syndrome, PEEP becomes an additional independent determinant. Tidal volume, the relationship of inspiratory time to expiratory time (I:E ratio), PEEP, and several other factors beyond the scope of this chapter all interact to affect $P\overline{aw}$. The interrelationships of those factors, as already discussed, must be considered when formulating the plan for mechanical ventilation.

B. Humidification

Gases delivered by mechanical ventilators are typically dry, and the upper airways of patients are bypassed by artificial airways. These circumstances result in loss of heat and moisture from the respiratory tract. Gases are routinely heated and humidified during mechanical ventilation to prevent mucosal damage and minimize inspissation of secretions. Available systems include passive humidifiers (artificial nose) or active, microprocessor-controlled heat and humidifying systems (heated humidifiers). The passive humidifiers are contraindicated in the presence of copious secretions, minute ventilation greater than 12 L/min, or blood in the airway.

C. Inspiratory Pressure

During positive pressure ventilation, airway pressure rises progressively to a peak inspiratory pressure (Ppeak), which is reached at end-inspiration. Peak inspiratory pressure may also be abbreviated as PIP or referred to as peak pressure or peak airway pressure. Peak inspiratory pressure is the sum of 2 pressures, the pressure required to overcome airway resistance and the pressure required to overcome elastic properties of the lung and chest wall. If a pause is set at the end of inspiration (zero gas flow with the airway closed), the pressure drops slightly below the Ppeak to the inspiratory plateau pressure (Pplat; see **Figure 6-2**). Inspiratory plateau pressure reflects the pressure required to overcome elastic recoil and is the best estimate of peak alveolar pressure, which is an important indicator of alveolar distension. Accurate measurement of Ppeak requires the absence of any patient effort during inspiration or exhalation.

Figure 6-2. Relationship of Peak Inspiratory Pressure and Inspiratory Plateau Pressure

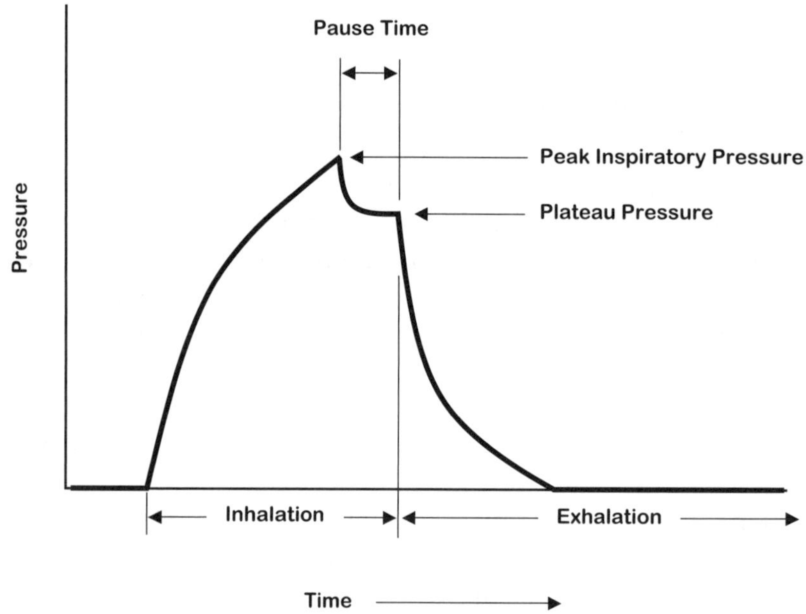

Potential adverse effects from high inspiratory pressure include barotrauma, volutrauma, and reduced cardiac output. Barotrauma (pneumothorax, pneumomediastinum) and volutrauma (lung parenchymal injury due to overinflation), although linked to high Ppeak, correlate best with Pplat, a better measurement of alveolar distension. An example of the relationship of Ppeak and Pplat to alveolar distension is demonstrated by the effect of ETT size on Ppeak and Pplat. As the internal diameter of the ETT is decreased in a patient receiving volume ventilation, the same VT will result in higher Ppeak, yet Pplat and alveolar distension remain unchanged as the pressure is dissipated across the ETT. The same VT, regardless of the type of breath, produces the same alveolar distension at end inspiration. Inspiratory plateau pressure should ideally be less than 30 cm H_2O.

Elevated inspiratory plateau airway pressure may be reduced by decreasing PEEP, which may also decrease oxygenation, or by decreasing VT, which may lead to a reduction in minute ventilation. Permissive hypercapnia and a controlled reduction in pH may be accepted when high Pplat must be reduced. Permissive hypercapnia should not be used in patients with elevated intracranial pressure (ICP) because Paco2 greater than 35 to 40 mm Hg (4.7 to 5.3 kPa) may increase cerebral blood flow and cerebral blood volume and further elevate the ICP.

D. Relationship of Inspiratory Time to Expiratory Time and Auto-PEEP

The total respiratory cycle time is calculated by dividing 60 seconds by the respiratory rate. The times for inhalation (inspiratory time) and exhalation (expiratory time) occur within the total cycle time and are termed the I:E ratio. During spontaneous breathing, the normal I:E ratio is ~1:2, indicating that for normal patients the exhalation time is about twice as long as inhalation time. In chronic lung disease and other conditions associated with obstruction to expiratory flow, such as asthma, the exhalation time becomes prolonged, and the I:E ratio changes (eg, 1:2.5 or 1:3). Such changes reflect the pathophysiology of the lung disease and directly influence techniques used during mechanical ventilation.

The inspiratory time during volume breaths (AC or SIMV modes) is often determined by the tidal volume and inspiratory gas flow rate (Flow × Inspiratory Time = Tidal Volume). A greater V_T takes longer to deliver if the flow rate remains constant, and the same V_T takes longer to deliver if the flow rate is reduced. In both cases, the inspiratory time is longer. However, given that the respiratory rate is constant, the total cycle time remains the same, and thus the time available for exhalation (the expiratory time) must be shortened to fit into the cycle time. In this situation the inspiratory time is actively set by adjusting V_T and inspiratory flow rate or by the use of inspiratory pauses on the ventilator. The expiratory time, however, is passively determined (ie, what is left over in the cycle time before the next inspiratory cycle of the mechanical ventilator or spontaneous breath) and varies inversely with the respiratory rate set on the ventilator.

If the expiratory time is too short to allow full exhalation, the next lung inflation is superimposed upon the residual gas in the lung and breath stacking occurs. This process will result in hyperinflation of the lung and the development of PEEP that exceeds the level of PEEP preset on the ventilator. This increase in end-expiratory pressure is called auto-PEEP, or intrinsic, inadvertent, or occult PEEP. Auto-PEEP can be quantified by using manual methods or through electronic programs available in some ventilators. However, it is most easily diagnosed qualitatively by the flow-over-time graphic waveform tracing available on most mechanical ventilators (**Figure 6-3**). The potentially harmful physiologic effects of auto-PEEP on Ppeak, Pplat, and mean airway pressures ($P\overline{aw}$) and on lung and cardiovascular function are the same as those of preset PEEP (**Table 6-5**). Auto-PEEP may also increase work of breathing because the difference between the set PEEP and auto-PEEP must be overcome on inspiration to allow for fresh gas flow.

Reduction in auto-PEEP can be accomplished through shortening the inspiratory time, thus extending the expiratory time to allow full exhalation of the V_T. However, this may cause alveoli with longer time constants to incompletely fill. The most effective way to decrease auto-PEEP is by decreasing the respiratory rate. Decreasing V_T may also be also effective. Increasing the inspiratory flow rate (volume breaths) is typically less effective unless flow rates are set inappropriately low. The influence of a decreased respiratory rate and V_T on the $Paco_2$, pH, and minute ventilation must be considered.

E. Minute Ventilation

The primary determinant of CO_2 exchange during mechanical ventilation is alveolar minute ventilation (V_A), calculated as

$$V_A = (V_T - V_D) \times f$$

where VD is dead space and f is respiratory rate. The VT, the respiratory rate, and their interrelationships with other ventilatory parameters have already been discussed. Physiologic VD represents, in general, lung units that are relatively well ventilated but underperfused. The physiologic effect of increased VD is hypercapnia. Increased physiologic VD may result from the pathologic process in the lung, high airway pressures associated with mechanical ventilation, low intravascular volume, or low cardiac output. If hypercapnia persists during mechanical ventilation despite use of appropriate VT and rates, as discussed earlier, consultation with a pediatric intensivist should be sought. It may be necessary to tolerate a higher $Paco_2$ to avoid high airway pressure and auto-PEEP. This permissive hypercapnia technique should be initiated only with the support of an appropriate consultant.

Figure 6-3. Flow-Over-Time Waveform Tracing Indicating Auto-PEEP

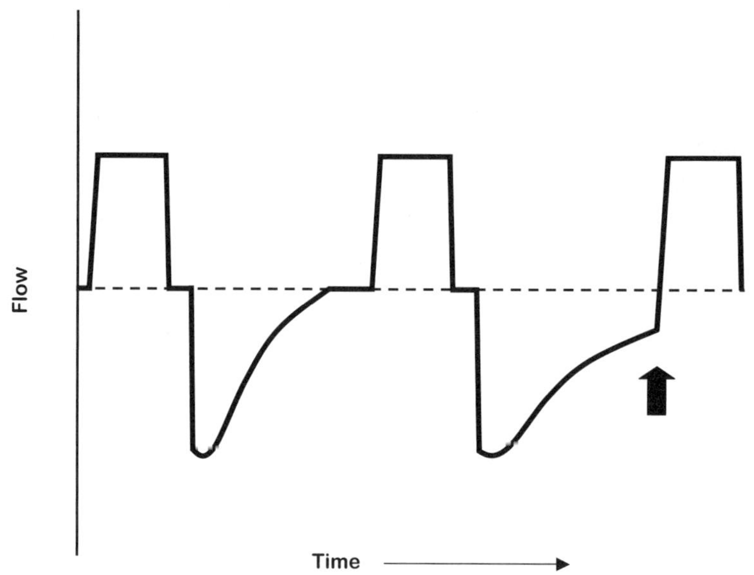

As previously discussed, adequate ventilation is assessed by consideration of both $Paco_2$ and pH. Hyperventilation resulting in a low $Paco_2$ may be an appropriate short-term compensatory goal during metabolic acidosis until the primary problem can be corrected. Similarly, a patient with chronic hypercapnia and increased $Paco_2$ at baseline, who maintains a near-normal pH by renal compensation (retention of bicarbonate), should receive only enough minute ventilation to maintain a normal pH. Driving $Paco_2$ to normal levels in the patient with chronic CO_2 retention will lead to severe alkalemia and loss of retained bicarbonate and may blunt the patient's respiratory drive.

Table 6-5. Use of Positive End-Expiratory Pressure in ALI/ARDS

Initiation of PEEP in ARDS

- Initiate PEEP at 5 cm H_2O and titrate up in increments of 2 to 3 cm H_2O.
- Full recruitment effect may not be apparent for several hours.
- Monitor blood pressure, heart rate, and Pao_2 during PEEP titration and at intervals while the patient is receiving PEEP therapy.
- Optimal PEEP settings are typically 8-15 cm H_2O.

Adverse Effects of PEEP

- Barotrauma
- Decreased venous return, decreased preload, decreased cardiac output, and hypotension
- Increase in $Paco_2$ (increase in dead space)
- Worsening oxygenation (especially with asymmetric ALI) as healthy lung is overdistended

Abbreviations: ALI, acute lung injury; ARDS, acute respiratory distress syndrome.

VII. SEDATION, ANALGESIA, AND NEUROMUSCULAR BLOCKADE

Endotracheal intubation and mechanical ventilation can be painful, frightening, and anxiety provoking. To improve patient comfort, relieve anxiety, and lessen the work of breathing, anxiolytics, sedatives, analgesics, and neuromuscular blocking agents are frequently administered. Guidelines for the use of these agents are outlined in **Table 6-6**. Administration of an opiate via continuous infusion and a benzodiazepine, either by intermittent bolus or continuous infusion, usually provides safe and effective analgesia and sedation. Neuromuscular blocking agents may be considered in consultation with a specialist experienced in their use. Certain agents, such as benzodiazepines, provide the added benefit of producing amnesia. Caution should be taken when using sedation in the nonintubated patient with acute respiratory insufficiency or impending respiratory failure in whom an intact native respiratory drive is required to prevent decompensation. The healthcare provider should be prepared to provide complete mechanical ventilatory support once sedating medications are given. Before administering neuromuscular blocking agents to a nonintubated patient, adequate ventilation with a bag-mask device should be assured.

Table 6-6. Guidelines for Commonly Used Analgesia, Sedation, and Neuromuscular Blocking Agents

	Agent	Usual Dose Range	Advantages	Disadvantages
Analgesia				
Opioids	Morphine sulfate	Bolus: 0.025-0.1 mg/kg Infusion: 0.05-0.1 mg/kg/h	Provides reliable analgesia, sedation, and some anxiolysis Reversal agent: naloxone	Adverse effects: respiratory depression, hypotension, bradycardia, pruritus, urinary retention, constipation
	Fentanyl	Bolus: 0.5-2 µg/kg Infusion: 0.5-2 µg/kg/h	Rapid onset of action; shorter acting; 100x more potent than morphine; less histamine release Reversal agent: naloxone	Adverse effects: respiratory depression, hypotension,[a] urinary retention, constipation, rigid chest (syndrome in which neonates receiving high-dose, rapid IV infusion cannot ventilate)
Non-opioid analgesics	Ketorolac	Loading dose: 1 mg/kg Maintenance dose: 0.5 mg/kg every 6 hours Maximum dose 30 mg/dose or 120 mg/24 hours	No respiratory depression; no risk of dependence Used with opiates to reduce the dose	Risk of gastritis and GI hemorrhage limit its use to 3-5 days
	Acetaminophen	15 mg/kg every 4 hours	Same as for ketorolac Minimal GI symptoms	An untreated overdose can result in organ failure requiring liver transplant
	Ibuprofen	10 mg/kg every 6-8 hours	Same as for ketorolac	Same as for ketorolac
Sedation				
Benzodiazepines	Midazolam	Bolus: 0.05-0.1 mg/kg Infusion: 0.05-0.1 mg/kg/h	Anxiolytic, amnestic Rapid onset (1-2 minutes) Short duration (1-4 hours) Can dose IV, IM, IN, IO Reversal agent: flumazenil	Frequent dose increases may be required when given as an infusion; may cause paradoxical agitation Involuntary jerking movements may be seen in neonates on infusions
	Lorazepam	Bolus: 0.05-0.1 mg/kg Infusion: 0.05-0.1 mg/kg/h	Anxiolytic, amnestic, anticonvulsant Onset: 5-15 minutes Duration: 2-6 hours Reversal agent: flumazenil	Continuous infusion may lead to anion gap acidosis, arrhythmias, and seizures due to propylene glycol preservative
Miscellaneous	Ketamine	Bolus: 1-4 mg/kg Infusion: 1-2 mg/kg/h	Dissociative anesthetic, amnestic, analgesic Potent bronchodilator	Adverse effects: elevated ICP, laryngospasm, hypersalivation May impair cardiac function in some patients Hallucinations are common on waking from the drug
	Propofol	Bolus: 1-3 mg/kg Infusion: 0.5-2 mg/kg/h	Rapid onset (1-2 minutes) Duration: dose dependent (5 minutes to 3 days [after 10-day infusion]) Amnestic, antiemetic, anticonvulsant	Adverse effects: apnea, bradycardia, and hypotension with rapid bolus dosing High-dose infusions may cause propofol infusion syndrome—refractory metabolic acidosis, bradycardia, and death

continued next page...

Table 6-6. Guidelines for Commonly Used Analgesia, Sedation, and Neuromuscular Blocking Agents (continued)

	Agent	Usual Dose Range	Advantages	Disadvantages
Neuromuscular Blockade				
Depolarizing agents	Succinylcholine	Bolus: 1-2 mg/kg	Rapid onset (~1 minute) Duration: varies with metabolism (3-5 minutes)	Rarely used in pediatrics outside of the OR May cause elevated ICP, dysrhythmias, hyperkalemia, malignant hyperthermia
Non-depolarizing agents	Vecuronium	Bolus: 0.1 mg/kg Infusion: 0.05-0.1 mg/kg/h	Onset: 45-90 seconds Duration: 30-90 minutes Minimal hemodynamic effects	Significant muscle weakness may persist after discontinuing the drug when used as a continuous infusion for a long period of time
	Rocuronium	Bolus: 0.6-1.2 mg/kg Infusion: 0.6-1.2 mg/kg/h	Onset: 30-60 seconds Duration: 30-60 minutes Agent of choice for intubation due to short duration of action	Same as for vecuronium, although rocuronium is not commonly used as a continuous infusion
	Pancuronium	Bolus: 0.1 mg/kg Infusion: 0.02-0.05 mg/kg/h	Onset: 2-4 minutes Duration: 75-90 minutes Longest acting	Adverse effects: tachycardia, bronchospasm (avoid in asthma) Mast cell degranulation causes histamine release

Abbreviations: IM, intramuscular; IN, intranasal; IO, intraosseous; IV, intravenous; NMB, neuromuscular blockade.
[a] Compared to morphine, fentanyl is associated with less histamine release, less hypotension, and less pruritus.

VIII. VENTILATORY GUIDELINES FOR SPECIFIC CLINICAL SITUATIONS

A. Acute Lung Injury/Acute Respiratory Distress Syndrome

Case Study

A 16-year-old male who underwent splenectomy 2 months ago presents to the emergency room with a 3-day history of fevers (38.8°C [101.8°F]), shaking chills, and increasing shortness of breath. Oxygen saturations are 86% while breathing room air and increase to 90% on 100% non-rebreather facemask. On exam, the respiratory rate is 24 breaths per minute, and coarse crackles can be heard throughout both lungs. All extremities are pale and cool, with a capillary refill of approximately 4 seconds. He is drowsy and disoriented. An arterial blood gas drawn while on the non-rebreather mask is pH 7.26; $Paco_2$ 54 mm Hg (7.1 kPa); Pao_2 62 mm Hg (8.1 kPa); base excess – 5; saturation 88%. The chest radiograph shows bilateral patchy infiltrates.

- What is the most likely diagnosis in this patient? What is the significance of his history of splenectomy?

- What should be the next intervention in the management of this patient?

- Is this patient a good candidate for NPPV? Why?

Compromised or inadequate oxygenation is the hallmark of acute respiratory distress syndrome (ARDS), thus the alternative name, acute hypoxemic respiratory failure. Infection and/or inflammation in the lungs triggers the release of chemical mediators that disturb normal lung function, cause capillary leak, and increase intrapulmonary shunting, thereby worsening ventilation-perfusion mismatch. Poor lung compliance and increased airway resistance require the use of high pressures during mechanical ventilation in order to restore adequate gas exchange, and the challenge lies in how best to support respiration while causing the least amount of trauma to the lungs. The landmark ARDS Network study, published in 2000, showed that the use of low VT (6 mL/kg) and high PEEP (~15 cm H_2O) compared to standard VT (12 mL/kg) resulted in decreased mortality and more ventilator-free days for adults with acute lung injury (ALI) and ARDS. A similar strategy has been widely adopted in PICUs throughout the world. Strategies borrowed from the neonatal experience with hyaline membrane disease, such as high-frequency oscillatory ventilation (HFOV), surfactant instillation, and inhaled nitric oxide, have also been employed in pediatric patients with ARDS, but to date, none has been shown to improve outcomes in large prospective randomized clinical trials.

Although the strategy for mechanical ventilation in patients with ARDS focuses on optimizing oxygenation, care must be taken to avoid the breath stacking and inadvertent PEEP that may result from the use of prolonged inspiratory time and inverse I:E ratios.

B. Obstructive Airway Disease

Case Study

A 19-year-old, 60-kilogram female with a history of mild intermittent asthma presents to the emergency department complaining of chest pain and shortness of breath that has worsened over the past 2 days. She is breathing at 36 breaths per minute, and oxygen saturations are 92% on room air. On exam, there are mild suprasternal retractions, and on auscultation, only minimal air entry is appreciated. Continuous inhaled bronchodilators and methylprednisolone are given without improvement, and she is rapidly transferred to the pediatric intensive care unit, where a terbutaline infusion is started, but her heart rate increases to 180 beats per minute with S-T wave elevations. Soon after arrival, the patient becomes drowsy and disoriented. As she is being prepared for intubation, an arterial blood gas shows the following values: pH 7.14; $Paco_2$ 80 mm Hg (10.7 kPa); Pao_2 76 mm Hg (10.1 kPa); base excess –8; saturation 88%. She is emergently intubated, and positive pressure ventilation is initiated in SIMV–volume-control mode with the following settings: rate 12 breaths per minute; VT 450 mL; Fio_2 1.0; PEEP 5 cm H_2O; inspiratory time 1 second; I:E ratio 1:4.

- What are the potential risks and benefits of endotracheal intubation and mechanical ventilation is this patient with severe status asthmaticus?
- What are some important considerations when setting the ventilator parameters in this patient?
- What is the indication for PEEP in a patient with obstructive lung disease whose lungs are already hyperinflated?

> !
>
> *The approach to ventilating the patient in status asthmaticus utilizes moderate VT, low respiratory rates, and prolonged expiratory times to allow the lungs to deflate between breaths*
>
> !

Intubation and mechanical ventilation of the patient with status asthmaticus should be an intervention of last resort, utilized only after all other measures have been exhausted. Laryngoscopy can trigger profound bronchospasm and should be performed by the most capable and experienced healthcare provider available. The lungs of patients with respiratory failure due to asthma are generally hyperinflated, and the risk of pneumothorax and pneumomediastinum is high.

The use of PEEP in these patients is controversial and stylistic. Large randomized controlled studies comparing the use of physiologic PEEP to no PEEP in the management of children receiving mechanical ventilation for severe asthma have not been done. When the patient with asthma is intubated for hypercarbic respiratory failure, it is likely due to air trapping rather than hypoventilation, and setting a high respiratory rate on the ventilator to blow off CO_2 will not result in the desired outcome. Bronchospasm and small airway obstruction should be treated aggressively with parenteral or inhaled bronchodilators and corticosteroids in order to relieve the obstruction and reverse the acute process. Patients intubated for status asthmaticus should be extubated as soon as their bronchospasm is under control and they meet clinical criteria for extubation.

Recent published cases describe pediatric patients who have developed cerebral edema in the setting of profound respiratory acidosis (with Pa_{CO_2} >100 mm Hg [13.3 kPa]) associated with status asthmaticus. Patients requiring intubation for hypercarbic respiratory failure should be monitored closely for signs of increased ICP.

C. Asymmetric Lung Disease

Asymmetric lung disease or injury that occurs after aspiration, contusion, localized pneumonia, or hemorrhage may cause abnormal distribution of ventilation and gas exchange during mechanical ventilation. Because the conditioned gas from the ventilator follows the path of least resistance along the bronchi, the VT is distributed primarily to the less-affected (more compliant) lung and may overexpand it. Overdistension of the less-affected lung and poor expansion of the diseased or injured lung worsen ventilation-perfusion relationships in both lungs, and hypoxemia and hypercapnia may occur, persist, or worsen. Standard settings and principles of ventilatory support should be initiated. However, if this attempt is unsuccessful, expert consultation should be obtained regarding further patient management. Positioning the patient so that the healthier, better-ventilated lung is in the gravitationally dependent position (sick side up) is a simple strategy for improving ventilation-perfusion matching and should result in improved oxygenation. Other techniques, such as differential lung ventilation, may be required.

D. Heart Disease

Case Study

A 3-month-old male with Down syndrome and a complete atrioventricular canal defect presents to his cardiologist 3 weeks after starting digoxin and furosemide. His mother reports he still requires 45 minutes to take 30 milliliters of formula and then is too exhausted to take any more. He has gained only 150 grams since birth and has fallen off his growth curve. On exam he is breathing at 72 breaths per minute with deep suprasternal retractions. His liver edge is firm and palpable 4 centimeters below the right costal margin. Extremities are pale and cool, and pulses are diminished.

- What is the reason for this patient's respiratory distress?
- What can be done to improve this child's condition?
- How would instating positive pressure ventilation impact this child's circulatory status?

The primary goal of ventilatory support in patients with myocardial ischemia or heart failure is to decrease work of breathing and ensure adequate oxygen delivery to the myocardium. Decreasing work of breathing reduces consumption of oxygen by respiratory muscles and increases the amount of oxygen available to the heart and end organs. Patients with cardiogenic pulmonary edema may also benefit from the increased thoracic pressure with positive pressure ventilation, which decreases biventricular filling (lowering pulmonary capillary pressure) and unloads the left ventricle (increasing stroke volume).

High $P\overline{aw}$ during mechanical ventilation may adversely affect cardiac performance by increasing right ventricular afterload and reducing venous return. Therefore, the parameters that affect $P\overline{aw}$ should be monitored and adjusted to maintain adequate cardiac function.

E. Neuromuscular Disease

Case Study

A 9-year-old boy is admitted to the pediatric intensive care unit for observation after falling down a flight of stairs. His parents report that his knees "just gave out from under him." His review of systems is significant only for a bout of "walking pneumonia" 2 weeks ago from which he recovered uneventfully. On exam, you note tenderness of both lower extremities, absent patellar reflexes, and decreased muscle tone. On the night of admission he develops difficulty swallowing, followed by respiratory distress requiring emergent intubation and positive pressure ventilation.

- What unique considerations that must be addressed when ventilating the child with neuromuscular disease?
- Would this patient be a good candidate for NPPV? Why?

Patients with peripheral neuromuscular disease typically have an intact respiratory drive and normal lungs. These patients may require a higher V_T to avoid the sensation of dyspnea. Adjustments may need to be made in other ventilatory parameters to ensure a normal arterial pH. Whenever possible, supported spontaneous breathing should be encouraged to prevent further deterioration in respiratory muscle function.

IX. MONITORING MECHANICAL VENTILATORY SUPPORT

Patients who receive mechanical ventilatory support require continuous monitoring to assess the effects of treatment (**Table 6-7**). Arterial blood gas measurements provide valuable information about the adequacy of oxygenation, ventilation, and acid-base balance. This information is mandatory during initiation of ventilatory support, periods of patient instability, and weaning from mechanical ventilation.

Table 6-7. Recommendations for Monitoring Mechanical Ventilatory Support

1. Obtain a chest radiograph after intubation and intermittently as needed to evaluate placement of endotracheal tube and deterioration in status.
2. Obtain arterial blood gas measurements after initiation of mechanical ventilation and intermittently based upon patient status.
3. Intermittently measure vital signs and frequently observe patient directly (including evaluation of patient-ventilator interaction).
4. Measure inspiratory plateau pressure as clinically appropriate.
5. Use continuous pulse oximetry to measure oxygenation.
6. Use ventilator alarms to monitor key physiologic and ventilator parameters.

Ventilators are equipped with sophisticated alarms and monitors to assist with patient management and the detection of adverse events. When initiating ventilatory support, the respiratory care practitioner usually establishes alarm parameters for low and high minute ventilation, high inspiratory pressures, and low exhaled volumes and pressures. In addition, many ventilators allow for the measurement of auto-PEEP.

The low-pressure alarm is intended to alert the clinician to a leak in the circuit or ventilator disconnection. A high-pressure alarm alerts the clinician that the set maximum peak inspiratory pressure has been exceeded. This alarm is usually set 5 to 10 cm H_2O above the patient's baseline peak inspiratory pressure. A high-pressure alarm for a patient receiving volume ventilation may indicate the presence of a mucus plug, a sudden change in airway or lung compliance due to an accumulation of secretions, or a change in ETT position. The patient may not receive the entire set V_T, since inspiration ends when the pressure limit is exceeded. For this reason, the frequent sounding of ventilator alarms should not be attributed to machine malfunction and should never be ignored or disabled.

X. HYPOTENSION WITH INITIATION OF MECHANICAL VENTILATION

A. Tension Pneumothorax

When hypotension occurs immediately after initiation of mechanical ventilation, one must entertain the possibility of a tension pneumothorax. Diagnosis of tension pneumothorax is based on a physical examination that finds decreased or absent breath sounds and tympany to percussion on the side of the pneumothorax. Changes in vital signs may include decreased oxygen saturations, tachycardia, and if the patient is breathing spontaneously, an increased respiratory rate. Tracheal deviation away from the side of the pneumothorax may be observed, although such a finding is uncommon after placement of an ETT. Treatment involves emergent decompression by insertion of a large-bore catheter or needle into the second or third intercostal space in the midclavicular line (see **Appendix 11**). Treatment should not be delayed to await radiographic confirmation. Decompression is both diagnostic and therapeutic and will restore blood pressure and vital signs to normal. The insertion of the catheter or needle must be followed by placement of a thoracostomy tube to prevent recurrence of the pneumothorax.

B. Conversion From Negative to Positive Intrathoracic Pressure

Normal intrathoracic pressure is slightly negative in relation to the atmosphere. When positive pressure ventilation is initiated, intrathoracic pressure becomes positive. As intrathoracic pressure rises, right atrial pressure rises, and the intravascular pressure gradient for return of blood from the large extrathoracic veins into the right heart decreases. As a result, systemic venous return to the heart is reduced. Left ventricular preload, stroke volume, cardiac output, and blood pressure may then decrease in sequence. The deleterious effects of increased intrathoracic pressure on cardiac output and blood pressure are exacerbated by underlying intravascular volume depletion. Treatment of this common complication involves volume resuscitation using rapidly infused fluid boluses, in aliquots of 10 or 20 mL/kg, to raise extrathoracic venous pressure and increase venous return to the right heart until the blood pressure increases. Oxygen saturation should be monitored to avoid overly aggressive fluid resuscitation. Use of ventilation techniques that incorporate high $P\overline{aw}$ may exacerbate the deleterious hemodynamic consequences of positive pressure ventilation.

C. Auto-PEEP

Auto-PEEP occurs when the lungs do not empty completely prior to the initiation of a new breath. Due to either obstruction to outflow of gas or a need for an excessively long inspiratory time, the combination of ventilator settings and patient physiology results in an inadequate expiratory time (see **Figure 6-3**). Excessive auto-PEEP may increase intrathoracic pressure and cause hypotension because of decreased venous return to the heart. Although auto-PEEP may occur in any patient, those with obstructive airway disease are particularly predisposed to this condition. Assessment and treatment of auto-PEEP is performed as previously described.

D. Acute Myocardial Ischemia/Infarction

Stress from acute respiratory failure, intubation, and the transition to positive pressure ventilation and β-adrenergic medications (ie, epinephrine, dobutamine) and some anesthetic agents (ketamine) may increase myocardial oxygen demand in patients with inadequate cardiac reserve. In older children and adults, this may lead to acute myocardial ischemia and subsequent hypotension.

XI. WEANING FROM MECHANICAL VENTILATION

No discussion of mechanical ventilation would be complete without a short review of current approaches to weaning the patient from the ventilator. This process should be considered as soon as pulmonary function begins to improve. Decisions concerning weaning from mechanical ventilation are separate and apart from decisions concerning extubation.

During weaning from mechanical ventilation, a patient gradually takes on more of the function of gas exchange while the ventilator contributes less to the patient's minute ventilation. As already mentioned, the circumstances that required the patient to be supported with mechanical ventilation need to be resolving. In addition, the patient must actively participate in the process, and objective and subjective criteria must be set to monitor the success or failure of the process.

Factors that influence weaning from mechanical ventilation include the patient's level of alertness, need for sedative medication, and respiratory drive, and the time elapsed since the patient's most recent episode of respiratory or hemodynamic decompensation.

Several approaches to weaning from mechanical ventilation have been proposed for adults and children. They share the demonstration of the patient's readiness for further weaning and ultimately for extubation, and almost universally include a spontaneous breathing trial. The conditions under which the trial takes place may vary, but an important component is the use of pressure support to prevent the patient's work of breathing from being hampered by the resistance of the ventilatory circuit. In small children with an ETT of 3.5 millimeters or less, unsupported spontaneous breathing may be akin to breathing through a straw. If respiratory muscles are deconditioned, the child's effort may be insufficient to overcome the resistance of the tube. Fatigue and respiratory distress may ensue unless pressure support is added.

> !
>
> *Goal-oriented protocols tend to be the most successful because they repeatedly challenge the patient to assume more of the function of breathing while monitoring for signs of failure to tolerate weaning.*
>
> !

The rate at which a patient is weaned from mechanical ventilation is based on a number of factors, including the physical condition of the patient and the duration of mechanical ventilation. A patient with normal lungs who is placed on mechanical ventilation for general anesthesia during an elective surgical procedure can be weaned and extubated rapidly, something that anesthesiologists often do in the operating room. This is in contradistinction to the patient who is intubated for several days or weeks for severe systemic illness, who requires a more gradual, closely monitored weaning regimen. Conditions should be optimized prior to initiating ventilator weaning; this includes adjusting sedatives and discontinuing neuromuscular blocking medications, optimizing nutrition and ensuring a positive nitrogen balance, and optimizing fluid and acid-base status. Patients with severe metabolic alkalosis (often the result of aggressive diuretic therapy) should have their acid-base status normalized to ensure optimal respiratory drive.

Once weaning has begun, a change in vital signs, such as increase in heart rate or respiratory rate, and an increase or decrease in blood pressure may indicate a patient's inability to tolerate the process. Clinical signs of fatigue, including paradoxical breathing or use of accessory muscles of respiration, diaphoresis, or agitation, suggest that the patient is not ready to be weaned further. Patients who become air hungry are easily recognized by their inability to attend to anything other than their next breath. The patient who becomes more tachypneic, develops retractions, and requires more oxygen to maintain the same saturations is failing to wean and should be placed back on a higher level of support until a later time. Arterial blood gases are a good objective indicator of how well a patient is tolerating weaning from mechanical ventilation. A need for more than 50% F_{IO_2} in order to achieve Pa_{O_2} greater than 60 mm Hg (8.0 kPa) or a Pa_{CO_2} greater than 50 mm Hg (6.7 kPa) usually indicates that the patient is not a candidate for further weaning. A chest radiograph should be obtained during the final stages of weaning to ensure there are no significant contraindications to extubation, such as atelectasis or pneumothorax.

XII. NEWER MODALITIES IN MECHANICAL VENTILATION

The increased overall survival rate of patients with respiratory failure, which has resulted from a better understanding of biomolecular and pathophysiologic mechanisms, has shifted the focus of attention to finding new approaches that will prevent or attenuate ventilator-induced lung injury (VILI). Although still not fully understood, the mechanisms for VILI are thought to involve 4 processes: barotrauma (from high pressure), volutrauma (as a result of overdistending alveoli), atelectrauma (from forcing open alveoli that have completely collapsed), and biotrauma (from inflammatory mediators released in response to the inciting process). The relative contribution of each of these processes to ALI remains to be fully determined, but there is a growing consensus that the shear forces generated as collapsed alveoli are forced open again result in damage to the alveolar-capillary interface, adversely affecting alveolar integrity and function. Supported by the results from the ARDS Network study (see the first suggested reading) and by multiple corroborative studies that followed, recent guidelines have promoted an open lung approach as a protective strategy to prevent VILI in patients with severe lung disease. Two modes of ventilation that offer promise in this area are airway pressure release ventilation (APRV) and high-frequency oscillatory ventilation (HFOV). Both are variations on a theme that might be described as new-and-improved CPAP.

A. Airway Pressure Release Ventilation

First studied in 1987 in animals, APRV underwent a trial in adults in 1988. In this time-triggered, pressure-limited, time-cycled mode of ventilatory support, a high level of CPAP is interspersed with short releases in the pressure. Airway pressure release ventilation is most helpful in patients with hypoxemic respiratory failure because the long periods of CPAP allow for recruitment of alveoli that require more time to reopen, thus improving ventilation-perfusion matching and increasing oxygenation. Unlike in other modes of positive pressure ventilation, patients are able to breathe spontaneously during all phases of ventilation and thus do not become dyspneic during the prolonged inspiratory positive-pressure cycle (see **Figure 6-4**).

Figure 6-4. Mechanical and Spontaneous Breaths During Airway Pressure Release Ventilation

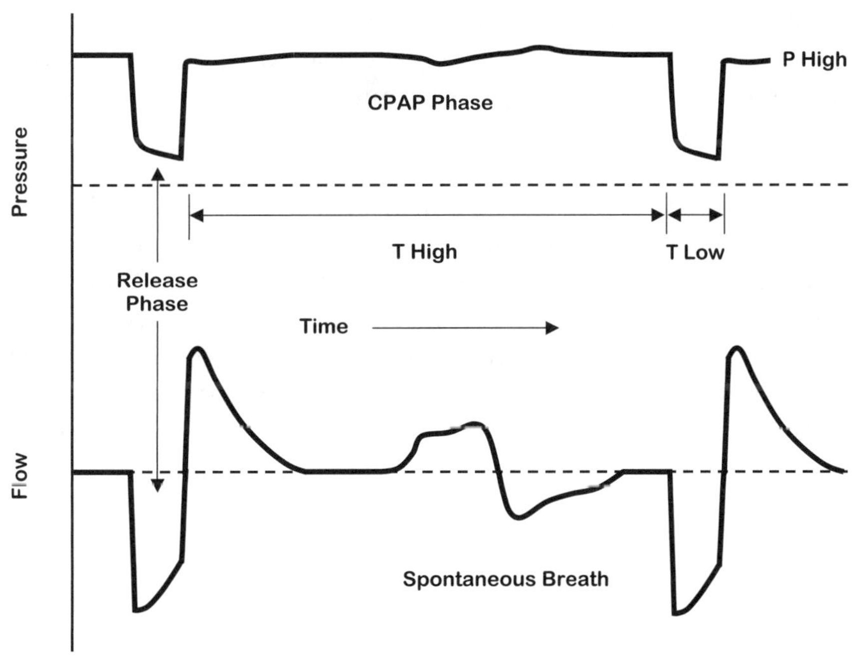

The parameters set in APRV include FIO_2; T-high—the time interval spent at high pressure, usually somewhere between 3 and 6 seconds; T-low—the time spent at low pressure, usually 0.3 to 0.8 seconds; P-high—the high pressure during T-high, approximately 75% of peak inspiratory pressure on conventional ventilation, approximating the plateau pressure; and P-low, often set at zero. Oxygenation is dictated by the T-high and P-high, and ventilation occurs during pressure release (P-low) and during spontaneous breaths. Increasing the differential between P-high and P-low has the effect of increasing the VT, and alveolar collapse is prevented by keeping the T-low very brief. This also results in a small amount of retained gas, which creates intrinsic PEEP.

Potential advantages of APRV are (1) it appears to be lung protective by maintaining higher mean airway pressures without introducing toxic peak inspiratory pressures, (2) it enhances cardiac performance by limiting high positive intrathoracic pressures that impair venous return to the right side of the heart, and (3) it promotes better patient-ventilator synchrony by allowing the patient to breathe spontaneously throughout the respiratory cycle, thus decreasing the need for high levels of sedation and continuous neuromuscular blockade. The use of lower doses of narcotics and sedatives has been shown to reduce morbidity and complications associated with mechanical ventilation in adults by decreasing the number of ventilator days, thereby shortening ICU length of stay. The data from several adult studies suggests that APRV may be helpful to patients with moderately severe respiratory insufficiency. Evidence to support the use of APRV in pediatric patients is limited.

B. High-Frequency Oscillatory Ventilation

High-frequency oscillatory ventilation provides many of the same advantages as APRV in that it enhances alveolar recruitment with an open lung strategy that is less traumatic to the lungs. This piston-driven system delivers VT of 1 to 2 mL/kg at breath rates of 180 to 900 per minute, thus maintaining high mean airway pressures without incurring any additional trauma. The exact mechanism of gas exchange is not completely understood, but extensive experience with HFOV in neonates and pediatric patients with ARDS provides support for the use of this mode of ventilation because high airway pressures are attenuated along the respiratory tree and are much lower at the small distal airways. Oscillatory ventilation is unique in that oxygenation and ventilation are uncoupled and can be approached and manipulated independently.

The parameters set on the oscillator are the FIO_2, mean airway pressure, amplitude, and frequency. (See **Table 6-8** for specific recommended settings.) Respiratory status is monitored with blood gases and chest radiographs (although the lungs may appear hazy while patients are on HFOV). Oxygenation can be controlled by adjusting the FIO_2 and mean airway pressure. The adequacy of amplitude is best judged by the degree of patient movement or wiggle visible from the torso down to the groin area or below. Changes in ventilation are made by adjusting the amplitude (increases augment ventilation) and frequency (increasing the frequency reduces ventilation because VT and frequency are inversely related).

Table 6-8. Recommended Parameters for High-Frequency Ventilation

FIO_2	Start at 100% and wean to less than 50%, if possible, to avoid oxygen toxicity
Mean airway pressure	Start at 5-8 cm H_2O greater than on conventional ventilator
Amplitude	Usually set at greater than 30 cm H_2O; titrate to patient's wiggle
Frequency	Usually set at 10-15 Hz for neonates and 5-10 Hz for infants and older children

Patients receiving HFOV, unlike those ventilated with APRV, require high levels of sedation and often need neuromuscular blockade in order to tolerate treatment. In addition, intravascular volume loading (fluid boluses) may be necessary to augment systemic venous return that may become inadequate in the setting of high intrathoracic pressures. Suctioning of the endotracheal tube is often kept to a minimum to avoid the derecruitment associated with breaking the circuit. However, accumulation of thick secretions or mucous plugs may obstruct the ETT, causing respiratory decompensation, pneumothorax, or ventilator malfunction. In addition, monitoring of the patient's clinical status is a significant challenge because breath sounds are masked by noise from the oscillator and acute changes in inspiratory pressures or volumes may go unnoticed until a blood gas is sent.

The pediatric experience with HFOV is better detailed and more convincing than the literature regarding adults. Adult studies have yielded mixed results, with a higher incidence of complications, probably due to the extremely high airway pressures that are utilized.

Key Points

Mechanical Ventilation

- In patients with acute respiratory failure, NPPV is more likely to be helpful as a transitional step following extubation than it is as a preventive measure to avoid progression to intubation and mechanical ventilation.

- Mechanical ventilation is indicated when less-invasive interventions for hypoxic or hypercapnic respiratory failure are unsuccessful.

- The primary goals of mechanical ventilation are to support ventilation and oxygenation and to reduce work of breathing while ensuring patient comfort.

- Various types of breaths and modes of ventilation are available to facilitate synchrony between the patient and the ventilator.

- The following guidelines may be used when initiating volume control ventilation: FIO_2 of 1.0; an age-appropriate rate, usually between 12 and 24 breaths per minute; a V_T of 8 to 10 mL/kg that results in adequate chest rise; and a PEEP between 2 and 5 cm H_2O. The inspiratory time, usually 0.5 to 1 second, is chosen based on patient age and disease process.

- The complex interactions between inspiratory pressures, I:E ratio, FIO_2, and PEEP must be appreciated in order to predict the potential beneficial and harmful effects in each patient.

- The primary determinants of oxygenation are FIO_2 and $P\overline{aw}$, whereas minute alveolar ventilation (respiratory rate and V_T) primarily affects CO_2 exchange.

- The importance of closely monitoring the patient during mechanical ventilation cannot be overstressed. This includes appropriate setting of and attention to ventilator alarm functions, continuous pulse oximetry, frequent bedside assessment of the patient, and obtaining arterial blood gases and chest radiographs as needed.

- Weaning from mechanical ventilation is an active process that should be started as soon as the indications for mechanical ventilation have begun to resolve. Objective criteria for assessing the patient's readiness for extubation should be considered frequently in order to liberate the patient from mechanical ventilation in a timely fashion. Close monitoring during the weaning process is required to avoid any additional stress and to ensure patient comfort.

- Airway pressure release ventilation (APRV) and high-frequency oscillatory ventilation (HFOV) are two more recent additions to the armamentarium available for the ventilator management of respiratory failure in children. Both utilize an open lung strategy to help recruit atelectatic lung while providing protection against ventilator-associated parenchymal injury. Whereas APRV encourages spontaneous breathing by the patient, thereby decreasing the need for heavy sedation, HFOV is poorly tolerated in the less heavily sedated, spontaneously breathing child.

Suggested Readings

1. Acute Respiratory Distress System Network. Ventilation with lower tidal volumes as compared with traditional tidal volumes for acute lung injury and the acute respiratory distress syndrome. *N Engl J Med.* 2000;342(18):1301-1308.

2. Arnold JH, Anas NG, Luckett P, et al. High-frequency oscillatory ventilation in pediatric respiratory failure: a multicenter experience. *Crit Care Med.* 2000;28(12):3913-3919.

3. Dekel B, Segal E, Perel A. Pressure support ventilation. *Arch Intern Med.*1996;156(4): 369-373.

4. Dick CR, Sassoon CSH. Patient-ventilator interactions. *Clin Chest Med.* 1996;17(3):423-428.

5. Fortenberry JD, Del Toro J, Jefferson LS, et al. Management of pediatric acute hypoxemic respiratory insufficiency with bilevel positive pressure (BiPAP) nasal mask ventilation. *Chest.* 1995;108(4):1059-1064.

6. Habashi NM. Other approaches to open-lung ventilation: airway pressure release ventilation. *Crit Care Med.* 2005;33(3)(suppl):S228-S240.

7. Jubran A, Tobin MJ. Monitoring during mechanical ventilation. *Clin Chest Med.* 1996;17(3):453-473.

8. Kaplan LJ, Bailey H, Formosa V. Airway pressure release ventilation increases cardiac performance in patients with acute lung injury/acute respiratory distress syndrome. *Crit Care.* 2001;5(4):221-226.

9. Keith RL, Pierson DJ. Complications of mechanical ventilation: a bedside approach. *Clin Chest Med.* 1996;17(3):439-451.

10. Padman R, Lawless ST, Kettrick R. Noninvasive ventilation via bilevel positive airway pressure support in pediatric practice. *Crit Care Med.* 1998;26(1):169-173.

11. Schultz TR, Costarino AT, Durning SM, et al. Airway pressure release ventilation in pediatrics. *Pediatr Crit Care Med.* 2001;2(3):243-246.

12. Venkataraman ST. Mechanical ventilation and respiratory care. In: Fuhrman BP, Zimmerman J, eds. *Pediatric Critical Care.* 3rd ed. Philadelphia, PA: Mosby, 2006;683-718.

Chapter 7:

DIAGNOSIS AND MANAGEMENT OF SHOCK

Objectives

- Define shock.
- Identify the 4 major categories of shock and their typical presentation.
- Determine the initial steps in the evaluation and management of a child in shock.
- Discuss the goals of fluid resuscitation for pediatric patients in shock.
- Describe the physiologic effects of vasopressors and inotropic agents.

Case Study

A previously healthy adolescent complains of severe malaise and shortness of breath. He describes the onset of an influenza-like illness and left knee swelling 2 days prior to his arrival in the emergency department. Upon examination, he is alert but clearly ill and severely tachycardiac, with a heart rate of 160 beats/min. He has brisk capillary refill, bounding pulses, and a blood pressure of 86/30 mm Hg. He receives 500 mL of normal saline over 1 hour and is then transferred to the PICU. On arrival, he is noted to be obtunded, with extremely poor perfusion and undetectable blood pressure. He is resuscitated with great difficulty and survives, albeit with renal insufficiency.

- What are the management priorities in patients presenting with shock?

- What are common pitfalls in the management of pediatric shock?

- Why is “cold shock” difficult to reverse?

I. INTRODUCTION

Shock, which may be simply described as inadequate provision of oxygen and other essential substrates to vital organs and peripheral tissues, is a common problem in acute care settings, including emergency departments, inpatient units, and intensive care areas.

Oxygen delivery (Do_2), which is by definition abnormal in shock states, is directly related to the arterial oxygen content (Cao_2) and cardiac output (CO). In turn, Cao_2 is the amount of oxygen carried bound to hemoglobin plus the amount of oxygen dissolved in arterial blood.

$$Do_2 = Cao_2 \times CO$$

$$Cao_2 = (Hgb \times 1.34 \times Sao_2) + (0.003 \times Pao_2)$$

$$CO = \text{Heart Rate} \times \text{Stroke Volume}$$

Stroke volume is a function of preload, afterload, and myocardial contractility. Therefore, cardiac output (and Do_2) can be augmented by optimizing preload, afterload, and contractility, and, in some cases, by increases in heart rate. In addition, Do_2 can be increased by optimizing hemoglobin oxygen saturation and by raising the circulating hemoglobin concentration.

Shock-related mortality has decreased dramatically over the last few years largely due to prompt diagnosis and management in accordance with established guidelines such as those published in 2002 by the American College of Critical Care Medicine (ACCM) and the American Academy of Pediatrics (AAP). Those guidelines emphasize the importance of prompt diagnosis and rapid, serial interventions with the goal of reversing the signs of shock and restoring vital signs to threshold values.

Reversal of shock within the first 75 minutes of a patient's presentation to a community hospital was associated with a 9-fold increase in the odds for survival, while each passing hour of persistent shock resulted in a 2-fold increase in mortality (**Figure 7-1**).

Figure 7-1. Survival Rates of Pediatric Patients With Shock Reversal Versus Persistent Shock

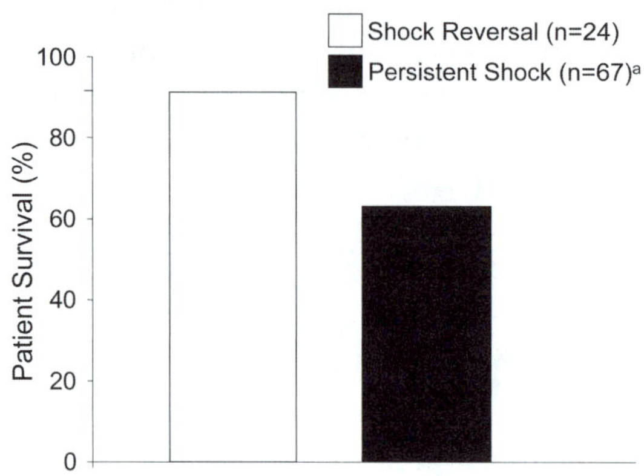

[a] $p < 0.05$.
Shock reversal from resuscitative efforts by community hospital physicians resulted in 96% survival versus 63% survival among patients who remained in a persistent state of shock.
Data from Han YY, Carcillo JA, Dragotta MA, et al. Early reversal of pediatric-neonatal septic shock by community physicians is associated with improved outcome. *Pediatrics.* 2003;112:793-799.

Developmental differences between pediatric and adult patients strongly influence diagnostic and therapeutic decisions. Although cardiac rate and contractility can increase in adult patients, ventricular function in infants is relatively fixed, so that any decrease in heart rate critically diminishes cardiac output. Infants and children also have higher baseline heart rates, which limits their hearts' ability to improve cardiac output by beating faster. Additionally, at any age, a child's systemic vascular resistance can markedly increase, which will maintain blood pressure (compensated shock) until the onset of decompensated shock. An elevated systemic vascular resistance may also compromise cardiac output in the presence of hypovolemia and decreased myocardial function.

> !
> *Tachycardia and tachypnea are early signs of shock in children.*
> !

Pediatric patients with early shock often have subtle presentations. Tachycardia and tachypnea may be the only abnormalities. Failure to detect and reverse these phenomena may allow a compensated, easily manageable shock state to progress to irreversible organ dysfunction.

II. TYPES OF SHOCK

A. Hypovolemic Shock

Case Study

A previously healthy 2-year-old child is brought to the emergency department. His family reports that he has had copious diarrhea and vomiting with an inability to tolerate any oral fluids. The child's heart rate is 172, and his blood pressure is 92/70 mm Hg. He is cool and mottled, and has thready pulses. His capillary refill is severely delayed, and he barely reacts when IV access is attempted. After fluid resuscitation and several hours of medical care, he is able to sit up and interact appropriately with caregivers.

> !
> *There are 4 main categories of shock: hypovolemic, distributive, cardiogenic, and obstructive.*
> !

– Which compensatory mechanisms are in place in this situation?

– How should this child's shock be addressed?

> !
> *The most common type of shock in children is hypovolemic shock.*
> !

Hypovolemic shock is without a doubt the most common type of shock seen in pediatric patients. Hypovolemic shock occurs when circulating intravascular blood volume decreases to a point at which adequate tissue perfusion can no longer be maintained. Hypovolemia causes a decrease in preload and adversely affects cardiac output. At first hypovolemia activates peripheral and central baroreceptors that promote catecholamine-mediated vasoconstriction and tachycardia. This initial response can maintain adequate circulation and blood pressure even after acute loss of as much as 15% of the circulating blood volume. However, acute losses in excess of 20% of the circulating blood volume result in a much more clinically obvious hypovolemic state that mandates prompt and aggressive treatment.

The typical case involves large losses of gastrointestinal fluid due to diarrhea, especially in patients unable to replenish ongoing losses orally due to concurrent emesis. Patients with other disease processes, such as traumatic injuries with severe and possibly ongoing blood losses are also encountered in the emergency setting. These patients typically present with tachycardia, a narrowed pulse pressure, delayed capillary refill, orthostatic changes, and in late stages, frank hypotension. They commonly manifest altered mentation and decreased urine output in the absence of an osmotic load.

B. Cardiogenic Shock

Case Study

An 8-month-old boy is being treated for presumed bronchiolitis. The nurses caring for him in the emergency department report that he appears to be getting sicker rather than better. His wheezing has not responded to several hours of continuous albuterol, and he is poorly responsive to his environment. A physician is called to the bedside when a wide-complex tachycardia is seen on the monitor. The child has barely perceptible pulses, markedly delayed capillary refill, and a gallop. Rales and hepatomegaly are noted. Further evaluation demonstrates cardiomegaly, ventricular tachycardia, and evidence of end-organ ischemia. The child arrests shortly after admission to the pediatric intensive care unit (PICU).

- What physical exam findings suggest the correct diagnosis?

- What are the general management principles for pediatric shock?

Cardiogenic shock is marked by a significant decrease in cardiac output. The inadequately low cardiac output can be caused by heart rate abnormalities, such as profound bradycardia in patients with complete heart block or tachycardia in patients with ventricular tachyarrhythmias or supraventricular tachycardias.

More frequently, however, cardiogenic shock is caused by a state of decreased myocardial contractility. Many etiologies can be implicated in the myocardial dysfunction of cardiogenic shock. These include primary or familial cardiomyopathies, infectious myocarditis, and systemic inflammatory processes such as sepsis, autoimmune diseases, impaired coronary perfusion, exposure to cardiopulmonary bypass, prolonged tachyarrhythmias, acidosis, hypoxic-ischemic events, and prolonged shock, to name a few.

A significant gradient in the blood pressure measured in the upper extremities compared to the lower extremities is typical of left-sided, ductus-dependent congenital cardiac lesions. In patients younger than 2 months who present with signs of cardiogenic shock, infusion of prostaglandin E1 to establish patency of the ductus arteriosus should be strongly considered until echocardiography definitively excludes a ductus-dependent lesion. Treatment centers on optimizing intravascular volume, improving myocardial contractility with inotropic agents, and reducing afterload with the use of vasodilators.

> **!** *Prostaglandin infusion should be considered for infants younger than 2 months who present in cardiogenic shock.* **!**

C. Distributive Shock

Case Study

A 13-year-old female ingests several medications, including tricyclic antidepressants after an argument with her parents. She is very sleepy, hypotensive (70/35 mm Hg), and flushed in appearance. Her capillary refill is quite brisk. She has mildly broadened QRS complexes and a prolonged QT interval. She improves rapidly after appropriate volume resuscitation , sodium bicarbonate , and vasoactive support.

- What are the important clues to this child's underlying physiology?
- How should this child be stabilized?
- What are common causes of distributive shock?

Distributive shock is a state of maldistribution of tissue blood flow due to decreased systemic vascular resistance. This type of shock may be observed in patients with early septic shock, anaphylaxis, toxic ingestions, spinal or epidural anesthesia, and spinal cord injuries. Patients with distributive shock typically have a flushed appearance, warm extremities with bounding pulses, and tachycardia with a wide pulse pressure. Capillary refill may be instantaneous. Distributive shock due to spinal cord injury may occur without significant compensatory rises in heart rate. Treatment should focus on reversal of the underlying etiology (whenever possible), rapid expansion of intravascular volume, and infusion of vasopressor medications.

D. Obstructive Shock

Case Study

An 8-month-old infant with pneumococcal sepsis is deteriorating rapidly. She has extremely poor perfusion, a narrow pulse pressure, and is hypotensive. She continues to worsen during transport to a tertiary PICU despite vigorous fluid and vasoactive support. A physician notes somewhat distant heart tones, and when her most recent chest radiograph is compared to the previous day's film, she is noted to have marked cardiomegaly. A fibrinous pericardial effusion is urgently decompressed under echocardiographic guidance and the patient improves rapidly .

- What are the clinical findings that suggest pericardial effusion?

- What general management principles must be observed?

Obstructive shock is relatively uncommon in pediatrics, thus requiring a high index of suspicion. This form of shock is caused by extrinsic forces acting on intrathoracic structures such as the great vessels or ventricles. Limitation of cardiac output occurs despite normal intravascular volume and myocardial contractility. Common causes include tension pneumothorax and hemopneumothorax. Additionally, tamponade physiology may occur when pericardial effusions form rapidly.

Clinical clues to the diagnosis include tachycardia, cool extremities with delayed capillary refill, a narrow pulse pressure, distended neck veins, distant heart tones, and asymmetric breath sounds, depending on the underlying process. Treatment is based on the prompt reversal of the underlying cause, such as evacuation of a tension pneumothorax or hemothorax, or drainage of a pericardial effusion. Isotonic crystalloid or albumin boluses, and the avoidance of any drug capable of causing hypotension are important therapeutic considerations while the etiology of the obstructive shock is addressed.

III. EVALUATION OF SHOCK

The evaluation of any significant problem in a pediatric patient, regardless of age, must begin with assessment of the airway, breathing, and circulation, including a complete set of vital signs, and rapid assessment of mental status with the use of a modified Glasgow Coma Scale.

A. ABCs: Assessment of Airway, Breathing, and Circulation

The child's airway should be evaluated on presentation and monitored closely. In addition to airway patency, the respiratory rate, pattern, and work of breathing should be noted. All children with suspected shock should receive supplemental oxygen, regardless of their baseline oxygen saturations. Children displaying severe respiratory distress may require immediate assisted ventilation. Any patient presenting with a modified Glasgow Coma Scale score of 8 or less is at risk for respiratory arrest, severe hypoxemia, and severe hypercarbia. These patients should have their airway secured as soon as possible. Ventilation can be assisted with careful bag-mask ventilation until preparations have been made for endotracheal intubation.

> ! *Oxygen should be provided to all children with suspected shock, regardless of their oxygen saturations.* !

Severe bradycardia (heart rate <90 beats per minute) or severe tachycardia (heart rate >180 beats per minute in ill-appearing children younger than 1 year or >140 in older children and adolescents) are markers of the severe systemic compromise that may precede circulatory collapse. Severe tachycardia in an obviously ill child may be quickly followed by hypotension and cardiac arrest. Any abnormality in heart rate should be confirmed with a rhythm strip, at the very least, or an electrocardiogram (ECG) to ascertain whether or not the child is in sinus rhythm. Early detection of rhythm abnormalities is imperative for the implementation of appropriate treatment following specialty consultation.

Hypotension is a late finding in pediatric shock, given children's capacity to increase systemic vascular resistance during the initial phase of decreased cardiac output. Children may be normotensive or even hypertensive in the presence of established shock. Blood pressure may fall precipitously in these patients. Failure to diagnose shock in a timely manner—before the onset of hypotension—may allow progression to an uncompensated and possibly irreversible state.

> ! *Hypotension is a late finding in pediatric shock.* !

Fever is common but not universal in pediatric patients with serious infections. In fact, hypothermia may be noted in infants and in septic patients of any age. Monitoring core temperature is of extreme importance. Infants commonly react with apnea and bradycardia to a cold environment. A significant difference in the temperatures of the torso and the toes suggests impaired perfusion and is a marker that can be easily followed as a child's resuscitation progresses.

Continuous pulse oximetry is usually very well tolerated, even by irritable children, and is mandatory in the evaluation and monitoring of any sick patient. Not only does pulse oximetry provide crucial information regarding oxygenation, but a poor signal may also prompt more aggressive management of a hypoperfused state. A child's perfusion should be assessed in a central location and in an extremity that has not been exposed to a cold environment. Under normal conditions, capillary refill is complete within 2 to 3 seconds. Deviations from the norm give important clues regarding the etiology of the circulatory derangement and response to treatment interventions. The quality of central and distal pulses should be compared at frequent intervals as well.

B. Blood Glucose

In addition to a complete initial set of vital signs, a bedside assessment of blood glucose is essential in any acutely ill child presenting for care. Infants are particularly vulnerable to hypoglycemia given their high metabolic rates and limited glycogen reserves. Failure to promptly diagnose and treat hypoglycemia may result in severe, permanent neurologic disability.

C. History and Physical Examination

A patient's history and physical examination will reveal important clues to the etiology of shock. Serial assessments of a child's vital signs, mentation, and perfusion are essential. The lung fields should be auscultated to detect new rales. A gallop rhythm may indicate underlying heart disease or hypervolemia due to overzealous fluid resuscitation. Palpation of the liver edge well below the costal margin may also indicate hypervolemia or cardiac failure. Rapidly evolving purpuric or petechial rashes may suggest an infectious origin. A careful secondary survey may demonstrate previously missed injuries in children with unclear or unknown histories.

IV. MANAGEMENT OF SHOCK

All patients presenting with shock should be placed on high-flow oxygen while their initial evaluation is being performed. Vascular access, control of the airway, fluid resuscitation and provision of appropriate vasoactive infusions, and appropriate antibiotic therapy are priorities to be addressed within the first few minutes of presentation.

A. Vascular Access

> **!** *Vascular access should be established early in children presenting with signs of shock.*

Vascular access must be obtained as soon as possible. Intravenous cannulas may be difficult to place in acutely ill children with poor peripheral perfusion. Common sites for catheter placement include the dorsum of the hands, the saphenous vein just anterior to the medial malleolus, and the veins in the antecubital fossae. Initial volume resuscitation may be readily accomplished through an infant's scalp vein. Care should be taken to avoid cannulating the temporal artery when these veins are utilized. The external jugular vein may be accessible to cannulation; however, care should be taken in the presence of respiratory distress or increased intracranial pressure to avoid further compromise with positioning, and the site should be monitored closely for evidence of infiltration.

Professionals caring for sick children should have a low threshold for placing intraosseous needles for initial or supplemental vascular access. Alternative sites, such as the distal femur, should be considered when indicated. **See Appendix 8.**

Central venous catheters are extremely helpful during complex resuscitations and should be placed by physicians with expertise in this procedure when a delay in transfer to a tertiary center is anticipated. Proper control of the airway, correct positioning, adequate analgesia and local anesthesia, and strict sterile technique with full barrier precautions are required. Obtaining subclavian venous access is much more treacherous in children than in adults, and a pneumothorax or vascular injury may be rapidly fatal in patients with preexisting hypovolemia. That site, therefore, should generally be avoided in children with shock, particularly in those with suspected coagulopathy.

Cannulation of the femoral vein carries less risk, although life-threatening retroperitoneal hematoma or injury to the femoral artery may occur. The right internal jugular vein can be cannulated blindly using the posterior approach. Other approaches to the internal jugular vein, such as the central or anterior, are facilitated by ultrasonography. Although the left internal jugular vein may also be accessed with these techniques, its cannulation carries the added risk of injury to the thoracic duct.

B. Fluid Resuscitation

Only isotonic solutions should be used in the rapid intravascular volume expansion of children in shock. The fluid of choice for initial resuscitation, a solution of 0.9% saline should be readily available and administered in aliquots of 20 mL/kg as quickly as possible. A common but dangerous error is to infuse boluses over 1 hour. Serial reassessment is extremely important to help guide initial fluid resuscitation, which should be continued until adequate perfusion is achieved and the child's vital signs and general appearance have improved.

> !
>
> *Start early fluid resuscitation with 20 mL/kg 0.9% saline solution as quickly as possible (<15 minutes). Continuous monitoring and frequent reassessment are recommended.]*
>
> !

Hypoglycemia diagnosed on presentation should be managed with 5 mL/kg boluses of a 10% dextrose solution as required to achieve a serum glucose level greater than 100 mg/dL, rather than with large volumes of dextrose-containing crystalloids, which may be relatively hypotonic and also carry the risk of inducing osmotic diuresis.

Patients in whom smaller aliquots of resuscitation fluid (5-10 mL/kg) should be considered include neonates and children with known or suspected heart disease. Frequent reassessment is mandatory so that adequate resuscitation is not delayed. Children, particularly those with septic shock or significant ongoing losses, may require enormous volumes of resuscitation fluid, sometimes well in excess of 100 mL/kg and up to 200 mL/kg. In fact, improved outcomes have been observed when at least 60 mL/kg of rapid intravascular fluid expansion are given to children with septic shock within the first hour of treatment (**Figure 7-2**).

Figure 7-2. Effects of Early Fluid Resuscitation on Pediatric Patients With Septic Shock

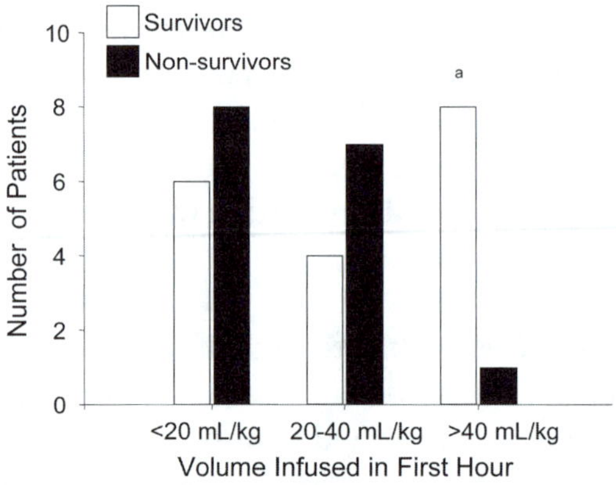

[a] Increased survival compared to all other groups.
Number of survivors and non-survivors among pediatric patients with septic shock stratified in groups according to volume of fluid resuscitation received within the first hour of presentation to the emergency department.
Data from Carcillo JA, Davis AL, Zaritsky A. Role of early fluid resuscitation in pediatric septic shock. *JAMA*. 1991;266:1242-1245.

Although vigorous fluid resuscitation does not correlate with adverse pulmonary or neurologic outcomes in children, there are some concerns when normal saline is used for resuscitation. One is that resuscitation fluid begins to redistribute to the extravascular space in as little as one hour. Other concerns include the frequent finding of hyperchloremic metabolic acidosis and the possible dilution of plasma proteins with development of ascites, pleural effusions, and anasarca. Lactated Ringer's solution, also known as Hartmann's solution, is used extensively in some countries and can be effective in the management of moderate to severe shock, particularly if albumin solutions are unavailable. It is less likely to produce hyperchloremic acidosis but must be used with caution in patients at high risk for hyperkalemia. Some experts advocate the use of 5% albumin, which remains in the intravascular space longer, as a strategy to possibly mitigate such problems. A reasonable approach is to use normal saline initially and to continue volume resuscitation using 5% albumin if more than 40 to 60 mL/kg are required to normalize perfusion.

Blood products may be required in special circumstances, such as the presence of injuries, and should be utilized as required to maintain a hemoglobin level of at least 10 g/dL in acutely ill patients. The risk of hypotension precludes the rapid infusion of fresh frozen plasma. Platelets and cryoprecipitate may be indicated in the presence of thrombocytopenia and hypofibrinogenemia, which underscores the importance of obtaining appropriate laboratory studies as soon as possible during the resuscitation.

Fluid resuscitation should be continued until clinical improvement is clear or there is clinical evidence of a hypervolemic state marked by the presence of new rales, a gallop rhythm, or hepatomegaly. Continued bolus administration of fluids at this point will cause excessive myocardial wall forces and depress function. Diuretic therapy with small doses of furosemide (0.3-0.5 mg/kg) may be considered in these children or in the presence of hypervolemia in an otherwise stabilizing child. This strategy may result in improved myocardial performance, enhanced urine output, and the possible mitigation of oliguric renal failure if acute tubular necrosis has developed. Higher doses of diuretics may be required in certain children, but it is prudent to administer a small dose first, particularly in the presence of hemodynamic instability.

Children who have required resuscitation and are felt to be close to a euvolemic state (neither wet nor dry) may be placed on maintenance fluids with additional boluses of normal saline or 5% albumin as required. Infants are at high risk of developing hypoglycemia and should, therefore, receive dextrose-containing fluids, such as 10% dextrose with appropriate sodium and potassium supplementation and hourly bedside glucose monitoring. A useful formula for calculating the infusion rate of maintenance fluids is to provide 4 mL/kg per hour for the first 10 kilograms of body weight, plus 2 mL/kg per hour for each additional kilogram up to 20 kilograms, plus 1 mL/kg per hour for each additional kilogram of body weight thereafter. Adult-sized children can be managed with maintenance infusions of 125 to 150 milliliters per hour.

> !
>
> *Infants at risk for hypoglycemia should receive dextrose-containing fluids after their initial fluid resuscitation is achieved.*
>
> !

Patients at risk for neurologic injury due to trauma or a hypoxic-ischemic insult are best managed with isotonic intravenous fluids. Although normal saline is commonly used, hypoglycemia is possible and may cause severe permanent injury. Hyperglycemia increases the risk of complications and must be managed meticulously.

C. Vasoactive and Inotropic Support

Although shock in adults, particularly septic shock, displays typical and relatively static hemodynamic patterns, shock in neonates and children varies significantly and requires frequent reassessment. Invasive hemodynamic monitoring with an arterial catheter and a central venous catheter should be used to provide continuous measurements and establish trends of cardiovascular performance during the initial phases of management. Vasoactive and inotropic infusions are extremely helpful in stabilizing the child in shock, but their use in patients who have not yet received adequate volume resuscitation has been associated with a poor outcome.

1. Dopamine

Dopamine, with its varied physiologic actions, is considered by most clinicians to be the first-line agent for the management of shock. Dopamine has dose-related effects. At high infusion rates, α_1-receptor-mediated effects predominate, with vasoconstriction and increases in systemic and pulmonary vascular resistance. At intermediate doses, β_1 and β_2 effects predominate, with inotropy/chronotropy and vasodilatation, respectively. At low infusion rates, dopamine1-receptor-mediated effect (renal vasodilatation) can be observed experimentally, although its significance in clinical practice is probably irrelevant.

Relatively small doses of dopamine, such as 5 µg/kg/min, may be all that is needed to provide inotropic support for a particular patient. However, when a child is hypotensive, this drug should be started at higher, α-receptor-activating doses of at least 10 µg/kg/min because an undesired β effect with vasodilation may predominate at lower doses. There is no benefit to increasing the dose of dopamine beyond 20 µg/kg/min. Additional considerations include that doses higher than 10 µg/kg/min may increase pulmonary vascular tone in young infants displaying a persistent fetal circulation pattern and that infants younger than 6 months may be relatively insensitive to the drug and may require directly acting catecholamines, such as epinephrine or norepinephrine (**see Table 7-1**).

Table 7-1. Hemodynamic Effects of Commonly Used Vasoactive and Inotropic Agents

Agent	α_1	β_1	β_2	D_1	V_1
Dopamine[a]	Vasoconstriction; ↑ SVR, PVR	Inotropy; chronotropy	Vasodilatation	Vasodilatation (renal)	
Dobutamine		Inotropy			
Epinephrine[b]	Vasoconstriction; ↑ SVR, PVR	Inotropy; chronotropy	Vasodilatation		
Norepinephrine	Vasoconstriction; ↑ SVR, PVR	Inotropy (minor)			
Vasopressin	Potentiates	Potentiates			Vasoconstriction
Non-receptor-mediated					
Milrinone	Inotropy, lusitropy, vasodilatation				

Abbreviations: D_1, dopamine receptor; PVR, pulmonary vascular resistance; SVR, systemic vascular resistance.

[a] Dose-related effects: at low dose, D_1–receptor effects might predominate; at intermediate doses, β_1 and β_1–receptor effects predominate; and at high doses, α_1-receptor effects predominate.

[b] Dose-related effects: at low doses β_1 and β_1–receptor effects predominate, and at high doses, α_1-receptor effects predominate on peripheral vasculature.

Adapted from Smith L, Hernan L. Shock states. In: Fuhrman BP, Zimmerman J, eds. *Pediatric Critical Care.* 3rd ed. Philadelphia, PA: Mosby Elsevier; 2006:394-410.

2. Dobutamine

Dobutamine has significant inotropic effects due to its preferential activation of the β receptor but usually trivial chronotropic and vasopressor activity. Although dobutamine may have a role in the management of infants with mild hypoperfusion, typically in doses of 5 mcg/kg/min, higher doses may be associated with unacceptable tachycardia. This agent is clearly not as helpful in older children, particularly in adolescents with septic shock, in whom a decrease in systemic vascular resistance and an increase in heart rate may compromise coronary perfusion. However, dobutamine is a useful agent when ventricular dysfunction plays a central role, such as in cardiogenic shock. This drug is commonly used following cardiac transplantation, surgery to repair congenital heart defects, myocardial revascularization, and in other conditions in which myocardial function is significantly depressed, but it has a very limited role in the contemporary management of pediatric septic shock.

3. Epinephrine

Epinephrine activates α and β receptors and is the principal stress hormone produced by the adrenal gland. Exogenously administered epinephrine has many important physiologic effects, including chronotropy, increased cardiac contractility, and increased systemic vascular resistance at higher doses, making it a very useful agent in the management of children with shock.

Epinephrine should be administered as a continuous infusion into a reliable peripheral vein or through a central venous catheter. Some experts suggest that nebulized racemic epinephrine can be used in the initial stabilization while vascular access is secured for volume resuscitation and vasoactive support. Epinephrine may increase myocardial oxygen consumption and cause a decrease in splanchnic perfusion. Because epinephrine also has the potential to decrease systemic vascular resistance under some circumstances, it may decrease coronary perfusion pressures, particularly in the presence of hypovolemia or severe tachycardia. These are important considerations in older children, who may be at greater risk for myocardial ischemia and dysrhythmias. A typical starting dose for epinephrine is 0.05 to 0.1 µg/kg/min, titrated to clinical effect (**see Table 7-2**).

Table 7-2. Suggested Infusion Doses for Commonly Used Vasoactive and Inotropic Agents

Agent	Inotropic	Pressor
Dopamine	2-15 µg/kg/min	>12 µg/kg/min
Dobutamine	2.5-20 µg/kg/min	
Epinephrine	0.05-0.5 µg/kg/min	0.1-1 µg/kg/min
Norepinephrine		0.05-1 µg/kg/min
Vasopressin		0.3 -2 milliunits/kg/min
Milrinone	0.25-0.75 µg/kg/min	

Adapted from Park MK. Use of digoxin in infants and children, with specific emphasis on dosage. *J Pediatr.* 1986;108:871.

4. Norepinephrine

Norepinephrine is extremely useful in the presence of warm shock unresponsive to high-dose dopamine. Some experts use it preferentially in patients presenting with septic shock, given its strong α-receptor selectivity, which results in increased vascular tone with minimal effect on the heart rate. This, in turn, translates into higher coronary and splanchnic perfusion pressures and, possibly, decreased end-organ dysfunction. The typical starting dose is 0.05 to 0.1 mcg/kg/min quickly titrated to the desired effect.

5. Milrinone

Milrinone is a bipyridine derivative of amrinone that causes inotropic and lusitropic effects and relaxation of vascular smooth muscle. Milrinone exerts its effects by selectively inhibiting phosphodiesterase 3. Unlike amrinone, milrinone does not appear to cause thrombocytopenia and, for this reason, is preferred over it in PICUs in North America.

Milrinone is commonly used in patients displaying signs of high systemic vascular resistance with low cardiac output and cold extremities. Although it is generally very useful in these patients, an important consideration is that milrinone has a long elimination half-life and duration of action. This drug also requires dose adjustment in patients with renal and hepatic failure. Significant and prolonged hypotension may be observed, particularly when a loading dose or doses in excess of 0.3 µg/kg/min are employed or in the presence of renal or hepatic dysfunction. Thus, milrinone is best used in an intensive care setting in the presence of continuous intravascular monitoring.

6. Nitroprusside and Nitroglycerin

Nitroprusside and nitroglycerin have vasodilator effects and much shorter half-lives than milrinone, making these agents more appropriate for short-term use prior to and during transfer to a tertiary center. They can be utilized at very low doses such as 0.05 mcg/kg/min to achieve desired decreases in systemic vascular resistance when administered in the presence of adequate volume loading and a readily available vasopressor agent, such as norepinephrine.

7. Vasopressin

Vasopressin is a potent vasopressor and a more recent addition to the standard formulary at the disposal of the pediatric intensivist for the treatment of shock with decreased systemic vascular resistance (SVR). Vasopressin exerts its hemodynamic effects via the V_{1a} receptor, promoting an increase in intracellular calcium in the peripheral vasculature, thus enhancing vasoconstriction and restoring systemic vascular tone. Vasopressin has been associated with improved blood pressure and urine output in patients with catecholamine-refractory vasodilatory shock and often allows weaning of catecholamines once treatment is initiated. Although a pediatric dose has not been established, some experts recommend starting with 0.5 milliunits/kg/min.

D. Endotracheal Intubation and Mechanical Ventilation

Mechanical ventilation, with careful preparation for intubation and meticulous attention to tidal volumes and pressures, may reduce or obviate the work of breathing, optimize oxygen transport, and improve hemodynamic performance by reducing left ventricular afterload. Subsequent planned and emergent procedures are significantly facilitated by a secure airway.

Due to the potential for deterioration during intubation in patients with shock, the most experienced person available should perform this procedure, preferably after volume resuscitation is well under way. A vasopressor infusion should be mixed and either infusing or available for immediate use. Preoxygenation with oxygen via a non-rebreathing face mask or application of a setup that ensures fresh oxygen flow, such as an anesthesia bag, is of extreme importance. A rapid-sequence intubation that includes cricoid pressure should be utilized in patients with recent oral intake or those at risk for delayed gastric emptying. A nasogastric tube in previously healthy children and careful venting of gastrostomy tubes in those with chronic disease will help prevent aspiration and excessive gaseous distention of the gastrointestinal tract caused by assisted ventilation.

Given infants' fixed myocardial contractility and their dependence on heart rate for adequate cardiac output, drug premedication should include atropine to prevent vagally mediated bradycardia. Atropine improves intubating conditions in patients of all ages by minimizing airway secretions and, possibly, decreasing airway tone. There are no contraindications to using atropine in appropriate doses, even in the presence of tachycardia. Therefore, it should be given to all children requiring intubation.

Drugs that may decrease systemic vascular resistance, such as large doses of midazolam or morphine, should be avoided in children with shock. Although many sources cite doses of midazolam of 0.1 mg/kg, that amount may have very significant effects in tenuous patients. Instead, this drug should be titrated carefully in small aliquots of 0.05 mg/kg or less, with the intention of using it as an adjuvant rather than the primary agent for intubation. Small doses of fentanyl (1-2 µg/kg) may be considered instead of other opioids, such as morphine, which has substantially more hemodynamic effects.

Ketamine, with its dissociative anesthetic properties and its minimal adverse effects on hemodynamics, is the drug of choice for intubating patients in shock. A dose of 1 to 2 mg/kg is usually effective and will ensure ability to ventilate the patient before administering neuromuscular blocking agents. Ketamine is usually avoided in patients known to have significant intracranial pathology and, by some practitioners, in patients suspected of having pulmonary hypertension, but is generally safe and effective in emergencies. Additionally, it can be given intramuscularly at a dose of 3 mg/kg with atropine in patients who do not yet have vascular access. The use of small doses of benzodiazepines may decrease the incidence of emergence phenomena such as hallucinations following ketamine administration. Atropine or glycopyrrolate should always be given with ketamine to mitigate the sialorrhea invariably associated with this drug.

Etomidate can cause a state of adrenal insufficiency and has been associated with increased risk of mortality in recent studies. This drug should not be used routinely unless there is a specific and compelling contraindication to the previously mentioned agents.

Rocuronium and vecuronium are neuromuscular blocking agents frequently utilized to secure the airway. Atracurium and cis-atracurium may have a relatively higher propensity to cause histamine release with consequent hypotension and bronchospasm and are best used in the PICU for specific indications.

The airway should be secured with an endotracheal tube of appropriate size. A useful indicator is the diameter of the child's fifth digit. Cuffed tubes are now preferred in children of all ages because worsening lung compliance may cause excessive air leak around the endotracheal tube, precluding adequate gas exchange.

Tidal volumes delivered during hand ventilation and during mechanical ventilation should be tailored to prevent pulmonary overdistention that could lead to decreased preload or intrathoracic air leaks. Most patients with shock but normal pulmonary mechanics can be ventilated with standard tidal volumes of approximately 8 mL/kg. For more information, please see **Chapter 6** on mechanical ventilation.

Specific problems, such as the presence of congenital heart disease or persistent pulmonary hypertension in the newborn, may call for specific advanced mechanical ventilation strategies. These, however, should be attempted only in consultation with the tertiary center.

E. Control of Acidosis

Metabolic acidosis, frequently offset by respiratory alkalosis in the initial stages of shock, may become evident as a child's condition worsens. Optimal management includes addressing underlying causes such as hypovolemia and abnormal organ perfusion and using volume resuscitation and vasoactive infusions as required. Adequate ventilation and oxygenation should be ensured by using cautious doses of sedation and analgesia, with neuromuscular blockade added only if absolutely necessary.

Sodium bicarbonate is indicated primarily for patients with hyperkalemia or intoxication with sodium-channel-blocking drugs, but it may also be considered in the management of selected profoundly acidemic (pH <7), adequately ventilated patients. Because the use of sodium bicarbonate may increase intracellular acidosis, this treatment is no longer routinely recommended. Agents such as tromethamine (THAM) given slowly, generally at 3 to 5 mL/kg over an hour, may be helpful in extreme situations, with the caveat that they can worsen hypokalemia, hyperkalemia, and hypoglycemia and should be avoided in the presence of established renal failure.

F. Laboratory Evaluation

Any child who is acutely ill should have a bedside glucose assay on presentation because significant time may elapse between sampling and report of laboratory results. The initial laboratory evaluation should also include a complete blood count (CBC), a complete chemistry profile, ionized calcium, blood gas analysis, and coagulation testing as the condition and presumed cause of shock warrant. A sample should be sent to the blood bank as soon as possible for blood typing and crossmatching to expedite the availability of blood products that may be required for ongoing resuscitation. Serial assessment of mixed venous oxygenation from a sample drawn from the superior vena cava may help guide clinical management in patients with severe shock when a central line has been placed for stabilization.

Although blood and urine cultures are of extreme importance in determining causal infectious agents, antibiotics should not be delayed due to difficulty in securing appropriate samples. Lumbar puncture should be deferred until a child has stabilized because it will not affect initial management and may instead result in significant deterioration with cardiopulmonary arrest, particularly in the presence of increased intracranial pressure, coagulopathy, or limited reserve, as may be found in patients who remain in shock without a secure airway.

> !
>
> *Early antibiotic administration is a priority in children presenting with septic shock.*
>
> !

Additional laboratory studies, such as an ammonia level, serum amino acids, and urine organic acids, may be called for in patients suspected of having inborn metabolic errors, which typically present in newborns but may present in older infants and even in older children. Toxicology screens are important in the differential diagnosis of any child presenting with shock and encephalopathy. Assays for endocrine dysfunction including cortisol levels and thyroid function tests should be considered in specific circumstances.

G. Radiographic Studies

A chest radiograph is essential to the complete evaluation of any child presenting with shock. Heart size provides important clues about the cause of shock and should raise concerns for cardiac etiologies if the silhouette is generous, particularly in patients beyond early infancy. A more extensive survey that includes radiographs of the chest, lateral cervical spine, and pelvis is required in patients who have sustained traumatic injuries. Careful consideration should be given to securing and maintaining the airway of a child requiring transfer out of the emergency department for radiology studies, such as computed tomography (CT), because deterioration may occur rapidly in settings not conducive to resuscitation.

V. GENERAL CARE

The treatment goals for the first hour of care for shock include complete initial and serial assessment of airway, breathing, and circulation. Adequate vascular access must be secured within the first few minutes of presentation. It may be necessary to control the airway to ensure adequate oxygenation and ventilation, normalize perfusion, and restore vital signs to threshold values. At a minimum, appropriate monitoring includes continuous oximetry and electrocardiography (ECG), very frequent (every 5 min) blood pressure measurements, hourly temperature and urine output measurement via an indwelling urinary catheter, and frequent assessments of glucose and ionized calcium.

Once arterial and central venous pressure monitoring catheters have been placed, which may not be possible at the primary hospital, continuous attention is paid to perfusion pressures and optimizing oxygen delivery. Additional laboratory data to be reviewed include indicators of end-organ dysfunction, coagulation, gas exchange, and endocrine function, including cortisol and thyroid function tests.

Further management is directed at optimizing oxygen delivery while minimizing oxygen consumption. A head-to-toe approach is generally very helpful. In most cases, sedation and analgesia can be safely and effectively accomplished using small, intermittent doses of benzodiazepines and fentanyl or ketamine. Continuous infusions of agents such as midazolam (0.1 mg/kg/h) and fentanyl (1-2 µg/kg/h) or ketamine (1-2 mg/kg/h) may be extremely useful in keeping the patient comfortable while reducing the risk of hypotension and inadvertent dislodgment of medical devices. Although propofol is used widely in adult medicine, it commonly causes hypotension in children, particularly in the presence of shock, and should be avoided. Neuromuscular blockade with vecuronium (0.1 mg/kg) may be necessary to ensure patient safety and ventilator synchrony, but it should be utilized only with adequate sedation and analgesia by individuals with excellent airway management skills. Soft restraints should be considered for all children, especially if neuromuscular blocking agents are not being used.

Continued meticulous attention to maintaining optimal preload, afterload, and contractility is essential. Adequate hemoglobin concentration and oxygen saturation should be maintained with a judicious transfusion strategy, inspired supplemental oxygen, and positive end-expiratory pressure. Ventilation and oxygenation should be assessed periodically with analysis of blood gases and ionized calcium. Lactate concentration, a surrogate marker of energy delivery to tissues and substrate utilization, should be followed at frequent intervals until shock has resolved. Targeted antibiotic therapy should be given within the hour of presentation to children of all ages when infection is suspected, even if suitable culture samples cannot be obtained in a timely fashion. Persistent hyperglycemia should be controlled using low-dose insulin, usually starting at 0.025 to 0.05 units/kg per hour. Loading doses are not recommended due to the risk of precipitating hypoglycemia. The infusion of insulin should be titrated to maintain a glucose level less than 150 mg/dL in small children and from 100 to 120 mg/dL in older children. Glucose levels must be measured hourly when insulin therapy is used.

Enteral nutrition should be delayed until the shock state has resolved. A nasogastric tube should be placed to gravity drainage unless there is a specific indication for continuous or intermittent suction, such as abdominal distention. Gastric protection with an H_2 blocker or proton pump inhibitor should be considered for every patient. If a child is oliguric or has evidence of renal dysfunction, pertinent adjustments to drug doses should be made based on creatinine clearance, and the trough levels of potentially nephrotoxic agents such as aminoglycosides should be monitored closely.

VI. ADDITIONAL CONSIDERATIONS

A. Neonatal Considerations

Very young infants with pulmonary and systemic circulations that are transitioning from the fetal to the neonatal pattern are at particular risk for developing right heart failure with progressive decreases in cardiac output. Acute right ventricular failure may rapidly ensue and may be manifested as shock with hepatomegaly and other indicators of worsening cardiac output and increased mesenteric and systemic vascular resistances. Echocardiography will demonstrate tricuspid regurgitation. Patency of the ductus arteriosus may result in pulmonary edema during volume resuscitation, mandating careful serial reevaluation and the use of discrete boluses of isotonic fluids in these infants.

While the cause of shock in the older child is generally easy to discover, the differential diagnosis is much more diverse in neonates. One of the most important causes to consider and treat until excluded is congenital heart disease, specifically ductus-dependent left-sided obstructive lesions that may have gone undetected until ductal closure and the onset of obvious shock. Any clinical suspicion of congenital heart disease should be addressed with appropriate support of ventilation and circulation with expansion of the intravascular space with isotonic fluids and administration of inotropic and vasoactive infusions. An infusion of prostaglandin E_1 must be started immediately at 0.05 to 0.1 µg/kg/min in neonates presenting with shock and should be continued with close attention to possible adverse effects, such as apnea or hypotension, until echocardiography can definitively exclude the presence of a lesion, such as coarctation of the aorta, interrupted aortic arch, critical aortic stenosis, or a constellation of malformations consistent with hypoplastic left heart syndrome.

Inborn errors of metabolism and congenital adrenal hyperplasia may present with hypoglycemia, metabolic acidosis, and evidence of end-organ dysfunction. These abnormalities must be treated aggressively while investigation progresses. Appropriate management prior to admission to a PICU includes close monitoring of glucose (at least hourly) and ionized calcium in addition to other general supportive measures.

B. Shock in the Injured Child

Once the airway has been secured and resuscitation has begun, a very careful secondary trauma survey is essential. Scalp lacerations may cause hypovolemia in patients of all sizes. Children younger than 2 years may develop hypovolemic shock from intracranial hemorrhage. Pelvic fractures may cause profuse internal hemorrhage until they are stabilized mechanically or bleeding is controlled by surgery or angiography. Rapidly completed CT scanning of suspected sites of injury (head, chest, abdomen, and pelvis) can complement the initial basic trauma imaging obtained in the emergency department. Administration of packed red blood cells, including uncrossmatched O-negative blood, may be lifesaving, especially in the presence of ongoing blood losses.

C. Septic Shock

Patients with septic shock often manifest elements typical of hypovolemic, distributive, and cardiogenic shock. Depending on the stage of presentation, patients in septic shock can have relative or absolute hypovolemia, abnormal vascular tone, maldistribution of blood flow, and myocardial dysfunction along with various complicating factors, such as refractory acidosis, coagulopathy, metabolic and endocrine derangements, and capillary leak syndromes, which may cause further compromise.

The inciting event is an invasive infection with the release of microbial toxins that, in turn, generate an intense host-mediated response. The resulting syndrome is a combination of the direct effects of microbial agents, toxins, and host inflammatory response to infection, including the release of pro- and anti-inflammatory mediators that can ultimately lead to multiorgan dysfunction and failure. In addition, septic shock is marked by abnormalities in energy utilization at the subcellular level.

The clinical features of septic shock vary greatly depending on the timing of presentation, the inciting organism, and the degree of host response to the infection. Approximately 80% of children who undergo invasive hemodynamic measurement for dopamine-resistant shock with appropriate volume resuscitation have clinical features of low cardiac output state, including tachycardia; altered mental status; poor peripheral pulses; mottled skin; and prolonged capillary refill. This presentation has often been referred to as *cold shock*. A more prevalent presentation in

> **!**
>
> *Hypotension may or may not be part of the initial presentation of cold or warm shock, and its absence should never be reassuring to the clinician.*

adults that is also seen in about 20% of children is a hyperdynamic state characterized by increased cardiac output, vasodilatation, tachycardia, bounding pulses, brisk capillary refill, and plethoric skin. This is often referred to as warm shock. A change from high to low cardiac output can occur rapidly as septic shock progresses. These patients go from a flushed, warm, well-perfused state to one marked by hypoperfusion with tachypnea, tachycardia, hypotension, prolonged capillary refill, weak pulses, and metabolic (lactic) acidosis.

Treatment goals include prompt identification of the shock state, rapid reversal of the cardiovascular dysfunction with adequate intravascular volume expansion, vasoactive and inotropic support, control of the infectious organism (antimicrobials or surgical debridement, if indicated), and advanced mechanical support in the form of extracorporeal membrane oxygenation (ECMO) in selected refractory cases.

D. Adrenal Insufficiency

Young infants are at increased risk of adrenal insufficiency, particularly if they have hypoglycemia, hyponatremia, and hyperkalemia on their initial laboratory screen. Also at risk are previously healthy children with profound shock refractory to conventional management and children with rapidly evolving rashes (especially if they are purpuric or petechial in nature), any exposure to etomidate, a history of systemic steroid use within the last year, severe head or abdominal injury, or a history of panhypopituitarism. Patients with known or suspected adrenal insufficiency should be treated with hydrocortisone, which will provide both mineralocorticoid and glucocorticoid support at stress doses of 2 mg/kg as a bolus, followed by intermittent dosing of 1 to 2 mg/kg every 6 hours. Higher doses are recommended by some experts. Additionally, enteral fludrocortisone may be required in children with congenital adrenal hyperplasia.

E. Shock in Children With Diabetes

Children with new-onset diabetes whose initial presentation is diabetic ketoacidosis may have severe hypovolemia and hypoperfusion. Hemodynamic instability in these children is appropriately addressed with volume resuscitation as described for any child with hypovolemic shock. However, once hemodynamic stability has been attained with normal saline or 5% albumin, most intensivists and endocrinologists recommend repleting the intravascular space more gingerly than when correcting hypovolemia stemming from another cause. Gradual control of the hyperglycemia is essential to controlling the catabolic state and ongoing fluid losses (**see Chapter 9**). Bedside glucose assays must be performed very frequently to avoid excessive decreases, particularly when the child must be transported.

F. Refractory Shock

Shock that is refractory to initial treatment should raise suspicions of alternative diagnoses, such as congenital cardiac disease, acquired cardiac disease (including blunt trauma to the heart), pericardial tamponade, pneumothorax, hemothorax, pulmonary hypertension, toxins, occult ongoing blood loss, inborn metabolic errors or adrenal insufficiency, abdominal catastrophe with evolving abdominal hypertension or compartment syndrome, and persistent infectious nidus.

Key Points

Diagnosis and Management of Shock

- Complete initial and serial assessment of airway patency, breathing, and circulation are essential for successful management of any seriously ill or injured patient.
- Oxygen should be administered to all patients at risk for shock, regardless of their initial saturation readings.
- Vascular access should be secured within the first few minutes of presentation, with prompt consideration of intraosseous needle placement.
- Fluid resuscitation should begin with isotonic crystalloid, such as 0.9% given in rapid boluses titrated to clinical response.
- Ketamine and atropine are the drugs of choice for airway control in the presence of shock.
- Antibiotics must be given within the hour of presentation.
- Careful physical examination will reveal clues to the underlying cause of shock.
- Avoid hypoglycemia, particularly in small infants.
- Hypotension is a late finding in pediatric shock of any etiology and may precede full arrest.

Suggested Readings

1. Carcillo JA, Davis AL, Zaritsky A. Role of early fluid resuscitation in pediatric septic shock. *JAMA.* 1991;266:1242-1245.

2. Carcillo JA, Piva JP, Thomas NJ et al. Shock and shock syndromes. In: Slonim AD, Pollack MM, eds. *Pediatric Critical Care Medicine.* Philadelphia, PA: Lippincott Williams & Wilkins; 2006:438-471.

3. Carcillo JA, Tasker RC. Fluid resuscitation of hypovolemic shock: acute medicine's great triumph for children. *Intensive Care Med.* 2006;32:958-961.

4. Colletti JE, Homme JL, Woodridge DP. Unsuspected neonatal killers in emergency medicine. *Emerg Med Clin North Am.* 2004;22:929-960.

5. Han YY, Carcillo JA, Dragotta MA, et al. Early reversal of pediatric-neonatal septic shock by community physicians is associated with improved outcome. *Pediatrics.* 2003;112:793-799.

6. Melendez E, Bachur R. Advances in the emergency management of pediatric sepsis. *Curr Opin Pediatr.* 2006;18:245-253.

7. Parker MM, Hazelzet JA, Carcillo JA. Pediatric considerations. *Crit Care Med.* 2004;32:S591-S594.

8. Pizarro CF, Troster EJ, Damiani D, Carcillo JA. Absolute and relative adrenal insufficiency in children with septic shock. *Crit Care Med.* 2005;33:855-859.

9. Smith L, Hernan L. Shock states. In: Fuhrman BP, Zimmerman JP, eds. *Pediatric Critical Care.* 3rd ed. Philadelphia, PA: Mosby Elsevier; 2006:394-410.

10. Vincent JL, Gerlach H. Fluid resuscitation in severe sepsis and septic shock: an evidence-based review. *Crit Care Med.* 2004;32:S451-S454.

Chapter 8:

Acute Infections

Objectives

- Recognize severe, life-threatening infections.
- Initiate timely, goal-directed management.
- Identify possible pathogens based on clinical findings and epidemiology.
- Select adequate initial antimicrobial treatment.
- Recognize and manage severe infections endemic in developing countries.

Case Study

A 2-year-old child is admitted to the ward with a 3 day history of fever, vomiting and irritability. On physical examination he is tachycardic (175 beats/minute) and his abdomen is tender with wall rigidity. White blood count reveals 18,500 leukocytes/mm_3. You suspect sepsis and initiate fluid boluses and antibiotic treatment.

- What site of infection would you suspect and how would you study it?

- Which would be your initial empirical antibiotic treatment?

- What other priorities should you consider?

I. INTRODUCTION

The spectrum of acute infections in the pediatric population is vast. Children may present with life-threatening symptoms, or they may present with subtle signs that may progress to severe conditions if undetected. Despite advances in the management of the critically ill children during the past decades, morbidity and mortality remain high in children with severe infections. The increase in morbidity and mortality is directly related to an increase in the at-risk populations: critically ill patients, patients with debilitating chronic conditions, and patients with immunosuppression stemming from cancer, immunodeficiencies, or organ transplants.

Early diagnosis and treatment of any type of infection is essential to a prompt recovery and improved outcome. Late diagnosis may result in organ dysfunction, shock, multiple organ failure, and death. The initial signs and symptoms, however, may be subtle, and astute clinicians need to proceed with thorough and frequent physical examinations. The management of neutropenia and fever is not within the scope of this chapter and is discussed in **Chapter 19**. Definitions of terms related to pediatric sepsis are presented in **Tables 8-1, 8-2, and 8-3**.

> *Early recognition and management of severe infections prevents life- threatening complications.*

Table 8-1. Definitions of Systemic Inflammatory Response Syndrome, Infection, Sepsis, Severe Sepsis, and Septic Shock

Systemic Inflammatory Response Syndrome

Systemic inflammatory response syndrome (SIRS) is characterized by the presence of at least 2 of the following 4 criteria, 1 of which must be abnormal temperature or abnormal leukocyte count:

- Core temperature (measured by rectal, bladder, oral, or central catheter probe) of >38.5°C (101.3°F) or <36°C (96.8°F).
- Tachycardia, defined as a mean heart rate >2 SD above the normal for age in the absence of external stimulus, chronic drug use, or painful stimuli, or otherwise unexplained persistent elevation over a 30-minute to 4-hour time period OR for children <1 year old, bradycardia, defined as a mean heart rate <10th percentile for age in the absence of external vagal stimulus, β-blocker drugs, or congenital heart disease, or otherwise unexplained persistent depression over a 30-minute time period.
- Mean respiratory rate >2 SD above the normal for age or mechanical ventilation for an acute process unrelated to underlying neuromuscular disease or the receipt of general anesthesia.
- Leukocyte count elevated or depressed for the patient's age (not secondary to chemotherapy-induced leukopenia) or >10% immature neutrophils.

Infection

A suspected or proven (by positive culture, tissue stain, or polymerase chain reaction test) infection caused by any pathogen OR a clinical syndrome associated with a high probability of infection. Evidence of infection includes positive findings on clinical examination, imaging, or laboratory tests (eg, white blood cells in a normally sterile body fluid, perforates viscus, chest radiograph consistent with pneumonia, petechial or purpuric rash, or purpura fulminans).

Sepsis

SIRS in the presence of or as a result of suspected or proven infection.

Severe Sepsis

Sepsis with cardiovascular organ dysfunction before treatment or corrected by fluid resuscitation of less than 40 mL/kg/h OR acute respiratory distress syndrome OR 2 or more other organ dysfunctions. Organ dysfunctions are defined in **Table 8-2**.

Septic Shock

Sepsis with cardiovascular organ dysfunction as defined in **Table 8-2**.

Modified from Goldstein B., et al. International Pediatric Sepsis Conference; definitions for sepsis and organ dysfunction in pediatrics. *Pediatr Crit Care Med.* 2005; 6:2-8.

II. DIAGNOSIS

An early diagnosis of severe infections is based on clear understanding of the risk factors, the epidemiology, and the findings of a meticulous physical examination. Complementary testing, though often nonspecific, can aid in the diagnostic process when used correctly. Adequately performed microbiology testing can be a diagnostic tool.

A. Clinical Findings

Infections have a variety of signs and symptoms. Some are easy to detect, whereas others can be subtle and should be sought carefully.

1. General Signs of Infection

Fever is the most frequent of the general signs. Rectal and oral temperatures are considered to be more accurate than axillary. A rectal temperature above 38°C (101.3°F) is usually considered to be abnormal. Most infections in children present with fever; however, some patients with severe infections may present with hypothermia (temperature <36°C [96.8°F]). In some other conditions, however, fever may not be caused by an infection, and additional differential diagnoses should be considered. Such possibilities include:

- Inflammatory disease (eg, Kawasaki disease)
- Reaction to drugs, blood, or blood-derived products
- Overheating, especially in neonates and young infants
- Neoplasms
- Surgery within the previous 24 hours
- Central nervous system (CNS) bleeding or thrombosis
- Endocrine disease (eg, thyrotoxicosis)

Other nonspecific signs of infection include chills, myalgia, tiredness, anorexia, and night sweating. Tachycardia and tachypnea are frequent, whereas hypotension is indicative of an advanced, severe infection. In young infants and neonates, irritability, poor feeding, lethargy, and mottled skin are possible findings. Specific signs vary according to thc affcctcd organ.

> !
>
> *Young infants with poor eye contact, irritability, feeding rejection, and perfusion changes should be considered at high risk of severe infection.*
>
> !

Table 8-2. Organ Dysfunction Criteria

Cardiovascular Dysfunction

Despite administration of isotonic fluid bolus ≥40 mL/kg in 1 hour

- Decrease in BP (hypotension) <5th percentile for age or systolic BP <2 SD below normal for agea

OR

- Need for vasoactive drugs to maintain BP in normal range

OR

- Two of the following:
  - Unexplained metabolic acidosis: base deficit 5 mmol/L
  - Increased arterial lactate >2 times upper limit of normal
  - Oliguria: urine output <0.5 mL/kg/h
  - Prolonged capillary refill: >5 sec
  - Core to peripheral temperature gap >3°C

Respiratory Dysfunction[b]

- Pao_2:Fio_2 <300 in absence of cyanotic heart disease or preexisting lung disease

OR

- $PaCo_2$ >20 mm Hg over baseline $PaCo_2$

OR

- Proven need or >50% Fio_2 to maintain saturation ≥92%

OR

- Need for nonelective invasive or noninvasive mechanical ventilation

Neurologic Dysfunction

- Glasgow Coma Score ≤11

OR

- Acute change in mental status with a decrease in Glasgow Coma Score ≥3 points from abnormal baseline

Hematologic Dysfunction

- Platelet count <80,000/mm3 or a decline of 50% in platelet count from highest value recorded over the past 3 days (for chronic hematology/oncology patients)

OR

- International normalized ratio >2

Renal Dysfunction

- Serum creatinine ≥2 times upper limit of normal for age or 2-fold increase in baseline creatinine

Hepatic Dysfunction

- Total bilirubin ≥4 mg/dL (not applicable for newborn)

OR

- ALT 2 times upper limit of normal for age

Abbreviations: ALT, alanine transaminase; BP, blood pressure; SD, standard deviation.

[a] See **Table 8-3**.

[b] Acute respiratory distress syndrome must include a Pao_2:Fio_2 ratio ≤200 mm Hg, bilateral infiltrates, acute onset, and no evidence of left heart failure. Acute lung injury is defined identically, except the Pao_2:Fio_2 ratio must be ≤300 mm Hg; proven need assumes oxygen requirement was tested by decreasing flow with subsequent increase in flow if required; in postoperative patients, this requirement can be met if the patient has developed an acute inflammatory or infectious pro cess in the lungs that prevents him or her from being extubated.

From Goldstein B, et al. International Pediatric Sepsis Consensus Conference: definitions for sepsis and organ dysfunction in pediatrics. *Pediatr Crit Care Med.* 2005;6:2-8.

Table 8-3. Age-Specific Upper Values (95th Percentile) for Heart Rate and Respiratory Rate, and Lower Values (5th Percentile) for Systolic Blood Pressure and Heart Rate

Age Group	Tachycardia Beats/min	Bradycardia Beats/min	Tachypnea Breaths/min	Leukocyte Count Leukocytes _ 103	SBP mm Hg
0 days-1 week	>180	<100	>50	>34	<65
1 week-1 month	>180	<100	>40	>19.5 or <5	<75
1 month-1 year	>180	<90	>34	>17.5 or <5	<100
2-5 years	>140	NA	>22	>15.5 or <6	<94
6-12 years	>130	NA	>18	>13.5 or <4.5	<105
13-<18 years	>110	NA	>14	>11 or <4.5	<117

Abbreviation: SBP, systolic blood pressure.
Adapted from Goldstein B, et al. International Pediatric Sepsis Consensus Conference: definitions for sepsis and organ dysfunction in pediatrics. *Pediatr Crit Care Med.* 2005;6:2-8.

2. Signs of Central Nervous System Infection

Central nervous system infections include meningitis and encephalitis. The clinical presentation of meningitis may vary depending on age. In young infants, fever, irritability, lethargy, anterior fontanel bulging, apnea, seizures, crying when handled, or poor eye contact may be present. Older children may present with fever, headaches, vomiting, and in later stages, irritability, mental status changes, or nuchal rigidity. Other signs in this group may include focal neurologic compromise or seizures. Encephalitis is characterized by disturbances of consciousness and may sometimes present with focal neurological signs, focal seizures, ataxia, or disturbances of speech. Ventriculitis is an inflammatory or infectious process affecting the brain's ventricular system. Signs of ventriculitis include headache, vomiting, strabismus, and sometimes seizures. General findings, such as lethargy and poor feeding, may also be present.

3. Signs of Respiratory Infection

Respiratory infections usually present with fever and symptoms such as cough, tachypnea, dyspnea, or chest pain. Other signs include abdominal pain, vomiting, chest pain, and asthenia. Chest auscultation may show decreased chest sounds, abnormal vocal resonance, crackles, or pleural rub. Signs of severe disease include nasal flaring, grunting, lower chest wall retractions, and central cyanosis.

4. Signs of Urinary Tract Infection

Urinary tract infection in neonates presents with general signs such as fever, irritability, feeding problems, vomiting, hyperbilirubinemia, or failure to thrive. Young infants usually have fever without focus; however, other signs, such as failure to thrive, vomiting, diarrhea, or irritability, may be present at this age. The older child may present with dysuria and voiding symptoms, such as urgency and increased frequency.

5. Signs of Cutaneous Infection

The classical manifestations of cutaneous infections are pain, erythema, indurated skin, and warmth. Fever may or may not be present, and signs of systemic involvement may occur in some cases. Preseptal cellulitis usually presents with eyelid swelling, erythema, local warmth, and tenderness. Fever is usually present, and in some cases children have a toxic appearance. The presence of abnormal eye movements or proptosis is suggestive of orbital cellulitis.

6. Signs of Septic Arthritis and Osteomyelitis

Septic arthritis and osteomyelitis may present with fever and local signs such as pain, swelling, erythema, movement limitation, and finger pain.

7. Signs of Abdominal Infection

Signs and symptoms of severe abdominal infection include high fever, diffuse abdominal pain, vomiting, rebound tenderness, rigid abdominal wall, and diminished or absent bowel sounds.

B. Laboratory Findings

A complete blood count (CBC) is done routinely in any patient suspected of having a severe infection. Leukocytosis (white blood count >12,000 mm^3) may be a reaction to an infectious or an inflammatory process, among other possibilities. Most bacterial infections cause leukocytosis with neutrophilia (neutrophil count ≥8000/mm^3 in adults and children older than 1 year); however, severe infections may present with leukopenia (leukocyte count <4000/mm^3), especially in young infants. The presence of leukocytosis or neutrophilia alone cannot accurately predict the presence or absence of bacterial infection. Platelets are acute-phase reactants; therefore, thrombocytosis (platelet count >450,000/mm^3) can be an indirect sign of infection. However, thrombocytopenia (platelet count <150,000/mm^3) and other clotting abnormalities are well-known complications of sepsis.

Alterations in the prothrombin time (PT) and activated partial thromboplastin time (aPTT) can be suggestive of disseminated intravascular coagulation (DIC) during severe sepsis. Elevated D-dimers and fibrin degradation products in association with low fibrinogen confirm the diagnosis. C-reactive protein (CRP) and erythrocyte sedimentation rate (ESR) are acute-phase reactants that can be elevated during severe infections. In the acute setting they do not contribute notably to clinical examination. Procalcitonin has been postulated to be useful to recognize severe infections or sepsis; however, there is no clear evidence about its benefits. When used together with other markers of inflammation and with clinical criteria, it may increase the sensibility and specificity of the diagnosis of sepsis.

In the evaluation of metabolic acidosis arterial blood gases are useful as a marker of poor tissue perfusion when accompanied by high lactate levels or low sodium bicarbonate levels. The partial pressure of oxygen (Pao_2) may be used to confirm impaired oxygen (O_2) diffusion and may help in the diagnosis of conditions such as acute lung injury or acute respiratory distress syndrome. Differences in arterial and central venous contents of O_2 can assess the adequacy of oxygen delivery. Partial pressure of carbon dioxide ($PaCo_2$) can be low during respiratory compensation ($PaCo_2$ <35 mm Hg [4.6 kPa]) or elevated ($PaCo_2$ >45 mm Hg [5.9 kPa]) during disease with ventilation impairment. Also, superior vena cava (SVC) or mixed venous oxygen saturation (SVo_2) when measured by co-oximetry are useful to guide treatment during severe sepsis.

Severe infections may affect renal function; therefore blood urea nitrogen (BUN) and serum creatinine should always be measured. During renal failure, drugs (antibiotics) should be adjusted to creatinine clearance.

Hypoglycemia (in neonates and young infants) or hyperglycemia may be present during severe infections. Hyperglycemia has been associated with increased mortality in critically ill adults, and the use of insulin to achieve normoglycemia seems to improve mortality and morbidity in surgical intensive care units. Evidence for the use of insulin therapy is controversial in pediatrics; however, it is standard to treat hyperglycemia in children when glucose values are >180 to 200 mg/dL (9.98 to 11.1 mmol/L). Blood glucose should be measured at the bedside during initial management, and frequent bedside controls should be utilized during the posterior management of severe infections in children.

Also useful during severe infections are measures of serum electrolytes (sodium, potassium, calcium, phosphorus, magnesium, or serum bicarbonate) and liver function tests, among others.

C. Microbiology Tests

Microbiology tests are essential in helping establish the final etiologic diagnosis. Clinicians must choose the correct laboratory tools in order to improve diagnostic sensitivity and specificity.

Routine cultures of any fluid collection or infected tissue or fluid should be obtained. Gram stain can quickly provide considerable information that can be applied immediately to patient care. It is particularly useful in the diagnostic confirmation of bacterial meningitis, urinary tract infection, or other fluid collections, such as abscess, empyema, and peritonitis. Specimens obtained during biopsy or bronchoscopy should be sent routinely for gram stain. Other stains should be considered (acid-fast bacilli, pneumocystis, fungal, etc) depending on the type of infection that is suspected. The growth of bacterial colonies in specific growth mediums (aerobe, anaerobe, fungal, mycobacteria) will help make the final microbiologic diagnosis and help test for antimicrobial susceptibility. Any material appropriately taken can be sent for culture.

Antigen-detection techniques with direct immunofluorescence and latex agglutination for rapid detection of bacterial antigens can be done in diverse specimens such as urine, sputum, or throat swab, among others. Antigen-detection techniques can give useful information; however, because the sensitivity of that information can be low, initial antibiotic management of severe infections should not be based on those techniques alone.

Polymerase chain reaction (PCR) for the detection of deoxyribonucleic acid (DNA) or ribonucleic acid (RNA) can be useful for the detection of diverse infections. It is now the standard technique to detect herpes virus and enterovirus in cerebrospinal fluid (CSF).

Serologic testing for the detection of antibodies is used mainly for the diagnosis of viral diseases (eg, adenovirus, influenza, Epstein-Barr virus, herpesvirus, dengue) and less frequently for some bacterial, parasitic, or fungal infections, such as *Mycoplasma pneumoniae*, toxoplasmosis, or histoplasmosis.

III. INFECTIOUS SYNDROMES

A. The Febrile Child

Fever is one of the most frequent causes of visits to the emergency department in infants and young children and can be a manifestation of infection. Most such infections are self-limiting viral diseases; however, some children will have bacteremia or other severe bacterial diseases such as meningitis. A frequent pediatric clinical dilemma is the evaluation of the healthy-appearing febrile child, especially if under 2 years of age, without localizing signs or symptoms, to establish the child's risk of developing occult bacteremia or severe bacterial disease. When studying children with fever who do not have an identifiable focus of infection, it is useful to group them by age. The younger the child, the more difficult it is to identify signs or symptoms suggestive of bacterial infection.

1. Newborns 0 to 28 Days Old

All neonates with fever should be hospitalized. Complete blood count, blood cultures, urine culture, lumbar puncture, and chest radiograph should be done. Empiric antibiotic treatment should be started with ampicillin and gentamicin or ampicillin and cefotaxime. Antibiotic doses are described in **Table 8-4**.

2. Infants 29 to 90 Days Old

When working with an infant 29 to 90 days old, it is important to decide whether the child has toxic appearance or not. Children with toxic appearance are at a higher risk of having bacterial disease. Characteristics of a toxic appearance may include poor eye contact, distal perfusion, cyanosis, and irritability.

Table 8-4. Antibiotic Doses for Sepsis

Age Group	Treatment
Neonates ≤7 days	Ampicillin 25-50 mg/kg/dose every 12 hours The higher doses are for meningitis or group B streptococcal sepsis. Gentamicin 4-5 mg/kg/dose every 24-48 hours, depending on gestational age Cefotaxime 50 mg/kg/dose every 12 hours
Neonates >7 days	Ampicillin 50 mg/kg/dose every 8-12 hours, depending on gestational age The higher doses are for meningitis or group B streptococcal sepsis. Gentamicin 4 mg/kg/dose; interval depends on plasma levels Cefotaxime 50 mg/kg/dose every 8-12 hours, depending on gestational age Vancomycin 10-15 mg/kg/dose every 8-18 hours, depending on gestational age Metronidazole 7.5 mg/kg/dose every 12-48 hours, depending on gestational age
Previously healthy infants and children	Ceftriaxone 50 mg/kg/dose every 12 hours Vancomycin 10-15 mg/kg/dose every 6 hours The higher dose is for CNS infection. Metronidazole 7.5 mg/kg/dose every 6 hours
Hospitalized or immunosuppressed children	Ceftriaxone 50 mg/kg/dose every 12 hours Gentamicin 2-2.5 mg/kg/dose every 8 hours Amikacin 5mg/kg/dose every 8 hours Ceftazidime 50 mg/kg/dose every 8 hours Metronidazole 7.5 mg/kg/dose every 6 hours Vancomycin 10-15 mg/kg/dose every 6 hours The higher dose is for CNS infection. Meropenem 20 mg/kg/dose every 8 hours; 60 mg/kg/dose every 8 hours for meningitis

All infants in this age group with toxic appearance should be hospitalized. Complete blood count, blood culture, urine culture and CSF should be taken. Empiric antibiotic treatment is started with ampicillin in combination with cefotaxime or gentamicin. Further, infants with low risk criteria can be admitted for observation without antibiotic treatment or cultured (blood, urine, and CSF), given ceftriaxone, and discharged home with close daily observation. Criteria for determining low risk are as follows:

- Lack of toxic appearance
- No infectious focus during physical examination other than upper respiratory viral infection
- No history of immunodeficiency
- White blood count (WBC) between 5000 and 15,000 mm3
- Band/neutrophil relation less than 0.2
- Normal urine test results

3. Children 90 Days to 36 Months Old

Like children 29 to 90 days old, children ages 90 days to 36 months may be classified into two groups, those who have a toxic appearance and those who do not. Children with toxic appearance should be treated in accordance with sepsis guidelines.

The management of the healthy-appearing child without a focus of infection depends on clinical assessment. A frequent approach is to base treatment on temperature. Children with a rectal temperature of less than 39°C (102.2°F) and a normal physical examination and urinalysis are discharged home with ambulatory control. For children with a rectal temperature of more than 39°C (102.2°F), CBC and urine tests should be obtained. A WBC greater than 15,000/mm^3 is an indication for obtaining a blood culture and performing a lumbar puncture when meningitis may not be ruled out by physical examination. One approach is to initiate antibiotic treatment with ceftriaxone after blood and urine cultures have been taken and if urinalysis is normal. Children are then discharged home with daily office controls.

Chest radiographs should be done in infants and young children with evidence of acute respiratory illness. It should also be considered in infants or children with high fever (≥39°C [102.2°F]) and WBC of 20,000/mm^3 or more.

B. Septic Shock

Sepsis is a systemic response to infection that can lead to high mortality if not treated adequately. The use of intensive care and goal-directed therapies have shown to improve outcome.

Early clinical suspicion should be based on the presence of hyperthermia or hypothermia, changes in mental status, and alterations in peripheral perfusion. Evaluation of children with suspected sepsis is based on meticulous and repeated physical examination. Heart rate, capillary refill, respiratory rate, mental status, urinary output, and alteration in the skin should be evaluated carefully.

> ! *Hypotension is a late manifestation in children with septic shock.*

> ! *Rapid initiation of adequate empiric antibiotic therapy is key to lowering mortality during severe infections.*

Management should be started as soon as sepsis is suspected. The goal of therapy is to avoid or to correct abnormalities that arise due to cellular hypoperfusion. As with all critically ill patients, assessment of the airway, proper ventilation, the establishment of adequate circulation, and rapid administration of antibiotics are the main priorities. Fluid and inotropic management of the septic patient is discussed at length in **Chapter 7**.

1. Steroids

There is continuous debate regarding the use of steroids in pediatric sepsis. Current guidelines recommend the use of hydrocortisone in the presence of catecholamine-resistant shock and risk of adrenal insufficiency. Risk factors for adrenal insufficiency include suspicion of meningococcemia, chronic use of steroids, and pituitary or adrenal abnormalities. Recommended doses vary from 1 to 2 mg/kg for stress coverage to 50 mg/kg for treatment of refractory shock followed by the same dose as a 24-hour infusion. When possible, blood cortisol concentrations should be obtained before the first dose of hydrocortisone.

2. Antibiotic Therapy

Antibiotics should be administered within the first hour of treatment, immediately after cultures have been obtained. However, if microbiology samples are difficult to obtain, treatment should be started without delay.

Choice of antibiotics depends on the type of infection suspected. Pathogens to consider vary depending on the patient's age, physical findings, immunological status, previous hospitalizations, previous antibiotic treatment, and presence of central catheters or other medical devices. Possible pathogens of sepsis are summarized in **Table 8-5**.

Table 8-5. Possible Pathogens of Sepsis

Age Group	Pathogens
0-30 days	Group B streptococci, enterococcus, enterobacteria, staphylococcus, and *L monocytogenes*
1-3 months	*S pneumoniae, N meningitidis, H influenzae*, and enterobacteria
3 months-5 years	*S pneumoniae, N meningitidis, H influenzae*, and staphylococcus
Older than 5 years	*S pneumoniae, N meningitidis*, streptococcus, and staphylococcus
Immunocompromised or hospitalized children	*S aureus*, staphylococcus epidermidis, gram-negative rods, and *Candida*

Antibiotic treatment depends on the suspected infection. In community-acquired sepsis, cefotaxime or ceftriaxone provides adequate coverage. In patients with risk factors or in hospitalized children, gram-negative coverage should be expanded with an aminoglycoside in combination with a third-generation cephalosporin (ceftazidime) or meropenem. If central lines are present or risk of resistant staphylococcal infection exists, vancomycin should be used. Antibiotic doses are identified in **Table 8-4**.

When a removable source of infection, such as an infected foreign body, an infected collection, or necrotic tissue, is present, that source should be eliminated after antibiotic treatment has been started.

3. Other Considerations

Useful blood tests during initial stabilization include blood gas, lactate, electrolytes, BUN, creatinine, glucose, CBC, and coagulation parameters (PT, aPTT, fibrinogen, and D-dimer). Hemoglobin levels of approximately 10 g/dL have been recommended to optimize oxygen delivery. Hypoglycemia and electrolyte abnormalities should be corrected.

Meningococcemia and toxic shock syndromes are two special situations of septic shock that are considered below.

a. Meningococcemia

Although management of meningococcemia is similar to that of sepsis, it has some distinctive features. Meningococcal disease is an important infectious cause of mortality in children. Even though some forms are less aggressive, the mortality rate associated with meningococcal disease can be as high as 50% in the most severe cases; however, there are recent descriptions of improved mortality using goal-directed therapies. Early recognition and management are essential to improving outcome.

Case Study

A 3-year-old boy presents to the emergency department with fever and vomiting after 6 hours of becoming progressively listless. Physical examination reveals heart rate 150 beats/minute, brisk capillary refill, mild tachypnea, and petechia in neck, face, and extremities.

– Which of the findings are suggestive of sepsis?

– What are the immediate priorities?

The characteristic finding during meningococcal disease is a non-blanching rash with or without signs of meningitis or sepsis. This rash is usually purpuric; however, during the initial phase of the disease, petechiae may be the only dermatologic finding. Differential diagnoses of petechiae include viral diseases, leukemia or other hematological diseases, idiopathic thrombocytopenic purpura, and hemolytic uremic syndrome, among others. In the most severe cases, fatal progression can be very fast regardless of whether the patient was severely affected on admission or not.

> **!** *Every child with fever and petechiae should be suspected of having meningococcemia until proven otherwise.*

If signs of sepsis are present, general management is similar to that of sepsis. Because myocardial dysfunction frequently occurs, inotrope support should be started promptly when response to initial fluid boluses proves inadequate. If there are signs of increased intracranial pressure (ICP), management should strive to decrease it. When patients are not severely affected, blood cultures should be taken. Lumbar puncture can be attempted only if there are no contraindications and there is diagnostic doubt. *Neisseria meningitidis* can be found in blood cultures, throat swabs, skin aspirates of purpuric lesions, and CSF cultures obtained from lumbar puncture. Antibiotic treatment with ceftriaxone (100 mg/kg/day) or cefotaxime (200 mg/kg/day) should be started immediately. Treatment can later be switched to penicillin G (250,000-400,000 units/kg/day) if there is microbiological confirmation of the disease.

Correction of hematological alterations with red blood cells, fresh frozen plasma (FFP), or platelets is frequently needed in severe cases and should be guided by the results of CBC and clotting tests. Hypoglycemia and hypokalemia should be sought and treated rapidly. Other abnormalities, such as hypocalcemia, hypomagnesemia, and hypophosphatemia, should also be corrected promptly.

> !
>
> *When meningococcal disease is suspected, management has to be started rapidly without waiting for laboratory investigations.*
>
> !

Chemoprophylaxis should be given to household, nursery, close school contacts or people exposed to the patient's oral secretions during the previous 7 days if the diagnosis is confirmed or strongly suspected. Health care workers directly exposed to secretions prior to antibiotic treatment (during intubation, mouth to mouth resuscitation or aspiration procedures) should receive prophylaxis as well.

Antimicrobial prophylaxis should be started with rifampin (10 mg/kg twice daily for a total of four doses or 5 mg/kg/dose in infants younger than 1 month), intramuscular ceftriaxone (125 mg in children younger than 12 years or 250 mg in those older than 12 years), or ciprofloxacin (500 mg as single dose) in adults.

b. Toxic Shock Syndromes

Case Study

You are called to evaluate a 7-year-old girl who was admitted 8 hours ago with diarrhea and high fever. Since admission she has developed a rash on the chest and abdomen, she has become progressively tachycardiac, and in the last control her systolic blood pressure was 80 mm Hg.

- What studies can contribute to the diagnosis?
- How would you start the treatment?

Staphylococcal toxic shock syndrome (STSS) and group A streptococcal toxic shock syndrome (GASTSS) are severe multisystem illnesses caused by toxins produced by *S aureus* or by group A streptococci (GAS). Staphylococcal toxic shock syndrome is more frequent in menstruating women, but it may also be secondary to any staphylococcal source of infection, including pneumonia, abscess, skin or wound infection, septicemia or osteomyelitis. Group A streptococcal toxic shock syndrome occurs in patients with any type of streptococcal infection, but it has been frequently associated with varicella lesions in children. Diagnosis can be difficult and is based on clinical criteria described in **Table 8-6** and **Table 8-7**.

> !
>
> *Toxic shock syndrome is a diagnosis to consider in children with fever, rash, and hemodynamic instability.*
>
> !

Table 8-6. Case Definitions of Group A Streptococcal Toxic Shock Syndrome

I. Isolation of group A streptococci

- A. From a normally sterile site (eg, blood, CSF, pleural fluid, peritoneal fluid)
- B. From a nonsterile site (eg, throat, sputum, skin lesion)

II. Clinical signs

- A. Hypotension (systolic blood pressure <5th percentile in patients younger than 16 years)
- B. Two or more of the following findings:
    1. Renal impairment (creatinine ≥twice the upper limit for age)
    2. Coagulopathy (platelets ≤100,000 mm^3 or disseminated intravascular coagulation)
    3. Liver involvement (transaminases or bilirubin ≥twice the upper limit)
    4. Acute respiratory distress syndrome (ARDS)
    5. Generalized erythematous macular rash that may desquamate or soft-tissue necrosis, including necrotizing fasciitis, myositis, or gangrene

Definite case: Criterion IA and criteria IIA and IIB are fulfilled.

Probable case: Criterion IB and criteria IIA and IIB are fulfilled.

Adapted from Hoge CW, Schwartz B, Talkington DF, Breiman RF, MacNeill EM, Englender SJ. The changing epidemiology of invasive group A streptococci infections and the emergence of streptococcal toxic shock-like syndrome: a retrospective population-based study. *JAMA.* 1993;269:390-391.

Table 8-7. Clinical Case Definition of Staphylococcal Toxic Shock Syndrome

1. Fever ≥38.9°C
2. Presence of a diffuse macular erythroderma
3. Desquamation 1-2 weeks after onset, particularly on the palms and soles
4. Hypotension, systolic blood pressure <5th percentile in patients younger than 16 years
5. Involvement of 3 or more of the following organ systems:
    - a. Gastrointestinal (vomiting or diarrhea at the onset of the illness)
    - b. Muscular (myalgia or serum CPK level ≥twice the upper limit for age)
    - c. Mucous membrane (hyperemia of the oropharyngeal, conjunctiva, or vaginal mucosa)
    - d. Renal (serum urea nitrogen or serum creatinine ≥twice the upper limit for age or ≥5 white blood cells per high-power field in the absence of a urinary tract infection)
    - e. Hepatic (transaminases or direct bilirubin ≥twice the upper limit)
    - f. Thrombocytopenia 100,000/mm^3)
    - g. CNS (alterations in consciousness or in orientation without focal signs in the absence of fever or hypotension)
6. Negative blood, throat, or cerebrospinal cultures with the exception that blood cultures may be positive for *S aureus*

Probable case: Presence of 5 clinical findings

Confirmed case: Presence of 6 clinical findings
If the patient dies before desquamation, the presence of 5 findings constitutes a definitive case.

Adapted from Wharton M, Chorba TL, Vogt RL, Morse DL, Buehler JW. Case definitions for public health surveillance. *MMWR Morb Mortal Wkly Rep.* 1990;39(RR-13):1-43.

It is essential to take a detailed history and to search for signs of *Streptococcus* or *Staphylococcus* during a thorough examination. Blood tests and cultures are necessary to fulfill the diagnostic criteria.

Management should include supportive therapy for respiratory failure, cardiovascular instability, and renal failure, and, when necessary, should also involve the correction of clotting abnormalities and blood replacement. Initial antimicrobial treatment for STSS should use oxacillin, cephalothin, or vancomycin. The antibiotic treatment of choice for GASTSS is penicillin G. Some experts have recommended a combination of penicillin G and intravenous clindamycin.

The use of intravenous immunoglobulin has been reported to be beneficial in severe cases of toxic shock syndromes. The recommended initial dose is 2 g/kg, followed by 0.4 g/kg for up to 5 days. Foreign bodies or the localized foci of infection should be removed.

C. Central Nervous System Infections

1. Meningitis

Bacterial meningitis is a life-threatening illness and should always be treated as an emergency. Neonatal pathogens include group B streptococci, *E coli*, other gram-negative rods, *S pneumoniae*, and *L monocytogenes*; less common pathogens include staphylococci, enterococci, *S viridans*, or *Candida*. In older infants and children, *N meningitidis* and *S pneumoniae* are the most frequent causes. *Haemophilus influenzae* type B (Hib) continues to be a common pathogen in young children who have not received adequate immunization.

The diagnosis of meningitis is confirmed by CSF analysis (**Table 8-8**); however, a lumbar puncture may place the patient at risk and may therefore be contraindicated. Lumbar punctures are contraindicated in cardiorespiratory instability, clotting abnormalities, signs of raised ICP (irregular pupils, absent doll's eye reflex, decerebrate or decorticate posturing, abnormal respiratory pattern, hypertension, bradycardia), recent (≤30 minutes) or prolonged (>30 minutes) seizure, local infection in the puncture site, Glasgow Coma Scale (GCS) score <13, with the presence of papilledema, localizing neurological signs, and intracranial mass or hydrocephalus. A normal computed tomographic (CT) scan does not rule out the possibility of cerebral herniation.

Empiric therapy is based on the age of the patient. Ampicillin combined with gentamicin or cefotaxime is the standard treatment in neonates. Ampicillin combined with cefotaxime or ceftriaxone is used in infants 1 to 3 months of age. Older infants and children can be treated with cefotaxime or ceftriaxone as well. Vancomycin should be considered when cephalosporin-resistant pneumococcus is suspected.

The use of steroids may be beneficial for *H influenzae* and pneumococcal meningitis. Steroids should be administered prior to starting antibiotics when bacterial meningitis is suspected. One recommended scheme is to administer 0.15 mg/kg of dexamethasone every 6 hours over the course of 4 days. Use of steroids is not currently recommended for neonates. Chemoprophylaxis in cases of *H influenzae* meningitis should be given to all household contacts with at least 1 susceptible contact (child <4 years of age who is incompletely immunized against Hib, child <12 months of age, or child who is immunocompromised). Chemoprophylaxis should also be given to nursery contacts in the presence of at least 2 cases of invasive disease within 2 months. Rifampicin 20 mg/kg/day for 4 days (maximum dose 600 mg) or 10 mg/kg/day in infants younger than 2 months is recommended. Pregnant women should receive ceftriaxone 125 mg IM. Chemoprophylaxis for meningococcal meningitis is the same as for meningococcemia. The recommended management for patients suspected of having increased ICP is described in **Table 8-9**.

> **!** *Antibiotic treatment should be started immediately in sick children with suspected bacterial meningitis even before a lumbar puncture is performed.* **!**

Table 8-8. Cerebrospinal Fluid Findings in Different Types of Meningitis

Type of Meningitis	Opening Pressure	Leucocytes mm^3	Glucose	Proteins
Bacterial	Elevated	100-10,000 (Usually >1000)	Low	++
Viral	Normal to elevated	10-1000 (Usually 100-500)	Usually normal	+
Tuberculous	Usually elevated	5-500	Normal to low	++++
Fungal	Usually elevated	5-500	Normal to low	++

2. Encephalitis

Acute encephalitis is characterized by changes in mental status. It is usually caused by a virus such as enterovirus, herpesvirus, Epstein-Barr, cytomegalovirus, arbovirus, or varicella zoster, among others. *Mycoplasma pneumoniae* and other etiologic agents may also be implicated.

Results of CSF investigation usually show some degree of pleocytosis but may also be normal. Polymerase chain reaction in CSF should be used to detect enterovirus and herpes simplex virus (HSV) infections. Central nervous system imaging with magnetic resonance imaging (MRI) is more sensitive than CT and may detect areas of inflammation or help rule out noninfectious causes. For instance, during HSV encephalitis, the MRI may show alterations in the temporal lobe, and the electroencephalogram (EEG) may show typical periodic lateralized epileptiform discharges (PLEDs). In patients with suspected HSV encephalitis, urgent treatment with acyclovir should always be considered until the infection can be ruled out with CSF PCRs. Ciprofloxacin, doxycycline, or azithromycin should be considered in patients with *M pneumoniae* encephalitis.

Table 8-9. Management of Children With Suspected Central Nervous System Infection and Signs of Increased Intracranial Pressure

Head of bed at 30°
Midline position of the head
Normothermia
Do not perform lumbar puncture if possibility of herniation exists.
Endotracheal intubation if GCS <8 or progressive deterioration of consciousness
Provide adequate sedation in ventilated patients.
Normoventilation. PCO_2 35 mm Hg
Osmotherapy if signs of cerebral herniation

Abbreviation: GCS, Glasgow Coma Scale.

3. Ventriculitis

Ventriculitis is an infection or inflammation of the ventricles usually associated with a ventriculoperitoneal shunt; it may present with or without shunt dysfunction. When shunt dysfunction is present, a CT scan may show ventricular enlargement. Cerebrospinal fluid should be obtained from the shunt reservoir in order to confirm an infectious etiology. The most frequent infecting organisms include coagulase-negative *Staphylococcus* species, *S aureus*, and gram-negative rods.

Initial antibiotic treatment usually includes vancomycin and a third-generation cephalosporin and is later adjusted according to the results of the CSF cultures. Rifampicin is sometimes used to improve CSF penetration. Removal of the ventricular shunt is mandatory in most cases, and intrathecal antibiotic treatment should be considered in some situations.

D. Pneumonia

Childhood pneumonia accounts for millions of deaths annually, most of which occur in developing countries. Most children with community-acquired pneumonia who are diagnosed in the early stages can be managed as ambulatory patients. Children with severe pneumonia or at risk of developing severe pneumonia should be promptly diagnosed and treated. The most frequently identified pathogens in children over 3 years of age include *S pneumoniae, M pneumoniae*, and *Chlamydophila* (formerly *Chlamydia*) *pneumoniae*. Less frequently found pathogens include *S pyogenes* and *S aureus*. Other pathogens, such as *Pseudomonas* species or *Pneumocystis jiroveci* (formerly *carinii*), may be present in immunosuppressed patients. Anaerobes should be suspected in those patients at risk for aspiration. The most frequent pathogens in younger children are viruses; other pathogens include *S pneumoniae* and *H influenzae*, although the latter is less frequent in immunized populations. Group B streptococci, *L monocytogenes*, and enteral gram-negative bacteria, among others, can affect neonates.

Chest radiograph is the main diagnostic tool; it helps to confirm the presence of pulmonary infection and its extension, and it is useful to rule out possible complications like empyema or atelectasis. Blood cultures may be positive in 20% to 30% of bacterial pneumonias. Nasopharyngeal aspirate helps to rule out or confirm a viral etiology when suspected. Antigen-detection tests for diverse pathogens can be performed using tracheal secretions, pleural fluid, blood, or urine. Bronchoalveolar lavage should be performed for microbiologic and histologic studies in immunocompromised children.

Children with respiratory distress or at risk of developing severe pneumonia should be observed closely. Frequent clinical evaluation of airway permeability and respiratory status is essential; blood gases should be used to evaluate ventilation and confirm oxygenation; and continuous monitoring of heart rate and rhythm, respiratory rate, and pulse oximetry should be used when possible. Support therapies include oxygen, intravenous (IV) fluids, and, in severe cases, advanced mechanical support.

Children with severe pneumonia need rapid initiation of antimicrobial treatment. The cause of the pneumonia is often unknown, and empiric treatment should be chosen in accordance with the clinical picture, risk factors, and epidemiology. Antibiotic options for neonates include ampicillin combined with gentamicin or cefotaxime. In young infants treatment may be started with cefotaxime. Clarithromycin, ampicillin, cefotaxime, or ceftriaxone are the antibiotics of choice in older children. Antipseudomonal antibiotics such as ceftazidime should be used in patients at risk for pseudomonas infections, including those with cystic fibrosis or with chronic respiratory failure on mechanical ventilation.

The treatment of children with pleural empyema should include evacuation of the pleural fluids and adequate antibiotic treatment. This is essential for the eradication of the infection and lung expansion. The fluid may be drained by means of needle thoracocentesis or, if it is purulent, by means of a chest tube. A chest ultrasound may be helpful in the diagnosis of a pleural effusion and in determining the best site for thoracocentesis.

E. Urinary Tract Infection

In children experiencing their first urinary tract infection (UTI), the most frequent pathogen is *E coli.* Other organisms, such as *Klebsiella, Proteus, P aeruginosa,* enterococci, *S epidermidis,* or *S faecalis,* may be present in children who have urinary tract obstruction or a urinary catheter.

The diagnosis of UTI is usually established with urinalysis and urine culture. The gold standard diagnostic technique is suprapubic aspiration; when this technique is used, any bacterial growth is indicative of infection. However, urine for a culture is most frequently obtained using the midstream, clean-catch technique. Brief catheterization may also be used, but it can introduce infection in a small percentage of children.

It can be difficult to differentiate upper urinary tract infection from lower urinary tract infection. High fever, leukocytosis and sometimes signs of bacteremia may be present in patients with acute pyelonephritis. The presence of enlarged kidneys in a renal ultrasound can help confirm the diagnosis.

Children with toxic appearance should always be treated with parenteral antibiotics. Cefotaxime, ceftriaxone, or the combination of ampicillin with an aminoglycoside are indicated in neonates and young children. Neonates with UTI should always receive parenteral treatment because of the high prevalence of concomitant bacteremia.

F. Peritonitis

Depending on the source of infection, peritoneal infections can be classified as primary peritonitis or secondary peritonitis. Peritonitis is considered primary when the peritoneal cavity is infected via hematogenous or lymphatic dissemination and the cause is a single organism. The bacterial organisms that most frequently cause primary peritonitis are *S pneumoniae*, GAS, and *E coli* or other enteric bacteria. The most frequent predisposing factor for primary peritonitis is the presence of ascites caused by cirrhosis, portal hypertension, or nephrotic syndrome.

Secondary peritonitis results from the rupture or extension of intra-abdominal viscus or abscess; therefore, it is usually polymicrobial. The most frequent pathogens are enteric gram-negative bacteria, such as *E coli, Klebsiella*, or *Enterobacter*, and anaerobes.

Any patient suspected of having peritonitis should be managed with the aid of a pediatric surgeon. Diagnostic techniques such as ultrasound or CT scan should help localize the focus of infection. Empiric antibiotic treatment for primary peritonitis is usually started with cefotaxime in combination with an aminoglycoside. Antibiotic treatment for secondary peritonitis should be aimed at treating anaerobic and gram-negative organisms. Ampicillin/sulbactam or ampicillin in combination with gentamicin and metronidazole or gentamicin in combination with clindamycin are used frequently. To improve gram-negative coverage in some patients, ceftazidime or meropenem should be considered.

G. Soft-Tissue Infections

Infections of the soft tissues are frequent in the pediatric population and can sometimes be the source of such severe diseases as toxic shock syndromes, sepsis, or meningitis. Superficial infections are usually monomicrobial. Deep infections are infrequent and can be monomicrobial or polymicrobial. Deep infections require imaging studies to confirm the diagnosis and to evaluate extension.

1. Cellulitis

Cellulitis is usually caused by *S aureus* and GAS. Complications associated with cellulitis include facial cellulitis, systemic involvement in immunodeficiency, rapidly spreading lesions, and areas of necrosis or gas formation.

Empiric antibiotic therapies include penicillinase-resistant penicillin, first-generation cephalosporins, clindamycin, cefuroxime, or ampicillin/sulbactam. Anti-pseudomonal and other gram-negative bacteria coverage should be considered in immunocompromised children or patients with hospital-acquired infections. Vancomycin should be used when resistant staphylococcal infection is a possibility.

2. Periorbital and Orbital Cellulitis

Case Study

A 2-year-old boy with edema of both eyelids of the right eye is referred from a community hospital. He has a 1 week history of nasal congestion and coughing, and a 2 day history of swollen eyelids. On examination he is febrile, with erythema and edema in the right upper and lower eyelids that do not allow proper examination of the eye. Nonetheless, the eyeball seems to be protruding mildly.

- What two clinical entities should be ruled out?
- What complementary studies are indicated?

Preseptal or periorbital cellulitis, which affects the eyelids and the preseptal space, is frequently seen in young children or infants. Orbital cellulitis may present as a direct infection of the orbit from wounds (*S aureus* and *S pyogenes*), hematogenous spread from bacteremia (*S pneumoniae*), or, more often, venous spread or direct spread from adjacent sites such as paranasal sinuses (*S pneumoniae, M catarrhalis, H influenzae*, or anaerobes). Children with periorbital cellulitis usually present with fever and a swollen and erythematous eyelid, and without systemic compromise. There is no pain on eye movement, and vision is not impaired.

Signs of meningitis must be ruled out. Orbital CT scan can be done to differentiate from orbital cellulitis. Antibiotic treatment for trauma or insect bites includes oxacillin or first-generation cephalosporins. Cefuroxime, third-generation cephalosporins, or ampicillin/sulbactam can be used in periorbital cellulitis secondary to sinusitis or hematogenous dissemination.

> **!** *Children with orbital cellulitis may appear irritable or toxic, with orbital pain that is exacerbated by eye movements.*

Orbital cellulitis is usually a complication of bacterial sinusitis spreading into the orbit. It presents with fever, eyelid edema, and induration, and may be difficult to differentiate from periorbital cellulitis. Later signs include headache, limitation of extraocular movement, proptosis, and decreased visual acuity. Imaging studies should be done to confirm the diagnosis, establish the presence of orbital collections that will need surgical drainage, and rule out epidural collections or cavernous sinus thrombosis. Cerebral CT should be considered in cases of orbital cellulitis due to the possibility of cerebral abscess. An ophthalmologist should always be consulted.

Treatment includes antibiotic therapy with cefotaxime or ceftriaxone and metronidazole if anaerobes are suspected. Surgical drainage should be performed when necessary.

H. Septic Arthritis and Osteomyelitis

Septic arthritis occurs more frequently during the first 2 years of life. The most frequent pathogen in all ages is *S aureus*. *Kingella kingae, S pneumoniae, N meningitidis*, or GAS may be found less frequently. *Haemophilus influenzae* can affect young infants with late immunization, whereas *N gonorrhoeae* may affect adolescents. Other pathogens, including enterobacteria, group B streptococci, *Candida*, and *Salmonella*, may be implicated in septic arthritis episodes in immunosuppressed children or neonates.

The treatment of septic arthritis should include an antistaphylococcic antibiotic, such as oxacillin, cefazolin, or cephalothin. Cefotaxime or ceftriaxone are the preferred initial treatments when other bacteria are suspected. Surgical treatment includes needle aspiration and, in some cases, surgical drainage.

Osteomyelitis is usually produced by *S aureus*. Less common pathogens include GAS, pneumococcus, *H influenzae*, gram-negative enteric bacteria, and *M tuberculosis*, among others. Antistaphylococcic coverage with antibiotics such as oxacillin, cefazolin, or cephalothin is the initial empiric antibiotic treatment. Cefotaxime or ceftriaxone is used when other pathogens are suspected.

IV. NOSOCOMIAL INFECTIONS

Nosocomial, or hospital-acquired, infections are localized or systemic illnesses that develop after hospitalization and are not incubating or present on admission. An infection that develops 2 days after admission may be nosocomial. Nosocomial infections are most frequently viral; however, bacterial and, less commonly, fungal infections are more closely linked to severe complications. Nosocomial infections produced by bacteria are often traced to the use of invasive devices: approximately half of all nosocomial infections are related to invasive procedures or associated with medical devices. Bacterial pathogens vary depending on the hospital flora, the specific area of the hospital, and the site of the infection. Isolated bacteria frequently include coagulase-negative staphylococci and gram-negative enteric rods.

Most common types of infection are bloodstream infections, pneumonia, urinary tract infections, surgical wound infections, and gastrointestinal tract infections. Other sites of nosocomial infection include the ear, nose and throat, eyes, skin, heart, and central nervous system. Among the conditions and situations associated with an increased risk of nosocomial infection are bone marrow or solid organ transplantation; oncologic disease; immunodeficiency; immunosuppressive therapy; the presence of a central venous line or other invasive device, such as an endotracheal tube, urinary catheter, or ventricular shunt; a history of antibiotic use; and burns or open wounds.

Signs of nosocomial infection vary depending on the organ affected and may range from readily evident (ie, skin infections) to difficult to detect (ie, intra-abdominal infection). Manifestations vary depending on the clinical condition of the patient.

Infections can be particularly difficult to detect in infants and patients who are receiving sedation. Thorough physical examination should include inspection of catheter insertion site and surgical wounds, and palpation of subcutaneous or tunneled medical devices, specifically looking for areas of tenderness. Investigations for nosocomial infections are summarized by site in **Table 8-10.**

Table 8-10. Investigations for Frequent Hospital-Acquired Infections

Infection	Investigation
Central line infection	Blood culture Semiquantitative or quantitative culture of each lumen
Pneumonia	Chest radiograph Tracheal aspirate: Gram stain and culture Nasopharyngeal aspirate Bronchoalveolar lavage if patient is intubated
Urinary tract infection	Urine analysis Urine culture Renal ultrasound if pyelonephritis is suspected
Wound infection	Percutaneous needle aspiration: Gram stain and culture
Gastrointestinal tract	Feces culture Identification of *Clostridium difficile* toxin

Special considerations when choosing empiric antibiotic treatment include patient's length of stay in the hospital; predominant hospital flora, particularly in the unit where the child has been admitted; etiology of previous infections; previous antibiotic treatment; source of infection, when evident; presence of any invasive medical devices (eg, central line, urinary catheter, endotracheal tube, or ventriculoperitoneal shunt); recent invasive procedures; host defenses and underlying disease; and transfused blood products or use of total parenteral nutrition (TPN).

Common empiric antibiotic therapy involves the combination of a third-generation cephalosporin and an aminoglycoside. Ceftazidime or meropenem should be considered for better gram-negative coverage. Vancomycin should be started in patients with suspected central-line infection if there is a high hospital rate of methicillin-resistant staphylococcus infection. The use of antifungal agents may be necessary in high-risk patients who have received broad-spectrum antibiotic treatment.

When a central venous catheter, urinary catheter, or other invasive medical device is the source of infection, it should be removed and any local purulent collections should be surgically eliminated.

V. ENDEMIC INFECTIONS

A. Dengue

Dengue is a viral febrile illness transmitted by mosquitoes, specifically, members of the *Aedes aegypti* species. It is produced by 4 closely related viruses of the Flaviviridae family. The regions with populations typically affected by this illness are Southeast Asia, Central and South America, Australia, Oceania, some Eastern European countries, and the northern border of Mexico.

The severity of dengue can range from an asymptomatic infection to the extreme forms of dengue hemorrhagic fever (DHF) and dengue shock syndrome. Clinical forms of dengue are characterized by a sudden onset of signs and symptoms that emerge after an incubation period of 3 to 14 days. In the less severe form of dengue, the signs and symptoms include fever, rash, myalgia, arthralgia, headache, nausea, vomiting, and bleeding complications, such as epistaxis, gum bleeding, or hematuria. The more severe manifestations of the disease include encephalitis, myocardial disease, pneumonia, hepatitis, and gastrointestinal bleeding. The most severe form of the disease is DHF. It is characterized by the presence of fever, bleeding manifestations, thrombocytopenia, and evidence of increased capillary permeability, such as increased hematocrit, pleural effusion, or hypoalbuminemia. If there are signs of shock, it is classified as dengue shock syndrome. Bleeding manifestations range from petechiae to diffuse bleeding, sometimes only evident with a tourniquet test. The tourniquet test is assessed by inflating an appropriately sized blood pressure cuff on the patient's arm to above venous pressure (70 mm Hg) for 5 minutes and then relieving the pressure. The test is considered to be positive when more than 20 petechiae are seen in an area 2.5 cm^2.

Laboratory diagnosis is made based on serology. The preferred serological test is detection of immunoglobulin M (IgM) by enzyme immunoassay. Specific IgM antibodies can be detected in most patients during the first week symptoms are present. Virus-isolation techniques and PCR to detect dengue RNA are effective, but they are not used routinely.

Management is supportive. Dengue hemorrhagic fever should be suspected in children who meet all of the following criteria:

- Fever (high and continuous, duration of 2-7 days)
- Hemorrhagic diathesis
- Thrombocytopenia (<100,000 platelets/mm^3)
- Hemoconcentration (increase in hematocrit of 20% or more in relation to baseline tests or other evidence of plasma leakage, such as pleural effusion or hypoproteinemia)

Children who meet the diagnostic criteria for DHF should be carefully examined for signs of shock. When shock is not present, management is based on adequate fluid administration (enteral or IV), treatment of fever with paracetamol, daily hematocrit determination, and careful monitoring of vital signs and fluid balance.

In patients with clinical signs of shock (tachycardia, weak pulses, cold extremities, narrow pulse pressure, hypotension, and restlessness or lethargy), early and aggressive management can avoid further deterioration and progression to multiorgan failure. The primary treatment is to replace fluids that have been lost as a result of increased permeability. Fluid boluses are given until vital signs improve. Maintenance fluids are started at a rate that is guided by hematocrit, urinary output, and vital signs. Fluid boluses containing 0.9% saline or Ringer's lactate at 10 to 20 mL/kg should be administered as quickly as possible and repeated as needed. Colloid boluses should be considered if there is no improvement after boluses totaling 60 mL/kg and hematocrit remains high. Blood transfusion should be given to patients with low hematocrit. The use of blood products is summarized in **Table 8-11**. Disturbances in electrolytes and acid base are frequent and should be treated and carefully monitored.

Table 8-11. Use of Blood Products in Dengue

Blood Product	Indication
Blood transfusion	Significant clinical bleeding Persistent shock with declining hematocrit after adequate volume replacement
Platelet transfusion	<50,000 platelets/mm^3 in the presence of bleeding <20,000 platelets/mm^3 without bleeding
Cryoprecipitate and fresh frozen plasma	Disseminated intravascular coagulation

B. Hantavirus

Hantavirus pulmonary syndrome is present in North and South America and in areas of Asia. Hantavirus epidemics are usually associated with an increase in rodent populations. This disease is characterized by severe pulmonary edema resulting from increased vascular permeability and shock. Hemoconcentration is a consequence of the loss of intravascular fluid. Early signs include severe myalgia and abdominal pain. The cardiovascular and respiratory support in the pediatric intensive care unit (PICU) allows for the recovery of the patient until the capillary leak syndrome resolves. The diagnosis is based in the detection of IgM and immunoglobulin G (IgG) antibodies measured by enzyme-linked immunosorbent assay (ELISA). Other diagnostic methods are reverse transcription PCR in blood or immunohistochemical staining of tissue samples. There is no specific treatment for this virus.

C. Malaria

Malaria is a parasitic infection that continues to cause the death of millions of people in endemic areas throughout the world. The infection occurs most commonly in Africa, Asia, Oceania, Central America, and regions of South America. Children between 6 months and 5 years of age are a heavily affected population. There are 4 species of *Plasmodium* that infect humans. Of these, the most common is *P falciparum.*

The clinical picture includes high fever with chills, sweat, rigor, and headache. Other signs and symptoms may include nausea, vomiting, diarrhea, abdominal pain, pallor, and jaundice. Fever is usually cyclic, appearing every other day or every third day.

Possible complications may include

- Hypovolemia, vascular collapse, and shock
- Hypoglycemia
- Metabolic acidosis, usually lactic acidosis
- Severe anemia
- Cerebral malaria characterized by signs that include seizures, increased ICP, confusion, or coma
- Respiratory failure with or without pulmonary edema
- Renal failure

The diagnosis is based on the presence of the parasite in a peripheral blood smear. Because of the potential for drug resistance, particularly in *Pfalciparum* malaria, every positive smear should be assessed and the parasitemia reported. When malaria is strongly suspected, blood smears should be repeated at least once daily for 3 days. Generally, the parasitemia will drop very quickly; however, in cases of drug resistance, the level may actually increase over time. Polymerase chain reaction has shown to be effective for early parasite detection.

The indicators of severity are

- Parasitemia greater than 20% in endemic areas or 10% in nonendemic areas
- Base deficit <–8
- Hypoglycemia
- GCS of 8 or less
- Respiratory failure
- Renal failure and oliguria

Complications must be treated aggressively. Patients with signs of shock should be resuscitated with fluids and vasoactive drugs. Blood glucose should be monitored closely, and corrections should be made if there is hypoglycemia. Mechanical ventilation is indicated for respiratory failure, refractory shock, and GCS of 8 or less. Children with severe cerebral malaria should be managed similarly to children with increased ICP.

Antimicrobial treatment for severe malaria includes quinidine gluconate combined with doxycycline, tetracycline, or clindamycin. Other antibiotics should be added if bacterial superinfection is suspected.

Key Points

Acute Infections

- Signs and symptoms of infection are multiple and vary with age. Detection of potentially severe infections is based on meticulous clinical examination.
- Adequate cultures should be taken before starting antibiotic treatment unless there are specific contraindications.
- The choice of antibiotics depends on the patient's age, the type of infection suspected, and risk factors such as immunosuppression, presence of invasive medical devices, or recent hospitalization.
- Severe infections and localizing signs of infection can be difficult to detect in young children, infants, and neonates. Management is based on risk factors, toxic appearance, and laboratory findings.
- Suspicion of sepsis implies rapid management with goal-directed therapy. Antibiotic treatment should be started within the first hour.
- *Staphylococcus aureus* and *S pyogenes* can produce invasive diseases such as toxic shock syndrome.
- Meningococcemia should be considered in all children with fever and petechiae.
- Meningitis should always be treated urgently. Lumbar puncture can be diagnostic, but there are contraindications for this procedure. Acyclovir treatment for HSV encephalitis should be considered in patients with fever and disturbances of consciousness.
- Pneumonia continues to be a cause of high mortality in some areas of the world. Pathogens vary depending on age. *Haemophilus influenzae* continues to be a leading cause of infection in geographic regions with little immunization available.
- Hospitalized children with fever should be suspected of having nosocomial infections. The most frequent bacteria involved in nosocomial infections include coagulase-negative staphylococci and gram-negative enteric rods.
- Infected lines or medical devices should be removed.
- Endemic infections, such as dengue and malaria, affect vast areas of the world and produce high mortality when not treated adequately. These infections should always be considered in patients from such regions.

Suggested Readings

1. American College of Emergency Physicians Clinical Policies Committee; American College of Emergency Physicians Clinical Policies Subcommittee on Pediatric Fever. Clinical policy for children younger than three years presenting to the emergency department with fever. *Ann Emerg Med.* 2003;42:530-545.

2. Carcillo JA. Pediatric septic shock and multiple organ failure. *Crit Care Clin.* 2003;19(3):413-440.

3. Carcillo JA, Field AI, Task Force Committee Members. Clinical practice parameters for hemodynamic support of pediatric and neonatal patients in septic shock. *Crit Care* Med. 2002;30:1365-1378.

4. Goldstein B, Giroir B, Randolph A, et al. International Pediatric Sepsis Consensus Conference: definitions for sepsis and organ dysfunction in pediatrics. *Pediatr Crit Care Med.* 2005;6:2-8.

5. Hart CA, Thomson AP. Meningococcal disease and its management in children. *BMJ.* 2006;30:333(7570):685-690.

6. Isturiz R, Torres J, Besso J. Global distribution of infectious diseases requiring intensive care. *Crit Care Clin.* 2006;22:469-488.

7. McIntosh K. Community acquired pneumonia in children. *N Engl J Med.* 2002; 7:346(6):429-437.

8. Melendez E, Bachur R. Advances in the emergency management of pediatric sepsis. *Curr Opin Pediatr.* 2006;18:245-253.

9. Pickering LK, Baker CJ, Long SS, McMillan JA, eds. *Red Book: 2006 Report of the Committee on Infectious Diseases.* 27th ed. Elk Grove Village, IL: American Academy of Pediatrics; 2006.

10. Pollard AJ, Britto J, Nadel S, et al. Emergency management of meningococcal disease. *Arch Dis Child.* 1999;80:290-296.

Chapter 9:

FLUIDS AND ELECTROLYTES

Objectives

- Summarize basic concepts in the maintenance of intravascular fluid homeostasis.
- Discuss the common electrolyte disturbances, their recognition, and management.
- Describe common endocrine emergencies, including those related to glucose metabolism, and discuss their management.

Case Study

A 12-month-old infant presents to the emergency department, via emergency medical service, with a 3-day history of vomiting, diarrhea, and temperature to 40°C (104° F). The patient is lethargic and has cracked lips and sunken fontanelle. Laboratory results are as follows: Na^+, 125 mEq/L; K^+ 4.8 mEq/L; Cl^- 89 mEq/L; Glu 89 mg/dL; CO_2 7 mEq/L; BUN 50 mg/dL; Creat 1.2 mg/dL.

- What is your diagnosis?
- After initial fluid boluses with isotonic saline, what is your plan for ongoing fluid management?
- If the sodium level drops to 117 mEq/L and the patient begins to seize, how will you respond?

Fluid and electrolyte disturbances are commonly seen in hospitalized children. An individualized approach to the fluid management of these children is required, based on the underlying diagnosis and severity of illness.

I. FLUIDS

A. Maintenance Fluids

The fluid intake required to maintain an euvolemic state is largely dependent on the patient's initial hydration status and underlying disease state.

The term *maintenance fluids* loosely denotes the quantity of intravenous (IV) fluids required to maintain hydration in an euvolemic child who is not experiencing abnormal ongoing loss of fluids as seen in gastrointestinal diseases, bleeding, and burns. The maintenance fluid calculations provide a rapid and convenient starting point for determining the amount of fluid required to maintain intravascular volume.

The Holliday-Segar method for calculating maintenance IV fluids is based on the caloric expenditure in fixed weight categories. Calculations are based on the patient's dry/baseline weight.

First 10 kg: fluid requirement is 100 mL/kg/day or 4 mL/kg/hr.

10-20 kg: for each kilogram of body weight above 10 kg, add 50 mL/kg/day or 2 mL/kg/hr to the initial 40 mL/hr (above).

Above 20 kg: for each kilogram of body weight above 20 kg, add 20 mL/kg/day or 1 mL/kg/hr to the 60 mL/hr (above).

EXAMPLE: A 26-kg child, who is NPO and awaiting surgery, would have a maintenance fluid requirement of 40+20+6 = 66 mL/hr of IV fluid.

> !
>
> *This method is not applicable to neonates younger than 2 weeks of age.*

Other methods are available and utilize nomograms for body surface area and caloric expenditure to determine fluid requirements. We have purposely limited ourselves to describing only one widely used methodology.

> !
>
> *Pediatric patients have been shown to develop hyponatremia when given hypotonic fluids within the hospital setting. The use of isotonic fluids (D5NS, D5LR) in hospitalized patients is advocated to prevent the development of hyponatremia.*

Maintenance fluids in children historically have been hypotonic (i.e., 0.225% normal saline [NS]). These are based on the daily electrolyte requirements in healthy children who require approximately 2-4 mEq/kg of sodium and 1-2 mEq/kg of potassium. This translates to approximately D5 .225% NS or ¼ % NS with 20 mEq/L of potassium chloride (KCl). This replacement fluid provides the required amount of sodium and potassium to keep these electrolytes within the normal range for patients without any significant additional losses or renal impairment. Traditional replacement fluids of ¼% normal saline may lead to hyponatremia in the ill child. Selecting a solution with ½% normal saline or 0.9% normal saline are the preferred maintenance solutions for the ill child.

Potassium in replacement IV fluids should be withheld until the patient has satisfactory urine output to avoid a risk of inducing hyperkalemia. The general practice of adding 20 mEq/L of KCl to the IV fluid solution and a "one-size-fits-all" approach to KCl concentrations in IV fluids should be avoided. The amount of KCl in the IV fluid should be individualized to the patient as urine and stool output and other parameters can affect potassium requirements.

B. Resuscitation Fluids

Resuscitation fluids in infants and children remain exclusively isotonic. Initial recommendations for treating hypovolemia include 20 mL/kg boluses of normal saline. Immediate reassessment and repeat boluses need to be done quickly (up to 60 mL/kg in 30-60 min). Most resuscitation protocols suggest that initial fluid resuscitation should begin with crystalloid (normal saline or Ringer's lactate). After 60 mL/kg of crystalloid has been administered, the use of colloid should be considered.

C. Fluid Resuscitation in Shock

Hypovolemia remains the most common cause of shock worldwide due to gastroenteritis. Rapid restoration of intravascular volume with fluid replacement remains the key to survival. Patients with inadequate or delayed fluid resuscitation are at risk of developing organ dysfunction or progressing to irreversible shock. Regardless of the type of shock, some degree of hypovolemia is usually present and IV fluid therapy is always part of the initial resuscitative measures. An exception to this is cardiogenic shock. These patients tend to be exquisitely sensitive to volume overload and administration of fluid in these patients must be done judiciously.

Rapid IV or intraosseous access should be established to provide a means of delivering the fluid and medications required during resuscitation.

Each bolus should be administered within 5-10 min or as rapidly as permitted by the vascular access. Reassessment of vital signs and clinical status must be conducted between boluses to assess for changes in clinical status and response to therapy.

II. ELECTROLYTE ABNORMALITIES

Electrolyte abnormalities are common in children. Occasionally these abnormalities are due to iatrogenic causes. Severe electrolyte disturbances can present with poor feeding or irritability and can result in dehydration, shock, seizures, coma, or even death.

> !
>
> *Serum osmolality can be measured in the laboratory and can also be calculated using the formula: (2 X sodium) + (glucose/18) + BUN/2.8 = serum osmolality. Normal serum osmolality range: 285-295 mOsm/L.*
>
> !

Osmolar Gap

- Osmolar gap = measured osmoles – calculated osmoles
- Calculated osmolality = $2Na^+ + \frac{Glucose}{18} + \frac{BUN}{2.8}$
- Sodium is measured in mEq/L, glucose and BUN in mg/dL.
- Normal osmolar gap is 3-10 mOsm/kg.
- A high osmolar gap is seen with toxins such as methanol, ethylene glycol, acetone, and isopropranol.

Normal Anion Gap Metabolic Acidosis (Bicarbonate Loss)

- Gastrointestinal losses of HCO_3
- Renal losses

High Anion Gap Metabolic Acidosis (MUDPILES)

- Methanol
- Uremia
- Diabetic ketoacidosis (DKA)
- Paraldehyde, phenformin
- Iron, isoniazid, isopropanol
- Lactic acidosis
- Ethanol, ethylene glycol
- Salicylates

> !
>
> *The anion gap is calculated as: Na^+ (mEq/L) – [Cl^- (mEq/L) + HCO_3^- (mEq/L)]. A normal anion gap ranges from 10 to 14. The anion gap is helpful in distinguishing various disease states in patients who present with metabolic acidosis. A high anion gap metabolic acidosis is due to the presence of anions, such as those from organic acids as seen in poisonings or ingestion of toxins.*
>
> !

A. Sodium (Na^+)

1. Hyponatremia

Hyponatremia is defined as a serum sodium level <135 mEq/L. The sodium level can be decreased due to a variety of causes: increased free water intake (dilute infant formula, polydipsia, infants drinking pool water), increased water retention (syndrome of inappropriate antidiuretic hormone [SIADH], renal failure), and increased sodium losses (gastroenteritis, diuretics, adrenal insufficiency).

a. Signs and Symptoms

Symptoms of hyponatremia include: irritability, poor feeding, nausea and vomiting, lethargy, seizures, and eventually coma and death.

> **!** *A change in mental status and other neurological signs are important clues to the need for emergent treatment.* **!**

b. Common Causes

Hyponatremia may occur because of significant sodium losses due to gastroenteritis, ostomy output, excessive sweating, cystic fibrosis, heatstroke, burns, or third spacing in pancreatitis or pleural effusions (**Table 9-1**). Children on diuretics are frequently hyponatremic. Renal diseases such as renal tubular acidosis can cause loss of salt and water. In hospitalized children, excess secretion of anti-diuretic hormone (ADH) leads to the development of the SIADH. Infants may present in the first few months of life with severe hyponatremia secondary to water intoxication from overly diluted formula or from swallowing large amounts of water in swimming or wading pools. Other causes include post-obstructive uropathy and losses secondary to ventriculostomy drainage.

Table 9-1. Causes of Hyponatremia

Normovolemia	Hypervolemia	Hypovolemia
SIADH	Congestive Heart Failure	Diarrhea
Adrenal Insufficiency	Renal Failure (Acute/Chronic)	Vomiting
Central Nervous System Disease	Nephrotic Syndrome	Burns
Pulmonary Disease	Cirrhosis	Pancreatitis

c. Treatment of Hyponatremia

Urgent treatment of hyponatremia should be initiated in all patients who exhibit neurological changes or seizures. If the serum sodium is <120 mEq/L a hypertonic saline solution should be administered, if available. Most frequently, 3% NaCl (513 mmol/L) is used. Ideally, 3% saline should be given through a central venous line. Administration of 3% saline through a peripheral IV or an intraosseous needle is acceptable during an emergency when establishment of central venous access is likely to take time to accomplish. The goal is to raise the serum sodium level to 120-125 mEq/L or until seizures stop. To raise the serum sodium level, administer the calculated amount of hypertonic saline over 15-20 minutes in order to gain rapid control of the seizures. A 1.2 mL/kg aliquot of 3% NaCl will raise the level by 1 mEq/L. If hypertonic saline solution is unavailable, a 20 mL/kg bolus of normal saline (0.9% NS) may be given.

Once the acute correction is completed or if the patient is not having neurological changes, correction of hyponatremia should proceed more slowly at approximately 12 mEq/L per day (0.5 to 1 mEq/L every hour). In adults, the syndrome of central pontine myelinolysis (osmotic demyelination) has been described in patients who had a rapid increase in serum sodium values.

> !
>
> *It is important to partially correct clinically significant hyponatremia rapidly (e.g., until seizures stop). However, the total correction should be done slowly and carefully.*
>
> !

Formula to calculate the amount of sodium required to correct to a desired mEq/L:
0.6 x (Wt in kg) x (target Na^+ – measured Na^+) =
Total mEq of Na^+ required to raise sodium level to target.

Example: A 6-week-old child (4 kg) presents with seizures and is found to have a sodium level of 114 mEq/L.

First step: acute correction

- You decide to give 3% saline to correct to 120 mEq/L.
- Amount of NaCl = 0.6 x 4 kg x (120-114)= 14.4 mEq of Na^+
- 3% NaCl = 0.5 mEq/L or approx 28 mL of 3% NaCl solution

or

- (1.2 mL/kg) of 3% NaCl raises the serum sodium approx 1 mEq/L
- 1.2 mL x 4 kg x (120-114) = 28 mL of 3 % NaCl solution

Second step: slower correction

- You need to raise the serum sodium level an additional 12 mEq/day from the 120 mEq/L.
- 0.6 x 4 kg x (132 desired Na^+ – 120 actual Na^+) = 29 mEq/L additional sodium needed over the remainder of the 24 hours
- A good fluid to start replacement is either normal saline or D5 ½% NS, with or without appropriate potassium at maintenance fluid rates. Additionally, the calculated deficit is added to this and administered over 12-24 hours.

d. Syndrome of Inappropriate Antidiuretic Hormone (SIADH)

i. Diagnosis

SIADH, by definition, is caused by an inappropriate release of ADH. When patients are hypertonic or significantly hypovolemic, there is an appropriate release of ADH with resultant decrease in urine output in an effort to maximize the circulating intravascular volume. In SIADH, the intravascular volume is normal or elevated and yet the urine output drops off. The diagnosis of SIADH requires three elements: low urine output, hyponatremia, and inappropriately concentrated urine (with elevated urinary sodium).

> ! *SIADH is a common cause of hyponatremia in the hospitalized patient.* !

ii. Causes

The causes of SIADH fall into four groups: central nervous system (CNS) [e.g., infection, trauma, surgery, tumors, shunts, hypoxic-ischemic injury]; pulmonary (e.g., pneumonia, effusions, positive pressure ventilation, asthma, tumors); drugs (e.g., carbamazepine [Tegretol], vinca alkaloids, narcotics, aspirin [ASA], ecstasy, selective serotonin reuptake inhibitors [SSRIs]); and tumors (e.g., leukemia, lymphoma, neuroblastoma).

iii. Treatment

The treatment for SIADH is water restriction. Reducing water intake to 50% maintenance will often allow a free water diuresis and improve the serum sodium measurement. It is occasionally necessary to correct the sodium level with salt supplementation and diuretic administration.

e. Hyponatremia due to Water Intoxication

Water intoxication occurs when powdered formula is diluted with an excessive amount of water, either inadvertently (not following directions) or purposely (to make the formula last longer), resulting in hyponatremia in the infant. This is a common occurrence and also is seen when formula or an electrolyte solution, such as Pedialyte, is being diluted with water when an infant has gastroenteritis and diarrhea.

Infant swimming is another potential source of hyponatremia. It follows after ingestion of large amounts of water by the infant playing in a bathtub, wading pool, or splash tub. The infant presents with irritability and poor appetite. A targeted history and check of the serum sodium level reveals the cause.

2. Hyponatremia and Hypovolemic States

a. Non-renal

i. Gastroenteritis

Worldwide, gastroenteritis is the leading cause of death in children between 1 and 5 years of age. Typically the history is that of large and frequent watery stools, and the patient presents in various stages of dehydration and possibly hypovolemic shock. Depending on the severity of the hypovolemia, the patient might require aggressive and timely fluid resuscitation with isotonic fluids.

ii. Third Spacing

Sepsis and peritonitis are examples of conditions where fluid can leak into the interstitial space. This can occur fairly rapidly over a matter of hours, leading to hypovolemia and hyponatremia because water as well as electrolytes move into the interstitial spaces. Patients present with clinical evidence of shock and hypovolemia. Serum electrolytes reveal hyponatremia, and potentially hypokalemia and hypocalcemia.

> !
>
> *Anytime a neonate presents with hyponatremia, hyperkalemia, hypoglycemia, and acidosis, a diagnosis of congenital adrenal hyperplasia must be considered. Immediate management includes a random cortisol measurement, correction of hypoglycemia, fluid resuscitation and replacement, and stress doses of glucocorticoid and mineralocorticoids.*
>
> !

iii. Fluid Losses

Burns result in rapid and excessive loss of fluid due to a capillary leak phenomenon. Fluid losses are both external (across the surface area involved in the burn) and internal (into the interstitial spaces). Rapid and ongoing fluid resuscitation is required in the management of burns/thermal injuries.

b. Renal

Diuretics can lead to hyponatremia with both short- and long-term use. Loop diuretics, such as furosemide and bumetanide, and drugs that interfere with renal tubular reabsorption, such as metolazone, can lead to significant hyponatremia. Other renal causes of hyponatremia are renal tubular acidosis, interstitial nephritis, and obstructive uropathy.

c. Other Causes of Hyponatremia

i. Cerebral Salt Wasting (CSW)

This is a poorly understood condition in terms of exact pathophysiology. Hyponatremia occurs in the setting of normal to high urine output, and urinary sodium excretion is elevated. Patients tend to be hypovolemic and exhibit symptoms of dehydration and hyponatremia. The condition is seen in conjunction with intracranial injury, intracranial tumors, and neurosurgical procedures. It is important to distinguish CSW from SIADH, which also presents with hyponatremia but without the hypovolemia seen in CSW. Treatment of SIADH includes fluid restriction, whereas fluid replacement and correction of hyponatremia is the therapeutic approach in CSW. Urinary sodium also tends to be higher in CSW (may be >100mEq/L) than in SIADH.

ii. Increased Total Body Sodium Associated with Serum Hyponatremia

Congestive heart failure (CHF), renal failure, and nephrotic syndrome are examples of hypervolemic conditions associated with hyponatremia despite an increase in total body sodium content. The hyponatremia is dilutional in these cases, and sodium intake restrictions are an important part of the management. Treatment is directed toward the underlying condition – diuretics and inotropes for CHF, steroids and diuretics in nephrotic syndrome, and dialysis in renal failure.

3. Hypernatremia

Hypernatremia is defined as a serum sodium of >145 mEq/L. At-risk groups for elevated sodium are infants, toddlers, and critically ill patients. Hypernatremia occurs when too much salt is ingested or too much free water is lost. Children who develop hypernatremia may have received concentrated formula, been breast-fed without supplementation, or been treated with salt supplements or sodium bicarbonate. Free water loss can be due to diarrhea, diabetes insipidus (central or nephrogenic), renal tubular disorders, or post-obstructive diuresis.

a. Signs and Symptoms

Signs and symptoms of hypernatremia include irritability, high-pitched cry, lethargy, seizures, fever, renal failure, and rhabdomyolysis. In infants, these symptoms mimic those of infections and sepsis.

b. Treatment

It is essential that hypernatremia is treated slowly and carefully. When the sodium goes up the serum osmolality increases, and fluid moves from inside the cells to the serum in an attempt to achieve balance. This increases the osmolality inside the cell. Administration of free water results in movement from low osmolality (i.e., serum) to higher osmolality (i.e., inside the cell), causing the cell to swell. This can result in cerebral edema.

It is essential to correct hypernatremia slowly. Most recommendations are to lower serum sodium values no more than 0.5 mEq/L/hr or 12 mEq/L/day.

To calculate the amount of free water necessary to correct the serum sodium:

> ! *4 mL/kg of free water will drop the sodium by 1 mEq/L.* !

Free water deficit = (Wt in kg x 0.6) x 1 – (desired Na^+/ actual Na^+) (1000 mL/L)

Example: 8-kg 10-month-old infant with serum sodium of 157 mEq/L

Free water deficit = (8 x 0.6) x 1 – (145/157) x (1000 mL/L)

365 mL = 4.8 x 0.076 (1000 mL/L)

> ! *D5 ½ normal saline with 20 mEq/L KCl is an excellent choice of replacement fluid (as long as urine output is adequate).* !

Quick Calculation:
4 mL x 8 kg x 12 mEq/L = 384 mL of free water

Maintenance fluid amounts for an 8-kg child are
(100 mL/kg x 8) = 800mL/24 hrs

1 L of ½ normal saline = 500 mL of free water
1 L of ¼ normal saline = 750mL of free water
1 L of D5 ½ NS will provide 400 mL of free water and is a good starting point.

Frequent measurement of the serum sodium is necessary to follow the gradual fall of the sodium level and make appropriate fluid changes.

4. Hypernatremia due to Diabetes Insipidus (DI)

Diabetes insipidus is an uncommon condition that results in severe hypernatremia and excessive free water loss. The etiology of DI is either CNS or nephrogenic (inherited or acquired). The diagnosis in the acute case is made by observing polyuria, a urine specific gravity <1.005, urine osmolality of <200 mOsm/L, serum hypernatremia, and hyperosmolality (serum osmolality of ≥295 mOsm/L).

The most common causes in the acute setting are CNS injuries, including severe head trauma and tumors (craniopharyngiomas). Elevated intracranial pressure can cause DI, and it is commonly seen in association with brain death. Nephrogenic DI is relatively rare, usually presents in a less acute setting, and is most commonly due to a hereditary defect. Treatment of DI consists of replacement of free water and administration of intranasal or intravenous DDAVP or vasopressin with strict monitoring of fluid balance and electrolytes.

B. Potassium (K^+)

Potassium, the most abundant cation in intracellular fluid, is involved in many cellular processes, including protein synthesis. Maintenance of a transmembrane potential results in an electrical gradient across cell membranes. Changes in this resting membrane potential result in muscle excitation and nerve conduction. In particular, potassium plays a key role in myocardial contractility and function.

Potassium levels in the body are tightly regulated by renal excretion – the main mechanism being distal tubular secretion; however, patients might develop hyperkalemia due to a combination of renal dysfunction and increased potassium release from injured tissue.

1. Hypokalemia

Hypokalemia, defined as a potassium level <3.5 mEq/L, may occur due to inadequate intake, renal losses, gastrointestinal losses, following insulin therapy and in association with metabolic alkalosis. Diuretics (especially furosemide and bumetanide), hyperventilation, mannitol, β- agonists (e.g., frequent use of inhaled bronchodilators), and amphotericin B can cause hypokalemia. Gastrointestinal losses via continuous nasogastric suctioning or diarrhea can also result in a significant drop in serum potassium levels.

a. Diagnosis

Signs and symptoms include fatigue and paresthesias. Electrocardiogram (ECG) changes, including U waves and ventricular dysrhythmias, can occur when the potassium level drops below 2.5 mEq/L. Treatment of hypokalemia may include oral or IV supplementation depending on the patient's status and the urgency of symptoms.

> **!** *The most important complication of hypokalemia is hyperkalemia! Potassium levels could end up being significantly elevated by vigorous or too rapid IV replacement of potassium.*

b. Treatment of hypokalemia

If the patient is receiving enteral feedings, the safest approach to correcting asymptomatic hypokalemia (no ECG changes) would be the gradual replacement of potassium by adding it to the dietary intake. Supplements of 1-3 mEq/kg/day can be administered enterally in three or four divided doses to correct hypokalemia or to prevent it in patients who are on diuretics without potassium-sparing properties. Potassium chloride can be an irritant to the gastric mucosa, might not be well tolerated, and may result in diarrhea.

A conservative protocol for IV replacement:

- For K^+ levels of 3.0-3.5 mEq/L, administer 0.25 mEq/kg of IV KCl over 1 hour.
- For K^+ levels of 2.5-3.0 mEq/L, administer 0.5 mEq/kg of IV KCl over 2 hours.

- For K^+ levels less than 2.5 mEq/L, administer 0.75 mEq/L of IV KCl over 3 hours. A potassium level should be checked halfway through this infusion.
- A conservative and safe aproach is to admister no more than 0.5 mEq/kg/hr of KCl in a single IV replacement dose, with a maximum dose of 10 mEq over 1 hr. These recommendations are considerably more stringent than what is employed in the care of adults.
- KCl infusion is recommended to be administered via a central venous line or a large bore IV with adequate intravenous solution dilution whenever possible.

2. Hyperkalemia

> !
>
> *Hyperkalemia (potassium levels> 5.5 mEq/L) can be a life-threatening emergency.*
>
> !

Hyperkalemia, or potassium levels >5.5 mEq/L, require urgent confirmation and rapid institution of therapy to lower the levels, especially if ECG changes are present. Since renal clearance of excess potassium is fairly efficient, hyperkalemia is unusual in the setting of adequate renal function. The condition can occur as a result of renal failure (acute or chronic), hypoaldosteronism, adrenal insufficiency, metabolic acidosis, muscle and tissue necrosis (rhabdomyolysis, burns, crush injuries), tumor lysis syndrome, and excessive intake or administration of potassium. Acidosis plays a role as well, increasing potassium levels by 0.5 mEq/L for every 0.1 decrease in the pH. Medications such as potassium-sparing diuretics (spironolactone [Aldactone]), angiotensin-converting enzyme inhibitors, and digoxin [Lanoxin] can also lead to hyperkalemia especially in the setting of concomitant renal dysfunction. Hemolysis from heel-stick blood sampling or tourniquet application is a common cause of spurious elevation of potassium levels. However, it should not be assumed that this is the cause without demonstrating a normal potassium on a repeated free-flowing sample without hemolysis.

a. Signs and Symptoms

Signs and symptoms of hyperkalemia are usually related to inadequate cardiac output due to arrhythmias. ECG changes include tall, peaked T waves, widening of the QRS complex, atrioventricular block, bradycardia, and eventually ventricular tachycardia or asystole. Weakness and paresthesias can occur when K^+ levels are >7 mEq/L.

b. Treatment

Hyperkalemia requires urgent intervention and therapy.

1. Place the patient on a cardiorespiratory monitor with rhythm strip and obtain a 12-lead ECG.

2. Recheck the electrolytes to confirm the hyperkalemia.

3. Discontinue any exogenous potassium being administered.

4. Administer one or more of the following therapies:

- Calcium gluconate,100 mg/kg over 3 min (1 mL/kg of 10% solution) intravenously to stabilize the myocardium and prevent arrhythmias.

- Sodium bicarbonate, 1-2 mEq/kg given IV over 10-15 min. Ensure the adequacy of ventilation prior to administration. Since calcium and bicarbonate will precipitate, the line must be flushed clear between these two medications.

- Insulin-glucose infusion to move potassium intracellularly. Insulin, 0.1 U/kg/hr, mixed with D25% solution equivalent to 0.5 g/kg/hr (2 mL/kg/hr). If more concentrated dextrose solutions are not available, 10 mL/kg/hour of D5% can be administered with the insulin infusion. The first hour's dose can even be administered rapidly (over 30 min) prior to initiating the continuous infusion. Glucose levels should be followed hourly for the duration of this infusion.

- An exchange resin, such as sodium polystyrene resin (Kayexalate), administered 1 g/kg rectally. If the patient's hemodynamics and airway are stable, it can be administered orally or by nasogastric tube at the same dose (1g/kg) every 6 hr. This agent exchanges sodium for potassium along the gastrointestinal tract in an approximate ratio of 1 g/kg resin to 1 mEq/L decrease in K^+ level. Sodium levels should be monitored if more than one dose of this agent is used due to the potential for hypernatremia.

5. Emergency hemodialysis should be initiated in addition to the above steps if the hyperkalemia is life-threatening and immediate correction is desired. Because it takes time to initiate this, particularly if a large-bore indwelling line is required, all other modalities mentioned above should be instituted as well.

C. Magnesium (Mg^+)

Magnesium is a co-factor for adenosine triphosphate (ATP) -related functions, such as oxidative phosphorylation, protein synthesis, and DNA transcription. It is abundant in most diets and daily intake is usually adequate. Intracellular magnesium is responsible for most of the physiologic functions requiring ATP and magnesium. Normal plasma levels are 1.6 to 2.4 mg/dL.

1. Hypomagnesemia

Hypomagnesemia (<2 mg/dL) occurs fairly frequently (20% to 50%) in intensive care unit patients, likely because of inadequate or absent dietary intake in the critically ill patient combined with increased gastrointestinal and renal losses. Pancreatitis can result in hypomagnesemia and concomitant hypocalcemia as well. Patients with renal dysfunction are less likely to develop hypomagnesemia as they have limited ability to excrete magnesium in the urine.

Hypomagnesemia is most commonly associated with hypocalcemia and may result in clinical features of hypocalcemia, such as neuromuscular weakness, muscle wasting, ECG changes (increased PR interval, QT prolongation, and flat T waves). Hypokalemia is also associated with hypomagnesemia. Laryngospasm and seizures may also be seen in severe cases.

a. Causes of Hypomagnesemia

NPO status and lack of IV supplementation.

Malabsorption due to familial hypomagnesemia, laxative use, short bowel syndrome.

Increased renal losses secondary to diuretic use, amphotericin B, aminoglycosides, intrinsic renal disease (acute tubular necrosis).

b. Treatment

Treatment of hypomagnesemia is accomplished with slow infusions of magnesium sulfate 25-50 mg/kg over 3-4 hours. Above a serum level of 2 mg/dL, the kidneys will waste the rest and therefore no additional benefit is gained from rapid IV replacement.

2. Hypermagnesemia

Excess magnesium is usually cleared by the kidneys, and hence hypermagnesemia is rarely encountered except in cases of renal dysfunction. Symptomatic hypermagnesemia is seen once levels are above 5 mg/dL.

a. Signs and symptoms

Signs and symptoms include nausea, vomiting, decreased tendon reflexes, and neuromuscular blockade. Cardiovascular effects include bradycardia, myocardial depression, and ECG changes, including prolonged PR interval and atrioventricular block. Neonates may present with hypotonia and apnea.

b. Treatment

Treatment consists of administering calcium gluconate, 50-100 mg/kg intravenously, followed by restriction of further intake and diuresis.

D. Calcium (Ca^+)

Calcium is a divalent cation, 99% of which is found in the skeleton; the remaining 1% is widely distributed throughout the body. Dietary sources of calcium include dairy products, green leafy vegetables, and seafood with bones. Calcium is essential for teeth, bone mineralization, and muscle activity, especially myocardial excitation-contraction coupling. It also plays a pivotal role in the coagulation cascade. Recent data also suggest a role in cellular mechanisms of injury and necrosis. Excessive use of calcium during resuscitation and post-resuscitation stabilization might be detrimental to the myocardium and other tissues.

Since almost 50% of total calcium is in the active, ionized form and most of the remaining calcium is bound to albumin and inactive, ionized calcium levels should be evaluated wherever available. Levels are closely regulated by interplay between parathyroid hormone, vitamin D, calcitonin, and renal excretion.

1. Hypocalcemia

Hypocalcemia is defined as total calcium <2.12 mmol/L (<8.5 mg/dL) or ionized calcium <1 mmol/L. Typically, calcium deficits occur as a result of low dietary intake and/or a lack of vitamin D or parathyroid hormone. The presentation of hypocalcemia is usually part of a more profound protein-calorie malnutrition but can occur as a stand-alone deficiency. It can occur as part of pancreatitis, but this is less common in pediatrics. The most common cause of hypocalcemia in infancy is due to congenital deficiencies of parathyroid hormone as seen in conditions such as DiGeorge syndrome.

Hypocalcemia is a common occurrence in critically ill patients, many of whom also tend to be hypoalbuminemic. It is more relevant to measure the ionized calcium levels rather than relying solely on total calcium.

a. Signs and Symptoms

Tetany, irritability, hyperreflexia, weakness and paresthesias, muscle fatigue, stridor, and laryngospasm are all common neuromuscular manifestations of hypocalcemia. Cardiovascular effects include hypotension, bradycardia, and arrhythmias.

i. Neonatal/Infant

Calcium levels in a term neonate drop after the first 24 hours and are then maintained by the regulatory hormones. Neonatal hypocalcemia can be encountered in association with maternal diabetes mellitus, toxemia of pregnancy, and maternal hyperparathyroidism. It can present with irritability, tetany, or seizures.

Neonates with DiGeorge syndrome (developmental anomaly of third and fourth pharyngeal pouches) can present with symptomatic hypocalcemia. These patients might exhibit lesions such as mandibular hypoplasia, hypoparathyroidism, T-lymphocyte deficiency (thymic dysfunction), and congenital heart disease (atrial septal defect, ventricular septal defect, aortic arch anomalies, pulmonic stenosis, and truncus arteriosus).

Hypocalcemia can occur in neonates as a result of hypomagnesemia. Correction of the hypomagnesemia is necessary to correct the low calcium.

ii. Child

Hypocalcemia in the older child is usually a result of a disruption of one or more of the regulatory mechanisms controlling calcium levels. Hypoparathyroidism, vitamin D deficiency, inadequate dietary intake, and renal losses are common conditions resulting in hypocalcemia, but it may also be seen in any critically ill or injured child.

b. Treatment

Aggressive calcium supplementation is reserved for symptomatic and documented hypocalcemia. It is important to evaluate renal function and check other electrolytes, particularly magnesium levels, in the evaluation and management of hypocalcemia. More detailed evaluation for the cause of hypocalcemia requires tests of parathyroid function, renal function (phosphate levels), and levels of vitamin D metabolites (25-hydroxyvitamin D and 1,25-dihydroxyvitamin D).

Therapy with IV calcium should ideally be administered through large-bore or central venous lines since calcium extravasation can result in a chemical burn with consequent tissue necrosis. Do not administer via scalp veins, intramuscularly, or subcutaneously.

Indications for IV calcium administration include hypocalcemia (low ionized calcium levels <1 mmol/L), hyperkalemia, calcium channel blocker overdose, hypermagnesemia, and post-arrest stabilization if there is laboratory evidence of hypocalcemia.

i. Calcium Chloride

Intravenous calcium chloride is the most readily bioavailable form of calcium. It is administered in a dose of 10-20 mg/kg IV over 5-10 minutes through a central venous line. Rapid administration can result in bradycardia and hypotension. A 10% solution of calcium chloride contains 1.36 mEq/mL of ionized calcium.

ii. Calcium Gluconate

Calcium gluconate is the preferred calcium salt in neonates and may be administered orally or intravenously in the older infant and child. A 10% solution of calcium gluconate contains 0.45 mEq/mL of ionized calcium. The dosage is 50-200 mg/kg IV over 5-10 minutes for neonates and in infants and children, the dosage is 50-125 mg/kg IV over 5-10 minutes.

2. Hypercalcemia

Hypercalcemia defined as a total calcium level >11 mg/dL (>2.75 mmol/L) or ionized calcium level >1.3 mmol/L, results from calcium release from bone. It can be seen following prolonged immobility, hyperparathyroidism, malignancies leading to tumor lysis, excessive intake of vitamin A or D, and granulomatous disease.

Though relatively rare in pediatric patients, hypercalcemia can present with signs and symptoms that might lead to a wrong diagnosis. Due to the presence of hypertension and decreased level of consciousness, a patient with hypercalcemia could be mistaken for one with impending intracranial herniation. Other signs and symptoms are seen as cardiovascular and neuromuscular effects and include hypertension, shortened QT interval, irritability, lethargy, seizures, coma, nausea, vomiting. and abdominal pain.

a. Treatment

The primary source of the hypercalcemia needs to be addressed and therapy directed specifically at lowering serum calcium levels. Acute hypercalcemia with total calcium levels >15 mg/dL requires aggressive attempts at lowering the levels.

Hydration with IV isotonic saline at 200-250 mL/kg/day in conjunction with furosemide-induced diuresis (1 mg/kg IV every 6 hours) provides a rapid response by increasing renal calcium excretion (calciuresis). Close monitoring of electrolytes, including phosphorus and magnesium, should be performed during diuresis.

Recombinant calcitonin has a rapid onset of action and acts by blocking bone resorption and promotes calciuria. The dose of calcitonin is 10 U/kg IV, and it can be repeated every 4 to 6 hours.

Mithramycin, aspirin, and indomethacin are alternative therapies that can be used to treat hypercalcemia.

Glucocorticoids can reduce calcium absorption from the gastrointestinal tract. Hydrocortisone, 1 mg/kg every 6 hours, is effective in curtailing calcium absorption but is less useful in acute hypercalcemia.

E. Phosphate (PO_4)

Phosphorus is present in adequate quantities in a regular diet. In the body, it is present as phosphate salts and is closely associated with calcium intake. Phosphate levels are closely regulated by renal filtration and proximal renal tubular reabsorption.

The main effects of phosphate occur in membrane phospholipids, bone, adenosine triphosphate, and 2,3-diphosphoglycerate. These four systems alone make phosphate homeostasis critical to many basic functions in the body.

1. Hypophosphatemia

a. Common Causes

Decreased intake and excessive excretion of phosphorus occur classically in DKA. Insulin therapy further reduces phosphate levels by driving it into the cells. Renal dysfunction, such as acute tubular necrosis, Wilson's disease, hypokalemia, and hyperparathyroidism all can lead to hypophosphatemia. Patients receiving IV fluids alone (without phosphorus supplementation), those ingesting aluminum-containing antacids, and the critically ill can become hypophosphatemic.

Signs and symptoms of hypophosphatemia in the acute setting include muscle weakness, hypoventilation, myocardial dysfunction, seizures, and coma.

b. Treatment

Treatment consists of addition of phosphate (as sodium and potassium salts) to the IV fluids when serum phosphorus levels are below 1 mg/dL. Sodium phosphate contains 3 mmol (94 mg) PO_4 and 4 mEq sodium/mL; potassium phosphate contains 3 mmol (94 mg) PO_4 and 4.4 mEq potassium/mL. Intravenous replacement is given at 0.16-0.32 mmol/kg IV over 4-6 hours, and either salt can be used. If renal dysfunction coexists and potassium phosphate is used, potassium levels need to be monitored closely. Also, phosphate infusions/supplements should not be administered in the presence of hypercalcemia.

2. Hyperphosphatemia

Excessive intake (rare) and reduced excretion, such as in renal failure, hypoparathyroidism, and pseudohypoparathyroidism, may all result in hyperphosphatemia, as may tumor lysis syndrome and rhabdomyolysis. A hemolyzed blood sample can result in an erroneous hyperphosphatemia.

The main effect of hyperphosphatemia is the occurrence of hypocalcemia due to chelation when the total calcium measurement multiplied by the inorganic phosphorus product is >60 mg/dL.

Treatment includes aluminum hydroxide antacids enterally and rehydration with isotonic fluids. Hypocalcemia should be treated aggressively as well.

III. Metabolic Disease

A. Glucose

Glucose is essential for tissue metabolism, and its levels are maintained within a tight range by the actions of insulin. Disorders of glucose metabolism can lead to hypoglycemia and hyperglycemia with fairly significant clinical consequences.

1. Hypoglycemia

Hypoglycemia is defined as a serum glucose level <40 mg/L.

a. Signs and Symptoms

Weakness, sweating, tachycardia, tremors and eventually seizures might develop with hypoglycemia. The CNS symptoms are particularly evident since the brain is dependant on a steady source of glucose for neural activity. Symptoms are varied, particularly in the neonate.

b. Causes

Hyperinsulinism, inborn errors of metabolism, endocrine disorders (including adrenal and pituitary dysfunction), ketotic hypoglycemia, and drugs/toxins are the broad categories of conditions leading to hypoglycemia. An extensive endocrine and metabolic workup is necessary to establish the diagnosis. Propranolol and other β-blockers might mask the symptoms (tachycardia, sweating) of hypoglycemia.

Laboratory tests, including cortisol, insulin, growth hormone, urine ketones, serum chemistry and liver function tests, should be obtained during the hypoglycemic episode if possible.

c. Treatment

Once hypoglycemia has been confirmed, immediate treatment with IV glucose should be initiated. Administration of 2-4 mL/kg of 25% dextrose IV will provide 0.5-1.0 Gm/kg of glucose. This solution can be diluted 1:1 so that a 12.5% solution is injected into a peripheral vein or intraosseously. Because dextrose is fairly hyperosmolar, neonates should not be given more than 12.5% dextrose. A bolus of 10 mL/kg of D5% will provide 0.5 Gm/kg of glucose.

2. Hyperglycemia

A blood glucose level >150 mg/dL is considered hyperglycemia. This condition is not unusual in the critically ill child. It is the result of a stress response and the presence of high levels of circulating epinephrine and other anti-insulin hormones. Glucose levels should be monitored in the post-resuscitation stabilization period.

B. Diabetic Ketoacidosis

This diagnosis sometimes may be missed, and the patient can present with a delay in diagnosis. DKA can lead to cerebral edema with catastrophic neurologic outcomes. A newly diagnosed diabetic child (approximately 30% present in DKA) or a known insulin-dependant diabetic patient can present in DKA and require prompt attention to fluid management and correction of metabolic abnormalities.

> ! *DKA constitutes a true endocrine emergency.* !

1. Signs and Symptoms

An intercurrent illness might trigger the episode of DKA. Patients present with headaches, emesis, abdominal pain, lethargy, and clinical signs of dehydration. The patients often present with a history of weight loss, polydypsia, and polyuria. The abdominal pain and emesis might lead to a mistaken diagnosis of an intra-abdominal process or "surgical abdomen." If the dehydration is severe, evidence of hypovolemic shock may be seen at presentation. The classic clinical signs of rapid/Kussmaul respirations have been mistaken for asthma and respiratory distress. The presence of a fruity (ketotic) odor to the breath is helpful in making the diagnosis.

2. Initial Stabilization

Once initial laboratory studies have been obtained and confirm the diagnosis, the mainstay of therapy is the administration of insulin by continuous infusion and correction of the dehydration. If the history is suggestive of an infection as the trigger, this should be investigated and appropriately treated.

An initial fluid bolus of 20 mL/kg of normal saline is administered, with an additional bolus given if the patient is hemodynamically unstable as a result of the dehydration. Only isotonic fluid should be administered during this initial bolus. Lactated Ringer's solution should be avoided if renal function is significantly impaired.

An insulin infusion without a bolus of IV insulin should be initiated at 0.05-0.1 U/kg/hr.

Subsequent IV fluids can be initiated as normal saline with 20 mEq/L of potassium chloride and 20 mEq/L of potassium phosphate at 1.5 to 2 times maintenance, for a total amount not to exceed 4,000 mL/m^2/day. Dextrose solution (D10% NS with potassium chloride and potassium phosphate) can be added once the blood glucose level is below 300 mg/dL.

Blood glucose levels should be brought down by no more than 100 mg/dL every hour. A more rapid decline in blood glucose might require the addition of dextrose to the IV fluid sooner, even if the serum level remains elevated above 300 mg/dL. Since insulin is responsible for correction of the acidosis, the insulin infusion should be maintained while adjusting the dextrose solution as required to effect an appropriate adjustment in blood glucose level.

Hourly monitoring of blood glucose, blood gases (every 1-2 hours), and frequent monitoring of electrolytes – including sodium, potassium, calcium, magnesium, and phosphate – should be performed.

3. Cerebral Edema

Most patients in DKA might already have some degree of cerebral edema at presentation. The main risk factors for the progression are administration of large quantities of hypotonic fluids, rapid hourly declines in blood glucose levels, and hyponatremia. The latter commonly occurs in DKA and is also a result of the hyperglycemia and hypertriglyceridemia (pseudohyponatremia). Na^+ corrected = Na^+ observed + [(Glucose in mg/dL - 100/100) x 1.6]

> **!**
>
> *There is NO indication for administration of sodium bicarbonate unless severe acidosis with resultant hemodynamic compromise or arrhythmias from hyperkalemia are present. Sodium bicarbonate is potentially harmful since it causes significant osmolar shifts and potentially worsens cerebral edema.*

C. Adrenal Insufficiency

1. Primary Adrenal Insufficiency

Congenital adrenal hyperplasia is often seen in the first 2-3 weeks of life, presenting as shock with associated hyponatremia, hypoglycemia, and hyperkalemia. It is characterized by a group of disorders that affect mineralocorticoid and glucocorticoid production due to enzymatic deficiency in the pathways leading to the synthesis of cortisol from cholesterol. The high levels of corticotropin lead to hyperplasia of the adrenal glands. Typically, neonates with or without ambiguous genitalia will present in shock out of proportion to the duration of symptoms. They have elevated levels of steroid metabolites. Partial enzyme deficiencies may also occur and require a corticotropin (ACTH) stimulation test to make the diagnosis.

2. Tertiary Adrenal Insufficiency

This is the most common form of adrenal insufficiency presenting in the pediatric intensive care unit. Patients present with a history of weakness, emesis, abdominal pain, and fever. Tertiary adrenal insufficiency may occur due to the patient being on long-term steroid therapy (such as for asthma), resulting in the suppression of the hypothalamic-pituitary-adrenal axis. An intercurrent illness might result in the patient presenting in shock out of proportion to the duration or severity of symptoms. Adrenal insufficiency should be suspected in the presence of hypoglycemia, hyponatremia, hyperkalemia, and metabolic acidosis together with azotemia. The presence of a random cortisol level of <25 µg/dL in a stressed, critically ill patient is highly suggestive of adrenal suppression or insufficiency. Both the corticotropin and cortisol levels are low in tertiary adrenal insufficiency.

Increasingly, adrenal insufficiency is being diagnosed early in a wide variety of critically ill children. It should be considered in any infant or child who remains hypotensive despite adequate volume resuscitation and initiation of appropriate vasoactive agents(Catecholamine resistant shock). A random cortisol level should be obtained and an initial dose of 2 mg/kg IV hydrocortisone may be administered and can be continued at 1mg/kg/dose every 6 hours if the cortisol level in a profoundly stressed patient remains below 25 µg/dL.

Treatment of adrenal insufficiency includes the following: fluid resuscitation with normal saline boluses of 20 mL/kg; correction of the hypoglycemia; administration of hydrocortisone, 50 mg/m^2 IV (provides mineralocorticoid effect as well), followed by 50 mg/m^2/day divided and given every 4 to 6 hours. Alternative dosing regimens include: 2 mg/kg IV hydrocortisone as the initial dose, followed by 1 mg/kg IV every 6 hours; or 0.2 mg/kg dexamethasone IV every 6 hours; or 1 mg/kg methylprednisolone IV every 6 hours.

Key Points

Fluids and Electrolytes

- Important conditions affecting sodium balance:
  - Syndrome of inappropriate antidiuretic hormone (SIADH): Low urine output, hyponatremia, and concentrated urine with high urinary Na^+ >30 mmol/L.
  - Cerebral salt wasting: Normal to high urine output, hypovolemia, and even higher urinary Na^+ >100 mmol/L.
  - Diabetes insipidus: High urine output, hypovolemia, hypernatremia, and dilute urine.
- Acute adrenal insufficiency: Occurs in congenital adrenal hyperplasia (neonates) or as tertiary condition in patients with long-term steroid use. Presents with hypovolemia (shock), hypoglycemia, hyponatremia, hyperkalemia, and azotemia.
- Symptomatic hyponatremia (hyponatremic seizures): Address the ABCs, then correct Na^+ level with IV 3% saline over 15-20 minutes. Once seizures are under control, continue to correct Na^+ slowly.
- Sodium should be corrected slowly (0.5-1.0 mEq/L change per hour). Too rapid drop can lead to cerebral edema, and too rapid increase can lead to central pontine myelinolysis.
- Hyperkalemia with associated electrocardiogram changes requires immediate therapy.
- Avoid hypotonic maintenance IV fluids, especially in patients at risk of SIADH.
- Potassium in IV fluids should be adjusted to real needs of patient, urine output and potassium levels. Avoid tendency to use 20 mEq/L of potassium chloride as a “standard” additive in IV fluids in all patients.
- With significant hypovolemia, ideally give >40 mL/kg in first hour of fluid resuscitation. Rapid IV fluid resuscitation with isotonic fluid (normal saline or Ringer’s lactate) should be accomplished with frequent reassessment of clinical status.
- In the management of diabetic ketoacidosis (DKA), do not drop blood glucose levels by >100 mg/dL/hr.
- Do not use an initial IV bolus of insulin in the treatment of DKA.

Suggested Readings

1. Arieff A, Ayus J. Treatment of symptomatic hyponatremia: Neither haste nor waste. *Crit Care Med.* 1991;19:748-751.

2. Bartter FC, Schwartz WB. The syndrome of inappropriate secretion of antidiuretic hormone. *Am J Med.* 1967;42:790-806.

3. Blaszak RT, Schexneyder SM. Fluid and electrolyte emergencies in critically ill children. Online Web resource available at: www.picucourse.org.

4. Bohn D. Problems associated with intravenous fluid administration in children: do we have the right solutions? *Curr Opin Pediatr.* 2000;12:217-221.

5. Carcillo JA, Davis AL, Zaritsky A. Role of early fluid resuscitation in pediatric septic shock. *JAMA.* 1991;266:1242-1245.

6. Holliday MA, Segar WE. The maintenance need for water in parenteral fluid therapy. *Pediatrics.* 1957;19:823-832.

7. Moritz ML, Ayus JC. Prevention of hospital-acquired hyponatremia: a case for using isotonic saline. *Pediatrics.* 2003;111:227-230.

8. Sarnaik A, Meert K, Hackbarth R, Fleischmann L. Management of hyponatremic seizures in children with hypertonic saline: a safe and effective strategy. *Crit Care Med.* 1991;19:758-762.

9. Singh S, Bohn D, Carlotti AP, Cusimano M, Rutka JT, Halperin ML. Cerebral salt wasting: truths, fallacies, theories, and challenges. *Crit Care Med.* 2002; 30: 2575-2579.

10. Werner H. Hyponatremia. Online Web resource available at: www.picucourse.org.

Chapter 10:

Traumatic Injuries in Children

✓ Objectives

- Rank priorities for the management of the injured child.
- Employ life-saving therapies in the injured child.
- Describe how children's patterns of injury differ from those of adults.

I. INTRODUCTION

Trauma remains an important cause of morbidity and mortality in children, whose injury patterns differ significantly from those of adults. Accidental and non-accidental injuries account for a significant proportion of emergency department visits and the use of healthcare resources.

II. THE PRIMARY SURVEY

The evaluation of an injured child begins with the primary survey, which is conducted in a systematic manner. The primary survey, which is remembered by the mnemonic ABCDE, involves evaluation and management of the airway followed by assessment of breathing, circulation, disability (neurologic status), and exposure (undressing and examining the patient while maintaining body temperature).

It is important to immobilize the cervical spine and back prior to moving a child after a traumatic event. Typically, the patient is placed in a cervical collar and on a long backboard at the location of the accident. If a collar is not placed at the scene, one should be placed as soon as possible. Prior to placement of a cervical collar, in-line immobilization should be provided.

A. Airway

Airway evaluation begins by assessing airway patency. Airway patency may be achieved by placing the patient in the sniffing position using a roll as an adjunct. In infants, the roll should be placed under the shoulders; in older children and adults, under the occiput. This difference is due to the infant's proportionally larger head and propensity to neck flexion in comparison to adults. If airway patency cannot be achieved by positioning the patient, several maneuvers, including a chin lift and a jaw thrust, may be used.

> **!**
>
> *Given the risk of cervical spine injury, a head tilt is contraindicated in trauma patients.*

> **!**
>
> *Nasopharyngeal airways should be avoided in patients with midface trauma, basilar skull trauma, evidence of cerebrospinal fluid rhinorrhea, or coagulopathy.*

Artificial airway adjuncts may also be useful. These are used to displace the tongue and pharyngeal tissue from the airway. An oropharyngeal airway should be used only in an unconscious patient as it may cause significant gagging and vomiting. The length of the airway is determined by measuring the distance from the mouth to the area just cephalad to the angle of the mandible. A nasopharyngeal (NP) airway may be used in a conscious, cooperative patient. The length of the airway is determined by measuring from the tip of the nose to the tragus.

Endotracheal intubation is indicated when a patient is apneic, in profound shock, unable to maintain an airway due to obstruction or trauma, has severe neurologic dysfunction (Glasgow Coma Scale score [GCS] <8), has inhalational injury, or requires airway protection from aspiration of gastric contents or blood. The correct size of endotracheal tube may be determined by either using the Broselow Pediatric Emergency Tape or the formula (16 + age in years)/4. Traditionally, uncuffed endotracheal tubes have been used for patients younger than 8 years. However, patients at risk for impaired gas exchange, such as those with acute respiratory distress syndrome, inhalational injury, or pulmonary contusions, can and should be intubated with a cuffed endotracheal tube regardless of their age because they may require high ventilatory pressures to achieve adequate oxygenation and ventilation.

All trauma patients are assumed to have a full stomach. Intubation should be performed using a rapid-sequence technique. Medications such as etomidate and midazolam should be used to avoid hypotension. Ketamine should be avoided because it carries the risk of elevating intracranial pressure (ICP). Succinylcholine is contraindicated in cases of hyperkalemia, neuromuscular disease, and burns.

Following paralysis, the endotracheal tube is inserted. The tube should be advanced to a depth of 3 times the internal diameter of the tube or to a depth derived from the formula (age/2) + 12. Placement is confirmed by auscultation, end-tidal carbon dioxide detection, and chest radiograph. Once the airway is secured, cricoid pressure may be removed. Inexperienced practitioners should not paralyze patients if they are not confident that they will be able to intubate. If intubation is unsuccessful, bag-mask ventilation should be used with application of cricoid pressure. Advanced airway techniques such as fiberoptic intubation may be required. If endotracheal intubation is not possible, an experienced practitioner should perform a cricothyrotomy.

B. Breathing

Once the airway is secured, breathing should be evaluated. The goal is normal oxygenation and ventilation. Pulse oximetry should be employed to monitor oxygen saturation with a goal of maintaining oxygen saturation greater than 94%. Oxygen may be provided by nasal canula, face mask, nonrebreather face mask, or mechanical ventilator. Ventilation may be provided by a bag-mask device or a mechanical ventilator. Routine hyperventilation is not recommended in trauma patients. In cases of suspected head injury, hyperventilation will decrease cerebral perfusion and potentially worsen secondary injury. However, hyperventilation should be employed in cases of impending cerebral herniation to decrease cerebral blood flow and lower ICP.

C. Circulation

The assessment of breathing is followed by assessment and stabilization of the circulation. Hemorrhage leading to hypovolemic shock is the most frequently encountered form of shock in trauma patients. Children may lose up to 30% of their circulating blood volume secondary to hemorrhage and continue to maintain normal blood pressure. Applying direct pressure to the wound may initially control hemorrhage.

Other types of shock that may be seen in trauma victims include cardiogenic shock resulting from trauma to the myocardium, neurogenic shock resulting from spinal cord injury, and obstructive shock resulting from tension pneumothorax or pericardial tamponade. Patients with signs of shock require volume resuscitation. Intravenous access should be obtained peripherally. After 2 unsuccessful attempts at gaining intravenous access, consideration should be given to placement of an intraosseous needle. Central venous catheter and venous cut-down by a skilled practitioner may also be considered. The preferred location for insertion of an intraosseous needle is the tibia.

Once intravenous or intraosseous access is established, 20 mL/kg of crystalloid solution should be administered and the patient should then be reassessed. If signs of shock persist, second and third boluses of 20 mL/kg should be administered. Once a patient has received 40 to 60 mL/kg of fluid and is still not hemodynamically stable, packed red blood cells should be administered. Urinary and central venous catheters should be placed to monitor urine output and central venous pressure. Urine output reflects renal perfusion, and central venous pressure reflects intravascular volume and preload. Ongoing hemodynamic instability may require operative intervention.

D. Disability

The evaluation of disability (neurologic status) follows stabilization of circulation. The level of consciousness, pupillary response, presence of localizing signs, and presence of paralysis should be assessed. The GCS should be tabulated during either the primary survey or the secondary survey. The GCS is used as a predictor of neurologic outcome. The score ranges from 3 to 15; 3 is the worst, and 15 the best. The components of the score are motor function (1-6 points), verbal response (1-5 points), and eye opening (1-4 points). Elements of the verbal score are modified to account for developmental differences in the verbal ability of young children and infants (**see Table 16-1**).

E. Exposure

Following assessment and stabilization of neurologic status, the patient should be exposed by removal of all clothing. This allows examination for any additional injuries. Patients should then be covered with warm blankets in order to prevent hypothermia.

F. Adjuncts to the Primary Survey

Depending on the nature of a patient's trauma, a number of additional tests, procedures, and devices may be used as adjuncts to the primary survey, including the following:

- Cardiopulmonary monitoring
- Pulse oximetry
- Blood pressure monitoring
- End-tidal carbon dioxide monitoring
- Arterial blood gases analysis
- Placement of a urinary catheter to measure output and assess renal perfusion
- Placement of a gastric catheter to decompress the stomach and prevent aspiration

> ! *Placement of a urinary catheter should be deferred if blood is visualized at the urethral meatus.*

> ! *A gastric tube should be placed orally if there is epistaxis, rhinorrhea, or signs of a basilar skull fracture.*

Radiographs of the chest, pelvis, and lateral cervical spine may be obtained during the primary survey or may be delayed until the secondary survey. Such radiographs may identify injuries that require immediate attention. A diagnostic peritoneal lavage or an abdominal ultrasound may be performed by a skilled practitioner to identify abdominal bleeding.

III. THE SECONDARY SURVEY

The secondary survey begins once the primary survey has been completed and the patient is stable.

> *The secondary survey involves a complete history and physical examination.*

A. History

Important components of the trauma history include past medical history, allergies, medications, pregnancy status, the events and environment surrounding the injury, and the patient's most recent meal. Knowing the mechanism of injury is extremely helpful in determining possible injuries.

B. Physical Examination

The physical examination should proceed from head to toe. In an infant, the anterior fontanelle should be evaluated. The patient's head is positioned at 30° (if not contraindicated) and the fontanelle is palpated. A full or bulging fontanelle is a sign of increased ICP, whereas a sunken fontanelle indicates intravascular volume loss. The head is examined for lacerations and step-offs indicating fractures. Raccoon eyes (periorbital ecchymosis) and Battle's sign (ecchymosis of the mastoid process) suggest a basilar skull fracture. The eyes are examined for pupillary response, subconjunctival hemorrhages, and extraocular movements. The nose is examined for epistaxis, rhinorrhea (suggesting leakage of cerebrospinal fluid [CSF]), and fractures. The oral pharynx is evaluated for lacerations and injury to the teeth.

> *Head and maxillofacial trauma are strongly associated with cervical spine trauma.*

In the secondary survey of the neck, the cervical collar is removed and in-line immobilization is applied. The neck and cervical spine are palpated for tenderness and crepitus. The carotid pulses should be assessed and the position of the trachea should be evaluated. Following neck examination, the cervical collar is replaced. The chest is inspected for deformity or obvious fracture and then palpated to determine the presence of tenderness. The lungs are auscultated for equality and clarity of breath sounds. Inequality of breath sounds may occur secondary to pneumothorax or hemothorax. The heart is examined with attention to the rate, rhythm, and quality of heart sounds. Distant, muffled heart sounds may represent pericardial effusion. Tachycardia with a narrow pulse pressure may be seen in pericardial tamponade. The abdomen is inspected for ecchymoses, auscultated for presence and quality of bowel sounds, and palpated for tenderness and rigidity.

The backboard is removed during the secondary survey. The patient is log-rolled off the backboard, and the back is inspected for deformities and ecchymoses and palpated for tenderness. Immobilization of the spine is extremely important in the management of possible spine injury. However, every effort should be made to remove the backboard within 2 hours to prevent the development of skin breakdown and pressure ulcers. Patients should be log-rolled every 2 hours thereafter to prevent pressure ulcers until the spine is cleared. The genitals are inspected for lacerations and blood at the urethral meatus; a rectal examination is performed with assessment of tone and presence of blood in the rectal vault. The musculoskeletal system is inspected and palpated to identify fractures or dislocations.

The patient's level of consciousness and pupillary response should be reassessed in the secondary survey. The GCS should be tabulated. Reflexes should be assessed, and the presence of sensory and motor deficits should be determined. Spinal cord injury should be localized by determining the level of motor and sensory function (**Tables 10-1 and 10-2**).

Table 10-1. Motor Levels

Nerve Root	Major Muscles Affected
C3-5	Diaphragm
C5	Elbow flexors
C6	Wrist extensors
C7	Elbow extensors
C8	Finger flexors
T1	Finger abductor (5th finger)
L2	Hip flexors
L3	Knee extensors
L4	Ankle dorsiflexors
L5	Long toe extensors
S1	Ankle plantar flexors

Table 10-2. Sensory Levels

Nerve Root	Major Sensory Area Affected
C4	Clavicle
C6	Thumb
C7	Second and third fingers
C8	Fifth finger
T4	Nipples
T10	Umbilicus
L1	Inguinal ligament
L3	Lower anterior thigh/knees
L5	Dig toe
S1	Lateral foot
S3-5	Perineum

C. Adjuncts to the Secondary Survey

During the secondary survey additional studies may be indicated to evaluate injuries. These include computed tomographic (CT) scans, completion of the cervical spine radiographs, radiographs of the thoracolumbar spine and extremities, angiography, and ultrasounds.

> !
>
> *Ongoing and repeated evaluation of the patient is imperative to ensure stability.*

IV. MANAGEMENT OF TRAUMATIC INJURIES

A. Traumatic Brain Injury

Traumatic brain injury (TBI) contributes to a significant number of trauma deaths in children and usually occurs secondary to motor vehicle collisions, falls, bicycle accidents, and sports injuries. Non-accidental trauma remains a significant cause of TBI in children younger than 2 years. Traumatic brain injury may be characterized as mild (GCS 13-15), moderate (GCS 9-12), or severe (GCS 3-8).

Children with mild brain injury generally do well. However, it has been shown that as many as 53% of these children have radiographic abnormalities on head CT despite their good appearance. Up to 57% of children and 85% of infants with epidural hematomas have no loss of consciousness at the time of impact, and 7% have no alteration of mental status at any time following the injury. These statistics underscore the likelihood that a life-threatening injury may exist despite a benign presentation. The concept of delayed deterioration has also been examined in this age group, and findings show that children with a normal neurologic examination and a normal head CT at presentation rarely deteriorate at a later point in time and can be safely discharged home.

The management of children with moderate to severe brain injury requires close attention to ventilatory and hemodynamic status as well as to ICP. Children with moderate brain injury may require intubation for other indications but not for the brain injury. Intubation and ICP monitoring are indicated in patients with a GCS of less than 8. When a patient with head trauma meets this criterion, the goals of mechanical ventilation are normal oxygenation and ventilation ($Paco_2$ 35-40 mm Hg [4.7-5.3 kPa]). Hyperventilation is indicated only in cases of impending herniation. Attention to respiratory and hemodynamic status is imperative because hypoxemia and hypotension have been shown to significantly increase morbidity and mortality in patients with TBI.

In patients with a GCS lower than 8, an ICP monitor may be placed in the brain parenchyma, subdural space, or lateral ventricle (ventriculostomy). Ventriculostomy catheters are preferred because they allow not only for monitoring of ICP but also for drainage of CSF as a means of lowering ICP. Normal ICP in adults is less than 10 mm Hg, and it is lower in young children and infants.

Cerebral perfusion pressure (CPP) must be monitored closely in patients with TBI. Numerically it is represented as the difference between the mean arterial pressure (MAP) and the ICP (CPP = MAP – ICP). In adults, a CPP of 60 to 70 mm Hg is usually targeted. There are no data documenting the appropriate CPP in children and infants. However, given their lower MAPs and ICPs, general ranges can be extrapolated. A reasonable range is 50 to 60 mm Hg in children and 40 to 50 mm Hg in infants. Other modalities that are utilized for control of ICP include sedation, neuromuscular blockade, elevation of the head, maintenance of mild hypothermia (~35°C [~95°F]), use of endotracheal or intravenous lidocaine prior to suctioning, maintenance of euvolemia, and titration of serum osmolality (serum sodium ~150 mEq/L, higher if needed). The use of mannitol as a means of decreasing ICP has fallen out of favor except in cases of intractable intracranial hypertension because mannitol is a potent osmotic diuretic that may cause hypotension. Hypertonic saline may be utilized to increase serum osmolality without causing intravascular volume depletion. In cases of intractable ICP elevation, inotropic or vasopressor agents may be used to optimize the CPP by increasing the MAP, even to the point of relative systemic hypertension. There is no role for the use of steroids in TBI.

B. Cervical Spine Injury

Case Study

A 17-year-old male presents to the emergency department after sustaining an injury during football practice. A hit under his chin resulted in severe hyperextension of his neck. He fell to the ground, unable to move his lower extremities and with significant weakness of the upper extremities. His vital signs were stable in the field, and he was immobilized with a cervical collar and backboard prior to transport. In the emergency department the patient is awake, alert, and afebrile, with a respiratory rate of 9/minute, oxygen saturation of 94% on room air, heart rate of 150/min, and blood pressure of 60/30 mm Hg.

- What is the first step in stabilizing this patient?

- Why is this patient hypotensive?

Cervical spine injury is uncommon in children. There is a mortality rate of 15% to 20%, largely due to its association with significant brain injury. Young children (<11 years) most frequently sustain cervical spine injury as the result of motor vehicle collisions, falls, and pedestrian accidents. They are at greater risk for high cervical injuries, cervical spine dislocations, and spinal cord injury without radiographic abnormality. Older children (>11 years) and adults are at higher risk for low cervical injuries and cervical spine fractures. A continuum exists in that children ages 10 to 11 years begin to show adult patterns of injury, and their transition to those patterns is eventually completed in late adolescence. Differences in injury patterns may be attributed to anatomical differences between the young child and the older child/adult. Young children have proportionally larger heads with relatively weak neck muscles, which makes them more susceptible to flexion and extension injuries. The vertebral bodies are incompletely ossified, and the ligaments are far more elastic than those of adults. The vertebral bodies of the upper cervical spine are anteriorly wedged in children, predisposing them to forward vertebral movement and anterior dislocation. The fulcrum for cervical motion is at C2 to C3 in the young child compared to C5 to C6 in adolescents and adults. The young child's spinal cord may be easily stretched, torn, or contused secondary to laxity of spinal ligaments. It may stretch up to 5 centimeters without rupturing, whereas the adult cord may rupture after only 5 to 6 millimeters of traction.

> **!** *Stretching of the spinal cord accounts for the occurrence of spinal cord injury without radiographic abnormality in children and its absence in adults. Spinal cord injury without radiographic abnormality may result in partial or complete spinal cord injury.*

C. Thoracic Trauma

Case Study

A 4-year-old girl presents to the emergency department after falling from a second-story window. She had a brief loss of consciousness at the scene but was awake, alert, and crying when EMS arrived. Her vital signs were stable and her spine was immobilized with a cervical collar and backboard. In the emergency department, the patient is awake and crying for her mother. She is afebrile, and her vital signs are respiratory rate 50/min, oxygen saturation 92% on room air, heart rate 120/min, and blood pressure 120/65 mm Hg. Her breathing pattern is paradoxical, with an asymmetric thorax.

- What is the source of this patient's hypoxemia?

- How will you treat her?

Thoracic injuries, which often occur as a result of blunt trauma, are the second leading cause of death due to trauma in children (behind head injuries). The overall mortality rate from thoracic trauma has been reported to be 5% and increases to 25% when accompanied by head and abdominal trauma. In infants and toddlers, thoracic injuries occur most commonly in the contexts of motor vehicle collisions and maltreatment. School-aged children are most likely to sustain thoracic trauma due to bicycle, scooter, and skating accidents, while teenagers are most commonly injured in motor vehicle collisions.

A chest radiograph should be the initial diagnostic test in the evaluation of thoracic trauma. Due to their extremely compliant chest walls, children suffer rib fractures much less frequently than adults do and are at higher risk for pulmonary contusions. Pulmonary contusions are the most common thoracic injuries in children and may be associated with hypoxemia, hypoventilation, ventilation-perfusion mismatch, and decreased pulmonary compliance. There may be consolidation, edema, and alveolar hemorrhage in the area of contusion. Contusions may not be immediately visualized radiographically. Treatment includes avoidance of fluid overload, supplemental oxygen, analgesia, incentive spirometry, and mechanical ventilation if required (**Table 10-3**).

Table 10-3. Diagnostic Evaluation

Type of Trauma	Diagnostic Study
Any	Complete blood count
	Prothrombin time/partial prothrombin time
	Complete metabolic panel, including aspartate aminotransferase/alanine aminotransferase, amylase, lipase
	Urinalysis
	Radiographs of the chest, cervical spine (posteroanterior, lateral, odontoid), and pelvis
Head	Head CT
	MRI: not indicated acutely; obtain later in the course to aid in prognostication
Cervical Spine	Cervical spine radiographs: posteroanterior, lateral, odontoid views
	Cervical spine CT: if plain radiographs are inadequate
	Flexion/extension radiographs: indicated when radiographs/CT scans are negative for bony injury but neck pain/tenderness is elicited; evaluates ligamentous injury[a]
	MRI: indicated when radiographs/CT scans are negative for bony injury but neck pain/tenderness is elicited; evaluates ligamentous injury[a]
Thoracic	Chest radiograph
	Chest CT
	Chest CT angiography: indicated when serious vascular injury is suspected
	Electrocardiogram
	Echocardiogram: indicated when pericardial effusion is suspected
	Esophagram: indicated when esophageal rupture is suspected
	Bronchoscopy/bronchography: indicated when injury to the tracheobronchial tree is suspected
Abdominal	Aspartate aminotransferase/alanine aminotransferase
	Amylase/lipase
	Urinalysis
	Focused abdominal sonography for trauma examination
	Abdominal CT with oral and intravenous contrast
	Diagnostic peritoneal lavage

[a] Flexion/extension films or MRI may be performed.

The presence of rib fractures, particularly posterior rib fractures, should raise suspicion of physical abuse. These fractures usually occur secondary to significant compression of the chest, as happens in shaking. Other potential etiologies include birth trauma and disorders of bone ossification, such as osteogenesis imperfecta and rickets. Fractures of the first rib are associated with a high incidence of intrathoracic injuries, including pneumothorax and hemothorax, and should prompt angiography (preferably CT angiography) for diagnosis of significant vascular injury. Multiple rib fractures have been shown to be associated with severe injury in children; mortality rates increase as the number of fractured ribs increases. Flail chest occurs when 2 or more contiguous ribs are fractured, resulting in paradoxical chest wall movement (inward movement with inspiration and outward movement with exhalation).

One-third of traumatic pneumothoraces occur in isolation, the other two-thirds in association with other injuries. Often pneumothoraces are asymptomatic and are only detected by chest radiography. Treatment is evacuation of air with a tube thoracostomy. Accumulation of a large amount of air in the pleural space may lead to collapse of the ipsilateral lung, with tracheal and mediastinal shift resulting in hemodynamic instability (tension pneumothorax). Signs of tension pneumothorax include tracheal shift, absence of breath sounds on the ipsilateral side, tachycardia, hypotension, dyspnea, and hypoxemia. Prompt evacuation of the pneumothorax is imperative to prevent hemodynamic collapse. Hemothorax can develop in the context of penetrating injuries to the chest with disruption of the thoracic vessels, intercostal blood vessels, or lung parenchyma. Evacuation of the hemothorax is important in the prevention of subsequent infection, chronic atelectasis, lung entrapment, and ventilation-perfusion abnormalities.

> !
>
> *Flail chest is often managed conservatively with analgesia but may require positive pressure ventilation and, less frequently, surgical repair.*
>
> !

Cardiac contusions most frequently occur as a result of blunt trauma and may present as chest pain, dysrhythmia, or hypotension. An electrocardiogram (ECG) may show ST-segment changes, atrial tachycardia, sinus tachycardia, or premature beats. Treatment is generally supportive, with cardiopulmonary monitoring required only if there is an abnormal ECG. Pericardial tamponade may occur if there is an accumulation of fluid in the pericardial space. Patients present with tachycardia, muffled heart sounds, and a narrow pulse pressure. Diagnosis is made by echocardiography. The treatment is removal of the fluid by pericardiocentesis.

Diaphragmatic injuries are uncommon. When they occur, they most frequently involve the posterolateral left hemidiaphragm. Upward turning of a nasogastric tube and herniation of the abdominal contents into the thorax may be visualized on the chest radiograph. Up to 50% of injuries are not diagnosed acutely.

Esophageal rupture occurs most frequently due to penetrating injury. Blunt trauma may also cause a tear at the gastroesophageal junction owing to acute movement of gastric contents into the esophagus. This may lead to spillage of gastric contents into the pleural space and mediastinum, resulting in mediastinitis. Diagnosis is made by esophagram, which reveals extravasation of contrast material. Treatment includes antibiotics and surgical repair.

Injuries to the tracheobronchial tree are rare in children but are associated with a mortality rate of 30%. They may be caused by blunt or penetrating trauma. Patients present with subcutaneous emphysema, pneumothorax, and hemoptysis. Diagnosis may be made by bronchoscopy; however, bronchography may be required to visualize tears in the distal bronchial tree.

D. Abdominal Trauma

Case Study

A 2-year-old girl is brought to the emergency department by her mother, who has found her to be irritable and difficult to console. There is no preceding history of fever, illness, ingestion, or trauma. The patient is afebrile, with respiratory rate 45/min, oxygen saturation 95% on room air, heart rate 170/min, and blood pressure 50/20 mm Hg. After stabilization and removal of clothing, you find a large ecchymotic area on her abdomen.

- What interventions would be made to stabilize this patient?
- What is the likely etiology of her injury?
- What is an appropriate diagnostic evaluation for this patient?

Due to their compliant chest walls and decreased abdominal-wall musculature and fat, children are at a higher risk of sustaining significant organ injury as a result of abdominal trauma than adults are. Also, owing to children's smaller size, multiple organs may be injured because a given force will strike a relatively larger proportion of body surface. Intra-abdominal injuries related to bicycle handlebars and car lap belts have a high likelihood or requiring surgical intervention. Physical findings include abdominal distention, abrasions, contusions, lap belt ecchymoses, and focal or diffuse tenderness. Hemodynamically unstable patients require emergent resuscitation and laparotomy; hemodynamically stable patients warrant further assessment.

Diagnostic evaluation of abdominal trauma begins with a laboratory evaluation. Decreasing hemoglobin should raise suspicion of abdominal hemorrhage. Several studies have shown that elevations in the serum aspartate aminotransferase and alanine aminotransferase may be associated with abdominal trauma. One study in particular showed that a serum alanine aminotransferase greater than 131 units/L together with abdominal tenderness is predictive of abdominal injury with a sensitivity of 100%. Serum amylase and lipase are variable predictors of pancreatic injury. Serum amylase may be normal when obtained soon after the occurrence of pancreatic injury, but at 3 hours or more following injury, serum amylase will be elevated 100% of the time. Elevations in serum amylase may also be seen in the presence of head injury without pancreatic injury. Serum lipase may also be predictive of pancreatic injury.

Indications for abdominal CT include abnormal physical examination, abnormal laboratory values, absence of a reliable physical examination due to distracting injuries or altered mental status, or an acute need to know (prior to undergoing general anesthesia). Abdominal CT is useful in detecting solid organ injuries, particularly those of the liver, kidney, and spleen, and is the diagnostic procedure of choice for evaluation of abdominal injury. It should be performed with intravenous contrast to best delineate these injuries. Pancreatic and intestinal injuries may be missed on abdominal CT, particularly if the test is performed soon after injury. Oral contrast may aid in the detection of pancreatic and intestinal injuries.

The focused abdominal sonography for trauma (FAST) examination is of limited utility in the pediatric population. The majority of abdominal injuries in hemodynamically stable children are managed nonoperatively. The FAST exam may be useful in 2 specific situations in pediatric patients: (1) in multiply injured, hemodynamically unstable patients, it may be used to detect abdominal hemorrhage as the source of instability, and (2) it may be used together with laboratory evaluation and physical examination as a screening tool to identify patients who would benefit from CT.

Diagnostic peritoneal lavage is of limited utility in children because it offers no information regarding specific organ injury or grade of injury. Identification of specific injuries and their severity is vital in determining whether surgery is indicated.

Splenic injury is the most common injury associated with blunt abdominal trauma. Abdominal CT with intravenous contrast is the most sensitive detector of splenic injury. Preservation of the spleen is the standard of care in children in order to prevent immunologic compromise. Splenectomy is indicated only in cases of hemodynamic instability with damage to the spleen that is not repairable.

Liver injury is the second most common injury associated with blunt abdominal trauma. Similar to splenic injuries, liver injuries are best diagnosed by abdominal CT with intravenous contrast. Most injuries may be managed without surgery.

Injury to the bowel occurs less frequently than solid organ injury in children. These injuries are more difficult to detect, and a high index of suspicion is required. Motor vehicle collisions in which children are restrained with poorly fitting lap belts may result in injury to the intestine. Pneumoperitoneum or extravasation of oral contrast may be detected on abdominal CT. Often, free abdominal fluid is the only abnormality and remains a very nonspecific finding.

> !
>
> *Abdominal CT findings and laboratory values are variable and may not be very sensitive soon after injury.*
>
> !

Pancreatic injuries occur much less frequently than other solid-organ injuries in children. They are often the result of accidents involving bicycle handlebars and may be an isolated injury. Abdominal CT is the diagnostic modality of choice for detection.

Near Drowning

Near drowning is defined as survival after suffocation by submersion in water. Drowning refers to death from asphyxia during submersion or within 24 hours of submersion. Drowning is characterized as dry or wet. Dry drowning occurs more frequently in adults. No fluid is aspirated into the lungs. Patients develop severe laryngospasm and often have significant mucous and froth in the upper airway. Death results from cerebral anoxia. Wet drowning involves the aspiration of fluid into the lungs with resultant pathophysiologic changes.

Following submersion, a period of voluntary apnea occurs. In young children, the initial contact with the water is accompanied by the diving reflex, which shunts blood flow from the skin and splanchnic circulations to the coronary and cerebral circulations. Blood pressure is increased and heart rate is decreased. Fear and cold water temperature amplify the diving reflex. This may partially account for the improved survival seen following long submersion in cold water. In warm water (above 15°C-20°C [59°F-68°F]), the submersion time to fatality in humans is 3 to 10 minutes. In cold water (0°C-15°C [32°F-59°F]), neurologically intact survival has been reported following up to 40 minutes of submersion. After the initial period of breath holding, a break point is reached, and the patient will take a breath resulting in aspiration of water. Secondary apnea will soon follow, leading to involuntary gasping breaths, respiratory arrest, and eventually cardiac arrest.

Management of patients after near drowning is similar to management of other trauma patients. Severe electrolyte abnormalities are uncommon, and antibiotics are generally not indicated. Emerging literature in adult and neonatal populations has suggested cooling the head as a treatment that may improve neurologic outcome in patients who have suffered a cardiac arrest.

Key Points

Traumatic Injuries in Children

- The primary survey consists of evaluation of ABCDE: airway, breathing, circulation, disability (neurologic status), and exposure.
- Adjuncts to the primary survey include cardiopulmonary monitoring, pulse oximetry, blood pressure monitoring, end-tidal carbon dioxide monitoring, arterial blood gas analysis, urinary catheter placement, gastric catheter placement, and radiographs of the chest, pelvis, and lateral cervical spine.
- The secondary survey, history and physical examination, covers past medical history, allergies, medications, pregnancy status, events and environment (mechanism of injury), and most recent meal. The physical examination proceeds from head to toe.
- Adjuncts to the secondary survey include computed tomography (CT) scans, completion of the cervical spine radiographs, radiographs of the thoracolumbar spine and the extremities, ultrasounds, and angiography.
- Pulmonary contusions are common in children, but rib fractures are rare due to chest-wall compliance. Because rib fractures are usually the result of significant trauma, their existence in the absence of significant trauma should raise suspicion of abuse.
- The incidence of abdominal organ damage is higher in children than in adults. Splenic injury is most common, followed by liver injury. Bowel injury is less common, and its diagnosis requires a high index of suspicion.

Suggested Readings

1. American College of Surgeons, Committee on Trauma. *Advanced Trauma Life Support for Doctors Student Course Manual.* 7th ed. Chicago, IL: American College of Surgeons; 2005.

2. American Heart Association. *Pediatric Advanced Life Support Provider Manual.* Chicago, IL: American Heart Association; 2006.

3. Dias MS. Traumatic brain and spinal cord injury. *Pediatr Clin of North Am* 2004; 51:271-303.

4. Fildes J, Cooper A, eds. American College of Surgeons National Trauma Data Bank. Pediatric Annual Report, 2005. Available at: HYPERLINK "http://www.facs.org/trauma/ntdbpediatric2005.pdf" http://www.facs.org/trauma/ntdbpediatric2005.pdf. Accessed 4/17/07.

5. Kokoska ER, Keller MS, Rallo MC, Weber TR. Characteristics of pediatric cervical spine injuries. *J Pediatr Surg.* 2001; (36)1:100-105.

6. Levin DL, Moriss FC, Toro LO, Brink LW, Turner GR. Drowning and near-drowning. *Ped Clin N Am.* 1993;40(2):321-336.

7. Pearn J. Pathophysiology of drowning. *Med J Australia.* 1985;142:586-588.

8. Pitetti RD, Walker S. Life-threatening chest injuries in children. *Clin Ped Emerg Med.* 2005;6:16-22.

9. Potoka DA, Saladino RA. Blunt abdominal trauma in the pediatric patient. *Clin Ped Emerg Med.* 2005;6:23-31.

Chapter 11:

PEDIATRIC BURN INJURY

Objectives

- Explain the pathophysiology of burn injury.
- Appropriately assess and initiate management of burn injuries in children.
- Recognize inhalation injury in children and initiate appropriate airway management.
- Recognize and appropriately manage the sequelae of burn injury.

Case Study

A 15-month-old is injured in a boiler explosion and partial building collapse. During initial assessment at a local emergency department she is awake and crying, her vital signs are remarkable for tachycardia and tachypnea, and physical exam demonstrates deep partial-thickness burns involving 20% of her body surface area (BSA) and full-thickness burns involving 40% BSA. Approximately 40 minutes after arriving in the emergency department the child produces black sputum and demonstrates wheezing, respiratory distress, and somnolence. An arterial blood gas reveals a normal Po_2 of 99 mm Hg (13.2 kPa)and a Pco_2 of 100 mm Hg (13.3 kPa).

- What are the priorities of assessment and management?

- What type of injury is this patient likely to have suffered?

I. INTRODUCTION

A burn is a traumatic injury to the skin that results from thermal energy or from chemical or physical agents. Annually in the United States, approximately 1.2 million people sustain burns, and one-third of burn unit admissions and deaths occur in children. Children under 4 years of age are the subset of the pediatric population at the greatest risk of burn injury, and it is also this population that suffers the greatest risk of abuse. Overall, scald injuries represent 65% of burns suffered by children, while contact burns represent 20% of pediatric burn injuries. Despite improvements in burn care over the past 20 years, burn injury is still the fifth leading cause of unintentional injury-related death in children. Mortality is closely related to the depth and extent of injury as well as age.

II. PATHOPHYSIOLOGY OF BURNS

The impact of a burn injury extends far beyond the involved areas of skin. The physiologic response to a burn can range from local inflammation in cases of limited injury to the systemic inflammatory response syndrome and burn shock with more extensive injury. Fluid loss from burned tissue is 5 to 10 times greater than that from healthy tissue and is accompanied by protein and electrolyte losses as well. Local edema is generated within 12 to 24 hours of injury and classically peaks between 24 and 48 hours. Some edema is always to be expected, but excessive fluid administration contributes to pathologic edema and to the development of compartment syndrome. The systemic inflammatory response syndrome can develop in response to burns of 15% to 20% body surface area (BSA) or greater. Temperature dysregulation, immuno dysfunction with an attendant increased risk of wound infection and sepsis, and hypermetabolism are among the short- and long-term sequelae of significant burns.

A. Approach and Initial Management

The approach to any emergency begins with an assessment of the airway, breathing, and circulation. The assessment of the airway and a critical appraisal of the risk of smoke inhalation and airway injury are particularly relevant to the house fire victim. Supplemental oxygen should be administered empirically until a thorough and definite evaluation is completed. Once the airway is assessed and stabilized, intravenous access should be established quickly, preferably with 2 relatively large bore catheters. The volume of fluid resuscitation required is dictated by the depth and extent of injury.

> *Signs of Inhalation Injury*
>
> - *Respiratory distress*
> - *Hypoxia*
> - *Stridor*
> - *Wheezing*
> - *Drooling*
> - *Tongue swelling*
> - *Oropharyngeal blisters*
> - *Singed nasal hairs and eyebrows*
> - *Production of carbonaceous sputum*

1. Airway Assessment

Signs of inhalation injury include respiratory distress, hypoxia, stridor, wheezing, singed nasal hairs and eyebrows, drooling, oropharyngeal blisters, tongue swelling, and production of carbonaceous sputum. If these signs are present, early intubation should be performed to protect the airway from progression to airway obstruction. Inhalation injury results from inflammation and edema that are generated in response to the inhalation of toxic products of combustion. The inflammatory reaction can lead to the formation of endobronchial casts and obstruction of the distal airways. Mucociliary clearance mechanisms are disrupted, and the accumulation of necrotic debris and products of inflammation provide an environment conducive to infection. These patients often benefit from bronchoscopy to enhance pulmonary toilet, and minimize the risk of pneumonia or, when pneumonia is present, facilitate its resolution.

Inhalation injury may or may not be associated with carbon monoxide (CO) poisoning. Any person exposed to fire in a confined space is at risk for CO poisoning, and CO poisoning may be responsible for as much as 80% of the mortality associated with inhalation injury. Carbon monoxide has a 250-fold higher affinity for hemoglobin than does oxygen. It diminishes the oxygen-carrying capacity and shifts the oxyhemoglobin dissociation curve to the left. It may also interfere with cellular oxygen metabolism at the mitochondrial level. Although measured partial pressures of oxygen are often normal in CO poisoning, there is relative tissue hypoxia. This is responsible for the delayed central nervous system sequelae of CO poisoning. Carbon monoxide poisoning is diagnosed by measuring carboxyhemoglobin (COHb) levels. Levels in excess of 5% are abnormal, and those greater than 25% mandate referral to an institution where hyperbaric oxygen therapy can be delivered. The half-life of COHb is 3 to 4 hours in room air, diminishes to 30 to 60 minutes at FIO_2 of 1.0, and further decreases to 15 to 20 minutes under hyperbaric conditions at 3 atmospheres.

> *Indications for Bronchoscopy*
>
> - *Diagnostic bronchoscopy is indicated in suspected inhalation injury to aid in definitive diagnosis*
> - *Therapeutic bronchoscopy facilitates removal of carbonaceous debris and the products of inflammation generated in response to inhalation injury*

A high index of suspicion is necessary to diagnose CO poisoning because patients may present with nonspecific signs such as nausea, vomiting, headache, or altered sensorium. Any patient who suffers loss of consciousness at the scene of a fire should be assumed to have CO poisoning. All patients at risk for CO poisoning should receive 100% oxygen. It should be remembered that

COHb levels do not reflect the tissue burden of CO. Therefore patients with significant neurologic abnormalities should be referred for hyperbaric oxygen therapy.

2. Fluid Resuscitation

The burn victim requires fluid resuscitation because the injury itself causes the elaboration of inflammatory mediators that produce local and systemic capillary leak and intravascular volume loss. Superficial burns involving 10% to 15% of BSA can be managed with oral rehydration alone or with intravenous (IV) fluids for supplementation. Burns in excess of 15% BSA typically require IV resuscitation, preferably with 2 IV lines. A bladder catheter should be inserted to facilitate accurate monitoring of urine output and to assess the adequacy of the resuscitation. Intravenous catheters can be safely placed through burn tissue, but placement distal to circumferential burns should be avoided.

> !
>
> *Guides for Fluid Resuscitation*
>
> *First 24 hours*
>
> - *Parkland formula: 4 mL/kg/% BSA burn over 24 h*
> - *Modified Brooke system: 2 mL/kg/% BSA burn over 24 h*
> - *Fluids ultimately titrated to*
>   - *Heart rate*
>   - *Capillary refill*
>   - *Blood pressure*
>   - *Urine output 0.5-1 mL/kg/h*
>
> *Second 24 hours*
>
> - *Maintenance IV fluids*
> - *Albumin 5%: 0.3-0.4 mL/kg/%BSA burn over 24 h*
>
> !

The volume of fluid resuscitation that is required is dictated by the depth and extent of injury and is most commonly guided by use of the Parkland formula, which estimates the fluid requirement of the patient to be 4 mL/kg/% BSA burn over 24 hours. Lactated Ringer's solution is the initial resuscitation fluid with 50% of the total volume delivered in the first 8 hours and the remaining 50% over the subsequent 16 hours. An alternative to the Parkland formula is the modified Brooke system, which recommends 2 mL/kg/% BSA burn over 24 hours. Ultimately, fluid administration should be guided by repeated evaluation of the patient's intravascular volume, which is reflected in the heart rate, blood pressure, capillary refill, and urine output. Adequate urine output for the child under 10 years of age is 1 mL/kg/h and is 0.5 mL/kg/h for children over 10 years of age. Crystalloid is typically employed during the first 24 hours of resuscitation. The use of colloid in the initial resuscitation has not been shown to be beneficial; however, albumin is often administered during the second 24 hours of burn resuscitation. In addition to maintenance IV fluids, during the second 24 hours, albumin is administered as a 5% solution at a daily dose of 0.3-0.4 mL/kg/%BSA divided over 24 hours. As fluid resuscitation progresses, care must be taken not to overload the patient as many burn victims receive a greater volume of fluid than that estimated by the above formulas.

3. Assessment of Burn Injury

The most appropriate tool to estimate the BSA involved in children under 15 years of age is the commonly published and frequently used Lund and Browder chart (**Figure 11-1**). The widely employed rule of nines is most appropriately applied to patients over 15 years of age (**Figure 11-2**). Careful assessment of the depth and severity of injury is important because these factors heavily affect healing. The grading of burns as first, second, and third degree is imprecise and fails to accurately reflect the depth of injury. The current classification scheme, while more precise, is similar to the former insofar as it is also based on depth of injury relative to the anatomy of the skin. The categories are superficial, superficial partial thickness, deep partial thickness, full thickness, and deep full thickness (subdermal).

!

Categorization of Burn Injury

Superficial partial thickness

- *Formerly first degree*
- *Red, wet, blisters*
- *Exquisitely painful*

Deep partial thickness

- *Formerly second degree*
- *White or yellow appearance*
- *Less pain and less blistering*

Full thickness

- *Formerly third degree*
- *White, yellow, black, or brown in color*
- *Firm and inelastic*
- *Distinctly not painful*

!

Figure 11-1. Lund-Browder Chart

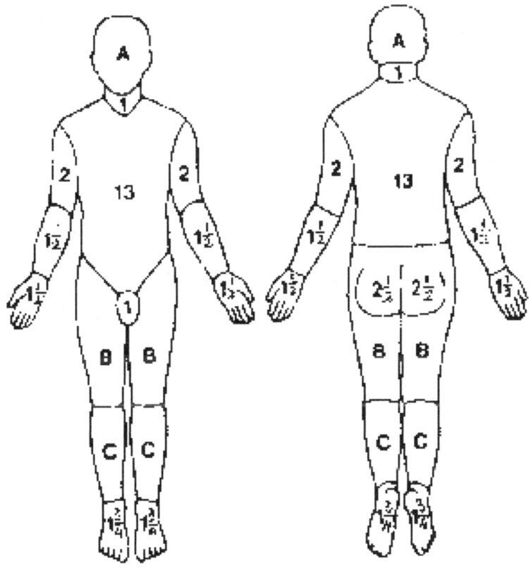

LUND-BROWDER CHART
Relative Percentage of Body Surface Area Affected by Growth

Age in years	0	1	5	10	15	Adult
A-head (back or front)	9½	8½	6½	5½	4½	3½
B-1 thigh (back or front)	2¾	3¼	4	4¼	4½	4¾
C-1 leg (back or front)	2½	2½	2¾	3	3¼	3½

The Lund-Browder chart is the most accurate method for estimating burn extent and must be used in the evaluation of pediatric patients under 15 years of age.

Figure 11-2. Rule of Nines

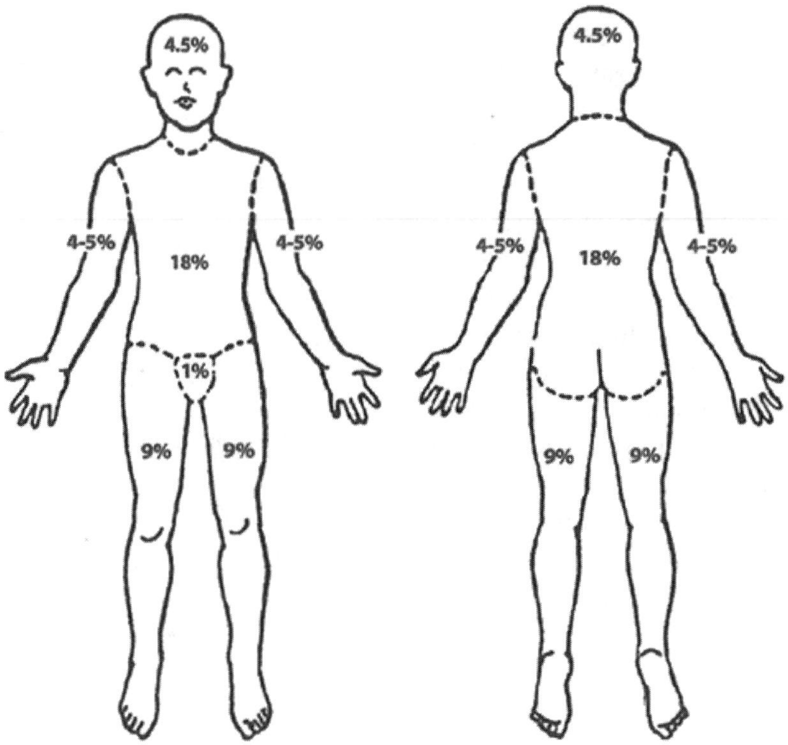

Most appropriate for children over 15 years of age

The skin is composed of 3 layers: epidermis, dermis, and subcutaneous tissue. The epidermis is the outermost layer and consists of stratified squamous epithelial cells known as keratinocytes. The epidermis is avascular and receives its blood supply and nutrients from the dermis. Basement membrane lies between the epidermis and dermis. The dermis is the most physiologically active layer of skin. It consists principally of fibroblasts but also contains basal epidermal cells, macrophages, and neutrophils, and is structurally supported by collagen, glycosaminoglycans, and fibronectin. The dermis contains blood vessels, lymphatic channels, sebaceous and sweat glands, and hair follicles.

The local response to burn is characterized by zones of coagulation, stasis, and hyperemia (**Figures 11-3** to **11-5**). The zone of coagulation is the most central area of injury and exhibits the necrosis that results from greatest contact with the heat source. The zone of stasis, or injury, surrounds the zone of coagulation (necrosis). The microvasculature of this tissue is disrupted, making it prone to secondary ischemic injury. Tissue within the zone of stasis has the potential for regeneration, but its circulation must be supported with fluid administration for the first 24 to 48 hours to maximize the survival of viable tissue. The zone of hyperemia, which surrounds the zone of stasis, is the minimally affected outer border of injury. Such areas heal spontaneously in 7 to 10 days.

Figure 11-3. Superficial Dermal Burn

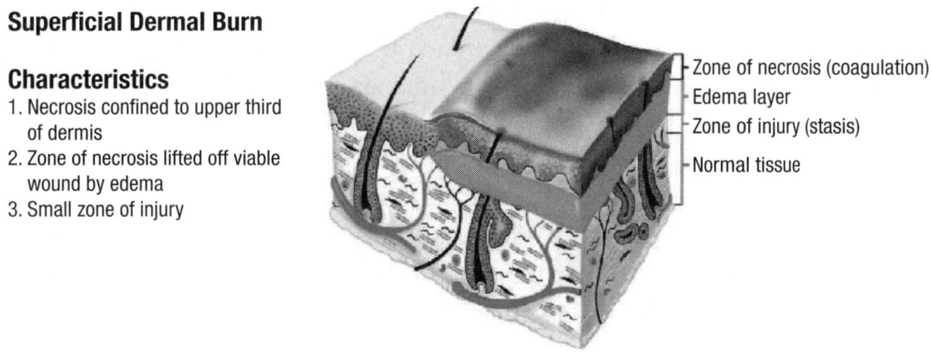
Superficial Dermal Burn
Characteristics
1. Necrosis confined to upper third of dermis
2. Zone of necrosis lifted off viable wound by edema
3. Small zone of injury
Zone of necrosis (coagulation)
Edema layer
Zone of injury (stasis)
Normal tissue

Figure 11-4. Deep Dermal Burn

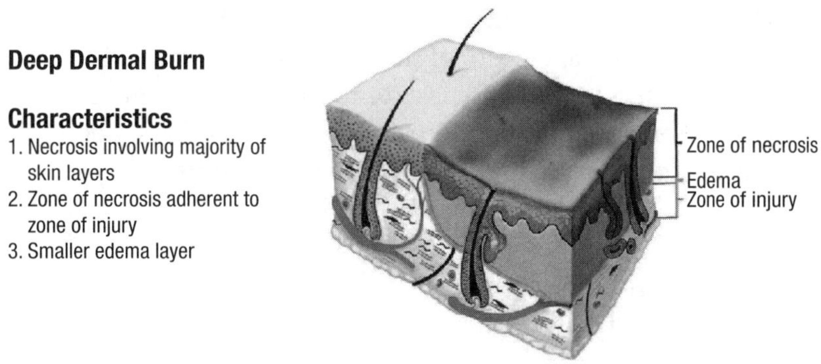

Figure 11-5. Full-Thickness Burn

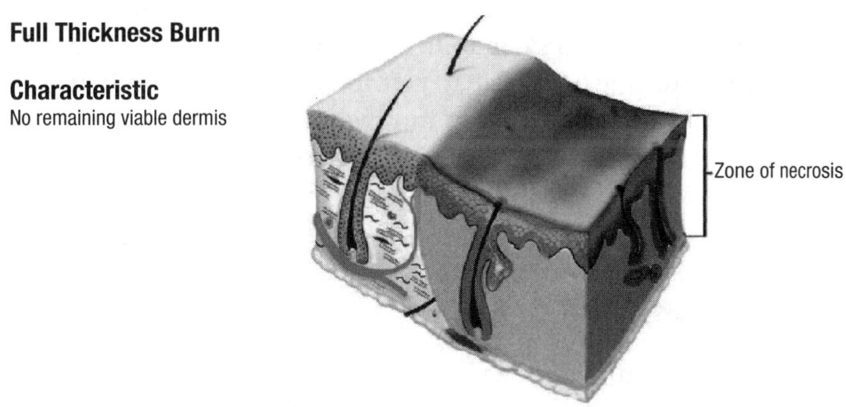

Superficial burns involve only the epidermis. They are typically dry and characterized by erythema and pain without bullae. The keratinocytes slough, and epithelial cells migrate to the surface to facilitate wound closure. These injuries typically heal spontaneously within 7 to 10 days. They are managed with topical analgesics and moisturizing creams. They are not customarily included in estimating the extent of BSA burned because they heal completely without intervention.

Partial-thickness burns extend through the epidermis and into the dermis. Scalding typically produces this type of injury in children. Because partial-thickness burns are not homogeneous and can evolve over hours to days, debridement is usually necessary to accurately assess the depth of injury. Superficial partial-thickness burns, or mid-dermal burns, are erythematous and moist, and the presence of blisters is a hallmark. They are exquisitely painful because of the exposed and injured nerves. Superficial partial-thickness burns heal via reepithelialization within 2 to 3 weeks.

Deep partial-thickness burns, characterized by a white or yellow appearance, may be less painful and demonstrate less blistering. As the depth of injury increases, the amount of pain decreases because more nerve endings are destroyed. Without intervention, deep partial-thickness burns can heal by epithelialization and contraction in 3 to 6 weeks. However, because the results are functionally and cosmetically poor, deep partial-thickness burns are typically managed with grafting.

Full-thickness burns, formerly called third-degree burns, usually result from flame, prolonged contact, or hot oil or grease. Scalding, without prolonged exposure to hot water, rarely produces such burns. Full-thickness burns are characterized by white, yellow, brown, or black discoloration. There is severe edema without blisters, the texture of the skin is firm and inelastic, and eschar may be present. Deep full-thickness, or subdermal, burns extend to the fascia and muscle with the potential to involve tendon and bone. Usually seen in victims of house fires, deep full-thickness burns absolutely require grafting, perhaps with musculocutaneous flaps.

III. TREATMENT OF BURNS

A. Criteria for Hospital Admission

The indications for a patient to be admitted to the hospital for burn care include superficial partial-thickness burns in excess of 10% BSA, inability to maintain adequate hydration or nutrition, caregivers who are unwilling or unable to provide burn care, burn injury in a child with a significant chronic medical condition, the need for intravenous analgesics or anxiolysis, and cases of suspected child abuse. The American Burn Association has established and published criteria for referring patients to burn centers (see **Table 11-1**).

B. Nonsurgical Wound Care

Among the goals of wound care are to minimize bacterial colonization and to prevent infection. A variety of topical agents may be applied to superficial partial-thickness burns and deep partial- or full-thickness burns prior to skin grafting to prevent wound infection. These include Bacitracin, silver sulfadiazine, mafenide acetate, and silver-impregnated antimicrobial dressings.

Bacitracin effectively prophylaxes against gram-positive and a few gram-negative organisms but may produce local irritation. Silver sulfadiazine is the most commonly used topical antimicrobial in burn wound management. It is bacteriocidal against gram-positive and gram-negative organisms and yeast. It is indicated for partial-thickness and full-thickness burns in anticipation of

Table 11-1. American Burn Association Indications for Referral to a Burn Center

- Any burn greater than 15% of the body surface area
- Any burn greater than 9% of the body surface area in patients with significant preexisting disease that may complicate or retard recovery
- Any burn greater than 9% of the body surface area in patients 5 years of age or younger or 60 years of age and older
- Any burn involving critical body parts, such as eyes, face, hands, feet, ears, or genital area
- Any third-degree burn of greater than 5% of the body surface area
- Inhalation injuries, electrical burns, and burn injuries complicated by underlying fractures or other trauma

grafting. However, silver sulfadiazine is to be avoided in patients with sulfa allergies and glucose-6-phosphate dehydrogenase deficiency. Due to permanent skin staining, it is contraindicated for facial burns in children under 2 months of age, and due to the association between kernicterus and sulfonamides, it is also contraindicated in late-term pregnant women. Mafenide acetate is a bacteriostatic agent effective against both gram-positive and gram-negative organisms, including pseudomonas and certain anaerobes. It is employed primarily in partial- or full-thickness burns because it can penetrate devitalized tissue. It is active in acidic (purulent) environments and is therefore particularly appropriate for eschars. Mafenide acetate can produce metabolic acidosis because it inhibits carbonic anhydrase.

A variety of relatively new, silver-impregnated, antimicrobial dressings with the ability to absorb exudate may be applied to burn wounds. The advantage of these dressings over the topical antimicrobials is that they can be left in place for several days, which eliminates the need for daily dressing changes and may in turn be associated with less pain and anxiety decreasing the need for sedation and analgesia. As yet there are no good comparative outcome data, but antimicrobial dressings appear to yield equal efficacy and cosmetic outcome when compared to topical antimicrobial agents.

!

Topical Agents Employed in Burn Care

Product	Application	Advantages	Disadvantages
Bacitracin	Deep partial thickness, small areas	Not water soluble, good on face	Not indicated for large surface area
Creams			
Silver sulfadiazine	Deep partial or full thickness	Soothing, good for range of motion	Possible neutropenia, little penetration
Mafenide acetate	Deep partial or full thickness	Penetrates eschar	Painful, metabolic acidosis
Solutions			
Aqueous silver nitrate (0.5%)	Deep partial or full thickness	Good antimicrobial	Hyponatremia, stains wound, little penetration
Mafenide acetate (5%)	Graft dressing and open wound soak	Broad activity, moist dressing	Not used for unexcised wound
Impregnated dressings			
Acticoat™	Deep partial thickness	Dressing change every 3 days	Only deep partial thickness
Aquacel® Ag	Deep partial thickness	May be left on for 21 days	Less flexibility and ease of motion, only deep partial thickness

!

C. Burn Wound Excision and Grafting

Although no controlled studies demonstrate improved outcomes with early excision and grafting of burn injuries, this practice may be responsible for the decreased mortality from burn injuries realized over the past 20 years. The rationale for early closure of deep injuries is to reduce local infection and fluid loss and their attendant complications.

Current practice calls for grafting within 1 to 2 weeks of the injury, performed by appropriately trained surgeons at a burn center.

For the young child with deep or large partial-thickness injury, it is often necessary to provide moderate to deep sedation in addition to analgesia to accomplish appropriate debridement and dressing changes. The depth of sedation necessary will be affected by the extent of the injury and debridement required, the patient's age, and respiratory and cardiovascular status.

D. Management of Inhalation Injury

Therapy for inhalation injury consists of aggressive pulmonary toilet, use of mucolytics, early identification and treatment of infection, and supportive care. Although there are no data supporting the routine use of mucolytics in patients with inhalation injury, many experts recommend N-acetyl-cysteine (3-5 mL of a 20% solution nebulized 3 or 4 times a day) or dornase alfa (2.5 mg nebulized once or twice daily) to help clear secretions. Routine prophylaxis with antibiotics is not used; corticosteroids are of no benefit and are potentially harmful.

The level of respiratory support that is required may range from supplemental oxygen to advanced modes of assisted ventilation and hyperbaric oxygen therapy. Supplemental oxygen should be provided via nasal cannula or simple facemask, both of which add additional humidification. If stridor due to upper airway inflammation and edema is present, racemic epinephrine may be employed to transiently relieve the obstruction to airflow. Helium-oxygen admixtures (heliox) reduce resistance to turbulent airflow and, in turn, improve work of breathing in situations of upper airway obstruction. When the airway is compromised, however, these patients should be intubated for airway control and to permit definitive assessment. Based on a recent survey of pediatric burn centers, approximately 12% of pediatric burn victims require intubation, with approximately 70% of those intubated having sustained inhalation injury.

Until quite recently, Pediatric Advanced Life Support (PALS) guidelines called for the use of uncuffed endotracheal tubes in children under 8 years of age. However, ample evidence suggests that cuffed endotracheal tubes are safe and more effective in critically ill and burned pediatric patients, especially those with restrictive lung disease, in whom the presence of a leak around the endotracheal tube would impair oxygenation and ventilation. Current PALS guidelines support the use of cuffed tubes in all children. Tube size may be calculated using the formula that has been employed for uncuffed tubes: (age + 16)/4. However, children with burns and/or inhalation injury frequently experience significant airway edema; therefore, the size of the endotracheal tube should be reduced by 0.5 millimeters when using a cuffed tube.

The prevalence of acute respiratory distress syndrome (ARDS) in mechanically ventilated adults with major burns has been estimated to be as high as 54%. Although the prevalence in pediatric burn patients is likely lower, acute lung injury and ARDS represent significant clinical challenges, especially in very young patients. The level of pulmonary dysfunction should govern the mode of mechanical ventilation employed in the care of the pediatric burn patient. Lung-protective ventilator strategies should be employed in patients at risk for acute lung injury. Low tidal volume/ high positive end-expiratory pressure (PEEP) is used initially and progresses to high-frequency oscillatory ventilation (HFOV) or airway pressure release ventilation (APRV) in patients who require PEEP in excess of 10 to 15 centimeters of H_2O.

1. Timing of Tracheostomy

Tracheostomy is classically utilized in patients following a prolonged course of endotracheal intubation. Although early tracheostomy (2-4 days after initiation of assisted ventilation) has also been used safely in a cohort of pediatric burn patients, tracheostomy is generally reserved for patients who have failed extubation or for those projected to require chronic mechanical ventilation, such as neurologically devastated patients.

E. Hypermetabolism and Nutrition

The classic description of the metabolic response to injury includes an early ebb phase that is characterized by low cardiac output and a decreased metabolic rate, followed by a hypermetabolic phase that starts at 24 to 36 hours after injury. Protein metabolism and energy expenditure increase by approximately 50% due to hypermetabolism, fluid losses, sepsis, and inflammation in children following a large burn injury, and this catabolic state can persist for 9 to 12 months. Early and aggressive nutritional therapy has been shown to reduce the elevated resting energy expenditure (REE) in burn victims. The most effective method of determining REE is by indirect calorimetry. When that is not available, nutritional therapy in the burn patient is usually guided by a formula, such as those used at the Shriners Burn Center (**Table 11-2**).

Table 11-2. Nutritional Therapy Formulas

Infants 0-12 months	2100 kcal/m^2 + 1000 kcal/m^2 burn
Children 1-11 years	1800 kcal/m^2 + 1300 kcal/m^2 burn
Children 12 years and older	1500 kcal/m^2 + 1500 kcal/m^2 burn

Source: Shriners Burn Center

The enteral route is preferred for administration of nutrition. A nasogastric or nasoduodenal tube should be placed as soon as the initial evaluation and burn resuscitation are complete, and in the absence of contraindications, enteral feeds should be initiated within 24 hours of injury. However, feeding intolerance as evidenced by significant gastric residual volume and diarrhea may limit use of the gastrointestinal tract for caloric delivery. Diarrhea is a commonly encountered problem in the burn population. The etiology is likely multifactorial, is usually noninfectious, and is not worsened by hypoalbuminemia. Factors associated with a decreased incidence of diarrhea in burn victims include fat intake less than 20% of overall caloric intake, vitamin A intake greater than 10,000 international units per day in adults, and early implementation of enteral feeds (within 48 hours of burn injury).

In addition to vitamin A, other vitamins, minerals, and trace elements may be required in excess of recommended daily allowances, including calcium, magnesium, vitamin D, zinc, copper, and other micronutrients. Supplementation of calcium and magnesium until serum levels are within the normal range is recommended.

In addition to early and aggressive nutritional support, attempts have been made to pharmacologically mitigate the hypermetabolic state that persists following burn injury. The hypermetabolism, which can be blunted to some extent by β-blockade, has led some to recommend the use of propranolol. This should be done only in a burn center experienced in the care of children.

F. Hypoalbuminemia

In burn patients, hypoalbuminemia is a frequent finding. The etiology is multifactorial. Increased losses of albumin occur directly via drainage from burn wounds and diffusely as a consequence of profound capillary leakage, which is ignited by the cascade of inflammatory mediators triggered by the burn injury. Albumin production is also reduced in critical illness, likely due to an increase in production of acute phase proteins. Additionally, in the immediate post-resuscitation phase, a dilutional contribution to hypoalbuminemia may occur if intravascular volume is increased. Chronic illness and malnutrition are other potential causes of nonacute hypoalbuminemia.

Albumin contributes 80% of the normal colloid oncotic pressure; therefore, hypoalbuminemia is associated with edema, particularly of the pulmonary interstitium and bowel wall. Albumin is often administered in an effort to avoid exacerbating acute lung injury, diarrhea, feeding intolerance, impaired wound healing, and the resultant complications. However, the preponderance of evidence demonstrates that mild-to-moderate hypoalbuminemia is well tolerated in previously healthy patients. Among burn patients with hypoalbuminemia, serum albumin gradually normalizes, especially in the context of aggressive nutritional therapy, and higher serum albumin concentration is seen in patients who receive enteral, as opposed to parenteral, nutrition. Therefore, routine albumin repletion may not be warranted. The current recommendation is to ensure appropriate caloric delivery, preferably by the enteral route, as quickly as possible, and in critically ill pediatric patients, 25% albumin should be added if the serum level is below 2 mg/dL.

G. Glycemic Control

As noted previously, protein metabolism and energy expenditure increase by approximately 50% in children following a large burn injury. The etiology of this catabolic state is multifactorial but favorably affected by insulin administration. Hyperglycemia in adult burn patients is associated with increased morbidity and mortality. Although it has not been demonstrated that intensive insulin therapy can be safely and effectively implemented in the pediatric population, its use in the pediatric burn population may lower infection rates and improve survival. Careful attention must be paid to avoiding hypoglycemia. Members of the healthcare team participating in the care of pediatric burn patients should be sensitized to the importance of glucose monitoring and the recognition of hypoglycemia, especially in very young or nonverbal children. Standing insulin orders should only be written for patients who demonstrate persistent hyperglycemia while they receive constant glucose delivery in the form of enteral tube feedings or parenteral nutrition and must be associated with frequent bedside monitoring of serum glucose.

IV. OUTCOME

Mortality from burns has improved over the past 20 years but may have reached a plateau in the past decade. The risk of mortality in children remains inversely proportional to age and directly proportional to extent of injury. In children over 2 years of age who suffer burns to greater than 50% BSA, mortality is approximately 20%, but in children under 2 years of age mortality is approximately 50%. Early excision and closure of injured tissue is believed to be the reason for improved mortality. Smoke inhalation and thermal injury remain risk factors for increased mortality; the risk of mortality increases by 20% with inhalation injury.

Care of the pediatric burn victim has advanced in parallel with advances in burn and critical care. The importance of early physical therapy, splinting of injured extremities, and advances in grafting techniques and skin substitutes are all contributing to improvements in quality of life following burn injury. Additional advancements in the elasticity of grafted tissues and microvascular reconstructive techniques promise to yield further improvements in cosmetic and functional outcomes.

Key Points

Pediatric Burn Injury

- Initial evaluation of the pediatric burn victim begins with assessment of airway, breathing and circulation as it would for any trauma patient. In addition, the extent and depth of burn injury should be assessed.
- SIRS is a common finding in burn victims, contributes to intravascular volume depletion and shock, and hence appropriate fluid resuscitation, in the first 24 hours and beyond is important to avoid early complications of serious burns. Fluid administration may be guided by the Parkland or Modified Brooke Formulas but ultimately must be titrated to urine output and perfusion.
- Early excision and grafting are now standards of care in the management of deep partial and full thickness burns and have impacted on mortality and morbidity associated with burns.
- Hypermetabolism is a significant long term (9-12 months) sequela of significant burn injury and appropriate management can significantly improve morbidity and mortality.
- Outcomes for burn injuries have improved over the past twenty years.

Suggested Readings

1. American Heart Association. Pediatric Advanced Life Support. *Circulation.* 2005;112(suppl 1):IV-167–IV-187.

2. Barrow RE, Wolfe RR, Dasu MR, et al. The use of beta-adrenergic blockade in preventing trauma-induced hepatomegaly. *Ann Surg.* 2006;243:115-120.

3. Cartotto R, Ellis S, Smith T. Use of high-frequency oscillatory ventilation in burn patients. *Crit Care Med.* 2005;33(3):S175-S181.

4. Duffy B, McLaughlin P, Eichelberger M. Assessment, triage, and early management of burns in children. *Clin Pediatr Emerg Med.* 2006;7:82-93.

5. Finfer S, Norton R, Bellomo R, et. al. The SAFE study: saline vs albumin for fluid resuscitation in the critically ill. *Vox Sang.* 2004;87(suppl 2):S123-S131.

6. Gottschlich MM, Warden GD, Michel M, et al. Diarrhea in tube-fed burn patients: incidence, etiology, nutritional impact, and prevention. *JPEN J Parenter Enteral Nutr.* 1988;12(4):338-345.

7. Greenhalgh DG, Housinger TA, Kagan RJ, et al. Maintenance of serum albumin levels in pediatric burn patients: a prospective, randomized trial. *J Trauma.* 1995;39(1):67-74.

8. Hart DW, Wolf SE, Ramzy PI, et al. Anabolic effects of oxandrolone after severe burn. *Ann Surg.* 2001;233(4):556-564.

9. Levine BA, Petroff PA, Slade CL, et al. Prospective trials of dexamethasone and aerosolized gentamycin in the treatment of inhalation injury in the burned patient. *J Trauma.* 1978;18:188-193.

10. Mlcak RP, Jeschke MG, Barrow RE, et al. The influence of age and gender on resting energy expenditure in severely burned children. *Ann Surg.* 2006;244:121-130.

11. Pham TN, Warren AJ, Phan HH, et al. Impact of tight glycemic control in severely burned children. *J Trauma.* 2005;59:1148-1154.

12. Sheridan RL, Prelack K, Cunningham JJ. Physiologic hypoalbuminemia is well tolerated by severely burned children. *J Trauma.* 1997;43(3):448-452.

13. Silver GM, Freiburg C, Halerz M, et al. A survey of airway and ventilator management strategies in North American pediatric burn units. *J Burn Care Rehabil.* 2004;25:435-440.

14. Suman OE, Mlcak RP, Chinkes DL, et al. Resting energy expenditure in severely burned children: analysis of agreement between indirect calorimetry and prediction equations using the Bland-Altman method. *Burns.* 2006;32:335-342.

15. Van den Berghe G, Wouters PJ, Bouillon R, et al. Outcome benefit of intensive insulin therapy in the critically ill: insulin dose versus glycemic control. *Crit Care Med.* 2003;31(2):359-366.

16. Voruganti VS, Klein GL, Lu H, et al. Impaired zinc and copper status in children with burn injuries: need to reassess nutritional requirements. *Burns.* 2005;31:711-716.

17. Yurt RW, Howell JD, Greenwald BM. Burns, electrical injuries, and smoke inhalation. In: M Rogers, ed. *Textbook of Pediatric Intensive Care.* 4th ed. Philadelphia, PA: Lippincott Williams & Wilkins; 2008.

Chapter 12:

NON-ACCIDENTAL INJURIES: DIAGNOSIS AND MANAGEMENT

Objectives

- Identify risk factors for abuse.
- Describe injury patterns suggestive of abuse.
- Discuss the appropriate evaluation of the child with suspicious injuries.
- Describe the initial resuscitation of a child with potentially abusive injuries.
- Review the healthcare provider role as a mandated reporter of suspected child abuse.

Case Studies

A 2-month-old, previously healthy baby girl is brought to the hospital for evaluation of apnea and lethargy after having choked during a feeding. The child's mother states that the child started to have episodes of colic over the past week but was otherwise well before the mother went to work earlier that morning, leaving the baby and an older sibling in the care of her boyfriend. On initial examination, the infant is tachycardic with cool extremities, and respirations are irregular. The infant is immediately intubated and given fluid resuscitation. Although the secondary survey does not show any bruises, her anterior fontanelle is tense. Retinal hemorrhages are noted.

- What is the possible diagnosis?

- What needs to be done to resuscitate this infant?

- What tests would be useful to evaluate the severity of the patient's condition?

I. INTRODUCTION

Child maltreatment is a tragically common cause of death, permanent disability, and suffering worldwide. Although many children present with histories and clinical findings that suggest abusive injuries, diagnosis and management may be complicated by atypical and delayed presentations, vague and misleading histories, and the patients' inability to communicate. In addition, inflicted injuries may be overlooked in children from prosperous, 2-parent families because suspicion tends to decrease in such circumstances. Child maltreatment must be considered in the differential diagnosis of any child presenting with injuries or a decreased level of consciousness.

Recognized risk factors for child maltreatment are varied, as can be seen in **Table 12-1.**

Table 12-1. Risk Factors for Child Maltreatment

Risk Factors
Intimate partner violence
Prior child abuse/neglect
Substance-abusing caregivers
Colicky/fussy child
Prematurity or prolonged neonatal hospitalization
Neurodevelopmental disability

Premature birth may interfere with infant-parent bonding. Babies discharged from the nursery after a prolonged hospitalization may have significant impairments, including developmental delays, feeding problems, and respiratory difficulties. These babies may be quite irritable and difficult to console, and may ultimately exhaust the ability of young, poorly supported caregivers to cope with them. Toileting mishaps and irritating behaviors may result in abusive injuries to toddlers and older children.

> ! *Non-accidental injuries are more likely to occur in stressed households, particularly when parent-child bonding is impaired.* !

II. INJURIES THAT RAISE SUSPICION OF CHILD ABUSE

Caregivers may report mechanisms of injury that are highly unlikely at the child's expected developmental stage. Preverbal siblings may be blamed for injuries. Caregivers with substance-abuse problems, particularly those involved in the production or sale of methamphetamine or other illegal drugs, may be reluctant to summon emergency medical services to the home and may opt to transport an injured child themselves despite the added risk to the child.

> ! *Inconsistencies relating to the circumstances of an injury and any delay in seeking care should raise concerns of child maltreatment.* !

A. Patterns Suggestive of Abuse

Although patterns of physical injury are not absolute, among the injuries consistently found in children with witnessed, accidental injuries are epidural hematomas, simple linear skull fractures, diaphyseal and spiral fractures in ambulatory children, and irregular, patternless, asymmetric thermal injuries that have splash marks and do not spare the popliteal or antecubital fossae. A comparison of some common accidental and non-accidental injuries is presented in **Table 12-2.**

Table 12-2. Accidental Versus Non-accidental Patterns of Injury[a]

Site of Injury	Accidental Injury	Non-accidental Injury
Head	Focal injuries at site of impact Clear history of causative accident Simple, linear skull fracture Absence of other injuries	Global/widespread Inconsistent description of injury Diastatic, depressed skull fractures from reported short falls Injuries to other body sites
Skeletal	Mid-shaft clavicular Diaphysis of long bones in ambulatory children	Posterior ribs Metaphyses of long bones in non-ambulatory children Vertebral body Multiple sites Varying ages of injury
Skeletal	Bruises over bony prominences in ambulatory children Burns with splash appearance	Bruises to face or head in non-ambulatory children Bruises over padded areas, ears, neck, genitalia Patterned injuries and bites Burns with well-demarcated edges Bruises or burns involving genitalia

[a] No pattern of injury is diagnostic of either accident or abuse without consideration of the supporting history and developmental stage of the child.

Although accidental impact injuries to the head can result in subdural hematomas adjacent to the site of impact, subdural hematomas are very uncommon in falls of less than 3 to 4 feet. Conversely, diffuse thin-rimmed subdural hematomas, retinal hemorrhages, posterior rib fractures, and metaphyseal fractures are more commonly found in children with inflicted injuries. Burns that are bilateral, symmetric, or of uniform depth; that have clearly defined borders, definable patterns, or evidence of healing or infection; or that include the anogenital areas should raise suspicion of maltreatment (see examples in **Figures 12-1 and 12-2**).

Figure 12-1. Burns Caused by Immersion in Hot Water

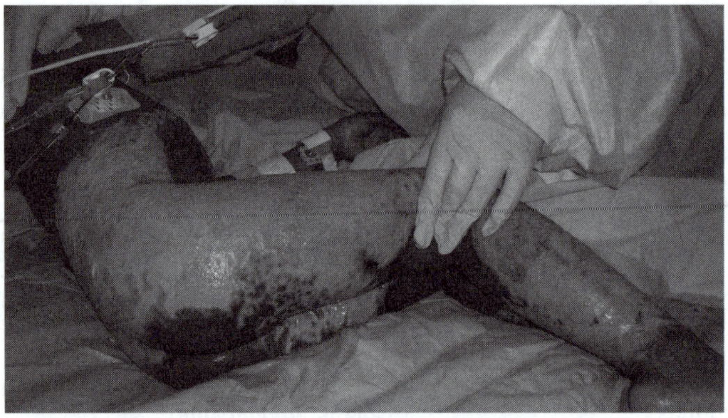

Full-thickness burns with flexure sparing due to immersion in hot water.

Figure 12-2. Small, Healed, Patterned Burns

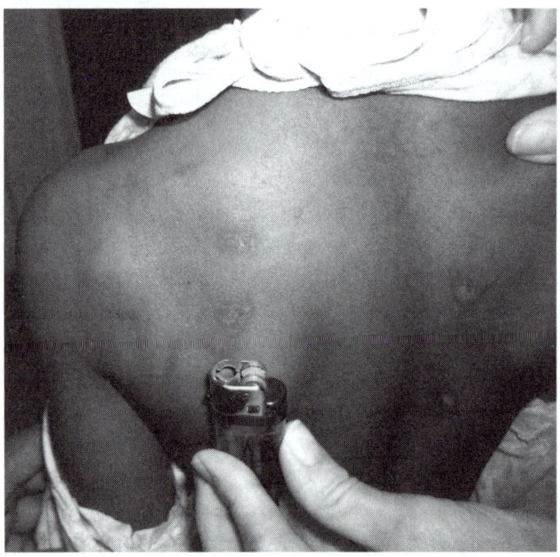

> *Although injury patterns may suggest either accidental or non-accidental injury, they must be considered in the context of the description of the mishap, the child's medical and developmental history, cultural factors, and clinical findings.*

B. Common Patterns of Maltreatment

1. Abusive Head Trauma

Abusive head trauma, also known as shaken-baby or shaken-impact syndrome, is a frequently incomplete triad consisting of inflicted head injury with extraaxial hematoma, retinal hemorrhage, and skeletal injury, including metaphyseal and posterior rib fractures (**Figure 12-3**). Young infants are at the highest risk, but toddlers may display this pattern of abuse as well. A frustrated caregiver's violent shaking of a child, with or without concomitant projection to a hard or soft surface, results in severe rotational and shearing forces capable of tearing bridging veins in the subdural and subarachnoid spaces.

Unlike children with accidental head injuries, who often present with clear histories and focal injury patterns, patients with inflicted head injuries will often present with more global cerebral findings, clinical features consistent with shock, and pallor. Caregivers commonly deny or minimize trauma. Soft-tissue swelling and bruising may or may not accompany severe inflicted head injuries, and bulging, tense fontanelles are noted. Loss of fontanelle pulsatility occurs as intracranial hypertension worsens. Cerebral edema may be fatal despite a relatively compliant infant skull.

Inflicted skull fractures may cross suture lines, be numerous, and be widely diastatic. Inflicted primary brain injury is compounded by secondary injury resulting from hypoventilation, hypoxia, and hypoperfusion. Neurogenic fever may occur within a few hours of injury. Seizures are extremely common in abused infants, may be subclinical, and are often very difficult to control. These secondary insults lead to profound, progressive, global cerebral edema and ischemia.

Figure 12-3. Radiograph From an Infant With Abusive Head Trauma

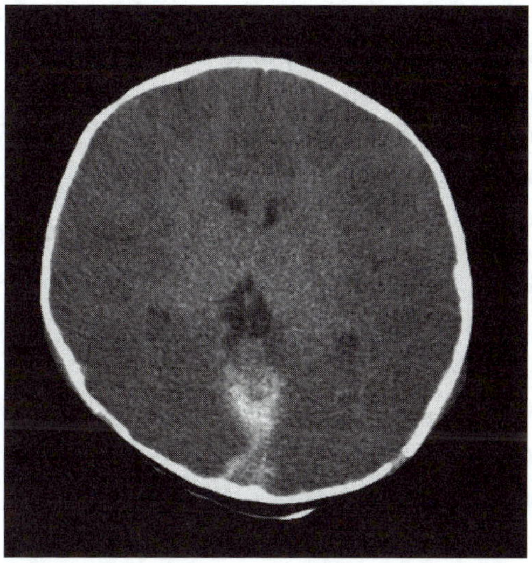

A radiograph reveals subarachnoid and subdural hemorrhages and cerebral edema consistent with abusive head trauma.

Other etiologies for intracranial pathology must be considered in the differential diagnosis of child abuse. Appropriate diagnostic testing and treatment, including antibiotics and possibly dexamethasone, should be rapidly initiated if bacterial meningitis is even a remote possibility. Acyclovir should be considered if the clinical picture suggests encephalitis. Nontraumatic causes of intracranial hemorrhage can be further investigated with neuroimaging and evaluation of coagulation or metabolic disorders.

Lumbar puncture should be reserved for infants who do not have any respiratory or hemodynamic abnormalities. In general, this procedure should not be performed in the emergency department during the initial evaluation and stabilization of critically ill children. Risks of lumbar puncture include cardiopulmonary arrest, herniation syndromes in the presence of intracranial hypertension, and spinal epidural hematoma if the child is coagulopathic. Thus, lumbar puncture is best not performed until all those problems have been corrected.

> ! *Lumbar puncture may precipitate cardiac arrest in the unstable child.*

2. Retinal Hemorrhages

> ! *Medications intended to facilitate funduscopy should be used with caution in children with evolving neurologic findings*

The retinal hemorrhages that frequently, though not always, accompany extraaxial hemorrhages in inflicted head injury are the result of shear forces disrupting vulnerable tissue interfaces. The vitreous body is adherent to the retina in young children, and traction on this structure during rotational injury results in retinal hemorrhages occurring in multiple layers and extending to the periphery of the retina. This pattern is distinct from the focal abnormalities noted in patients with increased intracranial pressure, those who have sustained prolonged resuscitative efforts, and those who have suffered an accidental traumatic brain injury. Medications that facilitate funduscopy should be used with caution in children with evolving neurologic findings because they may complicate the early diagnosis of worsening cerebral edema by precluding use of pupillary reactivity as a harbinger of evolving intracranial events.

> ! *Mydriatic drops may obscure early pupillary signs of increased intracranial pressure for many hours. A dilated ophthalmology exam may be safely deferred until this danger has passed.*

3. Blunt Abdominal Injury

Case Study

A 3-year-old boy is found on his doorstep by his grandmother. Paramedics called to the home note tachycardia and hypotension. He is resuscitated en route to the hospital. His abdomen is noted to be distended and tender to palpation.

- What is the possible diagnosis?

- What needs to be done immediately to resuscitate this youngster?

- What tests would be useful to evaluate the severity of the patient's condition?

Inflicted blunt abdominal trauma is most commonly seen in the larger and more mobile child, typically toddlers and children of preschool age. These injuries usually have a delayed presentation and extremely high associated morbidity. Although toddlers and older children may also suffer inflicted head injuries, these differ from the pattern seen in young infants in that they are usually due to direct impact or translational rather than rotational forces.

> !
>
> *Abdominal injuries typically present many hours after they occur. These injuries follow shaken-impact syndrome as the most common cause of death and severe morbidity in the abused child.*
>
> !

The combination of solid organ and hollow viscus injury in the absence of corroborated high-velocity impact is highly suggestive of child abuse. The following organs are the most commonly affected in inflicted abdominal injuries:

- Liver
- Spleen
- Hollow viscus
- Pancreas
- Kidney

Compressive forces may cause hematoma formation in the highly vascular duodenum. Although perforation may occur in any segment of the bowel, it is more common in the proximal jejunum due to that segment's relatively fixed position. Pancreatic contusion and transection may result in severe pancreatitis. Mesenteric disruption may compromise bowel perfusion, causing perforation. Hypovolemic shock may progress rapidly to uncompensated or even irreversible shock.

It is important to note that much like inflicted severe head injuries, fatal abdominal injuries may occur without cutaneous evidence. Children may demonstrate abdominal tenderness, peritoneal signs, and distention on presentation. The diagnosis of abdominal injury may be missed in the presence of severe neurologic injury when bruising is absent. Given the life-threatening nature of abdominal injuries, they should be suspected and excluded in children presenting with other abusive injuries. Although CT imaging readily demonstrates solid organ injury, hollow viscus injuries may escape detection until clinical deterioration occurs or a contrast study is performed.

4. Other Injury Patterns

a. Skeletal Trauma

Fractures involving the metaphyses in non-ambulatory children, posterior rib, scapula, sternum, and spinous processes are often associated with child abuse. However, any fracture that does not appear to coincide with a child's developmental stage, the related findings, and the reported mechanism of injury should raise suspicions of abuse and requires further evaluation. Posterior rib fractures in previously healthy infants indicate severe trauma to the skeletal system and, in the absence of a clear history of serious accidental trauma, are strongly linked to abuse. These fractures occur when a child is subjected to squeezing forces that cause disruption at the costovertebral junction, and they are often not visible on plain radiograph until they are in the healing phase of callus formation (**Figure 12-4**).

Figure 12-4. Radiograph Showing Numerous Healing and Acute Rib Fractures

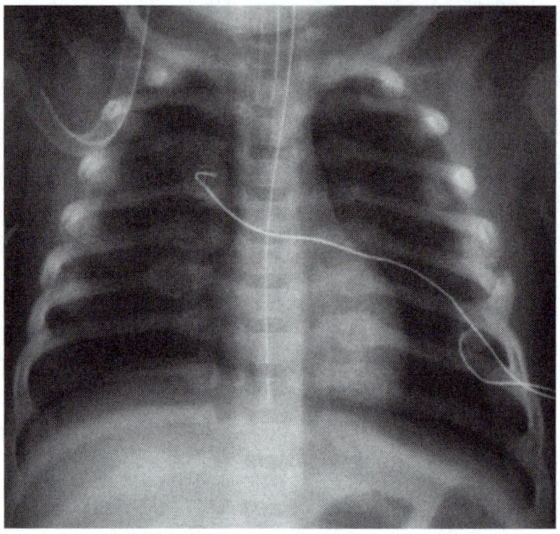

b. Cutaneous Injury

Bruises that occur in children who are not ambulatory, are clustered in pattern, occur away from bony prominences of the body, and involve the abdomen, buttocks, back, face, ears, and hands should be viewed with suspicion. Occasionally, bruising and other cutaneous injuries may have patterns that coincide with the object or implement used to inflict the injury. It should be noted that bruises cannot be accurately dated by appearance and that medical professionals should be cautious in handling requests from investigative personnel to do so. Child maltreatment specialists may help determine the significance of cutaneous abnormalities in patients with specific cultural backgrounds. When the distribution of bruising does not match the history provided by family members, a past medical and family history of easy bruising and bleeding should be obtained. Examples of patterned abusive bruising are presented in **Figures 12-5A and 12-5B.**

Figure 12-5A. Patterned Abusive Bruising

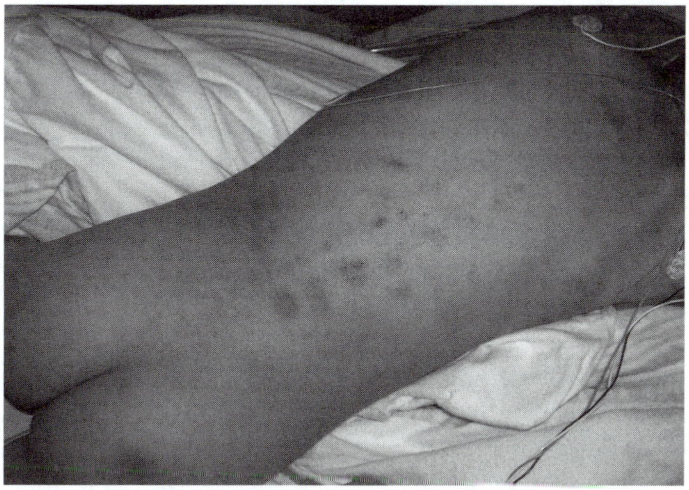

Many scratches and bruises over the back are present in this photograph.

Figure 12-5B. Patterned Abusive Bruising

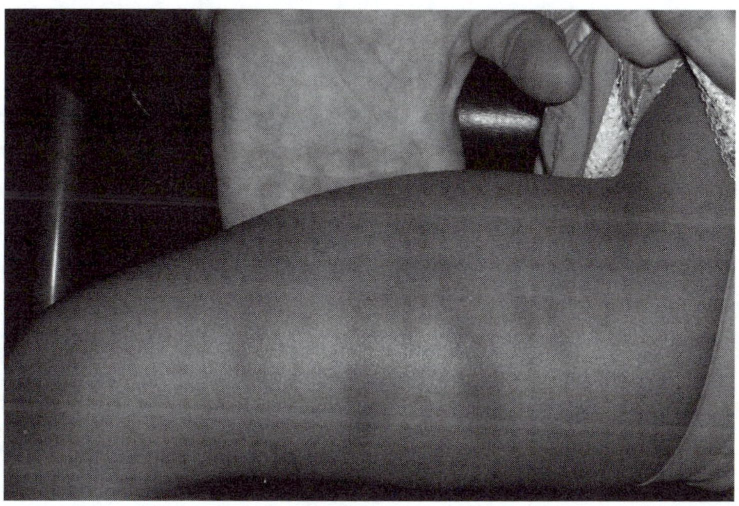

Clearly patterned bruising is visible on this child's thigh.

c. Sexual Abuse

Not only is sexual abuse distressingly frequent and underreported, but it also often goes undiagnosed until other injuries or even pregnancy prompt evaluation. Any patient presenting with perineal trauma with or without a history of sexual abuse should be carefully evaluated, and if the findings are suspicious, a report should be filed and an expert should be called in for further examination. Of course, even in the absence of obvious perineal injury, patients presenting with clear disclosures of abuse should still be reported and referred for expert evaluation.

> !
>
> *Life-threatening abdominal or pelvic injury must be carefully excluded in any patient with perineal trauma.*
>
> !

When a child has a history of sexual contact within the last 72 hours, an evidence-collection kit must be prepared using appropriate measures to ensure that the chain of evidence is not disrupted. Anal dilatation may be an incidental finding during the initial evaluation of deeply sedated, critically ill children and may mimic sexual abuse. This and any other troubling findings are best evaluated and excluded by a pediatrician experienced in the evaluation of sexual abuse. The possibility of sexually transmitted disease must be addressed in any child presenting with suspected sexual abuse.

d. Asphyxiation

Asphyxiation injuries may be very difficult to diagnose. Smothering may share some features of near-miss sudden infant death syndrome and presents as a global hypoxic-ischemic injury with varying degrees of neurological and multiorgan dysfunction. Careful questioning after the patient's initial stabilization may elicit a history suggestive of deliberate or accidental suffocation; however, the true etiology of the infant's collapse may never be disclosed.

e. Ingestions

Accidental ingestions are most common in children between 1 and 5 years of age. Ingestions in non-ambulatory or older preadolescent children should raise concern for abuse. All ingestions deemed to be accidental merit review of safety measures. Massive amounts of potentially lethal drugs may be forced upon children of all ages and may cause refractory hemodynamic instability with cardiac arrest. A comprehensive toxicology screen should be immediately sent during the evaluation of any child with disturbed consciousness. Positive results for illicit drugs on screening drug tests should be confirmed to avoid reporting a potentially false-positive test. Prompt consultation with a toxicologist or a poison control center for optimal antidote and decontamination advice may be lifesaving (**see Chapter 14**). Hemodialysis or other modes of extracorporeal support may be necessary, which underscores the importance of prompt referral.

Caustic ingestions that are more severe than expected based on history or developmental stage may indicate that a child is living in a home where illegal drug use or manufacture is occurring. This has become more common as the use of methamphetamine has increased.

f. Medical Neglect

Medical neglect is yet another tragic form of child maltreatment. The demands of caring for a chronically ill, technology-dependent child can become overwhelming. Substance abuse is a common comorbid factor in the negligent behavior of caregivers. Noncompliance with medical care may lead to near-fatal complications in children with diseases such as asthma, short bowel syndrome, and diabetes. Severe failure to thrive may present as a medical emergency when a child's weight is less than 70% of the predicted weight for length. Such children are at significant risk for refeeding syndrome with resultant life-threatening electrolyte disturbances and, thus, require extremely close monitoring during the initial stages of support.

III. ACUTE MANAGEMENT OF CHILD MALTREATMENT

Optimal care of any acutely ill or injured child begins with complete initial and serial assessments of the patient's airway, breathing, and circulation, aptly termed the ABCs. A complete set of vital signs and a score on the Glasgow Coma Scale (GCS) must be obtained on presentation and at frequent intervals thereafter. Specific stabilizing measures for the management of shock and pediatric trauma are described in depth in **Chapters 7 and 10**. In brief, the airway should be assessed for patency, respiratory rate, pattern and work of breathing. Continuous pulse oximetry is essential for ensuring adequate oxygenation. The child's circulation and perfusion are monitored with continuous electrocardiography and assessments of capillary refill in a central location.

> **!**
>
> *All principles of pediatric advanced life support and trauma management apply to abused children. These patients, however, may be more difficult to stabilize because their presentation to the emergency department may be significantly delayed.*
>
> **!**

Hypotension is a very late sign in pediatric shock; therefore, inadequate perfusion should be appropriately treated before frank hypotension develops. Hypoglycemia or hyperglycemia may both worsen neurological outcome and are easily treated. A rapid blood sugar determination is essential on presentation of all critically ill or unstable patients.

The modified GCS should be frequently monitored to track changes in mentation, particularly during transfers from one facility to another (**see Chapter 15**). Older infants and children incapable of making or maintaining eye contact are highly likely to have a severe injury with systemic and neurologic dysfunction. Intubation using neuroprotective strategies is indicated for patients with a GCS of 8 or a falling score. These patients may have inadequate airway reflexes and may rapidly progress to severe hypoxemia, hypercarbia, or complete respiratory arrest, all of which will adversely affect their neurological outcome.

Efforts to limit secondary brain injury by managing increased intracranial pressure, optimizing oxygenation and perfusion, controlling seizures, and maintaining body temperature are of key importance to inhibiting the progression of brain injury to cell death and encephalomalacia. Adequate analgesia and sedation must be provided. The head of the bed should be elevated 30 degrees, and the child's head should be positioned in the midline, avoiding flexon that could impair jugular venous return. Despite aggressive cerebral resuscitation, infants who survive an inflicted head injury often have worse neurologic outcomes than infants with accidental head injuries, presumably due to delays in presentation.

Cervical spine precautions must be implemented and maintained until cervical spine injury is excluded by appropriate clinical and radiological means, including MRI when indicated.

Once the child's impaired oxygenation, ventilation, and hemodynamics have been addressed and adequate analgesia and appropriate sedation have been provided, a systematic evaluation should be completed to diagnose any other potential injuries or underlying medical problems. A meticulous history should be obtained as soon as it is practical. All medications and alternative preparations to which the child has been exposed should be reviewed and reconciled in the medical record. The accidental omission of some medications, such as baclofen in chronically ill children, may result in life-threatening complications, including intractable seizures with hyperpyrexia and rhabdomyolysis.

IV. DIAGNOSIS OF CHILD MALTREATMENT

A thorough physical examination should be performed. Any abnormality should be investigated with indicated imaging and laboratory studies, and should be followed up with serial clinical examinations. Consultation with pediatric subspecialists, including neurosurgeons, surgeons, anesthesiologists, intensivists, and child maltreatment agencies, should be obtained as soon as possible, as some injuries require urgent attention in the trauma suite.

A. Laboratory Tests

Laboratory studies are directed toward rapidly identifying end organ injury and its sequelae as well as guiding critical care management (**Table 12-3**). A complete blood count with serial hematocrits is important in any child with a solid organ injury, such as a splenic, renal, or hepatic laceration. A rising white count, amylase, and/or lipase levels may be an important clue to an evolving pancreatic or bowel injury. A urine analysis will help exclude renal contusions or lacerations. Given that anemia from blood loss and clotting dysfunction from consumptive coagulopathy commonly occur in the critically ill patient, a blood clot for typing and crossmatch should be sent to the laboratory with the initial studies so that blood products can be given as soon as they are required.

Table 12-3. Laboratory Studies to Consider When Child Abuse Is Suspected

Problem	Laboratory Studies to Consider[a]
Skeletal injury	Complete blood count Serum bicarbonate, creatinine phosphokinase (CPK) Serum calcium, phosphorus, alkaline phosphatase 25-OH vitamin D
Bruising/bleeding	Complete blood count Coagulation studies Von Willebrand disease panel if bruising is unexplained or there is a family history of bruising/easy bleeding
Possible blunt-force abdominal trauma	Complete blood count with serial hematocrit Liver function tests Amylase and lipase Urine analysis
Altered level of consciousness	Bedside glucose and full electrolyte panel Toxicology testing Ammonia Liver function tests

[a] Other tests may be called for if the child's history, the family history, or the physical examination indicates other possible disease processes.

Serial blood gases are extremely important during the stabilization of any severely injured ventilated child. In general, P_{CO_2} should be maintained in the vicinity of 35 mm Hg (4.6 kPa) in children with brain injuries. Both hypercarbia and severe hypocarbia may worsen outcome by contributing to hyperemia or ischemic injury.

Calcium, phosphorus, and alkaline phosphatase levels can be obtained after stabilization to screen for systemic conditions affecting bone mineralization. Specialized studies and consultation are indicated if metabolic or genetic bone disease is suspected.

B. Imaging

1. Computed Tomographic Scan

Non-contrast computed tomographic (CT) scan is the preferred study in children with suspected abusive head injury. This study may be performed very rapidly and without sedation. Infants, toddlers, and children with decreased levels of consciousness should be immobilized for the scan in a manner that ensures airway patency. These children should be continuously observed during the study. Serial scans may be required in children with associated epidural hematomas, large evolving extraaxial collections, or worsening cerebral edema.

A CT of the abdomen and pelvis will complement careful serial clinical examinations, but findings of this examination may be subtle in hollow viscus injuries. The role of ultrasonography is less clearly defined in this setting.

2. Magnetic Resonance Imaging

Magnetic resonance imaging (MRI) is not as sensitive as CT in identifying acute hemorrhage, calls for additional transport of fragile patients, and requires sedation or general anesthesia with their attendant risks. Thus, for safety and optimal diagnostic yield, it is best delayed for 3 to 5 days. In general, initial neuroimaging should be limited to a plain CT of the head unless a spinal cord injury is suspected, in which case emergent MRI is required. Monitored sedation or general anesthesia is necessary to avoid any added hypoxic or ischemic insult. Special neuroradiology techniques may be indicated to evaluate other causes of subarachnoid hemorrhage.

3. Skeletal Survey

A complete skeletal survey should be performed in children less than 2 years of age when physical abuse is suspected. Protocols that follow the guidelines developed by the American College of Radiology should be used. Anteroposterior views of all extremities should be obtained, including anteroposterior feet and posteroanterior hands. This study should ideally be performed in the radiology suite; however, the risk of transport for an unstable patient may preclude this, and portable films may be initially obtained in the pediatric intensive care unit.

> !
>
> *Initial skeletal survey must include two-view skull, two-view chest with bone technique, anteroposterior pelvis and abdomen, and lateral lumbar spine images.*
>
> !

Acute fractures, particularly those involving the posterior ribs, may not be apparent on the initial skeletal survey in young children. A nuclear medicine bone scan is recommended in conjunction with the skeletal survey – once the child's condition has stabilized – because uptake of the radionucleotide tracer in areas of increased bone turnover allows for identification of injuries that may go undiagnosed using radiographs. A repeat skeletal survey in 2 to 3 weeks to disclose callus formation at fracture sites is an acceptable alternative to the bone scan in patients who cannot leave the PICU. Although rib and metaphyseal fractures may not require orthopedic intervention, long bone and spinal fractures may need stabilization. MRI should be performed only for indications during acute stabilization. Similarly, skeletal surveys should be deferred until the child is clearly improved from all standpoints.

4. Funduscopy and Medical Photography

Funduscopy and photo documentation by an ophthalmologist are important in establishing the extent and distribution of retinal abnormalities.

> !
>
> *Photographic documentation of physical findings and retinal abnormalities is an important part of a child's evaluation but should never delay necessary interventions.*
>
> !

V. MEDICOLEGAL ASPECTS OF CHILD MALTREATMENT

Child abuse is extremely upsetting to the healthcare team. The physician and other immediate care providers must concentrate exclusively on the child's immediate medical stabilization and subsequent care. Involving social workers early is extremely important. They can help gather vital information and can also begin notification of the local child protection agency, which may act in concert with law enforcement to remove other vulnerable children from a dangerous environment.

> !
>
> *The team's attention should be focused on stabilizing the child. All aspects of the investigation should be coordinated by social services and other child-advocacy professionals.*
>
> !

Interactions with parents or suspected perpetrators must remain civil. Remarks perceived as accusatory may hinder the child's medical care if protective custody is delayed. Unwise questioning may jeopardize the investigation.

The physician's role includes coordination of the child's medical care as well as complete, objective, and legible documentation of all relevant findings and events. Involvement in child-maltreatment cases is a stressful, time-consuming, frustrating, and unavoidable aspect of pediatric, emergency, and critical care medicine. Careful, clear documentation with appropriate medical imaging and photography during the child's hospitalization will be immensely helpful if a case proceeds to criminal trial, a process that may take several years. Complete, unbiased, accurate medical information must be presented clearly and understandably to facilitate judgments that are in the child's best interest, protect the innocent, and hold offenders accountable for their actions.

Every U.S. state mandates that injuries suspicious for maltreatment be reported by the professional caring for the child. Failure to report suspected non-accidental injuries might enable repetitive, possibly fatal injury to the patient and endanger other children. The laws protect the person making the report; therefore, reports made in good faith carry no liability. Conversely, failure to make a justified report can and has led to criminal prosecution and civil liability for physicians.

VI. ORGAN DONATION

Occasionally, children present to the emergency department in full cardiac arrest after an abusive injury. Other children may expire hours or days after admission to the PICU. In all cases, it is crucial to pay meticulous attention to all aspects of patient care, including hemodynamic and respiratory support in accordance with published guidelines

Hemodynamic instability may preclude full radiographic documentation of a child's injuries. A skeletal survey shortly after death occurs may reveal injuries that could be missed at autopsy. Close communication between the physicians and the medical examiner can make organ or tissue donation possible under such tragic circumstances.

> !
>
> *All children with fatal injuries should be considered—and managed—as potential organ donors.*
>
> !

Key Points

Non-accidental Injuries: Diagnosis and Management

- Complete initial and serial assessments of airway, breathing, and circulation (ABCs) are central to the management of any seriously ill or injured child.
- All principles of Pediatric Advanced Life Support and Advanced Trauma Life Support should be observed when evaluating potentially injured children.
- Initial evaluation includes a bedside glucose measurement as well as targeted laboratory and radiologic studies.
- Multidisciplinary consultation with anesthesiologists, pediatric surgeons, and pediatric intensivists should be obtained quickly.
- Children with non-accidental injuries typically present in a delayed fashion, complicating initial stabilization and eventual outcome.
- The team's efforts must be centered on the child's stability and comfort. Investigation of suspected abuse must be deferred to properly trained staff.
- Any negative factor –intrinsic to the child or the caregiver – raises the risk of neglect, abusive, and accidental injury.
- Patterns are suggestive, but never diagnostic, of abuse compared to accidental injury.

Suggested Readings

1. Aryan HE, Ghosheh FR, Jandial R, Levy ML. Retinal hemorrhage and pediatric brain injury: etiology and review of the literature. *J Clin Neurosci.* 2005;12:624-631.

2. Dubowitz H , Bennet S. Physical abuse and neglect of children. *Lancet.* 2007;369: 1891-1899.

3. Herr S, Fallat ME. Abusive abdominal and thoracic trauma. *Clin Ped Emerg Med.* 2006;7:149-152.

4. Hudson M, Kaplan R. Clinical response to child abuse. *Pediatr Clin North Am.* 2006;53:27-39.

5. Lonergan G, Baker AM, Morey MK, Boos SC. Child abuse: radiologic-pathologic correlation. *Radiographics.* 2003:23:811-845.

6. McGraw EP, Pless JE, Pennington DJ, White SJ. Postmortem radiography after unexpected death in neonates, infants, and children: should imaging be routine? *AJR Am J Roentgenol.* 2002;178:1517-1521.

7. Starling SP, Patel S, Burke BL, Sirotnak AP, Stronks S, Rosquist P. Analysis of perpetrator admissions in inflicted traumatic brain injury in children. *Arch Pediatr Adolesc Med.* 2004;158:454-458.

8. Trokel M, Discala C, Terrin NC, Sege RD. Patient and injury characteristics in abusive abdominal injuries. *Pediatr Emerg Care.* 2006;22:700-704.

Chapter 13:

PEDIATRIC EMERGENCY PREPAREDNESS

Objectives

- Identify the pediatric concerns involved in emergency preparedness.
- Describe the general concepts that need to be taken into consideration when caring for a pediatric patient during a disaster, a terrorist attack, or a public health emergency.
- Recognize the signs and symptoms of a patient exposed to chemical agents, biological agents, radiologic materials, or explosives and implement appropriate medical interventions.
- Describe the hospital pediatric preparedness considerations for disasters, terrorism, and public health emergencies.

I. INTRODUCTION

Since September 11, 2001, terrorism has become a new reality in the United States and worldwide. Although emergency preparedness is not a new idea, it has taken on new meaning. Understanding how to adapt and upgrade preparedness to enable effective response to potential attacks with chemical, biological, radiologic, nuclear, or explosive (CBRNE) weapons has become a significant national priority.

In a time of emergency, not only will pediatric healthcare providers have to provide direct care to children but they will also most likely need to orchestrate systems of care for children and advise governmental and nongovernmental agencies on children's needs. In addition to knowing how to care for patients directly and operate pediatric critical care units in times of disasters, terrorism, and public health emergencies, providers must understand the systems of emergency response and the unique needs of children addressed by these systems.

This chapter is designed to provide an overview of key issues related to preparedness for disaster, terrorism, and public health emergencies. It is not intended to cover every detail but rather to offer an approach to understanding the basic concepts of this difficult topic. Providers who will be responsible for the care of children during such events must become familiar with the following crucial areas of emergency preparedness:

- Aspects of terrorism and other disasters that relate uniquely to children
- Managing family concerns about terrorism and disaster preparedness
- Hospital preparedness
- Community, government, and public health preparedness

II. TYPES OF DISASTER

The World Association of Disaster Emergency Medicine and the Office of United States Foreign Disaster Assistance define a disaster as a situation or event that overwhelms local capacity, necessitating a request to national or international bodies for external assistance, or an unforeseen and often sudden event that causes great damage, destruction, and human suffering. Disasters are usually described as either natural, including earthquakes, hurricanes, tornados, and floods, or manmade, including fire, mass-transportation failures, environmental toxins, and civil unrest. More narrowly defined and distinct are mass casualty incidents, events that cause large numbers of injuries but do not threaten or harm large segments of the community.

The effects of each disaster are different. Consideration is given to the size of the area involved, the extent of damage, and the effect on community resources. The extent of damage includes physical injury to persons and wreckage of property, especially destruction of infrastructure (roadways, bridges, and communication lines). The effects on community resources include the absence of electricity, gas, sanitation, and potable water; the need to provide temporary shelter; and the potential for recurrence (eg, earthquakes with aftershocks).

III. LEVELS OF PREPAREDNESS

Emergency preparedness is important at many levels: personal, family, community, regional, state, and federal, with the state and federal governments playing pivotal roles. The federal government provides significant funding for disaster preparedness and response and also, to a large extent, establishes the framework that is then followed by states, regions, and communities. Federal, state and local government preparedness issues are beyond the scope of this chapter. This is material is covered in great detail in the Fundamemtals of Disaster Management (FDM) textbook (see recommended readings). In disaster response, the funding and planning tend to flow from the top down, whereas the response and use of resources tends to rise from the bottom up. In other words, as resources are exhausted at the local level, assistance is requested from the next level, such as the state, which then requests federal assistance. Recent approaches to disaster and aftermath response and planning include the involvement of neighborhoods and families and even have begun to address needs at the individual level. A successful response to a disaster requires personnel and resources from multiple agencies to function in an organized and coordinated manner according to a well-formulated plan. Although planning for disaster has increased in recent times, there has been little or no attention to the unique needs of children or inclusion of pediatric experts in the planning process.

IV. HOSPITAL PREPAREDNESS

The healthcare facilities responsible for treating pediatric victims in a biological, radiologic, nuclear, chemical, or explosive event may be strained or overwhelmed. Medical facilities can become inundated with patients if large numbers of victims appear without ambulance transport and pre-entry notification. This situation differs markedly from the usual hospital disaster-alert systems in which victims are triaged in the field and carefully distributed among available resources to prevent any single facility from being overwhelmed. Moreover, the arrival of victims without full hospital preparation could thwart attempts to isolate contaminated victims from other patients and hospital staff. Large-scale biological, chemical, nuclear, radiologic, or explosive incidents may necessitate the use of alternative healthcare sites (eg, auditoriums and arenas), which requires that pediatric healthcare resources be dispersed to areas where victims may not receive optimal care.

Children are difficult to care for by persons wearing the protective equipment that is essential in the management of biological or chemical events. Protective clothing is bulky and cumbersome; it impedes a provider's ability to perform procedures such as venipuncture on small children. It is imperative that hospitals and the healthcare community develop protocols and equipment that take into account the ways in which the wearing of protective clothing restricts the medical treatment of children. For example, given that providers find it difficult to secure intravenous access while wearing restrictive clothing, acceptable alternatives might include use of intraosseous access and intramuscular injections when appropriate.

Hospitals must have adequate plans to handle both disasters and terrorism, and those plans must take an all-hazards approach to ensure preparedness for any possible event. The plans must also establish an effective incident-command system that includes people capable of making decisions for the care of pediatric patients.

It is important that hospitals consider the needs of children in all aspects of emergency preparedness and hazard plans. Some of the matters to address include appropriate types and numbers of trained pediatric staff, equipment, medications, decontamination equipment, and how to handle nonambulatory children. Hospitals must be prepared to cope with situations in which patients are cared for as a family unit and children cannot be separated from adults, as in a quarantine situation. In a widespread emergency, all hospitals must have the capability to handle children, and all children's hospitals must be able to care for adult patients staying with their children.

A. Incident Command Systems

All emergency preparedness plans must establish an incident command system (ICS). The ICS works to avoid historical problems related to mass casualty incidents (MCIs), such as inadequate planning, poor communication, lack of on-scene needs assessment, and triage of patients. In addition to supplying a command structure, the ICS creates perimeters and areas to optimize responder safety and patient flow while preserving the evidence and environment.

An ICS may have many potential components and configurations depending on the magnitude of the event, location/terrain, weather, agencies that must involved, and available volunteer groups. For teaching purposes, we have kept our discussion simple, so it is important to keep in mind that approaches to disaster management should be tailored to the demands of the specific incident. Some guidelines for implementing an ICS within a hospital facility are presented in **Table 13-1**.

Table 13-1. Guidelines for an Effective Incident Command System

1. Common terminology avoids confusion by coordinating terms utilized with different agencies, allowing adequate identification of personnel, areas, equipment and procedures.
2. Modular organization is based on a top-down development approach. Beginning in the initial phases of the emergency, the Incident Commander will be responsible for the implementation and delegation of duties of the different functional areas as the situation develops.
3. Integrated communications allows the coordination of communications plans, operating procedures, terminology, and common frequencies.
4. Unified command structure with 1 Incident Commander or a Unified Command with more than 1 agency shares responsibility for the management of the situation. However, the Unity of Command should involve each person reporting to 1 supervisor.
5. Consolidated action plans, verbally or written, ideally follow established strategic goals, objectives, and activities.
6. Manageable span-of-control in which the number of individuals that report to a supervisor is established, ideally 5 with a range of 3 to 7.
7. Predesignated incident facilities or zones that clearly indicate areas for command post, search and rescue, staging, decontamination, transport, press, etc.
8. Comprehensive resource management that coordinates and consolidates independent resources, avoiding cluttering of personnel and communications.

One approach to hospital incident command is, the Hospital Emergency Incident Command System, or HEICS. In HEICS, a command staff is formed by appointing hospital personnel to serve as officers in charge of information, liaison, and safety and security. A fourth member, the medical officer, rounds out the command team.

B. The Two Phases of Care in a Mass Casualty Situation

There are 2 distinct phases of care in a mass casualty situation (MCS). Initially, during the arrival of casualties, the full magnitude of the event is unknown, and the key issue is conservation of limited hospital resources and facilities. Stable patients will temporarily receive only minimally acceptable care and will be transferred to other areas of the hospital to await subsequent definitive care. Only critical, treatable patients will have immediate access to key hospital resources, such as imaging techniques and operating rooms.

> ! *The key issue in mass casualty event is conservation of limited hospital resources and facilities*

The second phase of care in an MCS begins after the event has been contained and all casualties have arrived. Following secondary triage, a comprehensive, priority-oriented plan for definitive care of all patients can be devised.

C. Casualty Flow to the Hospital

The flow of casualties typically occurs in 3 waves. The first wave, shortly after the event, consists of casualties, usually with minor injuries, who evacuate themselves or are brought in by bystanders without previous triage. This wave arrives while the medical facility is still getting organized, and most of the casualties arrive in the hospital closest to the scene. This surge of new patients can overwhelm any hospital and practically block its emergency facilities. It is therefore vitally important that at the first notice of an MCS, an experienced physician be positioned in front of the emergency department to perform primary triage.

> !
> *The sudden increase of patients in a mass casualty event will overwhelm a hospital*
> !

The second wave consists of casualties with more serious injuries who were triaged at the scene, may have required extrication, received initial treatment, and were evacuated by EMS transportation. The third wave brings casualties with more minor injuries and people in emotional distress. These patients may continue to arrive for several hours or even several days after the initial event.

D. Casualty Flow Within the Hospital

A rapid, unobstructed flow of casualties within the hospital is crucial. Factors to be considered are the hospital layout, potential bottlenecks, and the number of available trauma teams, operating rooms, and hospital beds.

The basic goal is to establish a one-way, forward flow from the triage area into the final admitting ward. As patients are cared for they proceed only forward, with no possibility of backtracking. Backtracking or slow flow through the emergency department while the influx of casualties continues can have chaotic consequences.

E. Patient Triage

By definition a mass casualty situation is one in which the number of patients exceeds the availability of resources. As a result, the standard of care is temporarily altered. This often entails a reduction in the amount of individual care, with priority given to procedures aimed at saving the largest number of salvageable lives. There is an apparent correlation between the accuracy of triage and casualty outcome. The triage officer should be a physician experienced in trauma management and knowledgeable about the hospital's emergency preparedness triage system. The triage officer's role is to rapidly identify casualties who require immediate interventions and who have potentially reversible injuries.

> !
> *To ensure balance, the triage criteria should include physiologic and anatomic indicators rather than mechanism of injury only*
> !

In most systems casualties are triaged into 1 of 4 commonly recognized categories:

Red:	Immediate care
Yellow:	Delayed care
Green:	Minimal care
Black:	Deceased

1. Red Category

The immediate care category includes severely injured patients with a high probability of survival. They need procedures of moderately short duration to prevent death. Casualties with severe but potentially reversible injuries are the focus of medical efforts. Examples are airway obstructions, accessible hemorrhage, and, sometimes, emergency amputations (ABC's).

2. Yellow Category

Casualties in the delayed care category require operative interventions that may be postponed without compromising a successful outcome or endangering life. Temporizing measures include IV fluids, splints, antibiotics, pain management, catheterization, and gastric decompression. Some examples are large muscle wounds, severe bone fractures, uncomplicated major burns, head or spinal injuries, and intraabdominal and thoracic injuries.

3. Green Category

The minimal care group includes patients without serious injuries to vascular structures or nerves. The walking wounded can usually provide self-care or require only minimally trained personnel. Most casualties belong in this category.

The green designation also includes expectant patients. This category is the most difficult to describe because it includes victims for whom in other circumstances all available measures would be taken to give them a chance for survival. However, in an MCS their time-consuming or complicated requirements yield a low probability for survival and demand an excessive amount of manpower and supplies. This may compromise patients with a greater chance of recovery. These patients are supported with comfort measures and analgesics until the casualties in the red and yellow categories have been properly addressed.

4. Black Category

Patients found to be dead on arrival and casualties with terminal injuries are placed in the black category. Their treatment is given low priority and they are directed to a designated area.

F. Initial Management in the Hospital

Treatment priorities in a mass casualty situation are to save salvageable patients and to prevent complications and future handicaps. Generally, patient management should follow accepted guidelines (such as Advanced Trauma Life Support [ATLS]), though only essential interventions are performed in the first phase, and comprehensive treatment of all injuries is postponed.

Teamwork is crucial. Teams of 1 physician and, preferably, 2 nurses should be preassigned to every ED station. The ED director (or other position based on hospital ICS) plays the conductor's role. That person coordinates medical teams; oversees specialists' assignments; sets priorities for transfer to the operating room, intensive care unit, or ward; makes decisions regarding imaging; and ensures continuous patient flow through the admitting area. An important task is to prevent overcrowding and excessive commotion in the ED. Personnel not directly participating in patient care should be kept away to avoid havoc.

1. Use of Radiology

The radiology department is a common bottleneck during disasters and should be used judiciously. As a rule, mobile radiography and radiography of the chest, cervical spine, and pelvis are not performed on a routine basis. Focused abdominal sonography for trauma (FAST) is quick and beneficial but should be used conservative, for example, to confirm or rule out intraabdominal bleeding in unstable patients. Computer tomography (CT) scanning should be reserved for specific indications, and the ED director should make those decisions. Brain CTs are performed only to assist decision making about neurosurgery.

2. Use of Operating Rooms

Operating rooms may also become a serious bottleneck. Therefore, their immediate use should be reserved for a few absolute indications, such as compromised airway or control of active bleeding that endangers life or limb. Other surgeries are delayed to later phases.

Once a patient is in surgery, the fundamental goal is damage control. This approach demands that surgeons, accustomed to expending enormous resources and time on individual patients, reset their priorities to provide only the minimally acceptable care, moving patients quickly through the most-needed procedures in order to care for as many patients as possible.

3. Use of Secondary Transport

An important aspect of primary triage at the scene is allocating the patient load among available hospitals, taking into consideration specialty capabilities, such as neurosurgery, burns, and pediatric surgery. Secondary transport is the transfer of casualties from one medical facility to another. Secondary transport is indicated when the primary admitting hospital is unable to provide proper care due to lack of required specialties, overwhelming patient load, or inability to provide needed surgery within a reasonable time period, or when the hospital itself is compromised by the event.

4. Communication and Manpower Control

Rapid staff recruitment is crucial, and each hospital should have an effective paging system. Insufficient physician attendance in the ED of a large urban hospital was recorded in the first hours after a severe earthquake because physicians were helping their own families and because communication or transportation were lacking. On the other hand, data from disaster events have repeatedly shown that large numbers of hospital personnel arrive even without being paged. Emergency preparedness plans should identify a staff waiting area with communication to the event director, who will allocate personnel according to needs.

An emergency operations center should be rapidly set up in a preestablished, preequipped location. In addition to communication within the hospital, communication (preferably radio) with the EMS forces at the scene is critical.

5. Information Center and Public Relations

A public information center should be opened as soon as possible. Its telephone lines should be designated in advance, and their numbers should be announced by the media during and after the event. The information center should have software for creating a database of missing persons in a format prearranged by the hospital, local emergency management, and law enforcement agencies. In some cases those outside agencies may provide staff for this function. Because the hospital may be inundated with worried relatives, the information center should be located at a significant distance from the patient management area.

6. Communication and Information Technology

Two key elements cited in all evaluations of disaster, terrorism, and public health emergency events are communication and information technology systems. Forms of telecommunication, including telephone, radio, 2-way radio, video, fax, and digital imaging via satellite transmission, have been widely used in response to disasters. Telemedicine is one technology that can be used not only during the disaster phase but also before and after to educate the community, institute prevention programs, and establish emergency assistance, public health measures, and sanitation services. The use of the Internet and electronic mail can also prove effective.

G. Reassessment Phase

> !
>
> *Following the first phase of the event, all casualties should receive definitive, appropriate treatment as available resources allow*
>
> !

To avoid misdiagnoses and overlooked injuries, designated teams should perform the reassessment by reviewing every patient's chart and recommending further investigations or interventions. Once again, decision making and planning should be centralized to ensure consideration of individual priorities and the entire hospital's capabilities.

V. PEDIATRIC TRIAGE

Current triage systems, which are typically designed to allocate scarce resources to those who would benefit most from them and are usually based on assessment findings and physiological parameters, may not address children. These systems may either not triage children at all or may over-triage them. In either case, children are not given access to scarce resources or, in the case of over-triage, the resources go to the first-arriving patients and not those who would benefit most from them. For example, if the simply triage rapid treatment (START) system is used, a normal, healthy, and uninjured 6-month-old would be categorized as red and given the highest priority.

To avoid such problems, triage systems specifically designed for children are needed to adequately provide scarce resources to the children who would benefit from them. One example is the JumpSTART triage system, a variation of the adult START triage method that has been modified to provide values appropriate for pediatric triage.

VI. UNIQUE NEEDS OF CHILDREN IN MASS CRISIS SITUATIONS

The special needs of children have only recently begun to be considered and understood in disaster planning and terrorism preparedness. Planning must consider children who are at home, in school, at child care facilities, or in transit as well as children who cannot be reunited with their families. Children with special healthcare needs are particularly at risk, especially if their survival depends on technologic devices.

Children are uniquely vulnerable to disasters and acts of terrorism due to anatomic, physiologic, and clinical factors and developmental and psychological concerns. Although children may respond more rapidly to therapeutic intervention, they are more susceptible to various agents and conditions and more likely to deteriorate if not carefully monitored and appropriately treated,

The release of chemical or biological toxins would disproportionately affect children through several mechanisms. For example, because children become dehydrated easily and possess minimal reserve, they are at greater risk than adults when exposed to agents that may cause diarrhea or vomiting. Agents that might cause only mild symptoms in an adult could lead to hypovolemic shock in an infant.

Many of the agents used for chemical and biological attacks are aerosolized (eg, sarin, chlorine, or anthrax). Because children have faster respiratory rates than adults, they are exposed to relatively higher doses and will suffer the effects much more rapidly than adults. Children may also absorb more of the substance before it is cleared or diffuses from the respiratory tissues. Many chemical agents, including certain gases like sarin and chlorine, have a high vapor density and are heavier than air, which means they settle close to the ground in the air space used by children for breathing.

Many biological and chemical agents are absorbed through the skin. Because children have more surface area relative to body mass than adults and because young children, especially those younger than 6 months, have more permeable skin, they receive proportionally higher doses of agents that either affect the skin or are absorbed through the skin. In addition, because the skin of children is poorly keratinized, vesicants and corrosives result in greater injury to children than to adults. A further concern in children, given their relatively large surface area in relation to body mass, is that they lose heat quickly when showered. Consequently, skin decontamination with water may result in hypothermia unless heating lamps and other warming equipment are used.

Children are also more vulnerable to radiologic exposures than adults. Children have a disproportionately higher minute ventilation, leading to greater internal exposure to radioactive gases. Nuclear fallout quickly settles to the ground, resulting in a higher concentration of radioactive material in the space where children live and breathe. Children have a significantly greater risk of developing cancer even when they are exposed to radiation in utero.

Children are particularly vulnerable due to the limitations of their physical development. Infants, toddlers, and young children do not have the motor skills to escape from the site of a biological or chemical incident. Even children who are able to walk may not have the cognitive ability to understand the presence of a risk and may not seek escape or be able to decide in which direction to flee. Even worse, children may actually migrate toward the event out of curiosity about all the activity, sounds, colors, or other effects.

VII. TERRORISM PREPAREDNESS

Terrorism preparedness is one specific component of general emergency preparedness. Extending beyond the unique pediatric issues addressed in general emergency preparedness, terrorism preparedness takes into account several additional issues, including the unique vulnerabilities of children to various agents and the limited availability of age- and weight-appropriate antidotes and treatments.

Pediatricians must be knowledgeable about the following:

1. The classification and qualities of possible biological agents
2. The natural history and management of biological, chemical, and radiologic injuries and exposures
3. Chemical agents that may be used and their properties
4. Different types of radiologic terrorism
5. Decontamination procedures
6. Availability of antidotes and other therapies

A. Exposure to Biological Agents

Biological weapons are referred to as the poor man's nuclear bomb because they are easy to manufacture, can be deployed without sophisticated delivery systems, and have the ability to kill or injure hundreds of thousands of people.

Various biological agents may be used as weapons, and the actual clinical syndrome will vary depending on the type of agent, its virulence, the route of the exposure, and the victim's susceptibility to infection.

A covert release of a contagious biological agent has the potential for large-scale spread before detection, which is dependent on traditional disease-surveillance methods. For some infectious agents, secondary and tertiary transmission may continue for weeks or months after the initial attack. In an epidemic, overwhelming numbers of critically ill patients will require acute and follow-up medical care. Both infected persons and the worried well will seek medical attention, prompting yet further need for medical supplies, diagnostic tests, and hospital beds. Devices such as crop-dusting airplanes or small perfume atomizers are potential delivery systems for biological agents.

> **!**
>
> *Biological agents are often associated with delayed onset of illness and, therefore, may not be recognized in their initial stages. Chemical, conventional, and nuclear weapons generate immediate effects.*
>
> **!**

Biological infectious agents produce a marked diversity of injuries, with toxic effects ranging from incapacitation to death. Biological agents considered likely candidates for weaponization include: bacteria, viruses, rickettsia, fungi, and preformed toxins. The CDC separates bioterrorist agents into 3 categories, A, B, and C, in order of priority based on the combined factors of availability, potential for morbidity and mortality, and ease of dissemination.

Although virtually any microorganism has the potential to be used as a biological weapon, most would be difficult to weaponize and disseminate effectively. The biological agents most likely to be used in category A include: *Bacillus anthracis* (anthrax), *Clostridium botulinum* (botulism), *Francisella tularensis* (tularemia), *Yersinia pestis* (plague), Ebola virus, variola (smallpox) and the hemorrhagic fever viruses. The biological agents most likely to be used in category B include: *Brucella species* (brucellosis) and *Coxiella burnetii* (Q fever).

Children may be particularly vulnerable to aerosolized biological weapons that are inhaled or act through the skin as well as those that cause vomiting and diarrhea. They have lower circulating blood-volume reserves than adults and would be potentially more at risk for hemorrhagic shock if exposed to viral hemorrhagic fever.

In addition, children have shorter incubation periods for some of the biological agents and will become symptomatic earlier. That offers a window of opportunity for surveillance systems, although it must be remembered that children's symptoms may differ from those of an adult.

B. Potential Biological Agents of Terror

1. Anthrax

a. Signs and Symptoms

Anthrax is an acute infectious disease caused by the spore-forming bacterium *Bacillus anthracis.* The spores are the dominant form of the bacterium and may last for decades. In the right environment and conditions, such as within the human body, the spore germinates and produces infection. In nature, anthrax is most commonly found in herbivores, but it may also infect humans.

There are 3 forms of anthrax infection: cutaneous, inhalational, and gastrointestinal. The cutaneous form enters non-intact skin and is usually acquired by handling contaminated wool, hides, leather, or hair products of infected animals. Skin infection begins as an itchy papule that resembles an insect bite. Within 1 to 2 days, it progresses into a vesicle, then a painless ulcer, typically 1 to 3 centimeters in diameter, with a characteristic black necrotic area in the center. Adjacent lymph glands may swell. Patients may present with fever, chills, malaise, chest pain, and dry cough. Rapid clinical deterioration occurs as the bacteria overwhelm the body.

The gastrointestinal form of anthrax may follow the consumption of contaminated meat and is characterized by acute inflammation of the gastrointestinal tract. Initial signs of nausea, loss of appetite, vomiting, and fever are followed by abdominal pain, hematemesis, and bloody diarrhea.

Initial symptoms of the inhalational form may be mistaken for the flu or a cold, and an opportunity to initiate early, appropriate treatment may be missed. After several days, the symptoms progress to respiratory failure and shock. Without treatment, mortality rates for inhalational anthrax approach 100%, and usually result in death within 1 to 2 days after onset of acute pulmonary symptoms. Before the anthrax attacks of 2001, there had been only 18 cases of inhalational anthrax in the United States in the past century. The last case prior to 2001 occurred in 1976. Inhalational anthrax is not communicable.

b. Treatment

In the field, treatment of anthrax should be supportive and include the use of antibiotics. Due to their adverse effects, certain antibiotics are not recommended as first choices for children, but such concerns may be outweighed by the need for early treatment of children exposed to B anthracis. The methods of treating anthrax are summarized in **Table 13-2**.

Table 13-2. Recommended Therapy and Prophylaxis of Anthrax

Form of Anthrax	Category of Treatment (Therapy or Prophylaxis)	Agent and Dosing
Inhalation	Therapy[a]	Ciprofloxacin[b] 10-15 mg/kg IV (max 400 mg/dose) every 12 hours **or** Levofloxacin 10-15 mg/kg IV every 24 hours or Doxycycline 2.2 mg/kg IV (max 100 mg/dose) every 12 hours **and** Clindamycin[c] 10-15 mg/kg IV every 8 hours **and** Penicillin G[e] 400-600k units/kg/day IV divided every 4 hours Patients who are clinically stable after 14 days may be switched to a single oral agent (ciprofloxacin or doxycycline) to complete a 60-day coursed of therapy.
Inhalation	Postexposure prophylaxis (60-day course[d])	Ciprofloxacin[f] 10-15 mg/kg orally (max 500 mg/dose) every 12 hours **or** Levofloxacin 10-15 mg/kg IV every 24 hours **or** Doxycycline 2.2 mg/kg (max 100 mg/dose) orally every 12 hours
Cutaneous, endemic	Therapy[g]	Penicillin V 40-80 mg/kg/day orally divided every 6 hours **or** Amoxicillin 40-80 mg/kg/day orally divided every 8 hours **or** Ciprofloxacin 10-15 mg/kg orally (max 1 g/day) every 12 hours **or** Levofloxacin 10-15 mg/kg IV every 24 hours **or** Doxycycline 2.2 mg/kg orally (max 100 mg/dose) every 12 hours
Cutaneous (in setting of terrorism)	Therapy[a]	Ciprofloxacin 10-15 mg/kg orally (max 1 g/day) every 12 hours **or** Levofloxacin 10-15 mg/kg IV every 24 hours Doxycycline 2.2 mg/kg orally (max 100 mg) every 12 hours
Gastrointestinal	Therapy[a]	Same as for inhalational Abdominal CT with oral and intravenous contrast Diagnostic peritoneal lavage

This table was created from recommendations developed at the Consensus Conference and in part is based on reviewed reference materials from the American Academy of Pediatrics, Centers for Disease Control and Prevention, Food and Drug Administration, and Infectious Disease Society of America .

[a]In a mass casualty setting in which resources are severely limited, oral therapy may need to be substituted for the preferred parenteral option.

[b]Ofloxacin (and possibly other quinolones) may be acceptable alternatives to ciprofloxacin or levofloxacin

[c]Rifampin or clarithromycin may be acceptable alternatives to clindamycin as drugs that target bacterial protein synthesis.

[d]Assuming the organism is sensitive, children may be switched to oral amoxicillin (40-80 mg/kg/day divided every 8 hours) to complete a 60-day course. We recommend that the first 14 days of therapy or postexposure prophylaxis, however, include ciprofloxacin or levofloxacin and/or doxycycline, regardless of age.

[e]Ampicillin, imipenem, meropenem, or chloramphenicol may be acceptable alternatives to penicillin as drugs with good CNS penetration.

[f]According to most experts, ciprofloxacin is the preferred agent for oral prophylaxis.

[g]Ten days of therapy may be adequate for endemic cutaneous disease. We recommend a full 60-day course in the setting of terrorism, however, because of the possibility of concomitant inhalational exposure.

Adapted with permission from Markenson, D. Pediatric Emergency Preparedness for Natural Disasters, Terrorism and Public Health Emergencies: A National Consensus Conference. Executive Summary and Final Report, 2007.

At this time, anthrax vaccine is not recommended for children younger than 18 years but may still be indicated after a bona fide exposure based on assessment of the benefit versus the lack of indication. Consult with the CDC for current recommended treatments.

2. Plague

a. Signs and Symptoms

Plague has been reported throughout the western United States, but most human cases are seen in New Mexico, Arizona, California, and Colorado as isolated cases or in small clusters. More cases tend to occur during summers that follow mild winters and wet springs. In the United States, it is usually a rural disease. House cats are susceptible to plague and may directly transmit plague to persons who handle them. Dogs and cats may also bring plague-infected fleas into the home. Inhaling droplets expelled by the coughing of a plague-infected person or animal, especially house cats, can result in plague of the lungs, plague pneumonia.

Presentation of pediatric index cases in an urban setting or outside the normal geographic or seasonal distribution should be reported by medical providers.

b. Treatment

Treatment options in children include doxycycline or tetracycline (>8 years) (**Table 13-3**).

3. Tularemia

There are at least 9 species of domestic animals, including cats, that harbor tularemia and could be subjects of vector transmission by ticks, deerflies, and mosquitoes to children.

a. Treatment

In children, the same regimen of antibiotics is used in the treatment of tularemia as is used in the treatment of plague (**Table 13-3**).

4. Smallpox

a. Signs and Symptoms

The greatest difficulty for a medical provider approaching a potential pediatric smallpox victim may be in differentiating smallpox from the common childhood illness of chicken pox. Differences between the rashes of smallpox and chicken pox are listed in **Table 13-4**.

Table 13-3. Recommended Therapy and Prophylaxis of Additional Diseases Associated With Bioterrorism

Disease	Therapy or Prophylaxis	Treatment,[a] Agent, and Dosing
Smallpox	Therapy	Supportive care
	Prophylaxis	Vaccination may be effective if given within the first several days after exposure.
Plague	Therapy	Gentamicin 2.5 mg/kg IV every 8 hours **or** Streptomycin 15 mg/kg IM every 12 hours (max 2 g/day, although only available for compassionate usage and in limited supply) **or** Doxycycline 2.2 mg/kg IV every 12 hours (max 200 mg/day) **or** Ciprofloxacinb 15 mg/kg IV every 12 hours **or** Levofloxacin 10-15 mg/kg IV every 24 hours or Chloramphenicol[c] 25 mg/kg every 6 hours (max 4 g/day)
	Prophylaxis	Doxycycline 2.2 mg/kg orally every 12 hours **or** Ciprofloxacin[b] 20 mg/kg orally every 12 hours
Tularemia	Therapy	Same as for plague
Botulism	Therapy	Supportive care, antitoxin, and/or botulism immune globulin may halt progression of symptoms but are unlikely to reverse them
Viral hemorrhagic fevers	Therapy	Supportive care, ribavirin may be beneficial in select cases[d]
Brucellosis	Therapy[e]	TMP/SMX 30 mg/kg orally every 12 hours and rifampin 15 mg/kg every 24 hours or gentamicin 7.5 mg/kg IM every day [NA1]_ 5

Abbreviations: IV, intravenously; IM, intramuscularly; PO, per os; TMX/SMX, trimethoprim and sulfamethoxazole. This table was created from recommendations developed at the Consensus Conference and in part is based on reviewed reference materials from the American Academy of Pediatrics, Centers for Disease Control and Prevention, and the Infectious Disease Society of America.

[a]In a mass casualty setting, parenteral therapy might not be possible. In such cases, oral therapy (with analogous agents) may need to be used.

[b]Ofloxacin (and possibly other quinolones) may be acceptable alternatives to ciprofloxacin or levofloxacin; however, they are not approved for use in children.

[c]Concentration should be maintained between 5 and 20 mcg/mL. Some experts have recommended that chloramphenicol be used to treat patients with plague meningitis because chloramphenicol penetrates the blood-brain barrier. Use in children younger than 2 years be associated with adverse reactions but might be warranted for serious infections.

[d]Ribavirin is recommended for arenavirus or bunyavirus infections and may be indicated for a viral hemorrhagic fever of an unknown etiology, although it is not FDA approved for these indications. For intravenous therapy use a loading dose of 30 kg IV once (max dose, 2 g), then 16 mg/kg IV every 6 hours for 4 days (max dose 1 g), and then 8 mg/kg IV every 8 hours for 6 days (max dose 500 mg). In a mass casualty setting, it may be necessary to use oral therapy. For oral therapy, use a loading dose of 30 mg/kg orally once, then 15 mg/kg/day orally in 2 divided doses for 10 days.

[e]This is recommended for children younger than 8 years. For children older than 8 years, adult regimens are recommended. Oral drugs should be given for 6 weeks. Gentamicin, if used, should be given for the first 5 days of a 6-week course of TMP/SMX (trimethoprim/sulfamethoxazole).

Table 13-4. Differentiating Smallpox From Chicken Pox

Smallpox	Chicken Pox
All lesions in the same stage	Lesions appear in crops in different stages (papules, vesicles, crusted lesions)
Palms and soles involved	Palms and soles rarely involved
Patient appearing moribund or toxic	Patient rarely toxic or moribund
Increased concentration of lesions on face and extremities (centrifugal distribution)	Greatest concentration on face and trunk with relative sparing of the extremities
Lesions that develop into pustules and are deeply embedded in the dermis	Vesicles that are relatively superficial
Significant prodrome	Mild or no prodrome

b. Treatment

There is no effective treatment for smallpox. Infected patients should receive supportive care. Cidofovir has some activity for viruses in the same group and in vitro against smallpox. Exposed individuals should be immunized with smallpox vaccine. The CDC currently recommends against vaccinating children younger than 1 year. All contraindications to smallpox vaccination are relative. After bona fide exposure or known usage of weaponized smallpox, even the youngest exposed, at-risk infants should be vaccinated. Moreover, future studies of new-generation vaccines must include children (**Table 13-3**).

5. Viral Hemorrhagic Fever

Viral hemorrhagic fever (VHF) is a syndrome that may be seen in a diverse group of diseases, including Ebola, Marburg, yellow fever, Rift Valley fever, and Crimean-Congo hemorrhagic fever. The viruses are contagious and may be spread through direct contact with body fluids or inhalation of aerosolized droplets. Use of standard precautions for isolation of body substances has proven to be very effective in protecting healthcare workers from infection.

a. Signs and Symptoms

The presentation and progression of signs and symptoms vary depending upon the specific infecting agent and may include high fever, chills, headache, weakness, myalgia, nonbloody diarrhea, conjunctival hemorrhage, pharyngitis, epistaxis, hematemesis, hematuria, bloody stools, petechial hemorrhages, hypotension, bleeding from mucous membranes, and possibly central nervous system (CNS) and pulmonary effects.

b. Treatment

Care is primarily supportive and may include administration of fluids or vasopressors. It is commonly recommended to avoid intramuscular (IM) injections, aspirin, and other medications that could potentially inhibit coagulation. Patient isolation and strict infection control precautions are needed. Some of the hemorrhagic viruses may respond to antiviral agents such as ribavirin, although data regarding this is limited.

The recommended therapy and prophylaxis of diseases associated with bioterrorism are summarized in **Table 13-3**.

C. Toxins

1. Botulism

a. Signs and Symptoms

About 120 Americans get botulism each year. Approximately 90 of those victims are infants who obtained *C botulinum* spores from honey. Symptoms of botulism in adults and children usually begin within 18 to 36 hours of eating a contaminated food. However, symptoms can occur as early as 6 hours after eating food or as long as 10 days later.

b. Treatment

A licensed trivalent (types A, B, E) antitoxin for botulism is available through the CDC. This antitoxin is to be used in children of any age known to have been exposed to botulinum toxin of the appropriate serotypes. Licensed pentavalent (types A-E) botulism immune globulin was approved by the FDA in 2003. Although licensed specifically for use in infant botulism due to toxin types A and B, it may have a role in the treatment of bioterrorism victims who have been exposed to types C, D, and E as well. Antitoxin and/or botulism immune globulin may halt progression of symptoms but will be unlikely to reverse them.

2. Ricin

a. Signs and Symptoms

Ricin is a protein derived from the castor bean plant, which can be ground into a powder for inhalation, ingestion, or injection. Children may be exposed to toxic amounts of ricin by eating or chewing on castor beans. Severe crampy diarrhea and nausea, vomiting, CNS depression, shock, and seizures may occur. Hemolytic anemia and renal failure may develop.

b. Treatment

Children are managed with supportive therapy by maintaining patient comfort and administering fluids, oxygen, and pain medications. Gut decontamination with activated charcoal is utilized with ricin ingestion. Benzodiazepines are the drugs of choice for seizures.

D. Exposure to Chemical Agents

Although most physicians are unlikely to be involved in the frontline care of victims of a chemical attack, the possibility does exist. Several patients presenting with the same symptoms should alert physicians and hospital staff to the possibility of a chemical attack. If an attack occurs, most victims are likely to arrive at the hospital within a short time period. This situation differentiates a chemical attack from a biological attack involving infectious microorganisms. Toxic chemical agents have a high potential for secondary contamination from victims to responders.

Secondary contamination with even small amounts of these substances (particularly nerve agents such as VX) can be lethal. Medical treatment facilities must have clearly defined procedures for handling contaminated casualties, many of whom will transport themselves to the facility. Precautions must be used until thorough decontamination has been performed or the specific chemical agent is identified.

> !
>
> *Healthcare professionals must first protect themselves by using agent or risk appropriate personnel protective equipment, which may include protective suits, respiratory protection and chemical resistant gloves.*
>
> !

Chemical agents that have been used or are considered likely candidates for use in a chemical release are listed in **Table 13-5**, with examples of each class and possible antidotes if available.

Chemical agents are relatively easy to synthesize. They do not require sophisticated missiles, bombs, or other delivery devices for dispersion. Unlike most biological agents, they are capable of producing illness rapidly. Many of these agents could be stolen from industry or transport vehicles rather than manufactured by terrorists. Various chemical agents could be used as covert weapons, and the clinical syndrome will vary depending on the type, amount, concentration, and route of exposure.

The availability of adequate antidotes and treatments for children is problematic. Most treatments and antidotes were developed for military personnel (ie, adults) and have never been tested on children. Although there is ongoing development of new and improved antidotes and treatments to better protect our military and adult populations, there is no parallel process for developing appropriate agents for use in children.

Table 13-5. Recommended Treatment and Management of Chemical Agents Used in Terrorism

Agent	Toxicity	Clinical Findings	Onset	Decontamination[a]	Management
Tabun, Sarin, Soman, VX	Anticholinesterase: muscarinic, nicotinic, and CNS effects	Vapor: miosis, rhinorrhea, dyspnea Liquid: diaphoresis, vomiting Both: coma, paralysis, seizures, apnea	Vapor: seconds Liquid: minutes to hours	Vapor: fresh air, remove clothes, wash hair Liquid: remove clothes, copious washing of skin and hair with soap and water, ocular irrigation	ABCs Atropine[b,c,d]: 0.05 mg/kg IV, IM (min 0.1mg, max 5 mg), repeat every 2-5 min as needed for marked secretions, bronchospasm Pralidoxime[e]: 25 mg/kg IV, IM (max 1 g IV; 2 g IM), may repeat within 30-60 min as needed, then again every 1 hour for 1 or 2 doses as needed for persistent weakness, high atropine requirement Diazepam: 0.3 mg/kg (max 10 mg) IV; Lorazepam: 0.1 mg/kg IV, IM (max 4 mg); Midazolam: 0.2 mg/kg (max 10 mg) IM as needed seizures, or severe exposure
Vesicants					
Mustard	Alkylation	Skin: erythema, vesicles Eye: inflammation	Hours	Skin: soap and water Eyes: irrigation (water)	Symptomatic care
Lewisite	Arsenical	Respiratory tract: inflammation, respiratory distress, acute respiratory distress syndrome	Immediate pain	Both: major impact only if done within minutes of exposure	Possibly British anti-lewisite (BAL) 3 mg/kg IM every 4-6 hours for systemic effects of lewisite in severe cases
Pulmonary Agents					
Chlorine, phosgene	Liberate HCl,	Eyes, nose, alkylation Bronchospasm, pulmonary edema (especially phosgene)	Minutes throat, irritation (especially chlorine) Bronchospasm: minutes Pulmonary edema: hours	Fresh air Skin: water	Symptomatic care

continues next page…

Table 13-5. Recommended Treatment and Management of Chemical Agents Used in Terrorism (continued)

Agent	Toxicity	Clinical Findings	Onset	Decontamination[a]	Management
Pulmonary Agents, continued					
Cyanide	Cytochrome oxidase inhibition: cellular anoxia, lactic acidosis	Tachypnea, coma, seizures, apnea	Seconds	Fresh air Skin: soap and water	Airways, breathing, circulatory support; 100% oxygen Sodium bicarbonate as needed for metabolic acidosis Sodium nitrite (3%): Dosing (mL/kg) — Estimated Hgb (g/dL) For Average Child 0.27 — 10 0.33 — 12 0.39 — 14 Max 10 mL Sodium thiosulfate (25%) 1.65 mL/kg (max 50 mL)
Riot-Control Agents					
CS, CN (Mace_) capsaicin (pepper spray)	Neuropeptide substance P release, alkylation	Eye: tearing, pain, blepharospasm Nose and throat irritation Pulmonary failure (rare)	Seconds	Fresh air Eye: lavage	Ophthalmics topically, symptomatic care

Abbreviations: CNS, ; ABCs, airway, breathing and circulatory support; IV, intravenously; IM, intramuscularly; BAL, British anti-Lewisite; Hgb, hemoglobin concentration; est., estimated hemoglobin concentration; max, maximum; min, minimum.

[a]Decontamination, especially for patients with significant nerve agent or vesicant exposure, should be performed by healthcare providers garbed in adequate personal protective equipment. For emergency department staff, this consists of non-encapsulated, chemically resistant body suit, boots, and gloves with a full-face air purifier mask/hood.

[b]The intraosseous route is likely equivalent to intravenous.

[c]Atropine might have some benefit via endotracheal tube or inhalation, as might aerosolized ipratropium.

[d]As of September 2004, the FDA has approved pediatric auto-injectors of atropine in 0.25, 0.5, and 1 mg sizes.

[e]Pralidoxime is reconstituted to 50 mg/mL (1 g in 20 mL water) for IV administration, and the total dose is infused over 30 min or may be given by continuous infusion (loading dose 25 mg/kg over 30 min, then 10 mg/kg/h). For IM use, it might be diluted to a concentration of 300 mg/mL (1 g added to 3 mL water by analogy to auto-injector concentration), to effect a reasonable volume for injection. Pediatric auto-injectors of pralidoxime are not FDA approved or available.

Adapted with permission from Markenson, D. Pediatric Emergency Preparedness for Natural Disasters, Terrorism and Public Health Emergencies: A National Consensus Conference. Executive Summary and Final Report 2007.

1. Pulmonary Agents

a. Signs and Symptoms

Pulmonary (choking) agents, such as phosgene and chlorine, will have very similar effects in adults and children, except that children may become ill and more symptomatic at lower exposures. The difference in respiratory anatomy in young children can lead to unexpected upper-airway obstruction. Acute signs of exposure to pulmonary agents are usually seen first in the upper airway and include tearing, eye irritation, tachypnea, wheezing, and stridor. Effects on the lower airway may be delayed up to 24 hours after exposure.

b. Treatment

Appropriate airway management should include high-flow oxygen via a non-rebreather face mask. Early endotracheal intubation and positive pressure ventilation may be needed for the patient with depressed airway reflexes and signs of airway obstruction. Children with bronchospasm may be treated with β_2-agonists, and those with stridor may benefit from inhaled racemic epinephrine (**Table 4-4**).

2. Blood Agents

a. Signs and Symptoms

Inhaled cyanide is a rapidly intoxicating agent. The pediatric population, with their increased metabolic rate, will probably succumb to exposure at lower concentrations. Children may initially show hyperexcitability and tachypnea without cyanosis. Verbal children may complain of headache and nausea. High ambient concentrations of cyanide can quickly lead to unconsciousness and seizures, followed by apnea and death.

b. Treatment

Initial prehospital intervention is unchanged from adult therapy and involves removal of the child from exposure and placement in a clean atmosphere. The child should receive 100% oxygen by face mask. Use of the cyanide antidote kit is problematic. Although the kit may be lifesaving, the adult doses of the various agents may be toxic in children. The pharmacology of the antidote kit is to induce methemoglobinemia with amyl nitrite and sodium nitrite, then enhance cyanide elimination with sodium thiosulfate (**Table 13-5**). The iron moiety in methemoglobin binds cyanide more avidly than the iron in hemoglobin or in the cytochromes. The resultant cyanomethemoglobin then combines with sodium thiosulfate to form sodium thiocyanate, which is eliminated in the urine. However, if the level of induced methemoglobin is too high, the antidote itself will prevent oxygen utilization by cells and cause toxicity. The amount of sodium nitrite used is weight- and hemoglobin-dependent. Consider use of a lower dose for suspected anemia. Infants younger than 2 months have a physiologic anemia and require a lower dose of sodium nitrite than their weight would suggest. The same is true for children with anemia or a condition that would predispose them to reduced hemoglobin levels, such as sickle cell disease. Sodium thiosulfate dosing is also weight-dependent but less critical. Sodium bicarbonate can be used to treat metabolic acidosis.

3. Blister Agents

Blister agents, or vesicants, include mustard, lewisite, and phosgene oxime. All 3 are similar and can be addressed together, although the literature specific to children is limited.

Compared to adults, children have thinner, more permeable skin and an increased surface-to-mass ratio and are thus much more sensitive to the effects of blistering agents. As for adults, ambient temperature influences onset and severity of symptoms, with warmer temperatures producing more rapid onset. High humidity increases severity, and blistering tends to be more prominent in skin folds and damp areas. The perineum has much thinner skin and, in young children, is frequently damp and enclosed by diapers. This is an area where greater damage may occur. Young children may increase ocular and facial damage by rubbing their eyes and inadvertently spreading the agents to previously unaffected areas.

a. Signs and Symptoms of Mustard Agents

Mustard agents damage DNA in cells. They do their damage immediately, although onset of symptoms may be delayed for several hours. Initial signs and symptoms include reddened skin that is similar to a bad sunburn and eventually blisters. Eyes may itch or burn and redden. Children may cough, complain of difficulty breathing or swallowing, and be difficult to console. Noncardiogenic pulmonary edema may cause a persistent cough and hypoxemia. The speed of onset of signs and symptoms is an indicator of the severity of exposure. Nausea and diarrhea suggest significant systemic exposure and put the child at enhanced risk of dehydration, hypovolemia, and circulatory collapse.

b. Treatment of Mustard Agents

Treatment of mustard exposure is supportive. The skin needs to be decontaminated to limit further damage. Although damage occurs immediately, delayed irrigation may help symptomatically and may prevent further contamination by the child and healthcare worker. The pediatric patient with mustard burns who receives irrigation is at significant risk for hypothermia and should be immediately dried and placed in a warm environment. The blisters are quite fragile and should be protected with warm, dry dressings. Eyes should be irrigated profusely, and eyelids should be dressed with a water soluble lubricant to prevent the lids from adhering and healing together. Oxygen is necessary for respiratory difficulty, and endotracheal intubation is indicated for respiratory failure. Fluid replacement should be used for thermal burns. Analgesia should not be forgotten, and if respiratory status permits, doses of opioids may be needed (see **Chapter 22**).

c. Signs and Symptoms of Lewisite Exposure

Lewisite, unlike mustard, causes immediate pain on contact, but like mustard, it creates immediate tissue damage. Skin rapidly pales and becomes discolored as the outer layer undergoes necrosis. Blisters form within 12 to 18 hours. Again, damp areas such as skin folds, genitalia, and areas under diapers may be more affected due to humidity and the relative thinness of the skin. Contact with eyes leads to immediate pain and burning accompanied by ciliary muscle spasm and difficulty opening the eyelids. The respiratory tract may become inflamed and noncardiogenic pulmonary edema may occur. Systemic effects include nausea, vomiting, and diarrhea.

d. Treatment of Lewisite

Treatment of lewisite starts with irrigation and decontamination. Children exposed to lewisite are at high risk for hypothermia due to the magnitude of the denuded and damp injured surface area. Burns should be dressed with a neutral nonadherent dressing, and the eyes treated the same as with mustard exposure. If British anti-lewisite (BAL) ointment is available, it should be placed in symptomatic eyes. Fluid losses are greater with lewisite. Analgesia is very important because the burns produce immediate pain. Systemic toxicity is treated with BAL intramuscular injections, which may be especially painful in children with reduced muscle mass. There is also the potential for allergic response because BAL is dissolved in peanut oil (**Table 13-5**).

e. Signs and Symptoms of Phosgene Oxime Exposure

Phosgene oxime is an irritant that produces erythema, itching, wheals, and immediate pain. The skin blanches, then reddens. Eyes are immediately painful. Nausea and vomiting signify systemic effects.

f. Treatment of Phosgene Oxime

Phosgene oxide is treated in the same manner as mustard exposure and presents the same problems to children (**Table 13-5**).

4. Nerve Agents

a. Signs and Symptoms

Nerve agents are highly toxic: as little as 1 milligram can be lethal to an adult. Most nerve agents are highly volatile and are designed to produce gas clouds that are inhaled by victims.

There is almost no information about pediatric exposure to nerve agents. There is, however, a large body of literature about pediatric exposure to organophosphorus pesticides. Children are more sensitive to pesticides due to increased respiratory and cutaneous absorption and may thus become symptomatic prior to adults with the same exposure. Because these agents are heavier than air and are concentrated close to the ground, a child's exposure may be greater. Altered mental status and seizures may present early in children due to the immaturity of their blood-brain barrier and the hypersensitivity of their CNS receptors. Because young children have immature hepatic enzyme systems, they are less likely to have endogenous mechanisms to detoxify these agents.

Exposure to nerve agents may produce blurred vision, tearing, small pupils, respiratory insufficiency, cough, wheezing, pulmonary edema, diaphoresis, rhinorrhea, increased oral and respiratory secretions, vomiting, diarrhea, and urinary incontinence. If a child is still in diapers, the urinary and fecal incontinence is continual. The child may be weak and hypotonic, have trouble breathing, and experience twitching or fasciculations that lead to seizures and death.

b. Treatment

Treatment should be immediate. Once nerve agents bind to acetylcholinesterase and the acetylcholinesterase ages, the binding eventually becomes irreversible until new enzyme is formed. Clothing may harbor nerve agent and release gas into the environment, further poisoning the child or caregiver.

Symptomatic children should receive supportive care that includes 100% oxygen via a non-rebreather face mask. As with adult patients, the goal of treatment is to block the effects of acetylcholine excess and regenerate acetylcholinesterase. Atropine blocks the effects of acetylcholine at the postsynaptic nerve but works only for the effects that are muscarinic. It will not affect seizures, muscle weakness, fasciculations, or respiratory failure (nicotinic effects). Pralidoxime or 2-pralidoxime chloride promotes regeneration of acetylcholinesterase and improves both nicotinic and muscarinic signs. Benzodiazepines have been shown to reduce seizures and the secondary brain injury that may result from poisoning. In a mass casualty situation, these medications must be given rapidly to a large number of people, so intramuscular (IM) administration is preferred (**Table 13-5**).

Based on the dosing recommended in **Table 13-6**, an auto-injector kit may be used for children as young as 3 years and still be within the guidelines. In addition, research has shown that side effects from higher doses are mostly theoretical and, except for tachycardia, are rarely seen. Thus, after bona fide exposure the potential benefit of using an auto-injector kit for children of all ages far outweighs the risks.

Table 13-6. Pediatric Dosing of Nerve Agent Antidotes

Drug	Dosing
Atropine	0.05-0.1 mg/kg ETT, IV, or IM repeated every 2-5 minutes as necessary
Pralidoxime	25-50 mg/kg IV or IM repeated in 1 hour
Diazepam	0.05-03 mg/kg IV to a max of 10 mg/dose
0.3-0.5 mg/kg by rectum to a max of 20 mg/dose	

Other benzodiazepines such as lorazepam (0.1 mg/kg maximum 4 mg/dose) or midazolam (0.1-0.2 mg/kg maximum
10 mg/dose) may be used IM or IV.
Abbreviations: ETT, endotracheal tube; IV, intravenously, IM, intramuscularly.
Each Mark 1 kit contains 2 auto-injectors (0.8 inch needle insertion depth), 1 each of atropine 2 mg (0.7 mL) and pralidoxime 600 mg (2 mL) to be administered in 2 separate intramuscular sites. DuoDote provides the same medications, atropine 2.1 mg (0.7 mL) and pralidoxime 600 mg (2 mL) but as a single auto-injector with the need for only one intramuscular injection; while not approved for pediatric use, they should be used as initial treatment in circumstances for children with severe, life-threatening nerve agent toxicity for whom IV treatment is not possible or available or for whom more precise IM (mg/kg) dosing would be logistically impossible (especially prehospital). Suggested dosing guidelines are offered; note potential excess of initial atropine and pralidoxime dosage for age/weight, although within general guidelines recommend a total over first 60-90 min of therapy for severe exposures.
Adapted with permission from Markenson, D. Pediatric Emergency Preparedness for Natural Disasters, Terrorism and Public Health Emergencies: A National Consensus Conference. Executive Summary and Final Report 2007.

Children presenting without symptoms after exposure to aerosols, vapor, or gas may be watched for 4 to 6 hours and then discharged home.

E. Radiation Exposure

The likelihood that most physicians will ever have to treat radiation casualties may seem remote but is nonetheless real. A radiation emergency involves the release of potentially dangerous radioactive materials into the environment. Such incidents may occur anywhere radioactive isotopes are used, stored, or transported. Radiologic threats can be unintentional or intentional. Unintentional threats include power plant disasters (eg, Chernobyl and Three Mile Island). Intentional acts could be the result of military conflict or terrorism. Although the likelihood of a thermonuclear war is low, the possibility of either a single nuclear detonation or an incident involving accidental or deliberate radiologic contamination has increased.

There are 3 main types of radiation disaster threats:

- Detonation of a nuclear weapon, considered an unlikely terrorist action due to the sophistication and supplies required to build such devices
- Damage of a facility that contains nuclear material (eg, a facility that reprocesses nuclear waste, a medical facility with storage of nuclear material, a food-irradiation plant, or a nuclear power plant)
- Dispersal of nuclear material, either by detonation of a conventional explosive (a radioactive dispersal device, or dirty bomb) or the release of nuclear materials in transit via a dispersion device.

Given that radioactive dispersal devices are designed to use radioactive material obtained from relatively accessible sources, such as university research laboratories or hospital radiation therapy centers, the third situation is considered to be the most likely.

Radiation provokes a special fear, but with appropriate understanding and preparation, effective medical care can be provided to exposed victims. To decrease morbidity and mortality from a radiologic disaster or terrorist attack, pediatricians should have a basic understanding of radiation illness and its treatment. Key factors in the management of significant radiation exposure are:

- Knowledge of the type and dose of radiation received and the presence of concomitant injuries
- Recognition of the manifestations of radiation sickness
- Use of standard medical care
- Decontamination
- Decorporation techniques (removal of contaminated areas)

The principles of disaster management, including containment, decontamination, prehospital care, and field triage, are fully applicable. The first phase of managing pediatric radiation victims is to determine whether topical decontamination is warranted. Simple removal of clothing is responsible for more than 90% of effective decontamination after chemical or radiation exposure. Initial medical management includes careful assessment of airway, breathing, and circulation, particularly when there is the potential for blast or thermal injury. It is important to remember that most injuries caused by radiologic terrorism will be associated with a blast. Although decontamination is key, most initial therapy consists of standard trauma management. If warranted, surgical intervention should be performed as soon as possible, ideally within 48 hours of irradiation, before wound healing and immunity become impaired.

A 24-hour emergency response program at the US Department of Energy's Oak Ridge Institute for Science and Education, the Radiation Emergency Assistance Center/Training Site, is available to assist physicians and others in the response to all types of radiation accidents and incidents. For expert medical consultation and advice in the event of a radiation emergency, contact the Radiation Emergency Assistance Center/Training Site at 865/576-3131 or the 24-hour emergency number at 865/576-1005.

a. Signs and Symptoms

The signs and symptoms of acute radiation injury in the pediatric population are the same as those in adults and include damage to the gastrointestinal and nervous systems. However, the severity of injury in children may be greater due to their more rapidly replicating tissues. Symptoms in the gastrointestinal system are regularly seen at acute doses greater than 600 rads and result from damage to the epithelial cells lining the intestinal tract. The higher the exposure, the sooner the symptoms of nausea and vomiting develop. Even at lower doses (such as 100 rads), nausea and vomiting may be problematic for the pediatric patient owing to lower fluid reserves. The presence of these symptoms typically overlaps with dropping cell counts, and sepsis and opportunistic infections may complicate the picture. Persistently high fevers and bloody diarrhea despite adequate fluid and electrolyte replacement are ominous signs.

Central nervous system symptoms are seen with acute radiation doses in excess of 1000 rads and are probably due to diffuse microvascular leaks within the brain. Damage to these blood vessels results in the loss of fluids and electrolytes. The patient rarely lives long enough to suffer any hematologic or gastrointestinal symptoms. Cardiovascular collapse with shock may also occur in this patient population. In small children and infants, CNS symptoms may occur sooner and at lower doses than in adults because CNS development, including new cell formation, continues until approximately 2 years of age.

Long-term consequences and published epidemiologic studies demonstrate that children exposed to radiation have a higher susceptibility to cancers than adults exposed to the same dose. This is logical because the longer life expectancy of a child results in more time for the cancers seen from radiation exposure to manifest. The typical malignancies include thyroid and breast cancer and leukemia. The epidemiologic studies included children from the Hiroshima and Nagasaki atomic bombings, the Chernobyl nuclear reactor accident, and the fallout from atomic bomb testing in the Bikini Islands. The fact that children have higher respiratory rates and live closer to the ground (where radioactive particles may settle) increases their exposure rate when compared to adults.

b. Treatment

Decontamination for external contaminants should be performed. Airway, breathing, and circulation should be addressed as soon as safely possible. The remainder of care for the radiation-injured child is supportive. Antidotes should be used only in consultation with a specialist familiar with the clinical management of radiation-exposed patients. If a need for surgery is anticipated (such as to treat injuries from a blast), the operation should be conducted within 48 hours of exposure to reduce the effects of radiation on wound healing and immunity.

A multitude of agents could be used in a radiologic event. **Table 13-7** provides a summary of the most likely radiologic agents and their absorption, symptoms, and treatments.

Table 13-7. Radiologic Agents and Their Absorption, Toxicity, and Treatment

Element	Respiratory Absorption	GI Absorption	Skin Wound Absorption	Primary Toxicity	Treatment
Americium	75%	Minimal	Rapid	Skeletal deposition, marrow suppression, hepatic deposition	Chelation with DTPA or EDTA
Cesium	Complete	Complete	Complete	Whole body irradiation	Prussian blue
Cobalt	High	<5%	Unknown	Whole body irradiation	Supportive
Iodine	High	High	High	Thyroid ablation, carcinoma	Potassium iodide
Phosphorus	High	High	High	Bone, rapidly replicating cells	Aluminum hydroxide
Plutonium	High	Minimal	Limited, may form nodules	Lung, bone, liver	Chelation with DTPA or EDTA
Radium	Unknown	30%	Unknown	Bone marrow suppression, sarcoma	Magnesium sulfate lavage
Strontium	Limited	Moderate	Unknown	Bone	Supportive
Tritium	Minimal	Minimal	Complete	Panmyelocytopenia	Dilution with controlled water intake, diuresis
Tritiated water	Complete	Complete	Complete	Panmyelocytopenia	Dilution with controlled water intake, diuresis
Uranium	High	High to moderate	High absorption, skin irritant		Pulmonary, nephrotoxic Chelation with DTPA or EDTA, $NaHCO_3$ to alkalinize urine

Abbreviations: DTPA, diethylene triamine pentaacetic acid; EDTA, ethylenediamine tetraacetic acid; $NaHCO_3$, sodium bicarbonate.

Potassium iodide (KI) is typically used following radioiodine exposure. In the past, pediatric dosing was difficult because only an adult preparation was available. Recently, the FDA approved a liquid pediatric preparation of KI containing 65 milligrams of KI per milliliter. This is the preferred dosing form for young children. The adult preparation should be adapted in cases where the liquid preparation is not available. **Table 13-8** provides guidelines for KI dosing

Table 13-8. Guidelines for Potassium Iodide Dosing

Patient/Age	Exposure, GY (Rad)	KI Dose (mg)	KI Dose (Solution)
12-17 years	0.05 (5)	65	
4-11 years	0.05 (5)	65	1 mL
1 month-3 years	0.05 (5)	32	0.5 mL
Birth-1 month	0.05 (5)	16	0.25 mL
Pregnant/lactating	0.05 (5)	130	

Note: Children and adolescents weighing >70 kg should receive the adult dose (130 mg).
This table was created from recommendations developed at the Consensus Conference and in part is based on reviewed reference materials from the American Academy of Pediatrics, the Centers for Disease Control and Prevention, and the Food and Drug Administration.
Adapted with permission from Markenson, D. Pediatric Emergency Preparedness for Natural Disasters, Terrorism and Public Health Emergencies: A National Consensus Conference. Executive Summary and Final Report 2007.

Another agent used in certain radiologic exposures is Prussian blue, which was approved by the FDA in 2003 (as 500-mg capsules) for the treatment of internal 137Cs contamination. Treatment is not time-sensitive, and the dirty bomb that might be expected to provide the exposure to 137Cs would probably affect only modest numbers of people. The dosing recommendations are described in **Table 13-9**.

Table 13-9. Dosing of Prussian Blue

Prussian blue was approved by the FDA in 2003 (as 500-mg capsules) for the treatment of internal 137Cs contamination.

Dosing instructions are as follows:

Age	Dose[a]
Adults and adolescents	3 g (6 capsules) orally twice daily
Children 2-12 years	1 g (2 capsules) orally twice daily

[a]Capsules may be opened and the contents mixed with food or beverages.
Reprinted with permission from Markenson, D. Pediatric Emergency Preparedness for Natural Disasters, Terrorism and Public Health Emergencies: A National Consensus Conference. Executive Summary and Final Report, 2007.

F. Decontamination

Children exposed to biological or chemical agents are likely to require decontamination. Whether or not to use decontamination procedures for asymptomatic individuals after a known or suspected exposure must be decided before the agent has been identified. Current mass casualty decontamination procedures designed for adults are risky for children. Decontamination with room-temperature or colder water can lead to dangerous hypothermia. However, that is less risky than not decontaminating. Young children may be unable to understand the needs for decontamination and separation from their family. Clothing for children to be dressed in after decontamination must be available. This includes diapers.

Many shower systems are not suitable for children, who require the use warm water at high volume but low pressure. Shower decontamination units designed for young children and infants must be able to accommodate an adult (parent or caretaker) in addition to a child.

Questions to ask before proceeding with decontamination include:

- Is the water pressure appropriate for a child?
- Is the water temperature acceptable for the age of the child?
- Can the decontamination shower handle the non-ambulatory child (infants, toddlers and children with special needs)?
- Do the method and equipment allow decontamination of a child with a parent or caregiver?
- Have mental health concerns such as ability to follow instructions and long term effects been addressed?

VIII. THE IMPORTANCE OF SURVEILLANCE

One of the key elements in terrorism preparedness is early detection. Providers of healthcare to children must function as part of a bioterrorism surveillance system by becoming familiar with the types of agents that may be involved, referral procedures, and criteria for reporting to the local health department. Such reporting is based on local requirements but should be considered for all unusual cases, any suspicions of a terrorist agent, or an unusual number of patients presenting with similar symptoms. The 3 key steps in surveillance are

- Identify: Be aware of symptoms, know appropriate tests, and know some of the differential diagnoses.
- Report: Know correct agencies and be able to initiate a cascade of responses.
- Refer: Refer patients to providers who know how to treat their injuries, and refer the media to appropriate sources.

A. Public Health Emergencies

To enhance detection and treatment capabilities, practitioners should be familiar with the following:

- Warning signs of a potential public health emergency
- Mechanisms and procedures for reporting a suspicious case or cases that may suggest a public health emergency
- Indicators that patients should be referred to either a public health department or an emergency department

B. Reporting a Disaster, Terrorism, or Public Health Emergency

It is important that healthcare professionals know how and where to report an event, whether natural or manmade. In such cases, healthcare professionals should activate their local emergency system, which in most areas can be done by calling 911.

A practitioner who believes that someone has been deliberately exposed to a biological, chemical, or radioactive agent or that an intentional terrorist threat will occur or is occurring should immediately involve the public health authorities. This can be done by contacting the local health department, the local police or other law enforcement agency, or the CDC's 24-hour hotline at 770/488-7100. Any incident related to terrorism or possible terrorist activity also requires notification of local law enforcement and the National Response Center at 800/424-8802.

IX. HEALTHCARE PROVIDERS' LIABILITY DURING DISASTERS

Healthcare providers often volunteer their services during and after disasters. They may be called on to respond to community needs for assistance and to treat victims at the scene, casualty collection points, hospitals (where they may not have privileges), and shelters. Whenever possible, such activities should be coordinated through the local disaster plan or emergency medical services agencies. After a disaster or act of terrorism, offices or clinics may become sites for emergency care if area hospitals cannot provide adequate services. Local facilities may be unusable, and alternative sites for primary care may need to be identified. Recent experiences have demonstrated that healthcare may be administered in parking lots, malls, and tents. Pediatricians may need to provide urgent and routine care to their practice-based patients outside their usual practice locations.

In the past, many physicians provided care without affiliation with recognized government or volunteer agencies. However, during a disaster or terrorism event, it is important that healthcare professionals be a part of an organized program to avoid providing service that is not in concert with the organized response and placing themselves in a position that is not covered by professional liability insurance. Most malpractice coverage is limited to the healthcare professional's usual scope of practice and practice setting. Good Samaritan statutes provide some liability protection when medical care is rendered at the scene of an emergency to someone who would not otherwise receive care. However, although such statutes cover physicians at the scene of acute incidents, they vary from state to state and may not provide liability protection during or after disasters or terrorism events. In many states, for health care professionals to be covered for liability in a disaster, they must practice under the umbrella of an official disaster agency, such as FEMA, the US Department of Health and Human Services, a state or local health department, a state or local office of emergency management, the local emergency medical services authority, or some other recognized government or volunteer agency.

In some states, individual malpractice insurance policies do not cover out-of-office care or the expanded scope of practice that may be required during a disaster. Good Samaritan laws do not cover a physician if there is any payment for services or if there is an accusation of gross negligence.

Key Points

Pediatric Disaster Preparedness

1. All healthcare providers should:

    a. Understand that they may be the first to recognize a public health emergency and will be responsible for reporting to appropriate authorities.

    b. Protect themselves by having a general knowledge of personal protective equipment (e.g., by using protective suits, respiratory protection, and chemical-resistant gloves).

    c. Know decontamination procedures and the unique needs of children and be prepared to assist with the decontamination of children.

    d. Address immediate critical care needs (e.g., traumatic injuries, burns).

    e. Be available to participate in officially sanctioned and organized mass prophylaxis and points of distribution plans.

2. All hospital based personnel should:

    a. Be aware of the hospital disaster plan and their possible functional roles.

    b. Receive training in the incident command system.

    c. Participate in the hospital disaster plan, including drills and exercises.

d. Be prepared to deal with continued disruption of services in the context of the hospital disaster plan, which may include medical services in the community; supplies for their patients, their office, and hospitals; limited availability of pharmacy services; and altered utilities, such as telephone, electrical power, and water.

e. Ensure that the mental health needs of children and their families are being addressed, and when needed, provide appropriate referral for mental health services.

3. In the event of a biological emergency, healthcare providers should also:

   a. Be aware of infection control procedures to protect themselves and others from harm.

   b. Be knowledgeable of infectious disease diagnosis and treatment protocols.

   c. Avoid dispensing antimicrobials or administering immunizations that are not part of a public health program.

4. In the event of a chemical emergency, pediatricians should also:

   a. Protect themselves because secondary contamination with even small amounts of these substances (particularly nerve agents such as VX) can be lethal.

   b. Treat exposed persons by clinical syndrome rather than by specific agent.

5. In the event of a radiologic emergency, pediatricians should also:

   a. Wear protective gloves, protective clothing, and radiation dosimeters. Respirators or protective masks can prevent inhalation of radioactive particles. Use techniques to prevent contamination and radiation exposure of other health care workers.

   b. Be aware that removal of clothing and washing with soap and copious amounts of water are sufficient to remove most external radiation contamination.

   c. Remember that radiation treatment, other than decontamination, is a secondary concern. Persons being examined for potential radiation exposure may not exhibit significant symptoms when first examined (even if they received a considerable radiation dose) because of the characteristic delayed onset of symptoms after exposure.

   d. Ensure follow-up examination for patients over the ensuing hours and days to establish the true nature and extent of radiation exposure. Any externally contaminated casualty without respiratory protection should be evaluated for internal contamination.

   e. When concerned about a known or suspected exposure to radioactive iodine (e.g., nuclear power plant incident), facilitate potassium iodide administration as a thyroid-blocking agent to children, either the basis of either consultation with emergency management and public health agencies or preexisting plans.

Suggested Readings

Burklow T, Yu C, Madsen, J. Industrial Chemicals: Terrorist Weapons of Opportunity. *Pediatr Ann.* 2003;32(4):230-234.

Children More Vulnerable Than Adults In The Event Of a Chemical Spill or Chemical Weapons Attack. http://www.csmc.edu/pdf/Pediatrics-ChemicalWeapons&Kids.pdf. Cedars Sinai Medical Center Online. Retrieved August 1, 2005.

Henretig F, Mechem C, Jew R. Potential Use of Auto-injector-Packaged Antidotes for Treatment of Pediatric Nerve Agent Toxicity. *Ann Emerg Med.* 2002; 40(4)405-408.

Markenson D, Reynolds S. The Pediatrician and Disaster Preparedness. *Pediatrics.* 2006;117(2):340-362.

Markenson D, Redlener I. Pediatric Emergency Preparedness for Natural Disasters, Terrorism and Public Health Emergencies: A National Consensus Conference. Valhalla, NY: New York Medical College School of Public Health, Center for Disaster Medicine, 2008.

Pediatric Expert Advisory Panel. *Atropine Use in Children After Nerve Agent Exposure.* New York, NY: Columbia University Mailman School of Public Health, National Center for Disaster Preparedness. InfoBrief Spring 2004.

Rotenberg J. Diagnosis and Management of Nerve Agent Exposure. *Pediatr Ann.* 2003;32(4)242-251.

Rotenberg J, Newmark J. Nerve Agent Attacks on Children: Diagnosis and Management, *Pediatrics.* 2003; 112:648-658.

Rotenberg J, Burklow T, Selaniko J. Weapons of Mass Destruction: The Decontamination of Children. *Pediatr Ann.* 2003; 32(4);260-268.

Web Sites

American Academy of Pediatrics. www.aap.org/terrorism

Centers for Disease Control and Prevention. www.bt.cdc.gov

JumpSTART Pediatric Multiple Casualty Incident Triage. http://jumpstarttriage.com. Retrieved August 1, 2005.

Pediatric Preparedness Resources of the Center for Disaster Medicine. www.pediatricpreparedness.com

Report of the National Advisory Committee on Children and Terrorism, Department of Health and Human Services. www.bt.cdc.gov/children

Chapter 14:

Management of the Poisoned Child and Adolescent

Objectives

- Discuss the strategies to evaluate, resuscitate, and stabilize the poisoned patient.
- Compare indications and contraindications of decontamination and elimination techniques.
- Review common toxidromes, their presentations and therapies.
- Discuss two specific poisonings and therapy.

Case Study

A 2-year-old girl is brought to the emergency department with minimal response to painful stimuli. Her heart rate is 80 beats/min, blood pressure is 70/40 mmHg. Respiratory rate is 12 with normal pupillary size and response.

- What are the priorities of assessment and management?

- What is the etiology for the patient's altered mental status?

I. INTRODUCTION

There are two major groups of poisoned children; those younger than 6 years in whom 99% of poisoning is unintentional (the larger group), and adolescents in whom only 54% is unintentional. The younger children tend to ingest a single agent in a small amount, which is usually not toxic, and they present for medical attention shortly following the ingestion. Adolescent poisoning results in more fatalities than in the younger age group. Fatalities are due to suicide, mixed ingestions, experimentation, and intentional abuse, as well as delay in seeking medical intention. In all age groups, the most common class of substances resulting in fatalities is analgesics including acetaminophen and salicylate. Other classes of agents that result in fatalities include antidepressants, stimulants, and street drugs. In general the mortality is low with a case fatality rate of 0.007 for all children <19 years old, and even lower at 0.002 for the less than 6 years old group for the year 2005.

A. Resuscitation and Stabilization

> !
>
> *Maintain a low threshold for securing the airway and stabilizing the breathing in a poisoned child who has impaired airway reflexes or any respiratory insufficiency.*
>
> !

As with all acutely ill children, the first step is prompt recognition and intervention in life-threatening conditions. A primary survey or rapid cardiopulmonary assessment focuses on the **A** (*airway*), **B** (*breathing*), **C** (*circulation*), **D** (*depressed level of consciousness, disability, drugs, decontamination*) approach. Vital signs should be obtained immediately and age-related norms considered. Isotonic fluids such as normal saline should be first-line therapy for hypotension before the institution of vasopressors. Considerations for management of the patient with a depressed level of consciousness should include dextrose, naloxone, and flumazenil.

Following stabilization, a secondary survey is conducted, which includes a more focused history to determine substance, quantity, and time of ingestion. In addition to vital signs and general physical examination, mental status, whether agitated or depressed, pupillary size, presence of nystagmus, or seizure often suggests a specific toxicologic syndrome or toxidrome. Hypothermia, hypotension, or bradycardia suggests toxic ingestion of narcotics, sedative/hypnotics, or antihypertensives, while hyperthermia, hypertension, or tachycardia suggests anticholinergics, sympathomimetics, cocaine, or amphetamines. Dilated pupils are consistent with amphetamines, cocaine, anticholinergics, antihistamines, and sympathomimetics, while constricted pupils suggest narcotics, cholinergics, organophosphates, and phencyclidine. Nystagmus can be present with toxic ingestions of alcohols, carbamazepine, carbon monoxide, phencyclidine, phenytoin, or sedative/hypnotics, while seizures can be caused by a number of agents (**Table 14-1**).

Table 14-1. Toxic Ingestions Associated with Seizures

Amphetamines	Isoniazid
Anticholinergics	Lithium
Antihistamines	Nicotine
Caffeine	Organophosphates
Camphor	Phencyclidine
Carbamates	Phenothiazines
Carbon monoxide	Phenylpropanolamine
Cocaine	Salicylates
Cyanide	Strychnine
Cyclic antidepressants	Theophylline
Hypoglycemic agents	

With the possible exception of a blood glucose or arterial blood gas measurement, laboratory tests in poisoned patients are often not necessary for the initial management. At the start of treatment, the determination of the anion and osmolar gaps, electrolytes, renal function, and specific serum quantitative tests can provide valuable information in mixed or unknown ingestions as well as for assessing the need for antidotes or elimination therapies. Quantitative tests in pediatric toxicology **(Table 14-2)** should always include acetaminophen and salicylate levels as they represent common, treatable, and potentially lethal ingestions. Qualitative tests, such as those obtained using a urine toxicology screen, provide confirmation, assist in evaluation of the child with an altered mental status, and help determine the need for counseling. Other supportive tests include an electrocardiogram, co-oximetry, and pregnancy testing in older girls.

Table 14-2. Useful Quantitative Tests in Pediatric Toxicology

- Acetaminophen
- Anticonvulsants (e.g., carbamazepine, phenytoin, valproic acid)
- Barbiturates
- Carboxyhemoglobin
- Digoxin
- Ethanol
- Ethylene glycol
- Iron
- Lead
- Lithium
- Methanol
- Methemoglobin
- Salicylate
- Theophylline

Adapted from Hoffman RJ. Laboratory testing. In: Erickson TB, Ahrens WR, Aks SE, Baum C, Ling LJ, eds. *Pediatric Toxicology.* 1st ed. New York: McGraw Hill; 2005:151-159.

B. Gastrointestinal Decontamination

Gastric emptying procedures, such as emesis or lavage, for treatment of the acutely poisoned patient have been used for emergency management.

> !
>
> *Syrup of ipecac is no longer recommended for routine use in the home or hospital.*
>
> !

1. Syrup of ipecac

Syrup of ipecac, a potent agent producing emesis in greater than 90% of patients, has not been shown to demonstrate any benefit, and may interfere with charcoal administration. A number of contraindications and complications, including aspiration pneumonitis, further limit its use.

2. Gastric lavage

Gastric lavage, using a large orogastric tube and either saline or water, has no definite indications with studies demonstrating variable efficacy. Lavage may be considered under the following conditions: within 1 hour of ingestion, when emesis is contraindicated, when a rapid deterioration in mental status is expected such as with tricyclic antidepressants, or when even a minimal decrease in toxic exposure might be critical, such as may occur with ingestion of calcium channel blockers or lithium. The contraindications include caustic agents, large foreign bodies, sharp objects, inability to protect the airway, and when the agent is not expected to be in the stomach. Complications include aspiration, esophageal or gastric perforation, decreased oxygenation during the procedure, hyponatremia, and water intoxication.

> !
>
> *The contraindications to gastric lavage include:*
>
> - *caustic agents*
> - *large foreign bodies*
> - *sharp objects*
> - *inability to protect the airway*
> - *when the agent is not expected to be in the stomach*
>
> !

3. Activated Charcoal

Activated charcoal has increased particle surface area so that toxins adsorb to the charcoal. Early administration within 4 hours of ingestion at a dose of 1 g/kg is effective, except for small molecules and some other agents (e.g., iron, lithium, alcohols, strong acids and alkalis, cyanide, and hydrocarbons). Multiple doses of charcoal decrease absorption and enhance elimination.

C. Whole Bowel Irrigation

Whole bowel irrigation (WBI) using a polyethylene glycol solution produces a rapid catharsis with expulsion of the contents of the gastrointestinal tract. There are no established indications for use of WBI due to lack of demonstrated outcome benefit. This technique may be considered in potentially toxic ingestions of sustained release or enteric coated medications and drugs that are not well adsorbed by charcoal such as iron, lithium and lead. WBI may also facilitate removal of ingested packets of illicit drugs. The solutions used in WBI can liberate toxins from activated charcoal and potentially interfere with its efficacy; therefore, activated charcoal should be administered before WBI. Contraindications for use of WBI include the presence of ileus, bowel obstruction, bowel perforation, hemodynamic instability, and unprotected compromised airway.

D. Cathartics

Cathartic agents alone have not been shown to be beneficial and their routine use in children is not recommended. However, due to the constipating effects of charcoal and a desorption effect observed with salicylate overdose, whereby salicylate levels may increase due to the release of the drug from charcoal, it is recommended that a single dose of a cathartic be administered. Sorbitol results in shorter transit times than any magnesium preparation.

> !
>
> *Cathartics alone have not been shown to be beneficial and their routine use in children is not recommended.*

E. Enhanced Elimination

Forced diuresis, manipulation of urinary pH, hemodialysis, and charcoal hemoperfusion are attempts at enhanced toxin elimination with varying efficacies. Forced diuresis has been shown to be ineffective and is not recommended. Alkaline diuresis can increase the elimination of weak acids, such as salicylates and phenobarbital, and is indicated for toxicity with these agents. There are no indications for urine acidification.

> !
>
> *For patients with coma, renal failure or progressive instability, consider hemodialysis for:*
> - *Ethylene glycol*
> - *Methanol*
> - *Phenobarbital*
> - *Procainamide*
> - *Salicylates*

Hemodialysis uses a semipermeable membrane to remove specific toxins from the blood against a concentration gradient. It should be used for substances that have a small molecular weight, are water soluble, have a small volume of distribution, and are not highly protein bound. Patients poisoned with substances resulting in renal failure, coma, or progressive instability and who meet the appropriate pharmacokinetic criteria should be considered as candidates for hemodialysis. These substances include ethylene glycol, methanol, phenobarbital, procainamide, and salicylate.

Charcoal hemoperfusion uses a cartridge of activated charcoal to remove toxins from the blood and can be used for overdoses involving carbamazepine, phenobarbital, procainamide, and theophylline.

II. Toxidromes

A. Sympathomimetic

Sympathomimetic poisoning syndrome presents with hypertension, tachycardia, seizures, central nervous system excitation, and mydriasis. Cocaine and amphetamines are the typical ingestants. Additional findings on physical examination include tremor, warm skin, diaphoresis, hypoactive bowel sounds, restlessness, paranoia, hallucinations, mania, and insomnia. Treatment is mainly supportive with benzodiazepines and α- and β-blockade. Patients should be monitored for myocardial ischemia, stroke, and rhabdomyolysis.

B. Narcotic

Overdose with a narcotic agent presents with a triad of miosis, respiratory depression, and depressed level of consciousness. Ingestion of heroin, morphine, or clonidine can present with these findings, as well as hypotension, bradycardia, hypothermia, hypoactive bowel sounds, hyporeflexia, and confusion. Treatment for opioid and toxicity is supportive with nalaxone as an antidote.

C. Sedative/Hypnotic

Sedative or hypnotic poisoning presents with a depressed level of consciousness, respiratory depression, and hyporeflexia. Typical agents include benzodiazepines and less commonly in barbiturates. Additional findings could include confusion, delirium, ataxia, blurry vision due either to miosis or mydriasis, and nystagmus. The mainstay of therapy is observation and supportive care, with cautious consideration of flumazenil as it may induce seizures.

D. Anticholinergic

Anticholinergic toxidrome includes thirst, dry skin, hyperthermia, mydriasis, delirium, and tachycardia. Causative agents include atropine, diphenhydramine, antihistamines, tricyclic antidepressants, and antipsychotics. Other findings could include hypertension, psychosis, chorea, seizures, coma, depression, confusion, hallucination, and urinary retention. Treatment is supportive with a focus on cooling and antihypertensive therapy. Benzodiazepines can be helpful in the agitated patient.

E. Cholinergic

The cholinergic syndrome is classically explained by the mnemonic SLUDGE: **S**alivation, **L**acrimation, **U**rination, **D**efecation, **G**astrointestinal upset, and **E**mesis. Organophosphates, found in some insecticides and in nerve gases like sarin, are agents that inhibit cholinesterase so that acetylcholine accumulates in the affected tissues. SLUDGE represents the muscarinic receptor toxicity, in addition to bradycardia, tachypnea, hypothermia, miosis, and bronchorrhea, while nicotinic receptor stimulation produces tachycardia, hypertension, fasciculations, confusion, weakness, paralysis, drowsiness, coma, and mydriasis. Children may present only with the central symptoms and with tachycardia instead of bradycardia, as nicotinic predominates over the muscarinic effects; however, miosis is usually present, as well as a garlic odor, which may suggest the diagnosis. Atropine, a competitive inhibitor of only the muscarinic acetylcholine receptor, and pralidoxime (2-PAM), an enzyme that reverses cholinesterase inhibition at both muscarinic and nicotinic receptors, are effective antidotes.

III. Specific Agents and Antidotes

Common toxins and their antidotes are listed in **Table 14-3**; however, a more detailed discussion of acetaminophen and salicylate poisonings is warranted as they represent frequent, potentially fatal but treatable ingestions.

Table 14-3. Toxic Ingestions, Antidotes, Antagonists, and Specific Therapies

Agent	Therapy
Acetaminophen	*N*-acetylcysteine (NAC)
Amphetamine	Benzodiazepine
Anticholinesterase	Atropine, pralidoxime (2-PAM)
Benzodiazepine	Flumazenil
β-adrenergic blocker	Glucagon
Calcium channel blocker	Calcium, glucagon
Carbamate	Atropine, pralidoxime (2-PAM)
Carbon monoxide	Oxygen, hyperbaric oxygen
Cocaine	Benzodiazepine
Coumarin derivative	Vitamin K_1 Fresh frozen plasma
Cyanide	Amyl and sodium nitrite, thiosulfate, hydroxocobalamin
Cyclic antidepressant	Sodium bicarbonate
Digoxin	Digoxin-specific Fab fragments
Ethylene glycol	Fomepizole, ethanol
Heavy metal	BAL, DMSA
Heparin	Protamine
Hypoglycemic agent	Glucose, octreotide, glucagon
Iron	Deferoxamine
Isoniazid	Pyridoxine
Lead	British antilewisite (BAL), ethylenediaminetetraacetic acid (EDTA), penicillamine, 2,3-dimercaptosuccinic acid (DMSA)
Lithium	Hemodialysis
Methanol	Fomepizole, ethanol
Methemoglobin	Methylene blue
Nitrites	Methylene blue
Opioids	Naloxone, nalmefene
Organophosphate	Atropine, pralidoxime (2-PAM)
Phenothiazine	Diphenhydramine
Salicylate	Sodium bicarbonate, hemodialysis
Theophylline	Charcoal, hemoperfusion

A. Acetaminophen

Acetaminophen is the most commonly reported potentially toxic pharmaceutical agent and the cause of the greatest absolute number of fatalities from poisoning, given that it is a prevalent co-ingestant and has an increased incidence of therapeutic overuse. With the recognition of its role as a frequent cause of hepatotoxicity, liver failure, and death, and the availability of an effective antidote, it is strongly recommended that acetaminophen levels be obtained in all suspected ingestions.

> !
>
> *It is strongly recommended that acetaminophen levels be obtained in all suspected ingestions.*

Metabolism in the liver is predominantly by glucuronidation and sulfonation; when these systems are overwhelmed by toxic ingestions, the cytochrome P450 system produces a highly reactive and toxic metabolite, N-acetyl-para-benzoquinoneimine (NAPQI). This is usually reduced by glutathione into a nontoxic metabolite, but when glutathione stores are depleted, NAPQI increases and causes hepatocellular damage. Less lethal toxicity is seen in children as they have more glutathione than adults.

> !
>
> *Acetaminophen poisoning:*
> - *150 mg/kg may be lethal*
> - *Obtain serum level >4 hours post-ingestion*
>
> *RX:*
> - *Administer charcoal within 4 hours*
> - *Give N-acetylcysteine IV or PO within first 8 hours*

An acetaminophen dose of 150 mg/kg is potentially toxic. Drug levels should be obtained 4 hours after ingestion, or as soon as possible thereafter, to assess risk of toxicity using the Rumack-Matthew nomogram. The nomogram is not useful earlier than 4 hours post-ingestion as distribution following a single acute ingestion will not have occurred. A second level should be obtained 4 hours after the first when extended release formulations are suspected. The antidote for acetaminophen poisoning is *N*-acetylcysteine (NAC), which acts as a precursor for glutathione and increases non-toxic sulfation metabolism, among other mechanisms. NAC, available in both oral and intravenous forms, is most effective if administered within 8 hours of ingestion but should be given whenever acetaminophen toxicity is suspected. Activated charcoal binds to NAC, but the dose of NAC is such that losses due to charcoal binding are not clinically significant; therefore, charcoal should not be withheld in isolated acetaminophen ingestion presenting within 4 hours or with a potential co-ingestant.

B. Salicylates

Although the overall incidence of salicylate poisoning has declined and there have been no fatalities in children in 2006, these agents continue to be a major problem as they can be found in a number of oral and topical preparations, such as bismuth subsalicylate and oil of wintergreen. Physiologically salicylate poisoning causes a respiratory alkalosis by direct stimulation of the medulla and an increased anion gap metabolic acidosis through a number of mechanisms. Patients present with nausea, vomiting, tinnitus, cerebral edema, central nervous system disturbances, fever, coagulopathy, pulmonary edema, hepatotoxicity, rhabdomyolysis, hypoglycemia, hypokalemia, and dehydration. Infants and children may not demonstrate the initial respiratory alkalosis.

Ingestion of more than 150 mg/kg of aspirin should be considered toxic. A ferric chloride test, where 1 to 2 drops of $FeCl_3$ in 1 mL of urine produces a purple color change in the presence of any salicylate, may be performed as a screen. A quantitative test will be necessary to determine therapy. The Done nomogram is not considered useful. In acute ingestions, symptoms are typically present with levels greater than 30 mg/dL; patients with levels greater than 100 mg/dL should undergo dialysis. In long-term ingestions, serum levels are unreliable in predicting severity of illness; however, a level of greater than 60 mg/dL may be a relative indication for dialysis, as are seizures, altered mental status, refractory acidosis, or deterioration despite adequate supportive care.

The treatment plan should include gastrointestinal decontamination with gastric emptying in an acute overdose and activated charcoal for large ingestions. Aggressive fluid resuscitation is an important first step; however, urine alkalinization to trap ions and thereby prevent tubular absorption in the kidney should be instituted for serum levels greater than 40 mg/dL or in the presence of signs and symptoms of salicylism. Acetazolamide is not recommended; although it alkalinizes the urine, it acidifies the serum.

> !
>
> *Salicylate poisoning:*
> - *>150 mg/kg is toxic*
> - *Symptoms with blood levels >30 mg/dL*
>
> *RX:*
> - *Use GI emptying and activated charcoal*
> - *Alkalinize urine for serum level >40 mg/dL*
> - *Consider dialysis for serum levels >100 mg/dL*
>
> !

Suggested Readings

1. Watson WA, Litovitz TL, Rodgers GC, et al. 2004 annual report of the American Association of Poison Control Centers Toxic Exposure Surveillance System. *Am J Emerg Med.* 2005;23:589-666.

2. Abbruzzi G, Stork CM. Pediatric toxicologic concerns. *Emerg Med Clin North Am.* 2002;20:223-247.

3. Tenenbein M. Recent advances in pediatric toxicology. *Pediatr Clin North Am.* 1999;46:1179-1188.

4. Osterhoudt KC, Ewald MB, Shannon M, Henretig F. Toxicologic emergencies. In: Fleisher G, Ludwig S, Henretig F, eds. *Textbook of Pediatric Emergency Medicine.* 5th ed. Philadelphia: Lippincott Williams and Wilkins; 2006:951-1007.

5. Hoffman RJ. Laboratory testing. In: Erickson TB, Ahrens WR, Aks SE, Baum C, Ling LJ, eds. *Pediatric Toxicology.* 1st ed. New York: McGraw Hill; 2005:151-159.

6. Position paper: cathartics. American Academy of Clinical toxicology; European Association of Poisons Centers and Clinical toxicologists. *J Toxicol Clin Toxicol.* 2004;42:243-253.

7. Position paper: whole bowel irrigation. American Academy of Clinical Toxicology; European Association of Poisons Centers and Clinical toxicologists. *J Toxicol Clin Toxicol.* 2004;42:843-854.

8. Position paper: gastric lavage. American Academy of Clinical Toxicology; European Association of Poisons Centers and Clinical toxicologists. *J Toxicol Clin Toxicol.* 2004;42:933-943.

9. Mazor S, Aks SE. Antidotes. In: Erickson TB, Ahrens WR, Aks SE, Baum C, Ling LJ, eds. *Pediatric Toxicology.* 1st ed. New York: McGraw Hill; 2005:121-131.

10. Larson AM, Polson J, Fontana RJ, et al. Acetaminophen-induced acute liver failure: results of a United States multicenter, prospective study. *Hepatology.* 2005;42:1364-1372.

Chapter 15:

Transport of the Critically Ill Child

Objectives

- Describe factors that influence the method and mode of transport within and between hospital facilities.
- Identify potential high-risk problems for critically ill children during transport.
- Discuss transport considerations and practical issues.
- Specify the information that the referring institution should provide to the transport team and the accepting hospital facility to facilitate effective treatment, appropriate referral, and timely transfer.
- Identify the equipment necessary for a safe transport.

Case Study

A 2-year-old girl who is intubated secondary to smoke inhalation injury is being transported to the regional children's hospital. During transport, the ventilator alarm sounds for high pressure and the child's oxygen saturation drops below 90% despite the increase of FIO_2 to 1.0. The patient is suctioned, but the high-pressure alarms persist and oxygenation continues to deteriorate. The child is now becoming bradycardic and hypotensive, and develops poor perfusion.

- What are the priorities to stabilize the patient?

- What information should be communicated to the medical control person?

- What type of equipment should be accompanying this patient on transport?

I. INTRODUCTION

Critically ill pediatric patients are at increased risk of morbidity and mortality during transport, whether interfacility or intrafacility. Risk is not isolated to the patient but may extend to some degree to the accompanying personnel. The decision to transport a critically ill pediatric patient, either within the hospital facility or to another facility, is based on an assessment of the potential benefits versus the potential risks associated with the transport itself. The risks of transport can be minimized by careful planning, the use of appropriately qualified personnel, and selection and availability of appropriate equipment. Critically ill patients are transported to alternative locations to obtain additional care that is not available at the existing location. This may include care in a diagnostic department, operating room, specialized unit within the hospital, or another medical facility.

II. GENERAL CONSIDERATIONS

Many critically ill pediatric patients may require lengthy transport to an appropriate regional pediatric tertiary-care facility. Initially most critically ill or injured children are taken to the closest medical facility for primary stabilization if there is no regional pediatric tertiary-care facility in the vicinity. Once stabilized, these children will require transport to a facility with an appropriate level of care and expertise. Interhospital transport services are a vital link in the system of emergency and critical care for children, bridging the patient's initial stabilization with definitive care in the tertiary care center. This transport from one hospital to another should be from a lower level of care to an equal or higher level of care.

During transport, a patient is potentially at risk for instability and deterioration. Therefore, if a patient is being transported for a diagnostic test or a procedure that is unlikely to alter the management or outcome, the need for transport must be questioned. Whenever possible, diagnostic testing or simple procedures should be attempted bedside to avoid subjecting a patient to the risks associated with transport.

> !
>
> *Risk to the patient during transport can be minimized through careful planning, use of appropriately qualified personnel, and the selection and preparation of appropriate equipment.*
>
> !

The transport personnel (or transport team) are selected according to training and skills, and the available equipment and supplies are selected to provide for any ongoing or anticipated needs for acute care. There should be minimal disturbance in the monitoring or maintenance of the patient's vital functions during transport. Ideally, all transports of critically ill pediatric patients, both intrahospital and interhospital, would be performed by specially trained individuals, but that is not always possible.

Given that not all transferring facilities have access to a dedicated pediatric critical care transport team, contingency plans for using locally available resources should be developed. The standards for organized transport services as set forth by the American Academy of Pediatrics (AAP) and the

Society of Critical Care Medicine (SCCM) are considerably more rigorous. A comprehensive and effective interhospital transfer plan for facilities that do not have access to an organized pediatric critical care transport team can be developed in 4 steps:

1. A multidisciplinary team of physicians, nurses, respiratory therapists, hospital administrators, and local emergency medical services personnel is formed to plan and coordinate the process.

2. The team conducts a needs assessment that focuses on patient demographics, transfer volume, transfer patterns, available resources (personnel, equipment, emergency medical services, communication), and available receiving facilities.

3. A standardized transfer plan is written.

4. The transfer plan is regularly evaluated and refined after use and at periodic intervals using a standard quality improvement process.

> !
>
> *The mode of transport and the composition of the transport team should be based on the acuity and complexity of care required by the individual patient.*
>
> !

Transport and transfer to a tertiary care setting should be coordinated with the receiving providers to ensure that the patient is transported safely and arrives in stable or improved condition. Ideally, the transport is supervised in person or in communication with a physician who has experience and training in pediatric emergency medicine or pediatric critical care. The mode of transportation for a critically ill patient is an important aspect of comprehensive care.

Ground ambulances, helicopters, and fixed-wing aircraft are the principle vehicles available for pediatric interfacility transport. Depending upon geographic location and resources, other transport vehicles may be needed, including, but not limited to, boats, private vehicles, carts, and bicycles. The composition of the transport team will also depend upon the resources available but should include individuals with the skills and experience that best meet the needs of the patient during transport.

Pediatric transport medicine is a relatively new field of clinical interest that has developed rapidly over the past 3 decades. The AAP has stated that the goal of pediatric interfacility transport is to improve outcomes of critically ill or injured pediatric patients who are not in proximity to a hospital that provides the required level of care. Advances in technology and transportation have allowed dedicated pediatric critical care transport teams to offer many of the therapies that were previously restricted to use within the intensive care unit (ICU). This can minimize transport-associated risks and improve outcomes.

Every pediatric tertiary care facility should have an organized pediatric transport system. Ideally, the system is regional, with central medical control under the direction of a physician trained in pediatric emergency or intensive care.

III. INTRAFACILITY TRANSPORT

> !
>
> *The four key elements for transport are communication, personnel, equipment, and mode of transportation.*
>
> !

The basic reason for moving a critically ill pediatric patient within the facility is the need for additional care that utilizes technology and/or specialists not available in the child's current location. This may require a patient to be moved within the hospital to a diagnostic testing area, operating room, or pediatric intensive care unit (PICU). The transport process must be organized and efficient due to the potential risks it entails for the patient.

A. Pre-transport Communication and Coordination for Intrafacility Transport

Physician-to-physician and nurse-to-nurse communication regarding the pediatric patient's condition and treatment should occur both prior to and at completion of transport. Detailed hand-off communication should occur when a patient's management will be assumed by a different team, whether related to transfer from unit to unit or to testing or interventions performed outside the PICU.

> !
>
> *Communication occurs each time responsibility for patient care is transferred.*
>
> !

Pre-transport confirmation should be given indicating that the area to which the patient is being transported (radiology, operating room, nuclear medicine, etc.) is ready to receive the patient and immediately begin the specified procedure or test. Ancillary services and other members of the healthcare team (security, respiratory therapy, escort) should be notified of the timing of the transport and the equipment and equipment support that will be required. The responsible physician should either accompany the patient or be notified that the patient is out of the PICU and at risk of having an acute event in another area of the hospital. The medical record should document the indications for transport and the patient's status throughout the transport process.

B. Accompanying Personnel During Intrafacility Transport

It is strongly recommended that a minimum of 2 people accompany a critically ill pediatric patient. One should be a nurse who has completed a competency-based orientation and has met the prescribed standards for pediatric critical care nurses. Additional personnel may include a respiratory therapist, registered nurse, or critical care technician as needed. It is strongly advised that a healthcare professional (physician, nurse practitioner, physician assistant) with training in airway management, advanced pediatric life support, critical care, or the equivalent accompany intubated or unstable patients.

When a procedure is anticipated to be lengthy and the receiving location is staffed by appropriately trained personnel, patient care may be transferred to those individuals if acceptable to both groups. This allows for maximum utilization of staff and resources. If care responsibility is not transferred, the transport personnel should remain with the patient until transferred back to the PICU.

C. Accompanying Equipment During Intrafacility Transport

Certain equipment and resources accompany each and every patient during the transport process. All critically ill patients require a blood pressure monitor, a pulse oximeter, and a cardiac monitor/defibrillator.

> **!** *When a critically ill child requires transport, the same level of monitoring that occurs in the ICU should be maintained.* **!**

When available, monitors with the capacity for storing and reproducing patient bedside data should be utilized to allow for review of data collected during the procedure and transport. The minimum requirements are shown in **Table 15-1.**

Table 15-1. Minimum Monitoring Equipment Required for Transport
ECG monitor
Pulse oximeter
Defibrillator with battery backup and transcutaneous pacing capability
Oxygen analyzer and oxygen tank
Ventilator appropriate for infants, children, and adults
Infusion pumps
Noninvasive blood pressure monitor
Portable suction unit

Airway management equipment, including a resuscitation bag and facemask of proper size and fit for the patient's age and size, should accompany the patient. It is also important to have an oxygen source of ample volume to provide for the patient's projected needs while out of the PICU plus an additional 30 minutes of reserve.

Standard resuscitation drugs include epinephrine and antiarrhythmic agents. These are to be transported with each patient in the event of sudden cardiac arrhythmia or arrest. A more complete array of pharmacologic agents should either accompany the basic agents or be available from supplies in the emergency resuscitation carts or crash carts located along the transport route and in the receiving location. In many hospitals, pediatric patients share diagnostic and procedural facilities with adult patients, so it is imperative that a complete set of pediatric resuscitation equipment and medications accompany infants and children during transport and also be available in the diagnostic or procedure area. Supplemental medications, such as narcotics and sedative agents, are to be considered on a case-by-case basis.

An appropriate supply of intravenous fluids and continuous drip medications, administered and regulated on battery-operated infusion pumps, should be ensured. All battery-operated equipment must be fully charged and capable of functioning for the duration of the transport. Backup batteries and electric cords for the equipment should be included. If a healthcare professional capable of medical decision making will not be accompanying the patient during transport, protocols or communication mechanisms must be in place to permit the administration of medications and fluids by appropriately trained personnel under emergency circumstances.

Bag-mask ventilation is the most commonly employed ventilation method during intrahospital transports. However, portable mechanical ventilators are gaining in popularity and use because they are capable of more reliably administering prescribed minute ventilation and desired oxygen concentrations. In children, a default oxygen concentration of 100% is frequently used. However, oxygen concentration must be precisely regulated for neonates and patients with congenital heart disease who have single ventricle physiology or who are dependent on a right-to-left shunt to maintain systemic blood flow.

For patients with mechanical ventilatory support, equipment similar to that used in the PICU is preferably available at the receiving location. When that is not the case, the equipment used in the PICU is transported to meet the patient at the receiving location.

The position of a patient's endotracheal tube must be noted and confirmed radiologically prior to transport. The adequacy of oxygenation and ventilation is confirmed with either bag-mask ventilation or trial on transport ventilator. Occasionally, patients may require modes of ventilation or ventilator settings that are not replicable during transport or at the receiving location. In such cases, alternative modes of mechanical ventilation must be tested prior to transport to ensure appropriateness of therapy and patient stability. If a patient cannot be maintained safely with alternative therapy, the risks and benefits of the transport must be reexamined.

Transport ventilators must have alarms to indicate both disconnection and excessively high airway pressures. Pediatric patients with tracheostomy tubes must be transported with great caution because most home or transport ventilators are not capable of sensing disconnection and alarms will be delayed. All transport ventilators must have a backup battery power supply, and electrical cords must accompany the patient during transport.

D. Monitoring During Intrafacility Transport

> !
>
> *All critically ill pediatric patients who require transport must receive the same level of basic physiologic monitoring that they received in the ICU.*
>
> !

At the very minimum, monitoring should include continuous electrocardiography (ECG) monitoring, continuous pulse oximetry, and periodic measurement of blood pressure, pulse rate, and respiratory rate. Selected patients may also benefit from end tidal capnography, continuous intra-arterial blood pressure monitoring, and central venous pressure and intracranial pressure monitoring.

IV. INTERFACILITY TRANSPORT

The 2 general indications that a critically ill child requires interfacility transport are that the referring hospital lacks the inpatient resources to care for the patient beyond initial stabilization and that the patient has a diagnosis or severity of illness that would be best managed in a regional pediatric tertiary care center. The transport of a critically ill child has no strict contraindications when it is the judgment of the referring physician that the child cannot be adequately cared for in the referring hospital.

> ! *Transport of the critically ill or injured pediatric patient is best performed by a team experienced in such care, even if awaiting their arrival creates a delay at the referring hospital.*

Timely recognition of a child in need of transport is critical. Favorable patient outcomes depend on the expertise and availability of nursing and medical personnel and the technology available in the healthcare facility.

Delays are inherent in arranging an interfacility transport, particularly when a specialized team from the receiving hospital is necessary. Therefore, the clinical deterioration of the child must be anticipated and expected, and an appropriate team must be mobilized as early as possible during the patient's initial stabilization.

> ! *Difficulty in achieving and ensuring adequate stabilization in a patient may be considered a relative contraindication to transport. However, the problem may be that true stabilization is possible only at the receiving facility.*

Speed of delivery to the tertiary care center is rarely the sole concern in interfacility transport and rarely supersedes stabilization. The level of care that can be provided during transport is an equally important consideration. The transport team should be capable of providing an equal or higher level of care than the referring hospital and have the means to maintain that level of care during transport. The vehicle type, mode of transport, and team composition should be selected to best meet the needs of the patient during transport (see **Appendix 12**).

It is essential that healthcare practitioners be aware of their local, regional, and national laws regarding interfacility patient transfers. In the United States, there are federal regulations that define the legal responsibilities of the entities involved. In essence, financially motivated transfers are illegal and put both the institution and the individual practitioner at risk for serious penalty. Current regulations in the United States and best practices require that a competent patient or the legally authorized representative of a minor child or incompetent patient give informed consent prior to interfacility transport. This must include the disclosure of risks versus benefits of transport, with documentation in the medical record and a signed consent form. If circumstances do not allow for informed consent, both the indications for transport and the reason for not obtaining consent must be documented in the medical record. Transfer and transport agreements must be completed in advance to prevent needless transport delays. A transfer algorithm showing the sequence of events involved in an interfacility patient transport is presented in **Figure 15-1.**

Figure 15-1: Transport Algorithm

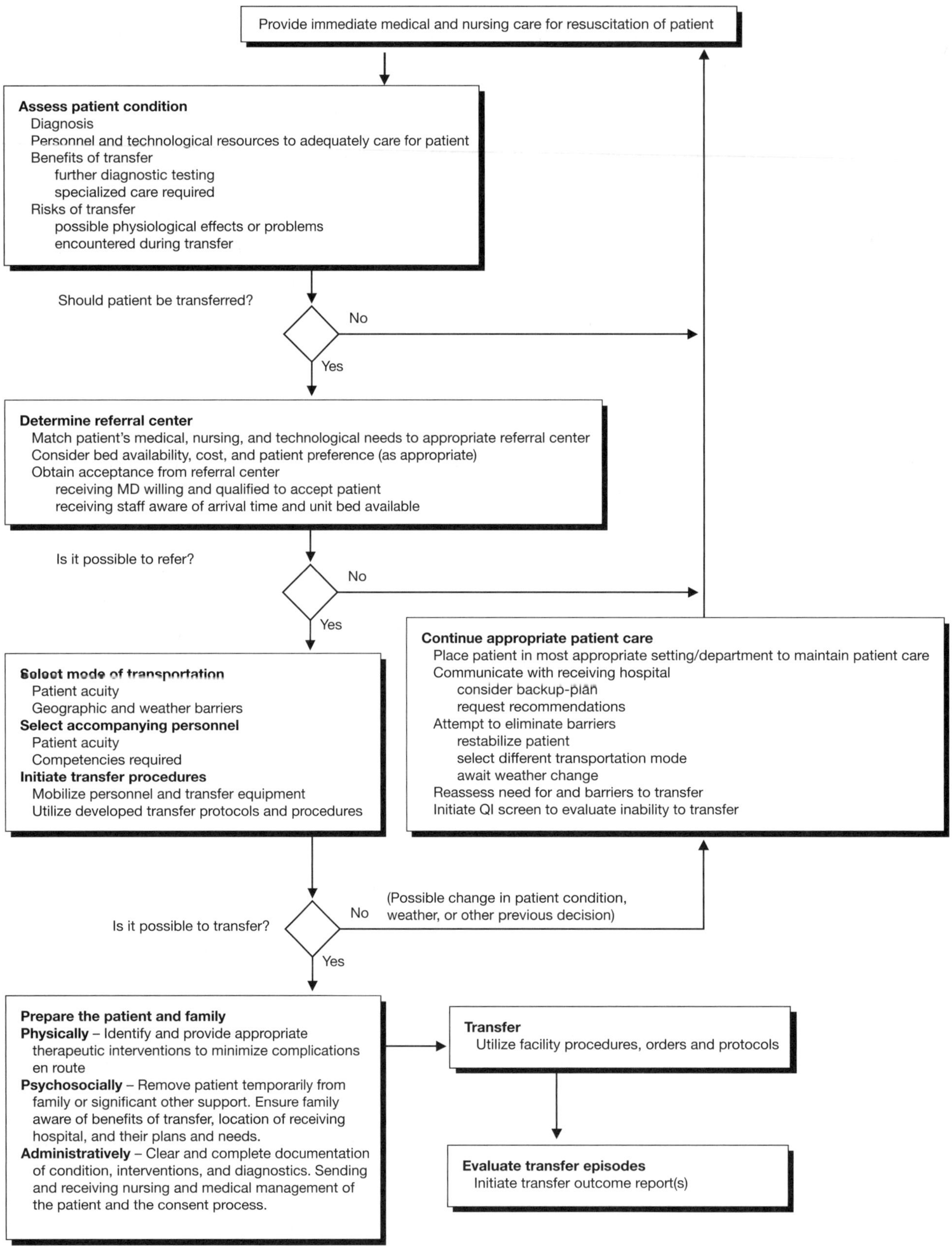

A. The Transport Process

Once the decision to transport has been made, the patient must be prepared. The goal is optimal stabilization. The patient's condition and the trajectory of illness or injury process must be considered. Whenever possible, medical interventions aimed at stabilizing the patient should be discussed with the receiving physician and the transport team. Airway patency must be assured.

> !
>
> *If there is any concern about maintaining airway patency for the duration of the transport process, the patient must be intubated.*
>
> !

Intubation should be performed at the referring institution by the most experienced individual available, whether it is someone at the referring institution or a member of the transport team. Once the airway is stabilized and secured, adequate ventilation and oxygenation are ensured. Circulation must be assessed and stabilized. Maintaining adequate intravenous access is important. In most circumstances, two functional intravenous lines are preferred during transport. Appropriate temperature control is also essential, especially while moving between buildings and vehicles and within transport vehicle.

While the patient is being stabilized, the medical record, laboratory reports, radiographs, and any additional imaging studies are copied to accompany the patient on transport. At least one parent or legal guardian should remain with the child during preparations. This will ensure that necessary information and consent are obtained prior to the actual transport. Often, at least one parent or legal guardian may accompany the child throughout the transport process.

B. Mode of Transport

To ensure a successful interfacility transport, the most appropriate vehicle type and the best team composition should be requested. The kinds of vehicles available vary greatly from one geographic region to another. Interfacility transport is typically accomplished through the use of a ground ambulance, critical care mobile ICU ambulance, helicopter, or fixed-wing aircraft, but other modes of transport may be dictated by regional or local resources. The following factors must be considered when selecting the optimal mode of interfacility transport for a critically ill pediatric patient:

- Diagnosis and severity of illness
- Risk of deterioration during transport
- Team capabilities
- Urgency to arrive at the tertiary care center and team response time
- Distance between the 2 hospitals
- Local geographic characteristics, current weather and traffic conditions
- Current availability of vehicles or aircraft

After all those factors have been weighed, the relative cost and availability of resources, both personnel and equipment, must be considered for each practical option.

As they prepare, the transport team must take into consideration the constraints of the transport environment (**Table 15-2**). The transport environment is small and confined, with finite resources. Consequently, team members' sensory perception, communication, and range of motion are limited.

Table 15-2. Comparison of Modes of Transport

	Ground Ambulance	Fixed-Wing Aircraft	Helicopter
Availability[a]	Excellent[a]	Fair[a]	Good[a]
Safety	Good	Good	Good
Cabin environment (space, noise, vibration)	Fair-Good	Good	Poor
Transport time	Fair	Good	Excellent
Range	<100 miles (typically)	200-2000 miles	100-150 miles
Special issues	Road and weather conditions	Need for multiple transfers	Weather conditions

[a] Depends upon local geographic characteristics and regional resources.

Adapted from Durbin DR. Preparing the child for interhospital transport. In: Henretig FM, King C, eds. *Textbook of Pediatric Emergency Procedures.* Baltimore, MD: Williams & Wilkins, 1997.

Compared to other modes of transport, ground ambulances are readily available, relatively inexpensive, and spacious. Ground ambulances are on average the most common mode of interfacility transport. They are operable in most weather conditions and can be brought to a halt if interventions or procedures are required. In some cases, weather may necessitate that a ground ambulance be used, even if the distance between facilities is significant. Ambulances are generally considered safer than either helicopters or fixed-wing aircraft. Disadvantages associated with ground transportation include increased transport time over long distances and the risk of traffic and weather-associated delays.

Helicopter transport is fast; it allows rapid transfer to the receiving facility and avoids traffic congestion. The distinct advantage of a helicopter over a ground ambulance is faster transport over a wider distance range. Helicopter transport is best utilized when speed of transport to a tertiary care center is the most critical factor in the management of a patient. Monitoring and evaluating the pediatric patient is extremely difficult during helicopter transport. The small space inside the helicopter cabin and the constant noise and vibration from the rotors limit the ability of transport personnel to perform procedures during flight. In addition, helicopter transport is more costly than ground transport. Weather conditions preclude flying up to 15% of the time and limit the availability of transport by helicopter.

> *Hypoxia is the single greatest stressor encountered during air transport. In an unpressurized aircraft cabin as altitude increases so does the risk for hypoxia.*

Fixed-wing aircraft are usually used for long-distance transports, typically more than 200 miles. Depending upon the type of aircraft, the cabin environment may permit excellent patient monitoring and assessment. Many of these aircraft are pressurized and land at controlled sites. Interventions can be performed more easily in fixed-wing aircraft than in rotor-wing aircraft. The disadvantages of fixed-wing transport are long start-up times (though this may be offset by the speed of the flight) and the need to move the patient multiple times, typically by ground ambulance, between the hospital and the aircraft. Multiple transfers increase the risk of such difficulties as airway deterioration, intravenous catheter malfunction, and equipment failure. Altitude may also increase the risk of adverse effects: hypoxia, gas expansion, and reactions to temperature, humidity, and gravitational forces are unique to air transport. All patients should be given nothing by mouth as soon as the decision is made to transport and should remain that way throughout the transport process.

A patient's initial compensatory response to hypoxia is an increase in respiratory rate and effort. Supplemental oxygen should be provided, especially when a child's pulmonary status may be compromised. Additionally, as altitude increases, gas volume proportionally increases. Physiologically a patient with a small pneumothorax may develop a clinically significant pneumothorax with increases in altitude. Similarly, a pneumocephalus may expand to further complicate a closed head injury. Nasogastric tubes must be connected to a functioning suction unit. Equipment that is under pressure may need adjustment at high altitude. The pressure in a cuffed endotracheal tube should be slightly deflated prior to flight and periodically checked and adjusted during flight to the minimal volume needed to maintain a seal. Nonetheless, despite the many added considerations, the time saved by flying may compensate for the potential risks.

C. Configuration of the Transport Team

The referring institution typically retains primary responsibility for a patient until arrival at the accepting facility, except when the transport team is sent from the accepting facility. During transport, a patient should not be put at increased risk by any decrease in level of care. Careful attention must be paid to the qualifications and experience of the transport personnel. A number of variations in team composition are possible, as shown in **Table 15-3.**

The composition of the transport team will be dictated by the patient's needs and the hospital's available resources. The team may include physicians, nurses, respiratory therapists, paramedics, and emergency medical technicians (EMTs). No single team composition is preferred over all others.

Table 15-3. Comparison of Transport Team Configurations

	Advantages	Disadvantages
Private vehicle	Cost, speed, readily accessible	No care en route, unreliable
Emergency medical services/ ambulance	Cost, speed, some monitoring	Limited skills/interventions
Emergency medical services + RN and/or MD	Improved skills/monitoring	Uses scarce resources
Broad-based critical care team	Cost, speed, improved monitoring, skills, and intervention	Limited pediatric critical care skills/knowledge
Specialized pediatric critical care transport team	Highest level of care, monitoring, and skills	Limited availability

Adapted from Durbin DR. Preparing the child for interhospital transport. In: Henretig FM, King C, eds. *Textbook of Pediatric Emergency Procedures.* Baltimore, MD: Williams & Wilkins; 1997.

Team members may be drawn from local EMS personnel, medical personnel from the referring hospital, hospital-based critical care teams that typically transport adult and trauma patients but can transport children when requested, and dedicated pediatric and neonatal transport teams. Patient safety and availability of needed medical care are factors to consider when creating a team for a specific transport. Although local EMS systems tend to offer rapid response times, their personnel usually do not have the training, experience, or equipment to transport a critically ill or injured child. Healthcare professionals from the referring hospital may be rapidly mobilized, but their absence due to inclusion in the transport team may place their facility at a disadvantage. Personnel with limited experience in pediatric pre-hospital or critical care will find patient management difficult in the mobile transport environment. Adult-based critical care transport services offer both ground and flight resources but often have limited expertise and equipment for the care of critically ill children.

Specialized pediatric and neonatal transport systems offer experienced personnel (nurses, respiratory therapists, nurse practitioners, physicians, and EMTs) who are skilled in the care of critically ill pediatric patients. These specialized teams offer the optimal level of care during transport and often provide continuity of care from transport to the PICU. They are usually based at the regional tertiary care center and have specific training and expertise in the transport of critically ill patients. Specialized teams are somewhat slower to arrive at the referring hospital because they must be mobilized from the regional center, and they may be costly in comparison to other ground transport methods. The advantage of specialized teams is their ability to deliver a high level of care and monitoring during transport. Unfortunately, such teams are not available in all areas, and they may not have access to all types of transport vehicles. When available, these teams should be used to transport the most unstable patients, even if they require more time to arrive or to stabilize a patient.

V. PREPARING A PATIENT FOR INTERFACILITY TRANSPORT

A. Pre-transport Coordination and Communication for Interfacility Transport

Every facility should establish a plan with protocols that outline the process for obtaining appropriate transport once it is determined that a seriously ill or injured child actually requires transfer. A list of names and telephone numbers of facilities equipped to manage critically ill children should be compiled and be readily available in the emergency department. There should also be a list of contact numbers for transport systems capable of accommodating a critically ill pediatric patient, if transport will not be provided by the tertiary care facility that will receive the patient.

> !
>
> *The most important determinant of a transport's success is effective communication between the referring and receiving hospital personnel.*
>
> !

One of the most important steps in the interfacility transport of a critically ill pediatric patient is the initial referral call. Based on the information exchanged, the receiving hospital must determine the most appropriate bed assignment and whether the patient would be best served in the PICU or on the general pediatric floor, and must anticipate the patient's need for specialized diagnostic or therapeutic modalities. If the decision to utilize a specialized pediatric transport team from the receiving hospital is made, the optimal team composition must be determined. The key patient information that must be provided by the referring facility during the initial referral call is listed below.

The following information should be initially provided to the receiving hospital:

- Patient's identifying information
- Referring physician's name
- Facility name, location, and contact telephone number
- Brief summary of the patient's condition
- Vital signs and weight
- Pertinent findings of physical exam
- Relevant laboratory and radiographic results
- Significant interventions performed and patient response

The receiving physician may provide advice about further evaluation or interventions. That physician must first accept the patient and confirm that the appropriate resources are available at the receiving hospital before transport can be initiated. The mode of transportation will be determined by the transferring physician in consultation with the receiving physician and based on patient acuity, time, weather, any medical interventions required for continued stabilization, and available personnel and resources.

If the transport team is not from the referring or receiving facility, the referring hospital must assist in the arrangements for efficient transfer of the patient. The provider that will transport the patient should be contacted to confirm availability and capabilities and to detail the patient's status and anticipated needs during transport. This should include an estimate of preparation and transport time (**Table 15-4**).

Table 15-4. Information Required by the Transport Team

Patient name, weight, age, sex, date of birth
Patient location (unit and hospital facility) at both the transferring and the receiving hospitals, including addresses and telephone numbers
Names and contact telephone numbers for both the transferring and the receiving attending physicians
Basic diagnosis
Method of transport (ground, fixed-wing aircraft, helicopter)
Nature of transport (isolette, pediatric stretcher, adult stretcher)
Team composition (number of team members)
Reason for mode of transport (patient acuity, traffic or weather conditions, etc.)
Equipment required or anticipated for transport
Patient status, including interventions already instituted

Adapted from Freedman SH, King BR. Aeromedical transport procedures. In: Henretig FM, King C, eds. *Textbook of Pediatric Emergency Procedures.* Baltimore, MD: Williams & Wilkins, 1997.

A nurse-to-nurse report should be given by the referring facility to the unit at the accepting facility. If the receiving facility is not involved in the transport process, the referring physician should telephone the receiving physician immediately before the patient's departure and report the patient's most recent vital signs, current clinical status, and estimated time of arrival at the receiving hospital.

While awaiting the arrival or coordination of the transport team, staff at the referring hospital should ensure that the patient is optimally prepared for transport. The medical record and laboratory and radiographic studies should be copied, monitoring and assessment should be continued, and necessary procedures should be performed by the most experienced personnel. If airway patency or ventilatory status is questionable, the airway should be secured with an endotracheal tube prior to transport. All intravascular lines should be checked for patency and taped securely in place. The cervical spine and any fractured bones should be stabilized and/or immobilized before transport. The patient should be given nothing by mouth for transport and throughout the transport process. Nasogastric tubes should be connected to a functioning suction unit. If clinically significant pneumothorax or hemothorax is present, a chest tube must be inserted and fluid or air collections must be evacuated prior to transport. In addition, the patient's parents and family should be prepared for the transport. Every attempt should be made to inform the family of the nature of their child's illness or injury and to explain why transport is being arranged so that they can provide consent. The responsibilities of the referring hospital are summarized in **Table 15-5.**

Table 15-5. Responsibilities of the Referring Hospital

Stabilize patient.
Communicate with accepting facility from the start.
Notify family and obtain consent for transfer/transport.
Secure vascular access and tracheal tube.
Stabilize cervical spine and any fractures (as indicated).
Copy all patient records and radiographic studies, including transfer summary, medication list, and laboratory results.
Provide transport team with telephone number to call for results of pending laboratory studies.
Prepare blood products, if indicated.

B. Accompanying Personnel During Interfacility Transport

A minimum of 2 people in addition to the vehicle operators are necessary to accompany the patient. At least 1 of the accompanying personnel must be a nurse, physician, or advanced EMS technician capable of providing advanced airway management, including endotracheal intubation, intravenous therapy, interpretation and treatment of dysrhythmia, and basic and advanced cardiac and trauma life support. When a physician does not accompany the patient on transport, there needs to be a mechanism available to communicate with a healthcare provider who is capable of providing advice and medical orders to manage changes in the patient's clinical condition. If this is not technically possible, the personnel accompanying the critically ill child should have standing orders to perform acute lifesaving interventions.

C. Minimum Required Equipment During Interfacility Transport

A list of the minimum necessary equipment should be reviewed and discussed regardless of who transports the patient. Ideally, transport packs containing correctly sized equipment and medications for pediatric patients should be prepared in advance and be readily available for emergency situations. **Tables 15-6, 15-7, and 15-8** list the recommended respiratory equipment, minimum transport equipment, and transport medications that should be available for the transport of a critically ill or injured pediatric patient. These items should accompany the patient during interfacility transport. The tables delineate the range of equipment and medications that may be necessary to care for the age spectrum that encompasses the pediatric population. Based on the team or system transporting the patient, the supplies may be adapted to meet the patient's clinical needs or mode of transport.

Table 15-6. Minimum Recommended Respiratory Equipment

500-mL resuscitation bag
1-liter resuscitation bag with oxygen reservoir
Oxygen supply tubing: #2
Manometer with tubing and adapter
Nasal cannulas: neonatal, pediatric, adult
Non-rebreather masks: pediatric, adult
Resuscitation face masks, 1 each: neonate, infant, toddler, pediatric, small adult, large adult
End-tidal carbon dioxide monitors (disposable): pediatric, adult
End-tidal carbon dioxide supplies, 1 each: ETT adapter, supply tubing, pediatric and adult cannulas
PEEP valve (adjustable)
Flexible adapters to connect bag-valve system to endotracheal/tracheostomy tube
Oral airways, 1 each: 5, 6, 7, 8, 9 (pediatric sizing); 0, 1, 2, 3, 4 (adult sizing)
Nasal trumpets, 1 each: 14F, 16F, 18F, 20F, 22F, 24F, 26F, 30F
Nebulizer setup with mask and ETT adapter
MacIntosh laryngoscope blades: #1, #2, #3, #4
Miller laryngoscope blades: #0, #1, #2
Endotracheal tube stylets, 1 each: small, medium, large
Magill forceps, 1 each: pediatric, adult
Laryngoscope handles: pediatric, adult
Extra laryngoscope batteries and light bulbs
Adhesive tape: 1-inch roll
Booted hemostat
10 mL syringes: 2
Endotracheal tubes, 2 each:
  uncuffed 2.5, 3.0, 3.5, 4.0, 4.5 (mm)
  cuffed 3.0, 3.5, 4.0, 4.5, 5.0, 5.5, 6.0, 6.5, 7.0, 8.0 (mm)
Water-soluble lubricant
Suction catheters, 2 each: 6F, 8F, 10F, 12F, 14F
Tonsil tip suction
Swivel adapter
Stethoscope
CPAP prong setup with tubing: extra small, small, large
Scalpel with blade for cricothyrotomy
Needle cricothyrotomy kit

Abbreviations: CPAP, continuous positive airway pressure; ETT, endotracheal tube; PEEP, positive end-expiratory pressure.

Table 15-7. Recommended Minimum Transport Equipment

Adhesive tape
Alcohol swabs
Arm boards: pediatric, adult
Arterial line tubing
Intraosseous needles
Blood pressure cuffs: neonatal, infant, child, small adult, large adult
Butterfly needles: 23-gauge, 25-gauge
Communications backup (eg, cellular telephone)
Defibrillator electrolyte pads (pediatric and adult) or jelly
Dextrostick or point-of-care testing capability for glucose
ECG electrodes: infant, pediatric, adult
Flashlights with extra batteries
Heimlich valve (chest evacuation valve)
Infusion pumps
Intravenous fluid-administration tubing: pediatric, adult
Y blood-administration tubing
Extension tubing
Microbore tubing for syringe pumps
3-way stopcocks
Intravenous catheters: 14- to 24-gauge
Intravenous solutions (plastic bags)
1000 mL, 500 mL of normal saline
1000 mL of Ringers lactate
250 mL of 5% dextrose
Irrigating syringe (60 mL), catheter tip
Kelly clamp
Hypodermic needles, assorted sizes
Hypodermic syringes, assorted sizes
Normal saline for irrigation
Pressure bags for fluid administration
Pulse oximeter with multiple-site adhesive or reusable sensors: neonatal, pediatric, adult sensors
Salem sump nasogastric tubes: assorted sizes
Soft restraints for upper and lower extremities
Stethoscope
Suction apparatus
Suction catheters
Surgical dressings (sponges, Kling, Kerlix)
Tourniquets for venipuncture/IV access

continued next page...

Table 15-7. Recommended Minimum Transport Equipment (Continued)
Scissors
Spinal and cervical spine immobilization devices
Thermometer
Sterile and nonsterile gloves
Chest tubes: 12F, 16F, 20F, 26F
Chest tube insertion kits
Nasogastric tubes: 8F, 10F, 12F, 14F
Urinary Foley catheters and urinary collection bags
Clear dressings for intravenous catheter sites

Table 15-8. Recommended Minimum Transport Medications
Pediatric emergency medication reference guide
Adenosine
Albuterol
Amiodarone
Atropine
Calcium chloride
Cetacaine/Hurricaine spray
Dextrose 25%, 10 mL
Dextrose 50%, 50 mL
Digoxin
Diltiazem
Diphenhydramine
Dopamine
Epinephrine, 1 mg/10 mL (1:10,000)
Epinephrine, 1 mg/1 mL (1:1000) multiple-dose vial
Fosphenytoin, (500 PE mg/10 mL)
Furosemide
Glucagon
Heparin, 1000 units/1 mL
Isoproterenol
Labetalol
Lidocaine, 100 mg/10 mL
Lidocaine, 2 g/10 mL

continued next page...

Table 15-8. Recommended Minimum Transport Medications (Continued)
Magnesium sulfate
Mannitol, 50 g/50 mL
Methylprednisolone
Metoprolol
Naloxone, 2 mg/2 mL
Narcotic analgesics (eg, morphine, fentanyl)
Neuromuscular blocking agents (eg, succinylcholine, pancuronium, atracurium, rocuronium)
Nitroglycerin injection
Nitroglycerin tablets
Nitroprusside
Normal saline, 30 mL for injection
Phenobarbital
Potassium chloride, 20 mEq/10 mL
Procainamide
Prostaglandin E1
Pulmonary surfactant
Sedatives/hypnotics (eg, lorazepam, midazolam, propofol, etomidate, ketamine)
Sodium bicarbonate, 5 mEq/10 mL
Sodium bicarbonate, 50 mEq/50 mL
Sterile water, 30 mL for injection
Terbutaline
Verapamil

D. Monitoring During Interfacility Transport

At a minimum, all critically ill or injured pediatric patients who require interfacility transport must have continuous pulse oximetry and ECG monitoring, intermittent or continuous blood pressure measurement, and respiratory rate measurement (**see Table 15-1**). Some patients, depending upon their clinical condition, may benefit from invasive arterial blood pressure, central venous pressure, intracranial pressure, and/or end-tidal carbon dioxide monitoring. Patients who require mechanical ventilatory support must have the position of their endotracheal tubes noted and secured prior to transport. The adequacy of oxygenation and ventilation must be reconfirmed frequently. The mode of mechanical ventilation must be evaluated before transport to ensure acceptability and patient stability during transport. The child's status, interventions, and management during transport must be documented in the patient medical record. The receiving facility should be given copies of all the transport documentation and the information from the referring institution.

Key Points

Transport of the Critically Ill Child

- Staff at the referring hospital should carry out all necessary interventions to stabilize a pediatric patient, including performing or assisting the transport team in any necessary procedures to prevent clinical deterioration during transport.
- To allow safe transport, patients should be transported only when sufficiently stabilized.
- Adequate information is required to determine a patient's optimal mode of transport and the composition of the transport team.
- Early contact must be established with the receiving physician and facility to ensure the most expedient transfer of a patient.
- Whenever possible, all appropriate materials (medical record, laboratory results, radiographic studies, and contact phone numbers) should be prepared prior to transport.
- The transport team and receiving physician/facility should be informed about any changes in the clinical condition of the patient.
- It is crucial that appropriate equipment accompany a patient during all inter- and intrafacility transports.
- The referring transport team should ensure provision of all necessary equipment and medications, including sufficient materials to sustain the patient for a minimum of 30 minutes beyond the expected transport time.

Suggested Readings

1. American Heart Association. *PALS Provider Manual.* Dallas, TX; 2002.

2. Henretig FM, King C, eds. *Textbook of Pediatric Emergency Procedures.* Baltimore, MD: Lippinocott Williams & Wilkins; 1997.

3. Kanter RK, Tompkins JM. Adverse events during interhospital transport: physiologic deterioration associated with pretransport severity of illness. *Pediatrics.* 1989;84:43-48.

4. McCloskey K, Orr R, eds. *Pediatric Transport Medicine.* St Louis, MO: Mosby; 1995.

5. Wallen E, Venkataraman ST, Grosso MJ, Kiene K, Orr RA. Intrahospital transport of critically ill pediatric patients. *Crit Care Med.* 1995;23:1588-1595.

6. Warren J, Fromm RE, Orr RA, Rotello RC, Horst HM. SCCM Guideline for the inter- and intrahospital transport of critically ill patients. *Crit Care Med.* 2004;32(1):256-262.

7. Woodward GA, ed. *Guidelines for Air and Ground Transport of Neonatal and Pediatric Patients.* 3rd ed. Elk Grove Village, IL: American Academy of Pediatrics; 2007.

Chapter 16:

Neurologic Emergencies

Objectives

- Describe the normal physiology of the intracranial vault and cerebral blood flow.
- Review the emergent neurological assessment of the pediatric patient.
- Summarize the acute management of seizures and status epilepticus.
- Describe the approach to the patient with altered mental status or coma.
- Explain how to manage intracranial hypertension.

Case Study

A 3-year-old girl presents to the emergency department after being found unresponsive by her parents in their living room. An open, empty bottle of pills was by her side. The paramedics found her apneic and bradycardic and began bag-mask ventilation en route to the hospital. She is now experiencing rhythmic, jerking movements on her right side and is febrile and unresponsive. You are called to assist in her evaluation and management.

- Does the patient need to be immediately intubated?

- What airway maneuvers and/or adjuncts should be considered?

- Should dextrose be administered?

I. INTRODUCTION

Although our understanding of neuronal physiology and response to injury continues to grow at the molecular and cellular levels, clinical data support few, if any, specific neuroprotective therapies. Therefore, prevention of secondary injury continues to be the paramount goal of neurointensive care. Because the homeostatic reflexes all serve to preserve cerebral function and neuronal survival under pathophysiologic conditions, altered or depressed neurologic function in a child should be considered an emergent situation. Functional recovery requires prompt resolution of the insult and minimization of secondary injury. Thus, maintenance of normal oxygen delivery to the central nervous system (CNS) while minimizing cerebral oxygen utilization remains the primary goal in patients with neurologic injury.

!

1. *Maintenance of adequate airway, breathing, and circulation (ABCs) takes priority in neurologic emergencies.*
2. *Early intubation protects against hypoxemia and hypercarbia.*
3. *The C-spine must often be immobilized during neurologic emergencies.*
4. *Fluids used for resuscitation generally should be isotonic or hypertonic.*

!

Establishing a patent airway and effective breathing and circulation (ABCs) takes priority in neurologic emergencies as in any other emergent situation. However, in neurologic emergencies, any known or suspected trauma requires C-spine stabilization during airway manipulation.

Patients with neurologic disease may suffer respiratory insufficiency for a variety of reasons, including hypoventilation and airway obstruction. Deteriorating neurologic status raises the possibility of impending respiratory failure, and establishment of an artificial airway should be promptly considered. Generally, elective intubation prevents hypoxemia and hypercarbia and is safer than emergent intubation. However, this consideration must be balanced by the level of skill of the provider and the nature of the circumstances. For example, an inexperienced caregiver in the field may chose to forgo a difficult intubation if the patient can be transported rapidly to a center with skilled pediatric airway physicians. Finally, fluids used for resuscitation should be isotonic or hypertonic to minimize the risk of cerebral edema.

II. BASIC PHYSIOLOGY OF THE INTRACRANIAL VAULT

Many neurologic emergencies share common pathophysiologic processes that affect the pressure within the cranial vault and/or impair cerebral blood flow (CBF). The human body has a number of regulatory mechanisms that help to reduce these changes and their impact on neurologic function. A basic understanding of these mechanisms, their perturbations, and the methods of improvement are imperative for persons treating children with neurologic conditions.

A. Intracranial Pressure

The Monro-Kellie doctrine states that the cranial vault contains a fixed volume consisting of 3 basic components—brain (80%), blood (10%), and cerebrospinal fluid (10%)—which are encased by the thick, inelastic dura mater and the semirigid cranium. These components exist in a state of volume-pressure equilibrium, and expansion of one induces a reduction in the volume of one or both of the others. **Figure 16-1** illustrates intracranial compliance. Between points 1 and 2, although there is an increase in intracranial volume (ie, by tumor, edema, or hemorrhage), the intracranial contents remain at a constant pressure. Displacement of cerebral spinal fluid (CSF) and intracerebral blood into the spinal space accommodates this increased intracranial volume. Point 2 on the curve represents an area where, although the intracranial pressure (ICP) is normal, any further increases in volume (such as may be seen with tumor, edema, obstructive hydrocephalus, or intracranial hemorrhage) will produce an exponential rise in ICP, which may be life-threatening. Point 3 represents a decompensated state and a neurosurgical emergency with dangerously high ICP.

Figure 16-1. Intracranial Compliance

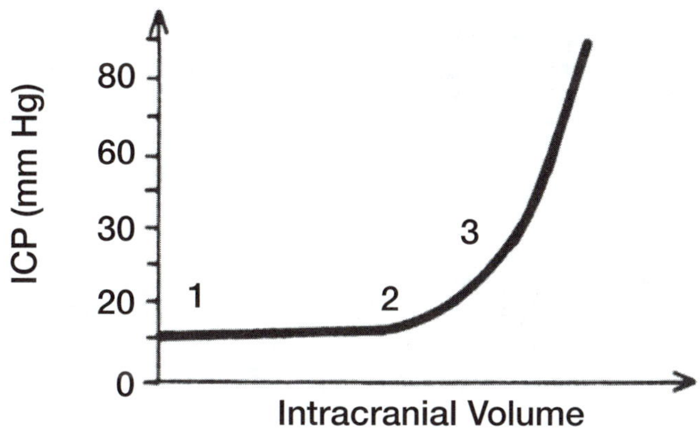

While infants with open fontanelles may be relatively protected against intracranial hypertension, this is by no means absolute. The inelastic dura mater, which encases the brain, limits expansion of the intracranial compartment, even in infants. Furthermore, the infant has a shorter craniospinal axis (measured from the cranial dura down the length of the spinal canal to the lumbosacral area) than the adult. This provides less potential space to allow for the displacement of CSV or cerebral blood volume (CBV) in the pediatric patient.

Figure 16-2 shows how the intracranial compartment compensates for a change in volume of 1 of its components. The top diagram demonstrates the 3 components of the intracranial vault in equilibrium (brain, CSF, cerebral blood volume [CBV]) with a normal ICP. The middle diagram represents an increasing mass lesion (ie, hemorrhage); the compensatory mechanisms include the extrusion of CSF and venous blood volume. This corresponds to a move from point 1 to point 2 in **Figure 16-1**, and the ICP remains normal. The bottom diagram illustrates the uncompensated state, which occurs following maximal compensatory fluid displacement from the intracranial space, producing an elevated ICP. This corresponds to a move from point 2 to point 3 in **Figure 16-1**. It is the interaction of these 3 components and the physiologic mechanisms controlling each of them that provides the framework for neurointensive care.

Figure 16-2. Interactions Between Intracranial Compartments

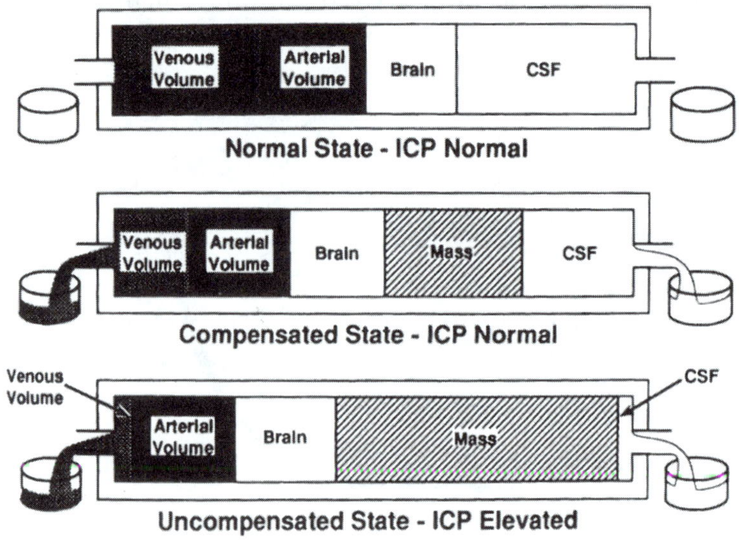

Mechanisms for compensation for an expanding intracranial mass lesion. Kanter MJ, Narayan RK. Intercranial pressure monitoring. *Neurosurg Clin N Am.* 1991; 2(2):257-65. Reproduced with permission from Elsevier, Amsterdam, Netherlands.

1. The Brain

The brain constitutes the largest volume (80%) of the intracranial vault. The brain parenchyma is composed of neurons (50%) and glial and vascular elements. Neurons require a significant amount of energy to produce neurotransmitters and maintain the transmembrane potential required as electrically active cells. Despite these significant energy requirements, the brain contains only a small amount of energy stores. Therefore, changes in CBF must occur in response to the metabolic needs of the brain. This results in an increase in CBV under conditions of increased metabolic demands, including during seizures and hyperthermia.

In addition to the metabolic demands of the brain and their effects on CBF, the brain's volume may increase when either the extracellular fluid (ECF) space or intracellular fluid (ICF) space expands. With the rapid lowering of ECF tonicity, ICF volume increases and may increase ICP. This certainly exacerbates any pathologic condition increasing ICP. The ECF volume of the brain increases with any process that increases the blood-brain barrier permeability (vasogenic edema). Cellular injury also produces edema (cytotoxic edema) due to a lack of intact membranes. Edema due to cellular injury (cytotoxic edema) responds particularly poorly to osmotic therapy and often portends a poor prognosis. Both forms of edema contribute to increased brain volume, and thus ICP, in many pathologic processes.

2. Cerebral Blood Volume

Blood in arteries, veins, and capillaries occupies approximately 10% of the intracranial space. Cerebral blood flow changes in response to brain metabolism, blood pressure, arterial $Paco_2$, and Pao_2. Arteriolar tone regulates these changes; therefore, to effect changes in cerebral blood volume, changes must occur in CBF. Although increased arteriolar tone (eg, by decreasing $Paco_2$ by hyperventilation) produces a rapid decrease in cerebral blood volume and therefore ICP, these changes place the brain at risk for ischemic injury. Because of this, recommendations currently support only brief manipulation of $Paco_2$ to reduce cerebral blood volume and consequently ICP.

> !
>
> *Acute lowering of ICP by hyperventilation increases the risk for ischemia by decreasing cerebral blood flow.*

3. Cerebrospinal Fluid

The third component of the intracranial compartment, the cerebrospinal fluid, composes approximately 10% of the intracranial volume. The brain essentially floats in the CSF, which provides a protective cushion and prevents traction on nerve roots, blood vessels, and delicate membranes. The actual intraventricular volumes are approximately 40 to 60 milliliters in infants, 60 to 100 milliliters in young children, 80 to 120 milliliters in older children, and 100 to 160 milliliters in adults. Approximately 70% of the CSF is produced by the choroid plexus, and the remainder is formed in the extrachoroidal sites, including the ventricular ependyma, Sylvian aqueduct, subarachnoid pial surface, and brain and spinal cord parenchyma. The rate of formation is approximately 0.35 to 0.40 milliliters per minute, or 500 to 600 milliliters per day, independent of age. The turnover time for CSF is approximately 5 to 7 hours.

> !
>
> 1. *CSF is produced at the same rate, independent of age.*
> 2. *Obstruction to flow, increased production, or impaired resorption of CSF all can increase ICP.*

Figure 16-3 shows the normal pathway of CSF flow, which is generated by pressure gradients as well as cilia on the ependymal surfaces. The arachnoid villi on the superior surface of the brain resorb the CSF and drain into the superior sagittal sinus.

Figure 16-3. Flow of Cerebrospinal Fluid

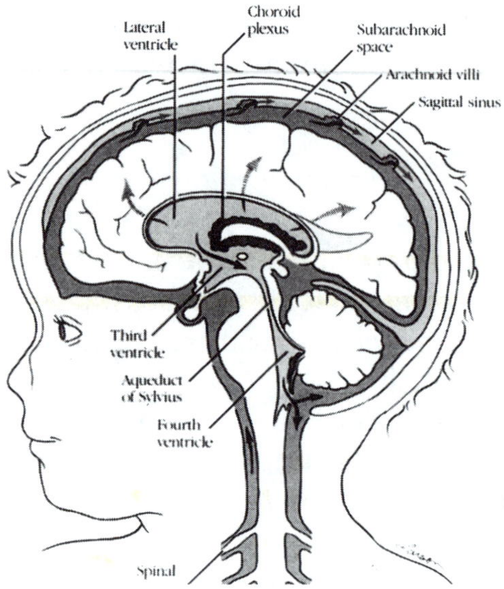

Normal cerebrospinal fluid production and pathways in the central nervous system. Reproduced with permission from Lynne Larson, BioVisual Communications, Menlo Park, CA.

Increased production of CSF, impaired resorption, or obstruction to CSF flow can all increase CSF volume and, ultimately, ICP. Cerebrospinal fluid provides a chemically appropriate environment for neurotransmission and the removal of metabolic by-products. As an ultrafiltrate of plasma, CSF contains the same electrolyte concentrations as serum and the rest of the ECF. However, glucose and other larger molecules are transported into the CSF across the impermeable blood-brain barrier. Alterations in the function of the blood-brain barrier can therefore perturb neurologic function. The use of osmotically active substances to reduce brain water in the treatment of intracranial hypertension also requires an intact blood-brain barrier.

B. Cerebral Blood Flow

The brain depends entirely upon exogenous glucose for its metabolic needs, and CBF is tightly matched to metabolic demands. Not surprisingly, CBF to gray matter (active neurons) exceeds that to white matter, which is less metabolically active. Other factors affecting CBF include mean arterial pressure, $Paco_2$, and Pao_2. Cerebral blood flow also varies with age; in adults the normal CBF is 50 mL/100g/min, whereas it is 40 mL/100g/min in neonates and 100 mL/100g/min in children. The critical threshold below which ischemia develops, producing electroencephalographic (EEG) changes, is 20 mL/100g/min in the adult and approximately 5 to 10 mL/100g/min lower in the infant.

As with all organs, the perfusion pressure of the brain is determined by the difference between the upstream and downstream pressures. In the brain, either the central venous pressure (CVP) or the ICP may provide the greater downstream pressure. Therefore,

cerebral perfusion pressure (CPP) = mean arterial pressure (MAP)– ICP or CVP, whichever is higher

The body maintains a stable CBF over a wide-range of arterial pressures through autoregulation, producing dilation or constriction of the precapillary arterioles as necessary. **Figure 16-4** depicts autoregulation in a normal adult. At extremely low cerebral perfusion pressure (CPP), CBF decreases and ischemia ensues. At CPP above the autoregulatory range, exuberant CBF produces cerebral edema. With time, the range over which autoregulation occurs adjusts to the patient's normal blood pressure. Generally, the lower limit for autoregulation is 25% below the patient's chronic mean arterial pressure (MAP), and this should be the maximal induced reduction in blood pressure used to decrease the risk of cerebral ischemia. Due to the lower prevailing MAP in young children and infants, the acceptable CPP is slightly lower than the value of 60 to 70 mm Hg targeted in adults.

Figure 16-4. Autoregulation of Cerebral Blood Flow

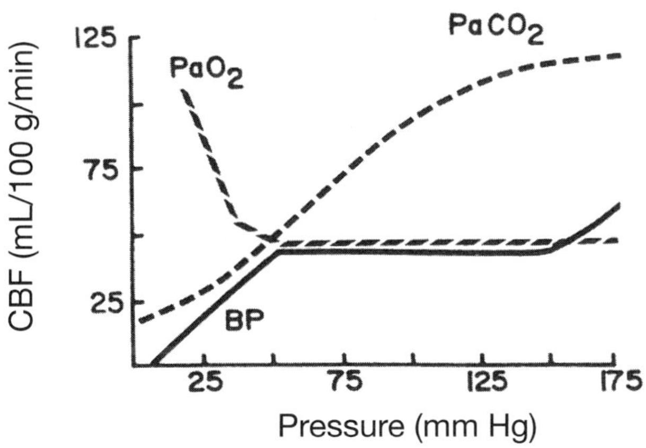

!

1. *Chronic hypertension shifts the autoregulatory curve rightward, so an acute drop in MAP >25% from baseline may place the patient at risk of ischemia.*
2. *Hypercarbia and hypoxia both dilate cerebral blood vessels.*
3. *Increased brain activity (including seizures) increases cerebral blood flow and, possibly, ICP.*

!

Cerebral blood flow correlates linearly with $PaCO_2$, ranging from 20 to 80 mm Hg. The changes in CBF with altered $PaCO_2$ occur independently of a change in arterial pH. Hyperventilation to lower $PaCO_2$ provides an effective means of rapid reduction of CBV and, consequently, ICP. However, as mentioned previously, this may place the patient at risk of cerebral ischemia. Hypoxemia below 40 to 50 mm Hg also dilates the cerebral blood vessels, resulting in increased CBF and maintenance of cerebral oxygen delivery to very low levels of oxygen content. However, this occurs at the expense of increased cerebral blood volume and possibly increased ICP. Finally, anything that increases the metabolic demands of the brain, including hyperthermia and seizures, increases CBF.

III. EMERGENT NEUROLOGIC ASSESMENT OF THE PEDIATRIC PATIENT

Certain aspects of a detailed neurologic exam cannot be assessed in young children due to their inability to follow commands or communicate verbally. However, careful, serial assessment of the level of consciousness is the most important component of this exam. Combative behavior may be appropriate for young children subjected to medical examinations and painful procedures, or it may be a sign of impaired neurologic function. A quiet child with eyes closed may simply be in a normal state of sleep or may have depressed consciousness. The response to noxious stimuli by such a patient often provides clues to the degree of altered consciousness. The Glasgow Coma Scale (GCS) is widely used in adult patients, and a modified pediatric scale exists for infants and children (**Table 16-1**).

Table 16-1. Glasgow Coma Scale Modified for Infants and Children

Clinical Parameter	Infants (Ages 0-12 Months)	Children (Ages 1-5 Years)	Points[a]
Eye opening	Spontaneous	Spontaneous	4
	Response to speech	Response to speech	3
	Response to pain	Response to pain	2
	No response	No response	1
Verbal response	Coos/babbles	Appropriate words	5
	Irritable cries	Inappropriate words	4
	Cries	Persistent cry	3
	Moans	Grunts	2
	No response	No response	1
Best motor response	Normal	Spontaneous	6
	Withdraws to touch	Localized pain	5
	Withdraws from pain	Withdraws from pain	4
	Flexor response	Flexor response	3
	Extensor response	Extensor response	2
	No response	No response	1

[a] Total Glasgow Coma Scale score = eye + verbal + motor points; best possible score = 15; worst possible score = 3.

Careful observation for asymmetric movements, both of the extremities and of facial/ocular muscles, may also provide diagnostic clues. Abnormal movements may indicate seizures (clonic, stereotyped), toxins or metabolic disease (tremors, asterixis, myoclonus), or basal ganglia injury (chorea, dystonia). Abnormal postures in response to stimulation, including that from suctioning and other procedures, consist of flexor posturing, extensor posturing, and flaccidity. Responses to placing a pen or similar object across the nail bed to apply pressure must be checked in all 4 extremities. While the terms "decorticate posture" and "decerebrate posture" are oversimplifications, progression along this spectrum generally indicates more severe, or more caudal, lesions. On the other hand, appropriate responses indicate intact sensory and effectors pathways. Care should be taken to ensure responses are not stereotypical, such as the triple-

> 1. *Motor and sensory function must be evaluated in all 4 extremities.*
> 2. *Pressure on the nail beds using a pen or similar object produces a strong stimulus without injury.*
> 3. *Evidence of a motor or sensory level strongly suggests a spinal cord lesion.*

flexion response in the lower extremities. In cooperative patients, careful assessment for a motor or sensory level may indicate a specific location of a spinal cord lesion.

Brainstem reflexes (cranial nerve exam) allow for localization of the lesion and provide diagnostic clues and indications about whether the airway reflexes and respiratory drive remain intact. Pupillary reflexes, corneal reflexes, oculocephalic reflexes (doll's eyes), vestibular reflexes (cold-water calorics), and the gag reflex should all be assessed in patients with depressed consciousness. These reflexes will help determine the location and severity of the lesion. However, in patients with possible cervical spine injury, occulocephalic reflexes should not be tested.

In patients treated with neuromuscular blockade, pupillary reactions may constitute the entire neurologic exam. Pupillary reactivity often persists in deep coma caused by metabolic disease. On the other hand, absence of pupillary reactivity indicates a lesion of the third cranial nerve or midbrain, including possible herniation syndromes. Obviously, an absent or diminished gag reflex places the patient at increased risk of airway obstruction.

Various respiratory patterns may indicate specific lesions (**Table 16-2**) or the potential need to secure an artificial airway. In Cheyne-Stokes respiration, a gradually increasing period of hyperventilation then diminishes to hypoventilation and apnea in a regularly alternating pattern. Sustained hyperventilation (with large tidal volumes) indicates rostral brainstem injury. This must be distinguished from the hyperventilation induced by pulmonary edema, which may also be induced by neurologic disease (neurogenic pulmonary edema). Patients with true central hyperventilation have elevated (or at least normal) arterial PaO_2 and increased arterial pH. On the other hand, patients may have Kussmaul respirations (large, rapid breaths) as compensation for a metabolic acidosis (such as with diabetic ketoacidosis). More caudal lesions produce apneustic breathing, which consists of inspiratory pauses, typically lasting 2 to 3 seconds. Ataxic breathing, the irregular alteration between deep and shallow breathing, occurs with lesions of the medulla. The lower the lesion, the more likely the patient will require mechanical ventilation, and patients with apneustic or ataxic breathing have a high likelihood of requiring complete mechanical respiratory support.

Table 16-2. Respiratory Patterns in Diseases of the Central Nervous System

Respiratory Pattern	Description	Lesion Localization
Cheyne-Stokes	Crescendo-decrescendo	Deep cortical or diencephalon
Central hyperventilation	Elevated PaO_2	Rostral brainstem
Apneustic	Inspiratory pause	Mid-caudal pons
Ataxic	Random deep/shallow	Central medulla

With herniation of CNS components into another compartment, several discrete syndromes may be seen. Any of these syndromes portends a poor prognosis and requires immediate intervention for recovery. Central herniation occurs when the hemispheres and basal nuclei are displaced downward through the tentorial notch. Initially, patients have depressed or altered consciousness, Cheyne-Stokes respirations, and small, reactive pupils. The eyes usually remain conjugate at this stage. With progression, patients may develop flexor posturing of the upper extremities. Further progression produces central hyperventilation, fixed, mid-position pupils, and extensor posturing. At this stage, patients may also have disconjugate eye movements in response to oculocephalic testing or cold-water calorics.

!

1. *Evidence of a herniation syndrome requires emergent therapy.*
2. *A unilateral, dilated pupil may be the only sign in early uncal herniation.*
3. *Posturing is a late sign in both uncal and central herniation.*

!

Uncal herniation occurs when a lateral lesion pushes the medial uncus and hippocampal gyrus over the lateral edge of the tentorium. The most consistent early sign is the unilaterally dilated pupil. Patients with uncal herniation may progress in an extremely rapid fashion to depressed consciousness with extensor then flexor posturing, typically of the contralateral extremities. They also develop disconjugate gaze.

IV. STATUS EPILEPTICUS

Case Study

While visiting with her grandparents, an 18-month-old child was noted to feel warm to the touch. She was not eating well and was put to bed for a nap. The grandparents heard a loud noise, and when they ran to check on the child, she was having generalized tonic-clonic movements. Emergency services responded and transported the child with a non-rebreather face mask and oxygenation saturations of 92% on $F{\rm IO}_2$ 1.0. Upon arrival, the child is febrile to 40°C (104°F) and lethargic.

- Which, if any, anti-epileptic medications should be considered?
- What are the indications for an imaging study?
- What are the indications for performing a lumbar puncture?

Status epilepticus (SE) is a common pediatric neurologic emergency. It is estimated to affect between 25,000 and 50,000 children annually, and 40% of all SE occurs in children under 2 years of age. Etiologies of SE are summarized in **Table 16-3**.

Table 16-3. Etiology of Status Epilepticus in Pediatric Patients

- Antiepileptic noncompliance
- Cerebrovascular accidents (stroke, AVM)
- CNS infections (meningitis, encephalitis)
- CNS tumors
- Head trauma (accidental, non-accidental)
- Hypoxic-ischemic injury
- Electrolyte disorders (glucose, sodium, calcium)
- Drug toxicity (penicillin, ciprofloxacin, theophylline, cyclosporine, amitriptyline, phenothiazines, lidocaine, imipenem, tacrolimus, cocaine, sympathomimetics, isoniazid, ethanol)
- Fever
- Drug withdrawal
- Malignant hypertension
- Underlying CNS disorders
- Neurocutaneous syndromes (Sturge-Weber, tuberous sclerosis, NF1)

Abbreviations: AVM, arteriovenous malformations; CNS, central nervous system; NF1, neurofibromatosis type 1.

The definition of SE has undergone many revisions but was previously defined as a single seizure lasting for more than 30 minutes or recurrent seizures lasting for more than 30 minutes without the patient regaining consciousness between seizures. The early definitions were based on animal studies that suggested that neuronal damage would occur if seizures persisted beyond an established timeline. Much has been learned since those early studies, and it appears that the underlying disorder certainly contributes to the morbidity and mortality seen in SE. But given that generalized tonic-clonic seizures are a well-recognized clinical phenomenon that may themselves promote neuronal injury (see below), a new operational definition of SE has been proposed: generalized convulsive SE in adults and older children (age >5 years) refers to ≥5 minutes of (1) continuous seizure or (2) 2 or more discrete seizures between which there is incomplete recovery of consciousness.

The authors of this new definition cite a paucity of pediatric data to make recommendations in children younger than 5 years. Although there is general agreement that seizures continuing for longer than 5 minutes should usually be treated, there exists a concern that overaggressive treatment may lead to avoidable morbidity.

A. Pathophysiology and Organ Dysfunction

Seizures result from abnormal synchronous electrical discharges (depolarization) of a group of neurons in the CNS. Depolarization stems from the influx of sodium into the neuron, whereas repolarization results from the egress of potassium from the cell, which restores the resting negative electrical potential across the cell. This potential is regulated by a sodium-potassium pump that is driven by adenosine triphosphate (ATP).

Prolonged seizures may cause selective neuronal loss in the hippocampus, cortex, and thalamus, areas rich in glutamate receptors. This calcium-mediated neuronal cell death is referred to as the excitotoxic theory, which is similar to that proposed to occur in CNS ischemia. Although prolonged seizures may be sufficient to cause neuronal damage, the superimposition of hypoxia, hypotension, acidosis, and hyperpyrexia exacerbate the degree of damage.

Status epilepticus may be divided into 2 stages. The first 30 minutes are characterized by increased autonomic activity: hypertension, tachycardia, hyperglycemia, diaphoresis, and hyperpyrexia. This is followed by a second stage after approximately 30 minutes, characterized by multi-organ involvement and includes respiratory failure (hypoxemia, hypercarbia), decreased CBF, increased ICP, and a dropping arterial blood pressure. Severe acidosis ensues, and the patients may develop a leukocytosis, hyperkalemia, and an elevated creatine kinase (secondary to increased muscle activity). The characteristics of early versus late SE are compared in **Table 16-4**.

Table 16-4. Physiologic Perturbations in Early Versus Late Status Epilepticus

	Early <30 Minutes	Late >30 Minutes	Complication
Blood pressure	↑	↓	Hypotension
Pao_2	↓	↓	Hypoxia
$Paco_2$	↑	Variable	↑ ICP
Serum pH	↓	↓	Acidosis
Autonomic	↑	↔	Arrhythmias
CK	Normal	↑	Renal failure
K^+	Normal	↑	Arrhythmias
CBF	↑ 900%	↑ 200%	CNS bleed
$CMRo_2$	↑ 300%	↑ 300%	Ischemia

Abbreviations: CBF, cerebral blood flow; CK, creatine kinase; $CMRo_2$, cerebral metabolic rate of oxygen consumption; ICP, intracranial pressure.
Adapted with permission from Dean JM, Singer HS. Status epilepticus. In: Rogers MC, ed. *Textbook of Pediatric Intensive Care Medicine*. Baltimore, MD: Williams & Wilkins; 1987, 610.

There is a relative decrease in CBF at a time when there are markedly increased demands for cerebral energy substrates (oxygen, glucose) and a loss of cerebral autoregulation. This signals the failure of adaptive mechanisms.

Respiratory failure associated with SE is multifactorial in origin. There is an increase in CO_2 production from the hypermetabolic state, a decrease in respiratory drive, and increased mechanical load on the respiratory muscles. The decrease in drive (hypoventilation) may be due to muscle fatigue or secondary to medications used to suppress the seizure. There may also be concomitant aspiration or neurogenic pulmonary edema, which can contribute to both hypoxemia and respiratory acidosis.

The cardiovascular changes and initial hyperadrenergic state are due to the release of endogenous catecholamines. Patients will have an initial increase in systemic vascular resistance that will decrease over time. As the duration of the seizure extends, it is imperative to prevent hyperpyrexia because it will contribute to neuronal cell death. Studies in adult patients have shown that there may be a CSF pleocytosis; however, any elevation in the CSF count in a pediatric patient should be considered suggestive of possible infection. Appropriate cultures should be obtained and therapy instituted. The prolonged muscle activity may lead to an elevation in creatine kinase (CK) and produce myoglobinuria; therefore, careful attention to the patient's hydration status and renal function is essential. The massive catabolic stress of SE may also lead to hyperkalemia, so attention to electrolyte status is required. Acidemia may be worsened by impaired ventilation, hypoxemia, and anaerobic metabolism. On the cellular level, amino acid excitotoxicity leads to cell injury and death through cascades, culminating in intracellular calcium influx.

B. Evaluation and Management of Status Epilepticus

The therapeutic goals for SE include (1) general supportive care, (2) termination of SE, (3) prevention of seizure recurrence, (4) correction of the precipitating causes, and (5) prevention and treatment of potential complications. Immediate attention to the airway, breathing, and circulation are essential. Status epilepticus is a situation that requires management and evaluation to be performed simultaneously. A suggested clinical approach to SE is outlined in **Table 16-5**.

Table 16-5. Treatment Algorithm for Status Epilepticus

1. Assess ABCs. Apply oxygen, establish airway and ventilation. Reassess throughout management.
2. Establish IV or IO access. Labs for initial studies. Administer dextrose if hypoglycemic. Isotonic fluid boluses for inadequate perfusion and/or hypotension.
3. Pharmacotherapy
    - **a.** Administer lorazepam 0.1 mg/kg IV; may repeat one time.
      Alternatives: diazepam 0.5 mg/kg PR; midazolam 0.2 mg/kg IM.
    - **b.** Administer fosphenytoin 20 mg/kg IV no faster than 150 mg/min immediately after initial dose of benzodiazepine. May give an additional 5-10 mg/kg prior to start of barbiturates if seizures continue. Monitor ECG, blood pressure, and IV site.
      Alternative: phenytoin 20 mg/kg no faster than 1 mg/kg/min with a maximum rate of 50 mg/min.
    - **c.** If seizures persist after initial benzodiazepine and fosphenytoin, administer phenobarbital 20 mg/kg IV no faster than 1 mg/kg/min up to a maximum rate of 100 mg/min. Monitor blood pressure and consider elective endotracheal intubation.
    - **d.** If seizures persist, initiate refractory SE treatment: midazolam bolus of 0.15 mg/kg and midazolam infusion beginning with 1 mcg/kg/min, increased every 15 minutes until seizure activity stops. Range: 1-18 mcg/kg/min. Monitor ECG, blood pressure, and EEG.
    - **e.** If seizures persist, administer pentobarbital 5 mg/kg IV up to a maximum rate of 50 mg/min. Begin infusion at 1 mg/kg/h. Additional boluses of 5 mg/kg may be given to achieve either burst suppression pattern on EEG or cessation of seizure activity. Monitor ECG, blood pressure, and EEG. Often, vasopressors are required for hypotension.
    - **f.** Clinical seizure activity may cease, but nonconvulsive SE may persist. EEG evaluation is warranted in patients who do not return to baseline neurological status.
4. Diagnostic evaluation. Treat underlying causes and systemic complications.

Abbreviations: ECG, electrocardiogram; EEG, electroencephalogram; IM, intramuscular; IO, intraosseus; IV, intravenous; PR, per rectum; SE, status epilepticus.

> *Management of Status Epilepticus (SE) includes:*
> 1. *General supportive care*
> 2. *Termination of SE*
> 3. *Prevention of seizure recurrence*
> 4. *Correction of precipitating causes*
> 5. *Prevention and treatment of potential complications*

Although most seizures are self-limited and stop in about 5 minutes or less, it is reasonable to assume that most children who arrive to the emergency department or pediatric intensive care unit (PICU) have been seizing for a significant length of time. This may include time seizing prior to discovery, time waiting for emergency personnel, and time spent en route to the hospital. Many patients may have already received potentially sedating medications by family members or emergency medical services (EMS) personnel, which may contribute to respiratory embarrassment on arrival.

The immediate assessment of the airway begins with a check for patency and reflexes. The airway may be secured by such simple maneuvers as suctioning, positioning, and the use of airway adjuncts (nasal trumpets). High-flow oxygen should be administered and pulse oximetry instituted to evaluate oxygenation status. The presence of nasal flaring, poor chest rise, retractions, cyanosis, abdominal paradoxical breathing, diminished breath sounds, or apnea suggests that the patient's trachea should be intubated. It is important to realize that some patients may require the administration of a neuromuscular blocker (NMB), and that one with a short half-life should be used. The NMB agent will stop the motor component of the seizure but will do nothing to stop the underlying seizure. Patients who are going to receive continued paralysis should be simultaneously monitored with continuous EEG. Patients may be hypovolemic, and the continued addition of medications and positive pressure ventilation may actually worsen hypovolemia and perfusion.

Tachycardia, cool extremities, delayed capillary refill, diminished pulses, and poor urine output suggest poor perfusion. The established Pediatric Advanced Life Support (PALS) guidelines should be followed to obtain vascular access, and once established, the patient may receive isotonic fluid boluses (20 mL/kg). Antipyretics should be administered early in the management of the patient in SE.

Specific studies should be tailored to match the patient history; however, serum glucose should be checked immediately, particularly in young infants. Other blood work may include testing serum electrolytes (sodium, calcium, and magnesium), liver function, arterial blood gas, urine toxicology, and antiepileptic levels. An imaging study (non-contrast computed tomography [CT] scan) should be done prior to a lumbar puncture. In the event that there is respiratory, cardiovascular, or neurologic concerns or other contraindications, such as a coagulopathy or elevated ICP, and a lumbar puncture is not done immediately, antibiotics and antivirals (if indicated) should be administered.

There is a possibility of nonconvulsive status epilepticus (NCSE) in patients who do not quickly return to their baseline. Electrographic seizure activity has been reported to occur in up to 15% of patients whose overt clinical seizures are pharmacologically controlled. Nonconvulsive status epilepticus presents with altered mentation and absent or very subtle motor findings (ie, finger twitch) and is therefore defined by EEG criteria. The incidence of NCSE in pediatrics is currently unknown; however, adult studies have shown a mortality rate between 30% and 50%.

C. Pharmacotherapy

The goal of administering an antiepileptic drug is to achieve rapid and safe termination of the event and to prevent recurrence. First-line medications commonly used include benzodiazepines (diazepam, lorazepam, and midazolam), and second-line agents include phenytoin, fosphenytoin, and phenobarbital. The pharmacology and routes of administration of these agents are presented in **Table 16-6**. Common errors in the management of SE include insufficient drug dosages, delay in advancing to a second-line drug, and inadequate supportive care.

Table 16-6. Pharmacologic Agents to Treat Status Epilepticus

Drug	Dosage	Onset	Duration
Lorazepam	0.1 mg/kg/dose IV/IO; may repeat once Maximum: 4 mg/dose	2-3 minutes	>6 hours
Midazolam	0.05-0.2 mg/kg/dose IV/IO/IM Maximum: 5 mg/dose Infusion: 1 mcg/kg/min (range 1-18 mcg/kg/min) PR: 0.5-1 mg/kg/dose	2-5 minutes	30-60 minutes
Diazepam	0.1-0.3 mg/kg/dose Maximum: 10 mg/dose PR: 0.3-0.5 mg/kg/dose	2-5 minutes	60-90 minutes
Fosphenytoin	20 mg/kg load IV/IM 3 mg/kg/min up to 150 mg/min	IV: 10-30 minutes IM: >30 minutes	>10 hours
Phenytoin	20 mg/kg load IV 1 mg/kg/min up to 50 mg/min	15-30 minutes	>10 hours
Phenobarbital	20 mg/kg load IV/IM 1 mg/kg/min up to 100 mg/min	20-30 minutes	>50 hours

Abbreviations: IM, intramuscular; IO, intraosseous; IV, intravenous; PR, per rectum.

> **!**
>
> *Common errors in the management of SE include (1) insufficient initial drug dosages, (2) delay in administering a second-line antiepileptic drug, and (3) inadequate supportive care.*

D. Refractory Status Epilepticus

Refractory status epilepticus (RSE) is defined as continued SE despite the administration of multiple agents, including benzodiazepines, fosphenytoin or phenytoin, and phenobarbital. Often these patients have had continuous (clinical and/or electrographic) seizure activity for several hours. The care of these patients should be a collaborative effort between intensive care specialists and neurologists, and requires standard invasive intensive care monitoring as well as 24-hour availability of EEG.

V. ALTERED MENTAL STATUS AND COMA

Case Study

A 15-year-old boy arrives at the emergency department after becoming combative and disoriented at school. He was involved in an altercation in the schoolyard and received minor facial trauma after being punched in the face. After he arrived in the emergency department, his mental status continued to deteriorate, and the staff called you to assist in his intubation and further management.

- What are the indications and techniques to consider in the management of the airway of a head injured patient?

- What medications should be considered for the intubation of a head-injured patient?

- What is the differential diagnosis of a patient with altered level of consciousness?

The differential diagnosis of coma and altered mental status includes all categories of neurologic and non-neurologic diseases and constitutes a true neurologic emergency. A systematic approach to these patients increases the likelihood of making the specific diagnosis. Maximal functional recovery depends upon removal of the primary insult, if possible, and prevention of any secondary injury.

!

1. *Altered mental status constitutes a medical emergency.*
2. *ABCs still receive top priority.*
3. *Don't forget D for "disability" (signs of herniation, c-spine, or other trauma) and "dextrose."*

!

A. Etiologies

Depressed consciousness results from either diffuse involvement of both cerebral cortices or involvement of the brainstem reticular activating system (RAS). This represents a medical emergency because prolonged exposure to an injury limits the likelihood of recovery. A wide variety of conditions produce alteration of consciousness in children. **Table 16-7** lists by category diseases that produce altered mental status. Trauma, including head trauma, both accidental and non-accidental, is a common cause of coma in the pediatric patient and is discussed in **Chapters 10 and 12**.

Table 16-7. Etiologies of Altered Mental Status and Coma in Children

Ischemic	Infection	Toxins
Cardiac arrest, cerebrovascular accident, near drowning, shock	Meningitis, encephalitis, brain abscess	Organophosphates, hypoglycemics, drugs of abuse and accidental ingestion
Metabolic	**Trauma**	**Neoplastic**
Diabetic ketoacidosis, hypoglycemia, sodium or osmolar abnormalities, hypoxia, hypercarbia, hyperammonemia	Accidental, non-accidental	Mass lesions, obstructive hydrocephalus, overproduction of cerebrospinal fluid (choroid plexus)
Inflammatory		
Systemic lupus erythematosus cerebritis		

Cerebral hypoxia and hypoxia-ischemia cause a significant proportion of coma in pediatric patients (see **Chapter 3** for a discussion of global ischemia). Cerebrovascular accidents (CVAs) producing focal ischemia occur much less commonly in pediatric patients than in adults, but patients predisposed to thromboembolic disease may present with focal ischemic CVA. Congenital heart disease both places patients at risk for paradoxical emboli and increases their risk for thrombosis formation. Thromboembolic CVA may also occur in patients with hemoglobinopathies and hypercoagulable states, including nephrotic syndrome, protein C, and protein S deficiencies. To result in coma, embolic CVAs must involve both cerebral hemispheres (uncommon) or the vertebrobasilar system, which supplies the RAS. Dural sinus thrombosis occurs in severely dehydrated neonates and following infections of the orbit or paranasal sinuses (particularly the sphenoid sinus). This may produce venous infarction of the brainstem and therefore result in coma.

Intoxication may result from either exogenous or endogenous toxins. Hypoglycemia, hyper- or hypocalcemia, hyper- or hypomagnesemia, and hyper- or hypo-osmolality may all produce altered mental status. Any cause of severe acidosis (lactate, inborn error of metabolism) or hyperammonemia (liver failure, inborn error) may also produce altered mental status. Toddlers may accidentally ingest any substance in the home, whereas teenagers may intentionally ingest a wide variety of substances. Sedatives (benzodiazepines, barbiturates, alcohols), tricyclic antidepressants, stimulants (PCP, amphetamines, cocaine), opiates, salicylates, organophosphates, and many other drugs may cause altered mental status.

Seizures from any cause may depress consciousness both during (ictal) and following (postictal) the actual seizure. Historic evidence for seizure may be subtle. Prolonged postictal states may occur due to persistence of the cause of the seizure (hypoglycemia, CVA, hyponatremia) or as a consequence of the seizure itself. Neuronal energy demands increase markedly with seizure, and inadequate augmentation of supply may produce an ischemic injury as noted.

Meningitis, encephalitis, brain abscess, and subdural empyema may all cause altered mental status. This may result from elevation of ICP, direct inflammation of the RAS, vasculitis, and subsequent infarctions and seizures. Collagen vascular diseases (systemic lupus erythematosus) may similarly affect the level of consciousness, as may tumors, particularly with acute enlargement (hemorrhage into the tumor) or acute obstructive hydrocephalus.

B. Evaluation

Serial examination of the level of consciousness is the most important aspect of the neurologic exam. As in all cases, assurance of adequate airway control, respiratory effort, and hemodynamic status is of paramount importance. Because hypoglycemia occurs more commonly in critically ill young children and infants than in adults, the ABCs should be expanded to include D for checking a dextrose (glucose) level and for disability—signs or symptoms of CNS emergencies, such as dilated pupils or Cushing's triad (hypertension, bradycardia, and abnormal respirations). Perturbations in any of these vital functions may in fact produce the patient's altered mental status. During the resuscitation of comatose patients, 2 key points must be considered. First, if trauma is known or suspected, c-spine immobilization must be maintained at all times, including during establishment of an artificial airway. One provider should use the jaw-thrust method to open the airway and stabilize the neck while a second provider performs laryngoscopy. An anesthesiologist may be required to use fiberoptic techniques for intubation. Second, as with any potential neurologic disease, fluids for resuscitation should be isotonic or hypertonic to minimize the possibility of cerebral edema and increased ICP.

> **!**
>
> 1. *If c-spine injury is known or suspected, intubation requires 2 people to provide c-spine immobilization. Fiberoptic techniques may be required.*
> 2. *Resuscitation should proceed with isotonic or hypertonic fluids.*
> 3. *Rule out life-threatening causes first and treat while the workup proceeds.*
>
> **!**

Once initial stability has been established and supported, specific evaluation for the cause of the altered/depressed mental status should begin. Many possibilities must be considered during the differential diagnosis of coma or altered mental status in children (**Table 16-7**). Life-threatening causes should be ruled out quickly with a careful history and physical exam, looking for signs of trauma, meningismus, elevated ICP (papilledema), or a toxidrome (see **Chapter 13**). Historical information may be limited or difficult to obtain. Specific considerations include the following: Is the patient's mental status worsening/improving? How/where was the patient found, and what was nearby? Were any medications given by family or emergency medical services personnel?

Emergent imaging using CT scan identifies significant intracranial hemorrhage, mass lesions, midline shift, skull fractures, or signs of intracranial hypertension, such as effacement of the sulci or basilar cisterns. The most important consideration prior to CT scan is whether the patient is stable enough for the procedure. Patients must be adequately resuscitated, and those with compromised airway protective reflexes or respiratory effort should have their airway secured before they are placed in the scanner.

!

1. *When elevated ICP is suspected, patients should not be sent for diagnostic procedures (CT scan, MRI, lumbar puncture) without adequate provision of airway and circulatory support.*
2. *Presumptive therapy for intracranial hypertension or CNS infection should be instituted expectantly if procedures necessary to diagnose them are delayed.*
3. *A negative head CT does not rule out possible herniation after lumbar puncture if clinical signs of intracranial hypertension are present.*

!

Lumbar puncture (LP) permits determination of the opening pressure, cell counts, protein and glucose levels, and culture with Gram stain. As with CT, cardiorespiratory function must be adequate prior to performing an LP, particularly in infants and small children whose respiratory function can be severely impaired by positioning for the procedure. There is controversy over whether a CT scan must be performed in all patients prior to LP. Concern exists that LP can precipitate herniation in patients with mass lesions or elevated ICP. However, negative CT scans do not rule out subsequent herniation. Patients with suspected CNS infection and contraindication to LP should be treated with empiric antibiotics (and antiviral agents when appropriate), and CSF should be obtained when deemed safe, with neurosurgical assistance if required.

In the patient with altered mental status, in addition to checking a whole-blood glucose, serum electrolytes (including calcium, magnesium, and phosphorous), liver and renal function, arterial blood gas, lactate, and ammonia should all be tested. A complete blood count (CBC) may provide evidence of an infectious process or anemia consistent with a chronic disease. Urine and serum toxicology screens should be obtained, ideally prior to the administration of sedatives or analgesics.

C. Therapy

Therapy for coma is directed at the underlying cause, while maintenance of normoxia, normocarbia, and normal perfusion is of paramount importance. Treatment of hypoglycemia with 25% dextrose 2 mL/kg or 10% dextrose 5 mL/kg rapidly restores serum glucose. Further glucose monitoring and maintenance of normoglycemia (80-150 mg/dL) appears prudent given adult literature showing improved outcome of critically ill patients who are kept normoglycemic. Therapy of symptomatic hyponatremia requires an initial, rapid increase in serum sodium to levels that do not produce symptoms. Usually, an increase of 5 mEq/L will suffice, and 6 mL/kg of 3% hypertonic saline will provide this increase.

VI. INTRACRANIAL HYPERTENSION

Case Study

A 2-year-old boy has presented to the emergency department after falling down a flight of stairs. Combative on arrival, he had a pulse oximetry value of 82%, and his trachea was intubated with C-spine precautions. You were called to assist in his management. During your exam he becomes stiff, his blood pressure increases to 150/90 mm Hg, and his heart rate decreases to 55 beats per minute.

- What are the clinical signs and symptoms associated with an elevation in intracranial pressure (ICP)?
- What is Cushing's triad?
- What are the indications for the administration of mannitol and/or hypertonic saline?

Although intracranial hypertension (increased ICP) has a number of different etiologies, specific management is imperative to promote adequate cerebral perfusion pressure and CBF.

A. Manifestations

As discussed earlier in this chapter, the Monro-Kellie doctrine states that intracranial hypertension results from any process that increases the volume of the brain, CSF, or CBV, without a compensatory decrease in the other components. **Table 16-8** lists some common diseases that may increase ICP. At least initially, an increase in ICP must be inferred from clinical manifestations. Increased ICP itself produces minimal findings (except papilledema and headache) unless mass effect produces local ischemia or herniation of intracranial components. Chronic, slowly progressive increases in ICP are particularly well-tolerated. Evidence of increased symptoms at night (increased $Paco_2$) or upon awakening (change in ICP with position changes) or with coughing (increased CBV) may all indicate an elevated ICP. Acute increases in ICP produce mental status changes and cranial nerve findings much more rapidly, and once intracranial hypertension is suspected, therapy should be instituted immediately and consideration given to monitoring the ICP.

Table 16-8. Diseases That Produce Increased Intracranial Pressure

Traumatic	Infection	Neoplastic
Accidental, non-accidental	Meningitis, encephalitis, brain abscess	Mass lesions, obstructive hydrocephalus, overproduction of cerebrospinal fluid (choroid plexus)
Ischemic	**Idiopathic**	
Cardiac arrest, cerebrovascular accident, near drowning, shock	Pseudotumor cerebri	

B. Monitoring Intracranial Pressure

Intracranial pressure can be monitored in a number of locations (intraventricular, intraparenchymal, subarachnoid/subdural, and epidural) and by different techniques. The gold standard is placement of an intraventricular catheter because such a system allows drainage of CSF, which provides a therapeutic option for increased ICP. The main disadvantages are the difficulty of placement, particularly in patients with compressed ventricles; the increased risk and consequences of infection; and the possibility of malfunction as the ventricles become progressively smaller. The ultimate goal is to recognize elevated ICP. Although an ICP of >20 mm Hg often triggers interventions, a cerebral perfusion pressure <65 to 70 mm Hg (and perhaps slightly lower in young children) also warrants therapy to raise MAP, lower ICP, or both.

> **!**
>
> 1. *An ICP greater than 20 mm Hg usually requires specific therapy to lower ICP.*
> 2. *Maintenance of CPP is the primary goal.*

C. Therapy

As stated multiple times in this chapter, assurance of adequate respiratory and circulatory function should receive top priority in all patients, including those with intracranial hypertension. Special attention should be paid during endotracheal intubation to use drugs that do not increase ICP and to provide adequate anesthesia to blunt ICP spikes with laryngoscopy. Fever should be aggressively treated to prevent increased cerebral metabolism and CBF. Similarly, seizures should be aggressively treated. Adequate analgesia and sedation during painful procedures also reduce ICP.

> **!**
>
> *Increased ICP with Intubation*
>
> 1. *Succinylcholine (without defasciculating non-depolarizer) and ketamine both may increase ICP.*
> 2. *Hypoxia and hypercarbia definitely increase ICP.*
> 3. *Inadequate anesthesia definitely increases ICP with laryngoscopy.*

Specific therapy for elevated ICP begins with midline neck positioning and elevating the head of the bed to 30° to maximize venous drainage. Other therapies aim to reduce the volume of the intracranial contents and/or to minimize cerebral metabolic demands.

One of the most difficult decisions when intracranial hypertension is suspected is when to electively sedate and intubate the patient who is otherwise maintaining adequate gas exchange. While sedation will obscure the clinical neurologic exam, elective intubation is much safer than emergent intubation when apnea or hypoventilation occurs. Once a patient is intubated, however, the need for ICP monitoring increases due to the lack of exam criteria of deterioration. As stated above, if a ventricular drain is present, CSF drainage is the next line of therapy. Placement of an extraventricular drain is particularly useful in the initial management of patients with ventricular shunt malfunction, infection, or obstructive hydrocephalus due to neoplasm. Neuromuscular blockade may further lower ICP, even in patients who appear adequately sedated, and has the added benefit of lowering systemic oxygen consumption.

Osmolar therapy constitutes the next line in medical therapy of intracranial hypertension. Either mannitol (0.5 g/kg IV as needed) or hypertonic saline (HTS) may be used to raise serum osmolarity. Controlled hypovolemia is *not* appropriate because it places the patient at risk for hypotension and decreased CPP. The diuretic effect of mannitol needs to be considered in this regard. However, diuretics do have a role in the euvolemic or volume-expanded patient with inadequate response to mannitol. Some evidence suggests that higher serum osmolality can be achieved with HTS (up to 360 mOsm) than with mannitol (320 mOsm) without increased risk of side effects. However, the choice of agent generally depends on rapid availability and the patient's volume status. The dose of HTS depends on the concentration of the solution. Because sodium distributes in the extracellular fluid space, 0.6 mEq/kg will raise the serum sodium by 1 mEq/L. Thus, 3 mEq/kg will raise the sodium by 5 mEq/L (corresponding to a dose of 6 mL/kg of 3% HTS). Infusions of HTS may be used to maintain the serum sodium (and osmolality) at a level that reduces ICP. Importantly, this setting differs dramatically from correction of hypotonicity in that increases in osmolality must often occur at rates greater than the 0.5 mEq/L/h. In the setting of increased ICP, normalization of ICP (and CPP) predominates over a specific target for the rate of increase in serum osmolality. Therefore, the frequency of HTS boluses and rate of infusions will depend on the response of the patient's ICP as long as serum osmolality remains below 360 mOsm.

Other medical therapies have beneficial effects in certain situations. Corticosteroids (decadron) reduce peritumor edema but have no beneficial effects in nonneoplastic causes of intracranial hypertension. Careful consideration should be given to gastrointestinal prophylaxis with antacid medications when using corticosteroids because these patients have an increased risk of intestinal ulceration and hemorrhage (Cushing's ulcer). High-dose barbiturates inducing pharmacologic coma have proven benefits in reducing ICP, though their effect on outcome remains less clear. In addition, they reduce cerebral oxygen consumption, providing another possible benefit. Barbiturate coma may also be necessary in patients with refractory seizures, which again increase ICP.

Two medical therapies deserve special mention. First, aggressive hyperventilation ($Paco_2$ <35 mmHg [4.7 kPa]), which may be required acutely for an acute increase in ICP, has no place in the chronic management of intracranial hypertension. As mentioned above, the reduction in CBF places the brain at risk of ischemia. Also, since the response depends on pH change in the CSF, accommodation occurs with sustained hypocapnia. Note that this also means that a patient with metabolic acidosis (ie, diabetic ketoacidosis) may require a lower $Paco_2$ to maintain a pH of 7.35 to 7.4 and normal CBF until the acidosis is corrected. Secondly, hypothermia theoretically promotes a number of conditions that reduce ICP. Various studies, mostly in animal models, have documented decreased cerebral oxygen consumption, decreased CBF, reduced inflammation, and altered intracellular signaling.

> !
>
> *Hyperventilation ($PaCo_2$ < 35 mm Hg [4.7 kPa]) has no place in the chronic management of increased ICP.*
>
> !

Surgical therapies for elevated ICP include removal of mass lesions (tumor, hematoma) or removal of cranial bones to increase the compliance of the cranial space (craniectomy). Again, limited comparative data exist to support the use of decompressive craniectomy in particular clinical conditions. However, in patients with medically refractory intracranial hypertension, craniectomy can reduce ICP. Another second-line surgical option is the placement of a lumbar drain in patients with slit-like ventricles and increased ICP but with open basilar cisterns. Limited data suggest that this lowers ICP and does not promote herniation.

VII. CEREBROVASCULAR ACCIDENTS

Case Study

Earlier in the day, a 5-year-old girl with sickle cell disease complained of headache; then her mother found her less responsive, with slurred speech and decreased movement of her left arm. She brought her to the emergency department, where you were consulted to assist in her care. She is dysarthric, hemiparetic on the left, with mildly decreased level of alertness. Her vital signs are significant for mild tachycardia and are otherwise normal.

- What are the common presenting signs and symptoms of a cerebrovascualr accident (CVA) in a pediatric patient?
- What laboratory studies should be obtained in a patient with a suspected CVA?
- What neuroimaging studies are required in a patient with a suspected CVA?

Although cerebrovascular accidents occur much less commonly in children than in adults, the reported incidence of about 2 cases per 100,000 children per year closely approximates that of childhood brain tumors. This incidence increases further in specific at-risk populations. Furthermore, CVAs rank among the top 10 causes of mortality in pediatric patients. Therefore, anyone providing emergency care for children must have the skills to recognize and manage CVAs. As in adults, therapies must be instituted rapidly to promote maximal functional recovery.

A. Manifestations of Cerebrovascular Accident

The manifestations of a CVA depend in part on the type of event (hemorrhagic vs thromboembolic) and on the location of the injury. The majority of pediatric CVAs involve the intracranial branches of the carotid artery and, specifically, the middle cerebral artery. Lesions in this distribution produce hemiparesis, hemianesthesia, hemianopia, and, when affecting the dominant hemisphere, aphasia. Because the motor and sensory cortex for the lower extremities resides on the medial aspect of the cortex, lesions of the anterior cerebral artery affect those functions. They also affect emotional control and intellectual function. Lesions of the posterior cerebral artery affect vision or the deep structures of the brainstem, producing motor and sensory defects, pupillary abnormalities, and depressed consciousness. Finally, the vertebrobasilar system (posterior circulation) supplies the lower brainstem and cranial nerves. Therefore, deep coma, cranial nerve abnormalities, and cerebellar signs all occur with CVAs in that distribution.

B. Hemorrhagic Cerebrovascular Accident

For hemorrhagic stroke, which has a higher mortality rate than ischemic stroke, the primary etiologies include both aneurysms and arteriovenous malformations (AVMs), although conversion of initially ischemic events may occur (particularly for venous infarctions). Aneurysms occur either with congenital defects in the muscular layer of arteries or in association with neurocutaneous syndromes and inherited defects of connective-tissue components (ie, Ehlers-Danlos syndrome). Nearly half of aneurysms occur in the posterior circulation, and many occur distally and deep within the brain substance.

Both the requisite increase in ICP and vasospasm contribute to the decreased CBF following aneurysmal bleeding. Blood in the basilar cisterns compromises blood flow to the hypothalamus, resulting in abnormalities of adrenergic tone. This likely contributes to the dysrhythmia and electrocardiogram (ECG) changes seen with subarachnoid hemorrhage (SAH). Increased sympathetic tone probably also produces the neurogenic pulmonary edema seen in these patients.

Several differences between SAH in adults and SAH in children deserve mention. First, the role of vasospasm in children remains less clear than that in adults. While some studies have suggested similar rates of vasospasm and others less vasospasm in children, children suffer fewer symptoms when vasospasm occurs. Generally, the therapy for vasospasm parallels that for CVAs, with maintenance of adequate CBF being the primary goal. However, in patients with untreated aneurysms, induced hypertension carries a significant risk of rebleeding and should be avoided. Also, calcium channel blockade probably has a limited role in the treatment of pediatric patients with SAH. Finally, children have a much lower incidence of rebleeding than adults, reducing the need for emergent surgical intervention in the absence of significant mass lesion or intracranial hypertension.

Arteriovenous malformations present most frequently in children in the second decade of life. Again, the vast majority are supratentorial, involving some component of the middle cerebral artery distribution. More than half of patients have intraparenchymal involvement of the hemorrhage, but while SAH may result from extension to the ventricular system or cerebral convexities, blood typically does not involve the basilar cisterns. Therefore, although other aspects of therapy for arteriovenous malformations are similar to aneurysmal bleeding, vasospasm is not a concern. Definitive treatment by surgical excision or, in some cases, embolization eradicates the 2% to 3% risk of rebleeding per year.

C. Thromboembolic Cerebrovascular Accidents

Thromboembolic disease, which produces bland, or ischemic, strokes, affects the middle cerebral artery distribution in the vast majority of cases. A wide variety of diseases predispose patients to thromboembolic disease. Cardiac disease, either acquired or congenital, is the most common of these factors. Sickle cell disease represents the well-studied predisposition and the only one for which controlled clinical trials have been performed. Infections, including meningitis and paranasal sinus infections, form another large category. Finally, a large number of metabolic and inherited hematologic disorders predispose to stroke to varying degrees.

Unfortunately, the majority of pediatric patients with ischemic CVA's present late. Thrombolytic therapy is contraindicated after 3 hours of symptoms. Therefore, the majority of therapy aims to prevent secondary injury by promoting adequate oxygen supply to marginal regions. As mentioned repeatedly in this chapter, decreased blood volume, hypotension, and hypocarbia all exacerbate cerebral ischemia. In fact, some authors recommend volume expansion with colloid to induce hemodilution and improve the microvascular rheology. Although this approach may remain controversial, prevention of hyperviscosity by limiting hematocrit to the normal range seems appropriate.

Generally speaking, thromboembolic CVAs should remain clinically static after presentation because the embolic event has already occurred. Therefore, deterioration of the neurologic exam should raise suspicion of a secondary insult. Possibilities include hyponatremia, hyper- or hypoglycemia, worsened perfusion, or hemorrhagic conversion. Also, edema surrounding the infarcted area typically increases over the first 24 to 48 hours before reaching its zenith. Prompt evaluation of each likelihood is required. Another possibility is recurrent embolism or extension of clot. Peak cerebral edema occurs later in patients suffering secondary insults, such as recurrent emboli, cerebral ischemia secondary to hypotension, or ECF hypotonicity. If other investigations fail to determine the etiology of the deterioration, consideration should be given to systemic anticoagulation with heparin. Heparinization should also be considered in patients with documented thrombus and acute thromboembolic CVA if the initial head CT determines there is no hemorrhage.

VIII. CEREBROSPINAL FLUID SHUNTS

Case Study

A 14-year-old male who was shunted at birth for aqueductal stenosis and underwent a shunt revision 3 months ago presents with a headache and complaints of just not feeling right. He has not gone to school in several days, and he vomited 3 times before presenting to the emergency department. His mother reports that he has a flulike illness. While being interviewed, the patient has a 1-minute right-sided seizure and seems a bit dazed as you try to continue your history and physical exam. He has a respiratory rate of 20 breaths per minute, heart rate of 70 beats per minute, blood pressure of 150/90 mm Hg, and temperature of 38.2°C (100.8°F). His mother asks what you think is going on.

- What are the common signs and symptoms of ventriculoperitoneal shunt (VPS) malfunction?
- What are the major complications which occur in patients with shunted hydrocephalus?
- What laboratory and neuroimaging studies should be performed?

Patients who present with shunt obstruction may show signs of increased ICP that include headache, nausea, vomiting, lethargy, and papilledema. It is crucial to involve the neurosurgeon early in the evaluation and management of these patients. Evaluation begins with a thorough history and physical exam. Following the ABCs, imaging studies are performed and include a head CT and a shunt series (lateral radiograph of the skull and an anterior-posterior view to include the neck, chest, and abdomen for evaluation of the shunt position and connections). After these images are obtained and reviewed with the neurosurgeon, an attempt to obtain CSF from the shunt is done in a sterile fashion. An inability to aspirate CSF or an elevated opening pressure suggests a shunt obstruction, and thus a surgical revision may be necessary. If CSF is obtained, it is sent to the laboratory for cell count, culture, Gram stain, and a glucose and protein determination.

Serious complications that may occur in patients with CSF shunts include mechanical failure (proximal or distal obstruction) and infection. The risk of shunt failure is greatest in the first several months following placement. Many, if not all, of these children are admitted to the PICU for observation preceding the surgical repair. Common signs and symptoms include headache, vomiting, nausea, altered mental status, lethargy, and a general feeling of malaise. It should always be remembered that in any patient with a shunt in place, the shunt is the source of the problem until proven otherwise.

> !
>
> *When a patient with a CSF shunt presents with any neurologic findings, it is important to assume that the shunt is the problem until proven otherwise.*

Obstruction is the most frequent cause of shunt malfunction, with proximal obstruction occurring more frequently than distal. The proximal end of the catheter may become occluded with choroid plexus, ependymal cells, glial tissue, brain debris, fibrin, or blood, or the tip of the catheter may migrate into the brain parenchyma. Distal obstruction may result from kinking of the tubing, disconnection of the tubing, migration of the catheter outside the peritoneum, intra-abdominal infection or pseudocyst formation. Regardless of the etiology of the obstruction, occlusion of the shunt will prevent the egress of CSF from the ventricular system, which will ultimately lead to a buildup of CSF in the ventricular system, which will ultimately lead to a rise in ICP.

The incidence of CSF shunt infections is between 5% and 8%. Infection may involve the shunt equipment, the wound, the CSF, or the distal site where the shunt drains. Approximately 70% of shunt infections occur within the first 2 months following surgery, and almost 90% will occur in the first 6 months postoperatively. The organisms most frequently isolated include *S epidermidis* (40%) and *S aureus* (20%), with the remainder caused by enterococci, streptococci, gram-negative rods, and yeast. Clinical signs of infection depend on the site of the infection. Wound infections manifest with fever and reddening of the incision or shunt tract, and as they progress, there is discharge of pus along the incision. Patients with ventriculitis and meningitis have fever, headache, irritability, and neck stiffness or nuchal rigidity. The treatment of choice is removal of the shunt hardware with placement of an external ventricular drain and administration of parenteral antibiotics. Infections of temporarily placed external ventricular drains are managed in the same manner.

Key Points

Neurologic Emergencies

- In the young child, irritability is an early sign of change in mental status.
- Acute changes in neurologic function, including change in mental status and weakness, require emergent evaluation and treatment to promote maximal recovery.
- Preservation of cerebral blood flow is of paramount importance in any neurologic emergency.
- Hypoxemia and hypercarbia should be aggressively prevented in a patient with any neurologic abnormality. In children, early signs of respiratory distress include tachypnea, grunting, and nasal flaring.
- Intracranial hemorrhage in the young infant can cause hemodynamically significant blood loss.
- Hypoglycemia is common in infants during stress and must be corrected promptly.

Suggested Readings

1. Adelson PD, Bratton SL, Carney NA, et al. Guidelines for the acute medical management of severe traumatic brain injury in infants, children, and adolescents. *Pediatr Crit Care Med.* 2003(suppl 4):S1-S75.

2. Ashwal S, ed. Section VII. Neurologic. In: Perkin RM, Swift JD, Newton DA, eds. *Pediatric Hospitalist Medicine: Textbook of Inpatient Management.* Philadelphia, PA: Lippincott Williams & Wilkins; 2003:289-326.

3. Avner JR. Altered states of consciousness. *Pediatrics in Review.* 2006;27(9):331-337.

4. Behrman RE, Kligman RM, Jenson HB, eds. *Nelson Textbook of Pediatrics.* 17th ed. Philadelphia, PA: Saunders; 2004:1973-2052.

5. Furhman BP, Zimmerman JJ, eds. *Pediatric Critical Care.* 3rd edition. Philadelphia, PA: Mosby Elsevier; 2006:767-928.

6. Issacman DJ, Trainor JL, Rothrock SG. Central nervous system. In: Gausche-Hill M, Fuchs S, Yamamoto L, eds. *The Pediatric Emergency Medicine Resource.* 4th ed. Sudbury, MA: Jones and Bartlett Publishers; 2004:146-185.

7. Mark PE, Varon J. The management of status epilepticus. *Chest.* 2004;126:582-591.

8. Ogden AT, Mayer SA, Connolly ES. Hyperosmolar agents in neurosurgical practice: the evolving role of hypertonic saline. *Neurosurgery.* 2005;57(2):207-215.

9. Posner JB, Saper CB, Schiff N, Plum F. *The Diagnosis of Stupor and Coma.* 4th ed. Cambridge, MA: Oxford University Press; 2007.

10. Stocchetti N, Maas AIR, Chieregato A, van der Plas AA. Hyperventilation in head injury: a review. *Chest.* 2005;127(5):1812-1827.

11. Vincent J-L, Beres J. Primer on medical management of severe brain injury. *Crit Care Med.* 2005;33(6):1392-1399.

12. Wheeler DS, Wong HR, Shanley TP. *Pediatric Critical Care Medicine: Basic Science and Clinical Evidence.* London: Springer-Verlag; 2007:865-1012.

Chapter 17:

ETHICAL AND LEGAL ISSUES

✓ Objectives

- Define core ethical principles.
- Identify the elements of informed consent.
- Describe the role of the surrogate decision maker.
- Explain how withholding and withdrawing treatment are morally similar.
- Discuss why effective communication skills are essential to the practice of ethics.

I. INTRODUCTION

A number of ethical concerns arise frequently in ICU practice. Professional caregivers often deal with patient-related dilemmas without identifying or fully understanding the ethical issues involved. Each participant (including caregivers, patient, and family members) brings his or her own values to the situation, and thus a number of viewpoints need to come together to inform a single decision. This chapter provides a basic framework for addressing the questions that commonly arise during patient care in the PICU. It is necessarily simplified because no single methodology can fully address the complex, considerations that may apply to a specific clinical case.

II. BASIC ETHICAL PRINCIPLES

Medical ethics is a branch of applied philosophy devoted to the identification, analysis, and resolution of problems that arise when the moral claims of medical staff, patient, and society at large fail to intersect. The discipline of ethics seeks to identify and apply fundamental precepts and transcend societal and religious institutions with the idea that people from different religious and cultural backgrounds can identify ethical choices and behavior to make judgments that are acceptable across cultures. However, differing opinions and interpretations exist even among the most thoughtful ethicists and healthcare professionals that are unlikely to be resolved and reflect deeply held beliefs or very different cultures.

In real life, ethical principles can and do conflict. No ethical rule can be constructed to incorporate all possible conflicts and exceptions. The dilemmas faced in clinical care occasionally stem from differing moral values but more often reflect conflicts between competing demands of ethical principles on which the participants fundamentally agree. For instance, although we generally respect patient autonomy, a patient's decision to refuse lifesaving care may conflict with a physician's obligation to act for their benefit. Ethical reasoning seeks to balance the weight of such compelling but competing claims.

Although most of the dilemmas to which we apply ethical reasoning stem from physician-patient interactions during severe illness and at the end of life, day-to-day interactions between patients and professionals also raise ethical questions. These less consequential interactions form the basis for the physician-patient relationship and shape the communication and trust on which more critical ethical decision making must depend. Meaningful application of ethical principles requires a set of core behavioral and communication skills that must be practiced throughout medicine. Skillful disclosure of information when making treatment plans, obtaining informed consent, assessing patient or surrogate understanding and decision-making capacity, discussing resuscitation status, communicating bad news, disclosing mistakes and apologizing, and resolving conflict requires training and practice. Very commonly, perceived ethical dilemmas are products of failed communication and are readily resolved when communication improves.

The guiding ethical principles of beneficence, nonmaleficence, autonomy, and justice form a basic conceptual framework to aid in identifying, analyzing, and resolving ethical dilemmas encountered in the practice of medicine. End-of-life care, medical futility, informed consent, and surrogate decision making will be discussed within the context of these principles.

> !
>
> *Meaningful application of ethical principles requires a set of core behavioral and communication skills. Very commonly, perceived ethical dilemmas are products of failed communication and are readily resolved when communication improves.*

A. Beneficence

The principle of beneficence relates to the obligation of the medical staff to take positive steps to improve the welfare of the patient or to maximize benefit to the patient. The benefit of greatest interest to physicians is health, but other benefits, such as comfort, maintaining independence, pleasing a loved one, or adhering to the tenets of a religion, may be more important to patients. When a patient's preference conflicts with a physician's advice, it is wise for the physician to work to understand the patient's assessment of what is in his or her best interest.

B. Nonmaleficence

The principle of nonmaleficence underlies the physician's duty to do no harm. Although this concept may seem obvious, its application is surely not. Physicians have the potential to harm patients by failing to consider the pain, discomfort, and inconvenience, as well as the potential risks, of medical treatment. Unintended harm may also result from physician or system error.

> ! *The principle of nonmaleficence underlies the physician's duty to do no harm.* !

Every medical treatment carries risk, which may range from minimal to life threatening. A child's hospitalization may lead to a parent's loss of control, family disruption, and economic hardship. Medical treatments that are broadly accepted as beneficial may violate a patient's strongly held beliefs and thus constitute harm to that person. Intensive care may be painful and terrifying, associated with multiple complications, and followed by long-term disability.

C. Autonomy

The principle of autonomy speaks to a patient's right to determine what is in his or her best interest and to make decisions about treatment according to a personal set of goals and values. Because children develop such values and an understanding of illness and goals of treatment only as they mature, and at different rates, physicians caring for infants and children generally consider the family's perspective.

> ! *The principle of autonomy speaks to the right of an individual to determine what is in his or her best interest and to make decisions about treatment according to a personal set of goals and values.* !

The principles of beneficence and autonomy are at odds when patients refuse treatments recommended by physicians. When a physician's need to benefit a patient is given priority over a patient's autonomy, the physician's actions are considered paternalistic. The degree of paternalism that is acceptable has declined over the last few decades as the emphasis on personal choice and liberty has increased in many regions of the world.

D. Justice

The principle of justice applies to the obligation to treat people fairly, that is, to treat patients in similar circumstances similarly, without considering factors extraneous to the medical condition. Discrimination based on race, religion, gender, socioeconomic status, and other factors violates this principle.

However, in reality, limited resources may prevent everyone from getting every possible service. In anticipation of such circumstances it is necessary to determine a set of criteria by which just allocation can occur. This determination is a huge challenge in modern medicine. Two broad strategies of resource allocation are most commonly used: egalitarian standards attempt to spread resources equally to all persons, regardless of need or projected benefit, whereas utilitarian standards seek to deliver services where the likelihood of benefit is the highest. Triage decisions in a disaster are classically based simply on medical utility. Determining which patients should receive ICU care when there is a shortage of beds or nurses is a related dilemma intensivists frequently face. Justice-related considerations often reflect public policy and are difficult for the individual provider to address at the bedside.

III. COMMON ISSUES IN INTENSIVE CARE

A. Consent

Current social trends and philosophy in North America and in many other regions of the world support patient and family autonomy and thus recognize the importance of informed consent in determining the course of medical treatment. Truly informed consent requires that a *competent* patient or surrogate with adequate *information* to *understand* the risks and benefits of available treatment alternatives make a *voluntary* decision, that is, a decision free from coercion. Successfully obtaining fully informed consent is difficult, however. Even when physicians put substantial effort into providing information, answering questions, and assessing understanding, they commonly overestimate how much the patient and family comprehend.

In addition, it is difficult to accurately predict the likelihood of benefit or the magnitude of burden for any individual patient. Ethical dilemmas arise when participants assign differing weights to the benefits and burdens of a given treatment. Competent adults whose personal assessment of a situation differs from that of their physician have almost unlimited entitlement to refuse medical care, even when the likelihood of benefit is great. As the number of young adults surviving illnesses of childhood increases and they continue to be hospitalized on pediatric services, recognition of their right to make their own decisions and is becoming more important.

The need for someone to speak for a sick child is a distinctive element of ethical decision making in pediatric medicine. Although parents have significant autonomy in deciding about their own medical care, their right to refuse medical care for their children is more limited.

B. Decision Making

1. Age-based Presumptions of Incompetence

Pediatric intensive care patients are typically unable to participate in decision making about treatment due to their level of intellectual development and the severity of their illness. By law, minor children are considered incompetent, regardless of their relative maturity. However, mature children with an understanding of their disease (as is often the case in children with chronic disease) should have an opportunity to enter into the decision-making process. Although children do not have legal decision-making capacity, in many instances they should be informed about and asked to assent to the treatments to which their parents have given formal consent.

Statutory and case law pertaining to the decision-making capacity of mature minors differs among states and countries. Ethical considerations aside, it is essential for medical care providers to know the law where they practice. In most instances, emancipated minor parents have the right of consent for their minor children.

2. The Role of Surrogates

Because children are considered incompetent, surrogate decision makers must authorize treatment for them. When an adult patient is incompetent, a surrogate attempts to make the same decisions that person would make under the same circumstances. To arrive at those decisions, the surrogate relies on written statements (eg, living wills) when they are available, previous conversations, or knowledge of the patient's values. This use of substituted judgment usually cannot be applied to children because they have never been competent, and because in most instances, their limited understanding precludes a meaningful sense of what they would want. Instead, decisions are based on what is thought to be in the best interest of the child, with the assumption that in most cases a child's parents or legal guardians are the most qualified people to determine those interests. Practitioners should, however, attend to older children's wishes when they are known.

Although parents' decisions may be flawed by incomplete understanding of the situation or their own emotional connection to the child, society supports the institution of parenting above the absolute best interests of the child. Under the law, application of the best-interest standard merely ensures that some reasonable, acceptable standard of care is met. Parents may also have some conflicts resulting from the impact of the child's illness on the family's or the parents' interests. The extent to which such concerns can be appropriately included in surrogate decision making remains an evolving topic.

The decision-making right of parents is protected but not absolute. Imprudent decisions that will endanger a child, such as refusing blood transfusion for hemorrhagic shock secondary to a splenic laceration or antibiotics for meningitis, may be overruled with the backing of the court.

3. Religious Beliefs in Medical Decisions

Religious beliefs sometimes underlie patient or family decisions that conflict with physicians' recommendations. As a rule, it is important for physicians to recognize patient autonomy in these settings. However, decisions to limit treatment for a child based on a parent's beliefs are problematic. Parents with strongly held beliefs usually feel that it is in their child's best interests to live and be treated in a manner that is consistent with the parents' beliefs. However, it is not clear that parents' religious views should prevent a child from receiving treatment that is clearly beneficial and that would allow the child to survive long enough to grow up and either endorse or reject the parents' belief system. Legal decisions have supported the position that children should be allowed to grow up and make their own choices.

The surrogate's ability to make a rational choice is rarely assessed. Concerns about competency and the validity of a decision tend to be triggered only when a patient or surrogate rejects medical advice. It is appropriate to use disagreements as grounds for further investigation into the understanding, goals, and relevant core values of patients and their families. However, disagreements are not themselves indications of incompetence. Sometimes referring an issue to an ethics consultant or committee can help to identify relevant principles, highlight differing opinions, and resolve the conflict.

C. Key Concepts Underlying Refusal of Treatment

Many attempts have been made to define circumstances in which it is permissible for a patient or surrogate decision maker to refuse treatment. The terminology frequently used as reasons for refusal of treatment has worked its way into both medical and lay parlance and deserves some attention.

1. Distinctions Between Ordinary and Extraordinary Care

As medical progress has led to improved outcomes, many treatments have come to be considered virtually obligatory. A distinction is sometimes drawn between those treatments and others that are extraordinary and thus not obligatory. The relationship of "ordinary" and "extraordinary" resembles that of other word pairs heard in medicine: routine/heroic, natural/artificial, invasive/noninvasive. As medical science progresses, the dividing line between ordinary and extraordinary changes. Consequently, the concept of ordinary versus extraordinary does not provide a very useful or precise distinction between obligatory and nonobligatory treatments.

> ! *A burdensome treatment with a low likelihood of benefit may be considered a form of extraordinary care.*

2. Distinctions Between Withholding and Withdrawing Care

> *Most ethicists believe that there is no moral distinction between withholding and withdrawing treatment. It is essential to define the desired benefit before concluding that a treatment is futile.*

Technological advancements in medicine have led to the point where a decision to allow death often must be made deliberately. Although both families and medical personnel often feel that discontinuing life-sustaining treatment is more momentous and consequential than a decision not to start such treatment, most ethicists believe that there is no moral distinction between withholding and withdrawing treatment. In fact, giving priority to withholding over withdrawing may lead to problems. On one hand, it may cause reluctance to start treatments that might prove to be beneficial or allow time for more accurate diagnosis and prognosis. On the other hand, it may encourage continuation of treatments beyond their usefulness, when they essentially constitute harm to the patient. The decision to withdraw a treatment is often a more informed decision than the decision to withhold.

3. Quality of Life

> *It is most useful to focus realistically on the value of a treatment itself with respect to the family's values and achievable goals for the patient.*

To the extent that the distinctions above fail to provide guidance about acceptable refusal of care, discussion often centers on quality of life. For most people, such discussions focus on the child's overall prognosis, pain or suffering related to the condition or its treatment, and similar issues. However, some people object to that approach, contending that it shifts the discussion from whether the patient is benefiting from treatment to whether continuation of the patient's life is beneficial to them and that it risks allowing doctors, parents, or the courts to make judgments based on some arbitrary continuum of individual worth.

When the benefit is marginal or very uncertain and the potential harm or burden is substantial, surrogate decision makers can reasonably refuse treatment for a child.

D. Futility

> *When a treatment cannot reasonably be expected to provide the hoped-for benefit, it may be considered futile. Futility is confirmed when the balance of benefits and burdens becomes unacceptable not to the medical team but rather to the patient and/or surrogate.*

When a treatment cannot reasonably be expected to provide the anticipated benefit, it may be considered futile. Physicians commonly disagree on the level of certainty that is necessary to claim medical futility. Futility is confirmed when the balance of benefits and burdens becomes unacceptable not to the medical team but rather to the patient and/or surrogate. Although concerns about benefit or burden to the larger community may also be important, they can rarely be addressed at the bedside.

It is essential to define the desired benefit before concluding that a treatment is futile. Clear communication about the goals and potential outcome of medical treatment is central to the definition of futility. For example:

- Administration of blood to a child with terminal cancer may be unlikely to accomplish the physician's goal of having the child survive to hospital discharge but may accomplish the family's goal of a few more weeks of life for their child.
- Providing nutrition by gastrostomy to a child in a persistent vegetative state may not accomplish the goal of allowing him to interact with family members but may satisfy the family's need to provide the care that seems synonymous with compassion.

There is no need to present futile or nonbeneficial treatment options to patients and families; in fact, doing so may give them the erroneous impression that meaningful choices can still be made. Skillful communication may obviate requests for futile care because families are most likely to make such demands when they have not received adequate information about treatment or prognosis.

> !
>
> *It is not necessary to present futile or non-beneficial treatment options to patients and families.*

E. Do-Not-Attempt-Resuscitation Orders

Decisions about resuscitation are based on the same set of principles as other crucial decisions in intensive care and on an assessment of the likely outcome. The benefit of effective resuscitation is survival, ideally without serious complications. However, the process of cardiopulmonary resuscitation itself is certainly not benign. For patients whose underlying problems are associated with significant suffering, resuscitation may serve only to increase or prolong that discomfort without significant hope of recovery. For patients who are already receiving maximal treatment, there may be nothing of benefit to offer following resuscitation. A decision not to resuscitate does not negate the value of other intensive care: for some patients a trial of full treatment with the exception of CPR may be effective, with the understanding that if cardiopulmonary arrest occurs, it would be evidence of inadequate response to therapy and the outcome would be acceptable.

> !
>
> *A decision not to resuscitate does not negate the value of other intensive care interventions.*

F. Sedation and Analgesia in the Care of the Dying

Addressing patient comfort is always appropriate, even following a decision to withhold or withdraw life-sustaining treatments. Providing sedation and analgesia is intended to relieve pain, anxiety, or air hunger; hastening death is not the goal. The distinction is important to the doctrine of double effect, which holds that an action (such as delivery of narcotics) may have both an intended effect (relief of suffering) and an unintended effect (respiratory depression and possible hastening of death).

> !
>
> *Care is never withdrawn; rather, the goals of treatment change.*

G. Provider Autonomy

Healthcare providers have their own ethical integrity that warrants respect. Patients and colleagues should not be allowed to compromise a provider's integrity, which is both personal (the beliefs that each person brings to the practice of medicine) and professional (the beliefs that the practice of medicine requires). Physicians may refuse to participate in a decision that goes against their conscience but generally should not unilaterally countermand a family's decision. Intractable disagreements may warrant ethics consultation, transfer to another physician's care, or judicial review.

> !
>
> *Providers may refuse to participate in a decision that goes against their beliefs but may not unilaterally countermand a family's decision.*

Nurses, who may have the most contact with families but are less empowered than physicians, may be distressed when they are unable to translate their moral choices into action. As the ultimate effectors of medical decisions, nurses should have a voice in decision making. The costs of unrelieved moral distress are high and include the loss of experienced critical care nursing staff, a resource already in short supply. Ultimately, as with all unresolved professional conflicts, the quality of patient care suffers. Because they spend most of their time at the bedside, nurses may have a privileged role in assessing patient or family understanding, identifying nonmedical influences on decision making, and recognizing situations in which medical opinion creates feelings of coercion. Their close contact with the patients gives them a unique opportunity to promote patient and family autonomy. The opinions of other team members who have been directly involved in the patient's care should also be considered.

> !
>
> *As the ultimate effectors of medical decisions, nurses should have a voice in decision-making.*

IV. ETHICS AT THE BEDSIDE

Application of ethics to intensive care practice requires skillful communication with patients and their families. The discipline of ethics usually does not provide answers but rather offers a framework for resolving problems. Each patient care situation is unique and requires continuous, caring communication and frequent reassessment of needs and goals. Education in ethics, clinical judgment, practical wisdom, common sense, compassion, and empathy are the key attributes required by clinicians involved in any ethically complex problem. A process for ethical decision making is outlined in **Table 17-1.**

Table 17-1. Process for Ethical Decision Making

Ensure that all end-of-life care decisions are made with full disclosure of alternatives and implications and potential conflicts of interest, are free of duress and coercion, and are made by persons with competence and capacity.
Assess the patient's and family's understanding of the situation and alternatives.
Communicate clearly and document extensively.
Whenever possible, initiate discussions with patients and/or families regarding their preferences for life support before a medical crisis occurs.
Know the legal standards pertaining to your practice in your region.
Develop consensus and a plan among the care team, and recognize the right of healthcare professionals to adhere to their own personal values.
When members of the healthcare team feel uncomfortable with a family's decision, involve support services such as clergy, an ethics committee or consultant, social services, or hospital counsel where indicated.

V. Case Studies

Case 1:

A 16 month-old boy was found in the family swimming pool after an uncertain amount of time. He was unconscious, pulseless, and apneic when the paramedics arrived approximately 10 minutes later. They intubated the child and initiated CPR. He was still unresponsive and asystolic on arrival in the emergency department after another 10 minutes but had return of spontaneous circulation after the first round of drugs there. He was admitted to the PICU, where he was initially unresponsive to verbal or noxious stimuli and had sluggishly responsive pupils but no other cranial nerve function except irregular respiratory effort. After 3 days of supportive care (including 24 hours of mild hypothermia) his condition is unchanged. An EEG reveals minimal burst-suppression activity. You tell the boy's parents that the likelihood of meaningful recovery is very small and recommend extubation and discontinuation of mechanical ventilation, which will allow him to die naturally. His parents feel that he has not been given enough time to recover and want everything done to support him.

> **!** *Whenever possible, initiate discussions with patients and/or families regarding their preferences for life support before a medical crisis occurs.*

Analysis

From the outset excellent communication with parents (and other family members they identify) is essential. Providers need to explain the devastating consequences of anoxia and the currently very limited ability to reverse its effects. Explaining the importance of an observation period after hypoxia and cardiac arrest before drawing conclusions about prognosis is consistent with current recommendations and helps assure parents that the physician intends to benefit their child if at all possible. Offering a bit of hope by explaining the possible benefits of hypothermia (without overstating its value) also may convey commitment to the best possible outcome.

Data about the outcome of out-of-hospital cardiac arrest, including after near-drowning, allow reasonable certainty about the child's prognosis, particularly when combined with the physical examination and EEG. Continued ventilatory support can be expected to sustain life, but the prognosis for neurologic recovery is very poor. It is critical to explain the expected outcome in clear terms, including the child's likely inability to recognize family members, walk, talk, go to school, or change significantly from his current status. Parents often are unable to imagine the severity of injury without very explicit examples.

Many providers and parents would conclude at this point that continued intensive care is of no benefit to the child, and that it may be associated with discomfort, indignity, risk of infection, and other complications, it could be considered a harm. However, in the absence of clear neglect or legal designation of another guardian, the parents have the rights and responsibilities of surrogate decision makers for their child. In general, providers allow parents to determine what is in their child's best interest, in this case continuing or withdrawing life support. Exploring their hopes and wishes for their child may suggest meaningful language for discussing the impact of the event.

Determining the parents' goals in maintaining life support is important: Do they not believe the prognosis? Are they convinced a miracle will occur? Or do they want the child to survive even with profound neurologic injury and on chronic ventilation? Although continued mechanical ventilation could be considered futile with respect to restoring the child to good neurologic function, it would not be futile if the parents' goal is simple survival. Allowing additional time to pass, may enable parents to comprehend the severity of the injury and face the loss of their child. Additional evaluation, may provide further information about prognosis that persuades parents to accept the recommendation to withdraw support. Other family members, friends, or clergy may help them accept the recommendation or at least consider the issues clearly. Ultimately, respect for the parents' autonomy and recognition of their values may require acquiescing to their wishes and continuing support, at least for a time. It is important to make sure that parents who elect to continue life support recognize that their decision does not have to be forever and that they may choose to withdraw support in the future. Although withdrawing life support in the present and withdrawing it in the future are morally equivalent, the parents should be aware that many families find it more difficult to withdraw support in the future.

If the parents do chose to withdraw life-sustaining therapy, it is permissible to provide sedation and analgesia. Although a child with this degree of injury may not be able to experience pain or anxiety, it is impossible to ascertain the nature of their experience. The potential for air hunger, in particular, cannot be eliminated. Administration of narcotics and sedative or anxiolytic agents decreases the chance of discomfort. Although such an approach may hasten death, the principle of double effect allows relief of suffering even when hastened death as a secondary effect can be foreseen.

Considerations of justice in this case are complex. Should this child's injury limit what is made available to him, or should he receive everything available to sustain him? Should costly resources be expended on this child when others do not have access to basic care? Should a child with such a grave prognosis take up precious nursing hours when there is a shortage of nurses? These are issues of enormous importance, but they are more a matter of public policy than of bedside care.

Case 2:

A 4 year-old boy with profound static encephalopathy due to near-drowning at age 16 months was admitted to the PICU in severe respiratory distress after an episode of vomiting associated with a gastrostomy feeding at home. He has had multiple previous prolonged hospital admissions for pneumonia and has required 3 to 4 days of mechanical ventilation on several occasions. Chest radiograph reveals a large right lower lobe pneumonia. His father and stepmother initially agree to intubation and mechanical ventilation. However, after a week, he has developed bilateral lung opacification and progressive hypoxemia despite increased ventilator support. When his parents are informed of a plan to switch him to high-frequency oscillatory ventilation, they request that his ventilatory support be discontinued instead.

Analysis

In this instance it is important to determine who the appropriate surrogate decision makers are. Do the father and stepmother have legal custody of the child, or does his mother continue to be involved? When custody is shared, it is important to try to reach consensus among all of those invested in caring for the child.

The potential benefit of continued ventilatory support and intensive care is resolution of the boy's pneumonia and discharge home again. However, there is also significant likelihood of a prolonged course of treatment with associated pain and discomfort. He may not recover sufficiently to wean from mechanical support. His history suggests that he is likely to have recurrent episodes of respiratory failure, and he may require tracheostomy and chronic ventilation.

Further discussion with the father and stepmother is important to clarify their sense of what is in his best interest.

The father states that following the boy's near drowning at age 16 months, physicians had recommended withdrawal of life-sustaining therapy. However, his mother and father had wanted to give him the best chance for recovery so they had cared for him at home and arranged for intensive rehabilitation. They subsequently divorced, and the father has remarried. The father has legal custody, the child's mother is no longer involved, and the stepmother supports the father.

Over time the child's neurologic status has not improved. Instead he has become more hypertonic and is often uncomfortable, which he expresses through long periods of moaning or crying. Moreover, he has required multiple hospitalizations that his father thinks have been accompanied by significant pain. He feels that his son has had enough and that his personal desire to keep him with him is no longer fair to the boy.

It appears that the father's request is based on recognition that his earlier hopes for the child's recovery are not realistic and that continuing treatment may not be in the child's best interest, given the evidence of discomfort and the likely frequent recurrence. A decision not to start mechanical ventilation at the time of admission might have been appropriate as well, but withdrawal of support is an acceptable alternative.

Some physicians might disagree with the father's decision on the grounds that the child might recover adequate respiratory function and should be given the opportunity to do so. They may feel that their duty to benefit the child requires them to continue treatment and outweighs the potential harm that the child's father foresees. Nonetheless, given both the substantial uncertainty of a good outcome in the short term and the poor outlook in the long term, the father's request is reasonable. In any case, the principle of autonomy would discourage the physician from unilaterally overruling the surrogate. The physician may identify another physician to assume responsibility for the child's care, seek ethics consultation to clarify the issues, or request that the courts become involved.

Case 3:

A 4-year-old girl with acute lymphocytic leukemia in remission has developed gram-negative septic shock that is most likely secondary to a bloodstream infection related to an indwelling catheter. Following appropriate antibiotic administration and fluid resuscitation she remained hypotensive and required initiation of a vasopressor. She has developed tachypnea and hypoxemia and is on increasing supplemental oxygen. When told that she may require intubation and mechanical ventilation, her very upset parents indicate they will not give consent. They feel that such treatment is too much for her and that she has been through enough.

Analysis

Decision making in the face of long-term uncertainty makes assessment of the relative benefit and burden of treatment difficult. An honest presentation of the child's prognosis with respect to her leukemia as well as the likely course of her septic shock is central to the discussion the physician needs to have with the parents. Unless there are special risk factors for this child, the likelihood of curing her leukemia is high (>80%), particularly given that she has entered remission. Septic shock presents an additional severe risk, but the possibility of a good outcome is greater than the possibility of death or long-term morbidity, at least given the child's current condition. Nonetheless, the child does face a very difficult and uncertain immediate future.

Understanding the nature of the parents' distress is critical. Are they simply overwhelmed with anxiety and grief? Do they have a good understanding of the optimistic outcome for her leukemia, or have they been so devastated by the diagnosis of cancer that they have been unable to process the information they have received? Are they aware of the potential for a good outcome even from the septic shock? Do they have previous associations with cancer or intensive care that make them especially pessimistic?

In this particular instance, statistics and the child's status suggest that the likelihood of a good outcome is high. The potential discomfort and risk of serious complications are also substantial, but refusing treatment will almost surely lead to the child's death. The balance at this moment appears to be strongly in favor of treatment, including intubation, but frequent reassessment of the child's course will be appropriate. Should she suffer severe, irreversible complications of the disease process, reconsideration of the decision might become appropriate.

Although parents have great latitude in making decisions about their child's care, refusing consent for treatment that is likely to have a good outcome can be challenged. In this case, it appears that their own distress is interfering with their ability to make a decision that is clearly in their child's best interest. Involving the oncologist who knows them best, other family members they trust, or other support may persuade them to accept the intensivist's recommendations. Requesting ethics consultation may help clarify important issues, and if necessary, a court order can be obtained.

If the child had had multiple relapses or a cancer with a poor prognosis, the balance between the benefits and burdens of treatment might be quite different. If a prolonged period of intensive care could only serve to extend the child's life very briefly before complications of the underlying malignancy led to her death, one might elect not to institute life-sustaining treatment. In this girl's case, once treatment is initiated frequent reassessment of its effectiveness versus associated problems is important. Should she develop complications (eg, severe multiple organ failure or central nervous system hemorrhage), continued treatment might no longer be in the child's best interest, and it could be withdrawn.

Key Points

Ethical and Legal Issues

- Healthcare professionals have an obligation to act in their patients' best interest based upon the ethical principles of autonomy, beneficence, nonmaleficence, and justice.
- Surrogate decision-making by the parent is based upon substituted judgment and is invoked in the best interest of the child.
- When faced with an ethical dilemma, consensus from the healthcare team and caregivers on the treatment plan and objectives facilitates consistent communication and documentation and minimizes liability risks.
- Most ethicists believe that there is no moral distinction between withholding and withdrawing treatment although the latter is more often emotionally difficult.
- It is important to remember that withdrawal of life support does not mean withdrawal of care, but, rather that the goals of treatment have changed.

Suggested Readings

1. Beauchamp TL, Childress JF. *Principles of Biomedical Ethics.* New York, NY: Oxford University Press; 2001.

2. Cooper R, Koch KA. Neonatal and pediatric critical care: ethical decision making. *Crit Care Clin.* 1996;12(1):149-164.

3. Downie RS, Randall F. Parenting and the best interests of minors. *J Med Philos.* 1997;22(3):219-231.

4. Kopelman LM. The best interests standards as a threshold, ideal, and standard of reasonableness. *J Med Philos.* 1997;22(3):271-289.

5. Ramsey P. *Ethics at the Edges of Life.* New Haven, CN: Yale University Press; 1978:172.

6. Ward, NS, Levy MM. Rationing and critical care medicine. *Crit Care Med.* 2007;35(2):S102-S105.

7. Youngner SJ. Medical futility. *Crit Care Clin.* 1996;12(1):165-179.

Chapter 18:

Management of the Child With Congenital Heart Disease

Objectives

- Identify congenital heart lesions that present with low cardiac output in neonates.
- Discuss initial management and diagnostic testing of a cyanotic infant.
- Review the evaluation and treatment of acyanotic congenital heart disease.
- State the most common causes of low cardiac output syndrome in the postoperative pediatric cardiac patient.
- Outline the evaluation and management of low cardiac output syndrome.
- Summarize the most common post-operative arrhythmias.

Case Study

A 6-day-old male presented to the pediatric unit with a 2-day history of decreased feeding and increasing tachypnea and lethargy. His vital signs are heart rate 195/min, respiratory rate 90/min, and pulse oximetry 87% on room air. He is tachypneic, but no retractions are noted. Pulses are difficult to palpate.

- What are the possible diagnoses?

- What are the most important initial evaluation and treatment?

I. INTRODUCTION

The purpose of this chapter is to consider the principal issues involved in the care of the pediatric cardiac patient. Although there are many facets of care common to all cardiac patients, the foundation of pediatric cardiac intensive care is an understanding of how specific lesions, operations, and types of cardiovascular physiology influence pre- and postoperative events.

II. NEONATES WITH LOW CARDIAC OUTPUT

A. Hypoplastic Left Heart Syndrome

Hypoplastic left heart syndrome occurs in 4% of children with congenital heart disease(CHD) and is characterized by stenosis or atresia of the mitral and/or aortic valves, coarctation of the aorta, and hypoplasia of the left ventricle. Neonates present within the first few days of life, typically with mild cyanosis and a shocklike state after the patent ductus arteriosus begins to close.

> !
>
> *Any infant in the first weeks of life with symptoms of shock and severely diminished to absent pulses must be suspected of having hypoplastic left heart syndrome.*
>
> !

An arterial blood gas will show a metabolic acidosis and a diminished Pao_2 (typically <100). Such children should be evaluated by echocardiography. Initial medical management is lifesaving. Prostaglandin E_1 (PGE_1) infusion should be promptly initiated.

> !
>
> *For children with hypoplastic left heart syndrome, PGE_1 infusion is the most important component of therapy and resuscitation. Oxygen therapy can be detrimental.*
>
> !

Prostaglandin infusion should be initiated rapidly to reopen the ductus arteriosus and restore perfusion to the distal aorta. The side effects of PGE_1 infusion include periodic breathing, apnea, and peripheral vasodilatation, so the clinician must be prepared to support the patient's airway, provide ventilation, and administer additional fluids.

Once the ductus has reopened, it is critical to avoid hyperventilation and hyperoxia. Both of these conditions will lead to preferential pulmonary blood flow through the ductus and will worsen systemic shock and distal perfusion. The result is increased pulmonary blood flow at the expense of systemic blood flow. When the diagnosis is made prenatally or before a state of profound shock develops, it is preferable for the infant to maintain spontaneous breathing, but when there is cardiogenic shock and critically low oxygen delivery, control of the airway and mechanical ventilation are indicated.

Judicious fluid administration (bolus 10-20 mL/ kg of 0.9% saline or 5% albumin) and inotropic support (dopamine 3-10 µg/kg/min, milrinone 0.25-0.75 µg/kg/min, or epinephrine 0.01-0.05 µg/kg/min) may be helpful or necessary in more severe cases of low cardiac output. Surgical treatment for this disease is variable and controversial. At some centers, but less commonly, no therapy is offered and the neonates die after intensive support is withdrawn. Cardiac transplantation has had some success at a few centers, but the limited number of donor organs and lifelong immunosuppression are significant concerns. In most centers, a staged surgical approach similar to that for children with tricuspid atresia is undertaken (**see Table 18-1**).

Table 18-1. Staged Surgical Repair of Hypoplastic Left Heart Syndrome

Procedure	Age of Patient	Actions Performed
Norwood procedure	First weeks of life	• PDA is ligated • Main pulmonary artery is separated from branch pulmonary arteries and used in the creation of a neo-aorta • Pulmonary blood flow is reestablished via modified Blalock-Taussig shunt or right ventricle to pulmonary artery conduit • Atrial septectomy is performed
Modified bidirectional Glenn anastomosis	3-6 months	• Modified Blalock-Taussig shunt or right ventricle to pulmonary artery conduit is taken down • Superior vena cava is sewn into the pulmonary arteries
Modified Fontan procedure	2-4 years	• Inferior vena cava is sewn into the pulmonary arteries

B. Aortic Stenosis

Aortic stenosis (AS) occurs in 3% of children with CHD. The commissures of the aortic valve are fused, resulting in a thickened, domed valve with a stenotic orifice. The presenting symptoms and findings on physical examination are variable and relate roughly to the degree of narrowing of the valve. Patients will have a systolic ejection murmur loudest at the upper right sternal border with radiation into the neck. Often a click will be audible. Patients with critical aortic stenosis have decreased systemic perfusion. They will have poor oral intake, tachypnea, and decreased urine output, and may be lethargic. Their peripheral pulses will be diminished throughout. Children with less severe stenosis are normally asymptomatic and present with a murmur.

Surgery is recommended for patients in whom the annulus and valve are very small and require valve replacement, and for those in whom balloon valvuloplasty was unsuccessful.

C. Coarctation of the Aorta

> *Infants with critical coarctation present with shock in the first week of life, after spontaneous closure of the ductus arteriosus.*

Coarctation of the aorta (CoA) occurs in 5% of children with CHD. It is a constriction of the descending aorta that usually occurs opposite the ductus/ligamentum arteriosus. The symptoms in these patients are variable. Typically, children with mild disease will present with hypertension or an asymptomatic murmur, while infants with critical CoA present with shock.

Infants with critical coarctation of the aorta are fussy, poor feeders, who will become lethargic with time. They will have decreased femoral pulses with normal to increased pulses in the upper extremities. If they are diagnosed late, they may have significant ventricular dysfunction and will present in shock, identical to patients with hypoplastic left heart syndrome.

> *Prostaglandin E_1 infusion (0.05 mcg/kg/min) is lifesaving for neonates with critical CoA who are in shock.*

Most children with CoA undergo surgical repair, although balloon angioplasty or stent implantation can be performed. Many older children with CoA have postoperative hypertension that is usually controlled well with β-receptor blockade or angiotensin-converting enzyme inhibitors. In the immediate postoperative period, esmolol (50-250 µg/kg/min) has the advantage of a very short half-life. We normally transition patients to oral therapy with either atenolol (0.8-2 mg/kg/day) or enalapril (0.05-0.25 mg/kg/dose given twice daily), titrating the dose as necessary to maintain a normal blood pressure.

D. Myocarditis and Cardiomyopathies

Myocarditis and cardiomyopathies may present in the neonatal period but are much more common at older ages. Both lesions are characterized by ventricular dysfunction. The patients typically present with varying signs and symptoms of heart failure (**see Tables 18-2 and 18-3**) but may also present in a shocklike state. Myocarditis typically occurs after a viral illness, whereas there is an extensive list of potential causes of cardiomyopathies (such as inborn errors of metabolism) that is beyond the scope of this chapter. Patients with either etiology may have significant improvement with appropriate medical therapy, or their condition may deteriorate necessitating heart transplantation.

Table 18-2. Common Symptoms of Heart Failure

In Infants	In Children
Tachypnea	Failure to thrive
Diaphoresis	Decreased energy
Feeding intolerance	Exercise intolerance
Decreased urine output	Frequent respiratory infections
Failure to thrive	

Table 18-3. Common Physical Findings of Heart Failure

Tachycardia
Displaced apical impulse
Gallop rhythm
Hepatomegaly
Tachypnea
Small stature
Pulmonary crackles and peripheral edema usually not present

The causes of low cardiac output in newborns are listed in **Table 18-4,** and a summary of the initial evaluation and treatment of low cardiac output is presented in **Table 18-5.**

Table 18-4. Causes of Low Cardiac Output in Newborns

Sepsis
Coarctation of the aorta
Hypoplastic left heart syndrome
Critical aortic stenosis
Interrupted aortic arch
Arrhythmia
Cardiomyopathy
Myocarditis
Pneumothorax

Table 18-5. Initial Evaluation and Treatment of Newborns with Low Cardiac Output

Initial Evaluation of Low Cardiac Output
Tests:
Blood culture
Arterial blood gas
Chest radiograph
Electrocardiogram
Echocardiogram
Initial Treatment of Low Cardiac Output
Antibiotics
Intravenous fluid resuscitation: 10 mL/kg IV bolus of normal saline solution or 5% albumin (packed red blood cells if anemic)
Prostaglandin E_1 if any concern for ductal dependent cardiac lesion: PGE_1 infusion at 0.05 µg/kg/min
Consideration that oxygen can be detrimental in hypoplastic left heart syndrome, causing increasing metabolic acidosis
Inotropic agents (see **Table 18-9**)
Treatment of underlying arrhythmia
Intravenous immune globulin for myocarditis: 500 mg/kg/day for 2-6 days

III. CYANOTIC CONGENITAL HEART DISEASE

Case Study

A 1-day-old female is noted to be cyanotic. She is mildly tachypneic but otherwise comfortable. She has a pulse oximetry reading of 70%.

- What are the possible diagnoses?
- What is the appropriate initial evaluation and treatment?

Either central cyanosis or acrocyanosis may be seen in newborns. Acrocyanosis involves the hands and the feet and does not represent true arterial hypoxemia. In central cyanosis there is more than 3 g/dL of deoxygenated hemoglobin.

A. Cyanotic Congenital Heart Disease with Decreased Pulmonary Vascularity

Patients with cyanotic CHD and decreased pulmonary vascularity have obstructed pulmonary blood flow and right-to-left shunting of blood at either the atrial or the ventricular level. In the neonatal period, children with this category of defects are usually intensely cyanotic, with hyperpnea but not dyspnea. This presentation is caused by the decrease in pulmonary blood flow and the absence of congestive heart failure.

1. Tetralogy of Fallot

Tetralogy of Fallot is the most common form of cyanotic CHD, occurring in 7% of children with CHD. The tetralogy consists of

- Pulmonary stenosis (subvalvar, valvar, and/or supravalvar)
- Ventricular septal defect (VSD)
- Aorta overriding the ventricular septum
- Right ventricular hypertrophy

Patients present with varying degrees of cyanosis, depending on the severity of the pulmonary stenosis. A hypercyanotic spell, or tetralogy spell, is a characteristic sequence of clinical events that begins with irritability and hyperpnea followed by a prolonged period of intense cyanosis leading to syncope.

!

Characteristic sequence of hypercyanotic spell:
- Irritability and hyperpnea
- Intense cyanosis
- Syncope
Treatment:
-Place child in knee-chest position
-Provide maximal supplemental oxygen
-If necessary, give morphine 0.1 mg/kg IM

!

Medical treatment is lifesaving in children with a hypercyanotic spell. Initially, the child should be calmed and placed in a knee-to chest-position. Maximal supplemental oxygen by facemask is then provided, and if the spell continues, morphine (0.1 mg/kg) is given intramuscularly. If the spell persists, more aggressive therapy is initiated. This includes rapid placement of an intravenous catheter followed by administration of intravenous fluid (10-20 mL/kg of 0.9% saline) and sodium bicarbonate (1 mEq/kg). Anemia (hemoglobin <10 g/dL), when present, often precipitates a hypercyanotic spell, and blood transfusion may be required.

Surgical repair of tetralogy of Fallot is indicated for any child with hypercyanotic spells or increasing cyanosis (typically oxygen saturation <75%). Until recently, the approach to these patients had been a palliative operation in infancy involving placement of a modified Blalock-Taussig shunt, which is a Gore-Tex tube connection between the innominate artery and the pulmonary artery. Historically, definitive repair with pulmonary valvotomy, resection of right ventricular infundibular muscle bundles, and VSD closure was performed in older childhood (ages 3-4 years). With advancements in the combined medical and surgical management of younger infants, definitive repair is often being performed in infancy as the only surgical procedure, and elective repair is most commonly performed at about 6 months of age.

2. Tricuspid Atresia

Tricuspid atresia (TA) with normally related great arteries is a rare form of CHD in which the tricuspid valve orifice is not patent. A patent foramen ovale or atrial septal defect (ASD) is present to allow systemic venous blood to shunt from right to left. The right ventricle and pulmonary outflow tract are typically hypoplastic unless a large VSD is present. When there is transposition of the great arteries in combination with TA and a VSD (not an uncommon constellation), the presentation is similar to hypoplastic left heart syndrome, and neonates present with shock when the ductus closes. Patients with TA and normally related great arteries present in the immediate neonatal period with marked cyanosis. Initial medical therapy includes the initiation of prostaglandin E_1 infusion (0.05 µg/kg/min) to maintain the patency of the ductus arteriosus. Palliative surgery is performed in the first week of life and consists of placement of a modified Blalock-Taussig shunt. A modified bidirectional Glenn anastomosis connecting the superior vena cava to the top of the right pulmonary artery is performed at 3 to 9 months as a staged approach, followed by the modified Fontan procedure at approximately 2 years of age. The modified Fontan procedure allows complete bypass of the right side of the heart by directing inferior vena cava and superior vena cava flow into the pulmonary arteries. This staged surgical repair is summarized in **Table 18-1.**

3. Pulmonic Stenosis

Pulmonic stenosis (PS), the second most common form of CHD, occurs in 9% of children with heart disease. Most children will present with a harsh crescendo-decrescendo murmur at the upper-left sternal border with radiation to the back. Infants with critical pulmonary stenosis will be cyanotic and have ductal-dependent pulmonary blood flow. Critical PS may also be considered to be in the category of cyanotic CHD with decreased pulmonary blood flow due to the large obligatory right-to-left atrial shunt. Newborns with critical PS may need to be treated with PGE infusion. Balloon valvuloplasty is usually successful in treating this lesion. Surgery is contemplated only in children with severely dysplastic and hypoplastic valves or those with additional obstruction at the subvalvar or supravalvar locations.

B. Cyanotic Congenital Heart Disease With Increased Pulmonary Vascularity

Cardiac lesions with cyanosis and increased pulmonary vascularity can be classified further into those with increased pulmonary arterial vascularity in which there is hilar prominence on chest radiograph (transposition of the great arteries and truncus arteriosus) and those with increased pulmonary venous vascularity in which the chest radiograph typically shows a ground-glass or white-out appearance (total anomalous pulmonary venous connection and hypoplastic left heart syndrome). In clinical practice these 2 groups often cannot be accurately distinguished from each other based on signs, symptoms, or radiographic findings, and echocardiography is needed to make the diagnosis.

1. Transposition of the Great Arteries

> *Transposition of the great arteries is the most common form of cyanotic heart disease to present on the first day of life.*

In transposition of the great arteries, the aorta arises from the right ventricle while the pulmonary artery arises from the left ventricle. The pulmonary and systemic circulations are configured in parallel rather than in series, resulting in cyanotic blood circulating back to the systemic circulation. Initiation of prostaglandin E_1 infusion (0.05 µg/kg/min) can help increase saturations while awaiting balloon septostomy as more definitive palliation. Septostomy is often necessary for the alleviation of cyanosis because mixing occurs most optimally between the low-pressure atria rather than at the ductus, where there is a large difference between systemic and pulmonary resistance. Furthermore, balloon septostomy is effective in decompressing the left atrium, which is often under high pressure owing to the massive amount of pulmonary blood flow in transposition of the great arteries. Failure to perform a septostomy in a timely fashion, even in the apparently stable neonate, can leave the infant at risk for pulmonary hypertension and relatively sudden occurrence of profound cyanosis fairly unresponsive to medical management. However, there is evidence that children who undergo balloon atrial septostomy are at increased risk of adverse neurologic outcomes, and some centers are performing the procedure only in unstable patients. The infants typically undergo surgical repair of the defect in the first week of life. The arterial switch operation, in which the aorta is connected to the left ventricle and the pulmonary artery to the right ventricle with transfer of the coronary arteries, is now the surgical procedure of choice.

2. Truncus Arteriosus

> *Truncous arteriosus*
> *-At risk for hypocalcemia*
> *- Use only irradiated blood*

Truncus arteriosus is a rare form of CHD in which a single-valved vessel is located above both right and left ventricles with a large VSD allowing for common egress of blood from both ventricles. This common vessel, the truncus arteriosus, gives rise to the aorta, coronary arteries, and pulmonary arteries. A significant percentage of these patients, particularly those with associated aortic arch anomalies, have a 22q11 microdeletion resulting in DiGeorge syndrome and should be evaluated immediately for hypocalcemia secondary to hypoparathyroidism and for T cell immunodeficiency. Only irradiated blood cells should be used for transfusions to prevent the development of graft versus host disease. Definitive surgical repair can usually be performed soon after diagnosis. A valved homograft conduit is placed from the right ventricle to the main pulmonary artery that has been separated from the truncus arteriosus, and the VSD is closed to direct the left ventricular blood into the truncus arteriosus. Subsequent surgical procedures are necessary to change the size of the conduit as the children grow.

3. Total Anomalous Pulmonary Venous Connection

Patients with total anomalous pulmonary venous connection, a rare form of CHD, have their entire supply of oxygenated pulmonary venous blood returning to the systemic venous circulation. This admixture of oxygenated and desaturated blood produces cyanosis. There are four subtypes of total anomalous pulmonary venous return based on the location of pulmonary venous return: supracardiac (to the innominate vein or superior vena cava), intracardiac (to the coronary sinus or right atrium), infracardiac (below the diaphragm to either the hepatic, portal, or umbilical venous system), or mixed (a combination of the above). The severity of the cyanosis increases if there is an obstruction to the return of the pulmonary venous blood, which promotes ductal and/or atrial right-to-left shunting. Neonates with obstructed total anomalous pulmonary venous connection frequently present in extremis with severe cyanosis. Patients without obstruction are less cyanotic and may be sent home from the nursery without diagnosis, but they are normally noted to be cyanotic or to have a pulmonary flow murmur in the first weeks of life. Surgical repair is done immediately upon presentation with very good long-term results.

> !
>
> *Neonates with obstructed total anomalous pulmonary venous connection present with severe cyanosis.*
>
> !

See **Table 18-6** for a list of causes of cyanosis in newborns and **Table 18-7** for a summary of the initial evaluation and treatment of cyanotic newborns.

Table 18-6. Causes of Cyanosis in Newborns

Cyanotic heart disease
- With decreased pulmonary vascularity
  - Tetralogy of Fallot
  - Tricuspid atresia
  - Critical pulmonary stenosis
- With increased pulmonary vascularity
  - Transposition of the great arteries
  - Truncus arteriosus
  - Total anomalous pulmonary venous return

Respiratory diseases

Hematologic disorders (methemoglobinemia)

Neuromuscular disorders (hypoventilation)

Table 18-7. Initial Evaluation and Treatment of Cyanotic Newborns

Initial Evaluation of Cyanotic Newborns
Tests:
Chest radiograph: will show possible lung pathology and cardiac silhouette
ECG
Hyperoxia test:
Obtain Pa_{O_2} on room air and after 10 minutes on 100% F_{IO_2}
If preductal Pa_{O_2} >150 mmHg then no cyanotic CHD
Cardiology consultation/echocardiography as appropriate for definitive diagnosis of suspected CHD
Initial Treatment of Cyanotic Newborns
ABCs: airway, breathing, circulation
Prostaglandin E_1 infusion at 0.05 μg/kg/min
Once diagnosis of cyanotic CHD is confirmed can wean O_2 to keep oxygen saturations in appropriate range for the specific lesion

IV. ACYANOTIC CONGENITAL HEART DISEASE

Case Study

A 2-month-old male presented to the emergency department with a several-day history of decreased feeding, tachypnea, diaphoresis, and decreasing energy levels. His vital signs include pulse of 180/min and respiratory rate of 75/min. There is a harsh systolic murmur. His liver is palpable 6 centimeters below the right costal margin.

- What are the possible diagnoses?

- What is the appropriate initial evaluation and treatment?

A. Acyanotic Congenital Heart Disease With Increased Pulmonary Vascularity

1. Ventricular Septal Defect

Ventricular septal defect (VSD) is the most common form of CHD. The ventricular septum is a complex structure that has 4 major embryologic regions:

- Inlet septum: located posteriorly and superiorly between the tricuspid and mitral valves

- Outlet septum: located anteriorly beneath the aortic and pulmonary valves
- Trabecular septum: located inferiorly
- Membranous septum: located in the subaortic region and beneath the septal leaflet of the tricuspid valve

The signs and symptoms of VSD are generally the result of the amount of left-to-right ventricular shunting. The shunt that occurs with a VSD is dependent on the relative pressures and/or resistances of both the systemic and the pulmonary circulations. Neonates are often asymptomatic until pulmonary vascular resistance drops at approximately 2 to 6 weeks of age, resulting in an increased shunt and the appearance of clinical symptoms. An infant with small to moderate VSDs will present with a holosystolic murmur and remain asymptomatic. The intensity of the murmur is inversely proportional to the size of the defect. Children with larger VSDs will have less impressive murmurs and typically develop signs and symptoms of heart failure (**Tables 18-2 and 18-3**). If the defect is large, right ventricle and pulmonary artery pressure will be systemic. Smaller defects will allow creation of a pressure difference between the left and right ventricles, and the amount of the shunting is dependent on the size of the VSD and the relative vascular resistances. In addition, other associated cardiac lesions may alter the amount and direction of shunting.

With advances in the medical and surgical care of children with CHD, cardiothoracic surgery is now being performed safely, even in small infants. Indications for surgical closure of a VSD include the following:

- Uncontrolled congestive heart failure
- Increased pulmonary vascular resistance with a risk for development of pulmonary vascular obstructive disease
- Failure to thrive despite maximum medical therapy (**see Table 18-9**)
- Recurrent pulmonary infections
- Endocarditis
- Paradoxical emboli

Eisenmenger syndrome develops when a significant shunt lesion is left unrepaired, and longstanding pulmonary hypertension progresses to irreversible pulmonary vascular obstructive disease with resultant right-to-left ventricular shunting and cyanosis. Death follows as a result of pulmonary hemorrhage, infections, and/or paradoxical emboli.

2. Atrial Septal Defect

Atrial septal defect (ASD) is the third most common form of CHD, occurring in 8% of children with heart disease. It is found more frequently in females than males (at a ratio of 2:1). Atrial septal defects occur in 3 separate locations in the atrial septum:

- Ostium primum defects are located in the lower third of the atrial septum, near the atrioventricular valves.
- Ostium secundum defects are found in the middle portion of the septum and are the most common.
- Sinus venosus defects occur in the posterior portion of the septum, adjacent to the vena cavae.

The direction and amount of atrial level shunting is determined by the relative compliances of the right and left ventricles and the size of the defect. Typically, the right ventricle is more compliant and, therefore, left-to-right shunting occurs more frequently.

With rare exception, patients with an ASD are asymptomatic. Asymptomatic patients classically have a fixed split S2 with a systolic ejection murmur at the upper-left sternal border due to relative pulmonary stenosis. They also may have a diastolic murmur at the lower-left sternal border due to relative tricuspid stenosis. If symptoms are present they develop later in childhood and are frequently related to arrhythmias. Indications for closure of an ASD are right ventricular volume overload, arrhythmias, paradoxical emboli, and elevated pulmonary vascular resistance. Closure is typically performed by cardiac catheterization or surgery, with very little morbidity or mortality.

3. Patent Ductus Arteriosus

An isolated patent ductus arteriosus (PDA) accounts for 2% of CHD, with an increased incidence in premature infants that is inversely proportional to their gestational age. The ductus arteriosus, a normal embryological structure connecting the main pulmonary artery to the descending aorta, normally closes within the first few days of life. Patients with a PDA have left-to-right shunting dependent on the same issues of anatomic shunt size and relative resistance that govern VSD flow. In the presence of increased pulmonary vascular resistance, a PDA is often noted to have bidirectional shunting with right-to-left flow in systole and left-to-right flow in diastole. Infants with a large PDA, especially premature infants, will have typical symptoms of heart failure. Patients with a small to moderate PDA will present with an asymptomatic continuous murmur over the upper-left sternal border.

Indomethacin is successful in closing most PDAs in premature infants. In older children or infants unresponsive to indomethacin, catheter-based closure and surgical ligation are extremely effective, with essentially no morbidity or mortality.

4. Atrioventricular Septal Defect

Atrioventricular septal defect (AVSD) occurs in 7% of children with CHD. It is commonly found in children with Down syndrome. The lesion consists of a large defect in the atrioventricular septum along with a common atrioventricular valve. Children with an AVSD are usually diagnosed in the first weeks of life due to a systolic murmur from atrioventricular valve insufficiency of a holosystolic murmur from a relatively pressure restrictive VSD. Often there is a large VSD, and right and left ventricular pressures will be equal, in which case there can be no murmur in the first weeks of life. If undiagnosed, patients with an AVSD will usually develop typical signs and symptoms of heart failure in the first months of life due to pulmonary vascular resistance decreasing and subsequent increase in the degree of left to right shunting. In order to avoid acute and long-term consequences of pulmonary hypertension, surgical repair is required in infancy, ideally at 3 to 6 months of age.

> !
>
> *Atrioventricular septal defect:*
> *- Commonly found in Down syndrome*
> *- Develops signs and symptoms of heart failure in first few months of life*
>
> !

To review the causes of acyanotic heart disease, see **Table 18-8.** An overview of the evaluation and treatment of acyanotic heart disease can be found in **Table 18-9.**

Table 18-8. Causes of Acyanotic Congenital Heart Disease

Acyanotic CHD with increased pulmonary vascularity (shunt lesions)
- Ventricular septal defect
- Atrial septal defect
- Patent ductus arteriosus
- Atrioventricular septal defect

Acyanotic CHD with obstructive lesions
- Pulmonary stenosis (valvar, supravalvar, subvalvar)
- Aortic stenosis (valvar, supravalvar, subvalvar)
- Coarctation of the aorta

Other causes of heart failure (arrhythmia, cardiomyopathy, myocarditis, coronary artery anomalies)

Table 18-9. Initial Evaluation and Treatment of Acyanotic Heart Disease

Initial Evaluation of Acyanotic Heart Disease

Tests:
- Echocardiography (the gold standard in diagnosis)
- Chest radiograph (can be helpful in assessing cardiac silhouette and pulmonary vascularity)
- ECG (to evaluate for arrhythmia)

Table 18-9. Initial Evaluation and Treatment of Acyanotic Heart Disease (Continued)

Initial Treatment of Acyanotic Heart Disease
Commonly used medications:
Diuretics
Loop diuretic (furosemide 1-2 mg/kg/dose orally or IV every 6-12 hours)
Thiazides (hydrochlorothiazide 2-5 mg/kg/dose every 6-12 hours)
Potassium sparing (spironolactone 0.5-3 mg/kg/day divided every 6-24 hours)
Afterload-reducing agents
ACE inhibitors (enalapril 0.05-0.25 mg/kg/day every 12 hours)
Milrinone 0.25-0.75 mcg/kg/min IV
Nitroprusside 0.5-10 mcg/kg/min IV
Nitroglycerine 0.5-5 mcg/kg/min IV
Inotropic agents
Digoxin 8-10 mcg/kg/day divided every 12 hours
Dopamine ≤5 mcg/kg/min (β-Adrenergic agonist)
Dobutamine 5-15 mcg/kg/min (β-Adrenergic agonist)
Epinephrine ≤0.05 mcg/kg/min (β-Adrenergic agonist)
Milrinone 0.25-0.75 mcg/kg/min (Phosphodiesterase inhibitor)
Minimize use of oxygen (can increase left to right shunting)

V. LOW CARDIAC OUTPUT SYNDROME

Case Study

A 4-year-old male presents to the emergency department with lethargy 2 weeks after an uncomplicated surgical repair of an atrial septal defect. He is found to be tachycardiac and tachypneic. An arterial blood gas is obtained and shows a metabolic acidosis.

- What are the possible diagnoses?
- What is the appropriate initial evaluation?

In the postoperative patient, metabolic acidosis should be considered an indication of low cardiac output and inadequate tissue perfusion until proven otherwise. Low cardiac output syndrome (LCOS) is an inability of the heart to provide oxygen delivery adequate for demand. It is similar to the older terminology of cardiogenic shock, although it may have etiologies other than poor myocardial contractility. Common causes of low cardiac output are presented in **Tables 18-10** and **18-11.** The findings associated with LCOS are listed in **Table 18-12,** but a patient need not have all of those findings to be diagnosed with LCOS. The goal is to make the diagnosis early in order to identify treatable causes and institute therapy in a timely fashion to prevent irreversible end-organ injury.

Table 18-10. Causes of Postoperative Low Cardiac Output

Arrhythmias
Hypovolemia
Anemia
Myocardial dysfunction
Residual cardiac lesions (see **Table 18-11**)
Pulmonary hypertension
Cardiac tamponade

Table 18-11. Possible Residual Lesions After Surgery

Valvular stenosis
Valvular insufficiency
Arterial stenosis
Residual shunt lesions
Outflow tract obstructions

Table 18-12. Signs and Symptoms of Low Cardiac Output Syndrome

The following reflect poor tissue oxygen delivery:
Tachycardia
Poor peripheral effusion
Decreased urine output
Metabolic acidosis
Elevated or rapidly rising lactate levels (>0.75 mm/L/h)
Widened arterial-mixed venous oxygen saturation difference (>30-40%)
Hypotension
Late findings
Increased creatinine
Increased liver enzymes
Seizures
Other indicators of end organ damage

!

The development of LCOS after surgery should prompt a reevaluation for the presence of residual hemodynamic lesions, tamponade, or arrhythmia.

!

A. Arrhythmias

It is essential to determine the cardiac rhythm when assessing an unstable postoperative patient. A 12-lead electrocardiogram (ECG) should be performed as soon as possible. Descriptions of the most common arrhythmias following congenital heart surgery and their usual modes of treatment are presented in **Table 18-13.** It is important to note that these rhythms can also occur in patients without any underlying structural heart disease.

Table 18-13. Common Arrhythmias Following Congenital Heart Surgery and Usual Treatments

Arrhythmia	Signs/Symptoms	Circumstances	Treatment
Junctional ectopic tachycardia	Narrow (normal) complex tachycardia Rate ≥180 VA relationship is 1:1 (with retrograde P wave) or greater	Most common after surgeries involving the ventricular septum: Tetralogy of Fallot VSD Atrioventricular septal defect Truncus arteriosus Fontan (much less frequently)	Pace the atrium to restore AV synchrony Cool the patient Wean β adrenergic agonists as much as hemodynamically possible Amiodarone (2-5 mg/kg/dose IV given over 20-60 minutes) Procainamide (3-6 mg/kg/dose IV)
Heart block	First degree: prolonged PR interval Second degree: Type I/Wenkebach: progressive prolongation of the PR interval until AV conduction is lost Type II : AV conduction that occurs in a fixed ratio other than 1:1 Third degree: complete loss of AV conduction	Most common after surgeries around the AV node: VSD repairs Mitral valve replacement Enlargement of left ventricular outflow tract (Konno procedure) L-looped heart (ventricular inversion) is additional risk factor	None (first degree and Wenkebach often asymptomatic) Temporary or permanent pacing First degree and Wenkebach: in setting of tachycardia and very prolonged AV interval (can be similar to junctional ectopic tachycardia) Second degree, type II, and third degree block: always require dual chamber pacing If dual chamber pacing is not possible ventricular pacing will prevent ventricular asystole
Orthodromic reciprocating tachycardia	Reentrant tachycardia (normal conduction from atria to ventricles across AV node with reentry into atria via a bypass tract) with P in T wave VA relationship always 1:1 Sudden onset and cessation of tachycardia	Wolff-Parkinson White Syndrome Hidden Accessory Pathway	Adenosine (50-300 μg/kg IV rapid push) Synchronized direct current cardioversion (0.5-2 joules/kg) Amiodarone or β-blocker (atenolol) for recurrent episodes Atrial overdrive pacing

Table 18-13. Common Arrhythmias Following Congenital Heart Surgery and Usual Treatments

Arrhythmia	Signs/Symptoms	Circumstances	Treatment
Atrial flutter	Reentrant tachycardia within the atrium Narrow QRS complex usually with 2:1 or 3:1 AV conduction	Most common with severe right atrial enlargement or extensive atrial surgery: Fontan patients (atriopulmonary connection or lateral tunnel) years after surgery Ebstein's anomaly Mustard procedure (for transportation of) the great arteries) Senning procedure (for transportation of) the great arteries)	Adenosine (does not alter atrial rate, but can help in diagnosis) Synchronized cardioversion (0.5-2 joules/kg) Rapid atrial pacing (at rate greater than the atrial rate) Amiodarone or other antiarrhythmics for recurrent episodes
Ventricular tachycardia	Wide complex tachycardia Rare in pediatrics	Most common in: Sick ventricles with poor hemodynamics Severely hypertrophied ventricle	Direct current cardioversion (2-4 joules/kg) Amiodarone (5 mg/kg IV) Lidocaine (0.5-1.5 mg/kg IV)

!

An unstable patient with a wide complex tachycardia should be presumed to have ventricular tachycardia and treated immediately with direct-current cardioversion at 2.4 joules/kg.

!

B. Cardiac Tamponade

!

Cardiac tamponade must be considered in all patients with LCOS after open heart surgery.

!

One important cause of LCOS that requires immediate recognition and management is cardiac tamponade. Echocardiography can confirm the diagnosis by demonstrating a collection of pericardial fluid with associated atrial compression or collapse during ventricular systole. It is imperative to consider the diagnosis of tamponade in any postoperative patient with LCOS, even in the absence of high filling pressures, radiograph, or echocardiographic changes, because even a small amount of blood can cause tamponade if it is located in an area that results in impairment of myocardial filling. Cardiac tamponade is treated by attempting to clear occluded chest tubes, by pericardiocentesis, or by mediastinal reexploration. Rapid fluid resuscitation may also be necessary and can help support the circulation until adequate mediastinal drainage is achieved.

C. Myocardial Dysfunction

Myocardial contractility can be enhanced by using β-adrenergic agonists or phosphodiesterase inhibitors (see **Table 18-9**). Cardiomyocyte contractility and relaxation occur due to rapid calcium cycling within the cells. β-Adrenergic agonists work by increasing intracellular cyclic adenosine monophosphate, which subsequently increases calcium cycling in both systole and diastole. Given that cyclic adenosine monophosphate is degraded by phosphodiesterases, phosphodiesterase inhibitors also increase cyclic adenosine monophosphate. Milrinone at 0.75 μg/kg/min has been shown to prevent LCOS following repair of congenital heart disease. One particular advantage of phosphodiesterase inhibition is that it is not receptor dependent and, therefore, not altered by receptor down regulation that occurs during chronic adrenergic stimulation. Another advantage of these drugs is that they promote afterload reduction for the systemic (and perhaps pulmonary) ventricle. At higher doses β-adrenergic agonists stimulate vascular α-adrenergic receptors, resulting in vasoconstriction.

Blood pressure is determined by both the cardiac output and the systemic vascular resistance, and there is an inverse relationship between systemic vascular resistance and cardiac contractility. Therefore, use of vasodilators for afterload reduction results in an increase in cardiac contractility, cardiac output, and oxygen delivery, albeit often at a lower blood pressure. When vascular tone is high, either intrinsically or secondary to the use of higher doses of adrenergic agonists, and cardiac output is low, pure vasodilating agents can be used to improve oxygen delivery. Nitroprusside (0.5-10 μg/kg/min), and nitroglycerine (0.5-5 μg/kg/min) are commonly used for this purpose, particularly in combination with epinephrine or norepinephrine to boost contractility.

When blood pressure is too low to maintain adequate organ perfusion, it is preferable to maximize preload and contractility before resorting to increasing systemic vascular resistance. Such an approach is preferred due to the inverse relationship between afterload and cardiac function and the likelihood that the increase in blood pressure will come at the cost of a decrease in cardiac output and oxygen delivery. An exception to this relationship occurs when coronary perfusion has become critically low and an increase in blood pressure can increase myocardial function. Despite the inverse relationship between ventricular function and afterload, it is sometimes necessary to increase systemic vascular resistance to achieve an acceptable blood pressure. Commonly used vasopressors include epinephrine and norepinephrine (both of which also have significant β-adrenergic agonist effects), phenylephrine (0.1-0.5 μg/kg/min), and, more recently, vasopressin (0.0003-0.002 units/kg/min). Persistent hypotension refractory to catecholamines should lead to the consideration of abnormalities in adrenal or thyroid function. Supplementation with steroids, in particular, has shown some promise in treating refractory hypotension.

> **!** *Consider evaluating adrenal and thyroid function in patients with hypotension refractory to catecholamines.*

The neonatal heart has an immature calcium-handling system and is more dependent on extracellular calcium for contractility than is the mature heart. There is much laboratory and anecdotal evidence to suggest that maintenance of ionized calcium levels 20% to 30% above the normal physiologic range is associated with improved hemodynamics soon after neonatal cardiac surgery. Hypocalcemia, either secondary to genetic issues, such as chromosome 22 deletions, or as a result of citrate in packed red blood cells or fresh frozen plasma, should be aggressively treated.

The management of the pediatric cardiology patient requires a comprehensive understanding of the basic principles of oxygen delivery, cardiovascular physiology, and the anatomy and physiology of congenital heart disease. Signs and symptoms of LCOS should be treated aggressively, and diagnostic and therapeutic strategies should address both universal and lesion-specific problems.

The tests used to evaluate patients with low cardiac output are summarized in **Table 18-14.**

Table 18-14. Evaluation of Patients With Low Cardiac Output

Tests and monitoring:
Chest radiograph
EKG
Arterial blood gas
Complete blood counts
Serum electrolytes
Echocardiogram
Central venous and arterial blood pressure monitoring

Key Points

Management of the Child With Congenital Heart Disease

- Any infant in the first weeks of life presenting with low cardiac output or a shock like state must be suspected of having congenital heart disease.
- Most forms of congenital heart disease can be appropriately categorized into 2 groups—acyanotic and cyanotic—and a presumptive diagnosis can be made by integrating information obtained from the history, physical examination, chest radiograph, and pulse oximeter.
- Initiation of Prostaglandin E_1 infusion can be life saving in children with congenital heart disease and ductal dependent blood flow.
- Prompt recognition and appropriate treatment for low cardiac output syndrome is essential in pediatric cardiac critical care.

Suggested Readings

1. Chang AC, Hanley FL, Wernovsky G, Wessel DL, eds. *Pediatric Cardiac Intensive Care.* Philadelphia, PA: Lippincott Williams and Wilkins; 1998.

2. Garson A Jr, Bricker JT, Fisher DJ, Neish SR, eds. *The Science and Practice of Pediatric Cardiology.* 2nd ed. Baltimore, MD: Williams and Wilkins; 1998.

3. Hoffman TM, Wernovsky G, Atz AM, et al. Efficacy and safety of milrinone in preventing low cardiac output syndrome in infants and children after corrective surgery for congenital heart disease. *Circulation.* 2003;107:996-1002.

4. Kolovos NS, Bratton SL, Moler FW, et al. Outcome of pediatric patients treated with extracorporeal life support after cardiac surgery. *Ann Thorac Surg.* 2003;76:1435-1441.

5. McQuillen PS, Hamrick SEG, Perez MJ, et al. Balloon atrial septostomy is associated with preoperative stroke in neonates with transposition of the great arteries. *Circulation.* 2006;113:280-285.

6. Nichols D, Greeley WJ, Lappe DG, Wetzel RC, eds. *Critical Heart Disease in Infants and Children.* 2nd ed. Cambridge, MA: Elsevier Science; 2006.

7. Schroeder VA, Pearl JM, Schwartz SM, et al. Combined steroid treatment for congenital heart surgery improves oxygen delivery and reduces postbypass inflammatory mediator expression. *Circulation.* 2003;107:2823-2828.

8. Wernovsky G, Wypij D, Jonas RA, et al. Postoperative course and hemodynamic profile after the arterial switch operation in neonates and infants: a comparison of low-flow cardiopulmonary bypass and circulatory arrest. *Circulation.* 1995;92:2226-2235.

9. Wheeler D, Wong H, Shanley T, eds. *Pediatric Critical Care Medicine: Basic Science and Clinical Evidence.* New York, NY: Springer-Verlag; 2007.

Chapter 19:

Oncologic Emergencies And Complications

Objectives

- Describe risk factors unique to the immunosuppressed pediatric patient.
- Recognize and treat causes of shock in the pediatric cancer patient.
- Recognize and treat causes of respiratory failure in the pediatric cancer patient.
- Review metabolic abnormalities associated to tumor lysis syndrome and list treatment priorities.
- Describe risk factors associated with hyperleukocytosis.
- Recognize and treat spinal cord compression.

Case Study

A 12-year-old patient with acute lymphocytic leukemia who was recently released from the hospital after induction chemotherapy, presented to a referring hospital with a 2-hour history of fever, shaking, and chills after having her routine central-line flush with heparin. On admission the patient's temperature is 39.2°C (102.6°F), heart rate (HR) is 156/min, blood pressure (BP) is 82/35 mm Hg, and respiratory rate (RR) is 28/min. Laboratory data obtained on admission show a white blood cell (WBC) count of 0.1 mm^3, Hgb 7.2 g/dL, platelet count of 15,000 mm^3. Her electrolytes are normal except for a K^+ 2.8 mmol/L. Blood culture 12 hours after admission is positive for gram-positive cocci.

- Should this patient receive fluids or blood?
- What antibiotics are indicated in this patient?
- What are the risk factors for this patient?

I. INTRODUCTION

This chapter is designed to provide the pediatric team with essential information on aspects of care that may be critical in the early course of treatment of oncology patients.

Recent evidence supports the use of aggressive therapies early in the course of the patient's illness. These may include broad-spectrum antimicrobial coverage, fluid resuscitation, and early respiratory and inotropic support. The therapeutic goals should be discussed with the primary attending, the patient's guardian, the patient if appropriate, and the intensive care unit (ICU) team. Decisions concerning continuation or limitations of care should be frequently reexplored based on the patient's primary diagnosis, oncologic prognosis, and clinical course.

II. FEVER AND NEUTROPENIA

A. Definitions

Fever and neutropenia are common complications of the treatment of pediatric malignancies. Fever is defined as a single oral temperature measurement ≥38.3°C (100.9°F) or a temperature of ≥ 38°C (100.4°F) persisting for more than 1 hour. Rectal temperature measurements are contraindicated in febrile neutropenic patients, since these may cause disruption of the rectal mucosal barrier, thus creating a nidus for infection. Neutropenia is defined as an absolute neutrophil count (ANC) of either <500 cells/mm^3 or <1000 cells/mm^3 with a downward trend of the ANC on 2 separate peripheral blood counts.

B. Risk Factors

The risk of sepsis increases with the degree and duration of neutropenia. The risk of bacteremia and septicemia increases with an ANC of <200 cells/mm^3. Episodes of neutropenia lasting more than 7 days are associated with a worse outcome. Children with leukemias, including patients in relapse as well as patients who have undergone bone-marrow or stem-cell transplantation, are at a greater risk of severe and prolonged neutropenia due to the intensity of their chemotherapeutic regimens. Certain clinical and laboratory risk factors are also associated with serious infection. These include shock, myeloablative chemotherapy, bone-marrow and stem-cell transplantation, relapsed leukemia, pneumonia, neutropenic enterocolitis, oral mucositis, invasive fungal infections, temperature >39°C (102.2°F), C-reactive protein >10 mg/L, absolute monocyte count <100 cells/mm^3, and gram-negative bacteremia.

C. Treatment

The current standard of care for patients with fever and neutropenia requires early empiric inpatient intravenous antibiotic therapy. In such situations, a full workup is recommended and should include blood culture, urine culture, chest radiograph, and lumbar puncture, if clinically indicated. Early drainage of fluid collections (abscess, empyema) for culture and symptom relief is highly recommended.

The organisms associated with serious infections in children and the suggested antimicrobials and dosages are summarized in **Table 19-1**. Febrile neutropenic patients without a focus of infection may be treated with a broad-spectrum antibiotic with antipseudomonal coverage, such as cefepime or ceftazidime. The addition of a broad-spectrum gram-positive antimicrobial, such as vancomycin, is recommended in patients with clinical and laboratory risk factors. Further changes to the patient antibiotic coverage should be based on documentation or high suspicion for a particular infectious agent, subsequent susceptibility results, and resistance patterns.

!

Fever and Neutropenia

- *Blood and urine culture, CXR*
- *Early empiric intravenous antibiotic therapy:*
  - *Cefepime: 150 mg/kg/24 h ÷ every 8 h IV/IM*
  - *Vancomycin: 60 mg/kg/24 h ÷ every 6 h IV*
- *G-CSF: 5-10 µg/kg/day SC*
- *Close monitoring*

!

Colony-stimulating factors (CSFs) may be used to shorten the duration of neutropenia. These agents have been utilized with increasing frequency for patients with neutropenia and multiple-organ-system failure (MOSF), sepsis or septic shock, and/or invasive fungal disease. Granulocyte colony-stimulating factor (G-CSF) given subcutaneously in a dose of 5 to 10 mcg/kg/day stimulates the release of neutrophils. It should be considered in patients with neutropenia and bacterial sepsis. Granulocyte-macrophage colony-stimulating factor (GM-CSF), dosed at 5 mcg/kg/day subcutaneously, enhances the release of both neutrophils and macrophages. Granulocyte-macrophage colony-stimulating factor should be considered for patients in whom fungal disease is confirmed or strongly suspected. Either medication should be continued until the absolute neutrophil count exceeds 1000 for 3 consecutive days. A recent study showed a reduction in the duration of neutropenia, length of antibiotic treatment, and number of hospital days with the use of colony-stimulating factors.

Table 19-1. Treatment Recommendations for Serious Infections in Immunosuppressed Children

Organism	Treatment[a]
Gram-positive organisms: coagulase-negative Staphylococcus, α-hemolytic Streptococcus, Enterococcus, Coryneform	Vancomycin[b]: 15 mg/kg every 6 hours IV Linezolid: 10 mg/kg every 8 hours IV; max dose 1200 mg/24 h Daptomycin[b]: 4-6 mg/kg every 24 hours IV (not approved for children <18 years)
Gram-negative organisms: Klebsiella, Bacillus, Pseudomonas, E coli	Cephalosporins[b]: - Cefepime: 50 mg/kg every 8 hours IV/IM; max dose 6 g/24 h - Ceftazidime: 50 mg/kg every 8 hours IV/IM; max dose 6 g/24 h Aminoglycosides[b]: - Gentamicin: 2.5 mg/kg every 8 hours IV - Tobramycin: 2.5 mg/kg every 8 hours IV Carbapenems[b]: - Imipenem-cilastatin: 25 mg/kg every 6 hours IV; max dose 4 g/24 h - Meropenem: 40 mg/kg every 8 hours IV; max dose 6 g/24 h
Fungi: candida, aspergillus	Fluconazole[b]: Loading dose 12 mg/kg IV; maintenance 6 mg/kg IV every 24 hours after loading dose; max loading dose 400 mg Liposomal amphotericin B: 3-5 mg/kg every 24 hours IV Caspofungin: Loading dose 70 mg/m² IV; maintenance 50 mg/m² IV every 24 hours after loading dose; max loading dose 70 mg. Voriconazole: loading dose of 6 mg/kg every 12 hours IV x 2 doses; 4 mg/kg every 12 hours IV
Anaerobes	Clindamycin: 10 mg/kg every 6-8 hours IV/IM; max dose 2800 mg/24 h Metronidazole: 7.5 mg/kg every 6 hours IV/PO; max dose 4 g/24 h
Antivirals	
- RSV (respiratory syncytial virus)	Ribavirin: 6 g by aerosol (small-particle aerosol generator, or SPAG-2) over 12-18 hours daily for 3-7 days (6 g in 300 mL preservative-free sterile water)
- Influenza type A	Amantadine: - 1-9 years: 5 mg/kg PO once daily; max dose 150 mg/24 h - >9 years (<40 kg): 5 mg/kg PO once daily; max dose 200 mg/24 h - >40 kg: 200 mg once daily Rimantadine: - 1-9 years: 5 mg/kg PO once daily; max dose 150 mg/24 h - >10 years (<40 kg): 5 mg/kg PO once daily; max dose 150 mg/24 h - >40 kg: 100 mg PO twice daily

continued next page…

Table 19-1. Treatment Recommendations for Serious Infections in Immunosuppressed Children (continued)

Organism	Treatment[a]
- Influenza types A and B	Zanamivir: >7 years and adults - Day 1: 2 doses (5 mg/inhalation) at least 2-12 hours apart - Days 2-5: 2 inhalations (5 mg/inhalation) every 12 hours for 4 days; initiate within 2 days of symptom onset Oseltamivir[b]: - <15 kg: 30 mg PO twice daily - >15-23 kg: 45 mg PO twice daily - >23-40 kg: 60 mg PO twice daily - >40 kg: 75 mg PO twice daily - >12 years and adults: 75 mg PO twice daily for 5 days
- Parainfluenza	Ribavirin may be beneficial if used early (see RSV treatment for dose)
- CMV pneumonia	Ganciclovir[b]: 5 mg/kg every 12 hours IV OR Foscarnet[b]: 90 mg/kg every 12 hours IV AND Immunoglobulin: 0.5 g/kg/day IV
Pneumocystis carinii	Trimethoprim-sulfamethoxazole[b]: 5 mg/kg of trimethoprim component every 6-8 hours IV

[a]These recommendations are general guidelines only. Specific antibiotic choices should be individualized, taking into consideration clinical circumstances (renal function, liver function), patient age, immunization status, and local microbial virulence, sensitivities, and patterns of resistance. The antibiotic dosing, interval, and frequency should be discussed with a pediatric intensivist or pediatric infectious disease expert.
[b]Adjust for renal failure.

D. Complications of the Febrile Neutropenia State

1. Bacteremia

Up to 40% of febrile neutropenic patients will have documented bacteremia. Catheter-related infections are the most frequent cause of bacteremia. The most common infective agent is coagulase-negative staphylococci, although enterococci and *Staphylococcus aureus* may also be present. Certain patient populations, such as those with acute myelogenous leukemia, are at risk for *Streptococcus viridans* infections. The rate of infections caused by gram-negative organisms appears to be increasing. The causes for this change are not clear, but it may be related to the use of more aggressive chemotherapeutic techniques that lead to periods of prolonged profound neutropenia, increased use of indwelling devices, and selective antibiotic resistance.

2. Lower-Respiratory-Tract Infections

Case Study

An 11-year-old male who underwent peripheral stem cell transplant 100 days ago is admitted to the ICU from the emergency department for respiratory distress and hypoxia, Spo_2 on 50% oxygen 89%. A chest computed tomographic (CT) scan shows a diffuse ground-glass pattern. The WBC is 5.2 mm^3.

- Should this patient be intubated?
- What is the most likely etiology for his deterioration?

The immune deficiency that results from the primary disease, the toxicity of the therapy, or both make pediatric cancer patients susceptible to a wide range of infectious and noninfectious problems that may progress rapidly to respiratory failure. Initiation of broad-spectrum antibacterial, antifungal, and antiviral therapy is often indicated in patients with rapid clinical or radiologic deterioration. High-resolution CT to identify pulmonary pathology should be utilized in all patients with respiratory symptomatology, irrespective of the plain radiograph findings. Bronchoscopy with bronchoalveolar lavage or open lung biopsy should be considered early in the course of the patient's illness. This may help differentiate infectious from noninfectious etiologies (diffuse alveolar hemorrhage), particularly in patients who have undergone bone marrow and stem cell transplantation.

Community-acquired viral infections such as influenza, respiratory syncytial virus (RSV), and parainfluenza can have devastating effects in pediatric oncology patients, and transplant patients in particular. Patients with RSV infections may benefit from ribavirin, palivizumab, and RSV immunoglobulin. Patients with influenza infections will benefit from the early use of antiviral medications (amantadine, rimantadine, zanamivir, or oseltamivir). No effective therapy exists for parainfluenza pneumonia. Mortality from cytomegalovirus (CMV) pneumonitis in bone marrow transplant patients is high. Current recommended initial treatment for CMV pneumonia is a combination of IV ganciclovir and immune globulin. *Pneumocystis jiroveci* (formerly *Pneumocystis carinii*) pneumonia should be in the differential of any immunocompromised patient who presents with respiratory symptoms, hypoxemia, and diffuse patchy infiltrates shown on the chest radiograph. The treatment of choice is intravenous trimethoprim-sulfamethoxazole (pentamidine in allergic patients). Corticosteroids (methylprednisolone 1-2 mg/kg/day IV ÷ every 6 hours) should be initiated in patients with moderate or severe Pneumocystis *jiroveci pneumonia* (Pao_2 <70 mm Hg (9.3 kPa)on room air) within 72 hours of initiating antibiotic therapy.

Pediatric oncology patients presenting with respiratory failure should promptly receive noninvasive positive pressure ventilation (BiPAP) or be intubated and mechanically ventilated as indicated. Recent data support placing pediatric stem cell recipients with acute respiratory failure on high-frequency oscillatory ventilation within 6 hours of initiating mechanical ventilation. These data demonstrate potential for improved outcome with early application of lung-protective strategies in the acute lung-injury process.

3. Neutropenic Enterocolitis

Another complication found in febrile neutropenic patients is neutropenic enterocolitis or typhlitis (when it involves the cecum). The precise incidence or prevalence is unknown. Most patients survive and are never diagnosed. The pathogenesis is not clear but may be related to a combination of factors, including neutropenia and mucositis, direct cytotoxic effect of chemotherapy on the intestinal mucosa, altered enteric bacterial flora, and fungal overgrowth. The typical presentation of neutropenic enterocolitis mimics acute appendicitis. Most patients present with fever, abdominal pain, watery or bloody diarrhea, nausea, and vomiting. The diagnostic modality of choice is CT scan. Ultrasonography may also be useful as a bedside diagnostic tool, particularly in critically ill patients. It may also be used as a follow-up tool to assess the evolution of changes to the bowel wall. Barium enemas are usually contraindicated. Sepsis and perforation are the most common associated complications. Early diagnosis is essential for a good outcome. Treatment includes both medical and surgical modalities. The medical management of neutropenic enterocolitis includes bowel rest with nasogastric decompression, platelet and red cell infusions, parenteral nutrition, and broad-spectrum antimicrobial therapy, such as anaerobic (metronidazole), gram-negative, and antifungal coverage in critically ill patients. Surgical intervention may be needed in patients with perforations, clinical deterioration despite adequate medical management, abscess formation, or continued bleeding.

4. Invasive Fungal Infections

Recurrent episodes of prolonged neutropenia, immunosuppressive agents, and chronic steroid use place the pediatric oncology patients at high risk for developing invasive fungal infections. Populations at risk include patients with an acute leukemia and patients who have undergone bone marrow and stem cell transplantation. Mortality from disseminated fungal infection is high. The most common fungal infections are caused by *Candida albicans*, non-*albicans* species, and *Aspergillus fumigatus*. The use of prophylactic antifungals (in particular fluconazole) is likely responsible for a recent shift from invasive candidiasis toward invasive aspergillosis and non-*albicans* species infections. Neutropenic patients with persistent fever lasting longer than 3 to 5 days should receive empiric antifungal coverage. Combination antifungal therapy with caspofungin and liposomal amphotericin B followed by voriconazole maintenance after completion of caspofungin and liposomal amphotericin B has proven to be a safe regimen for immunosuppressed children with invasive pulmonary aspergillosis.

The management of infectious complications in the febrile neutropenic pediatric patient requires an aggressive multidisciplinary approach. The emergency department physician, nurse, respiratory therapist, hospitalist, and intensivist should work in conjunction with the pediatric oncology and infectious disease teams to develop the best management strategy for these patients.

III. SHOCK IN THE PEDIATRIC ONCOLOGY PATIENT

A. Risk Factors

Case Study

A 5-year-old with a history of acute lymphocytic leukemia is brought into the pediatric intensive care unit (PICU) from a referring hospital where he presented 24 hours ago with fever, neutropenia, and thrombocytopenia. He was treated with ceftriaxone and acetaminophen. He became oliguric, tachycardiac, and hypothermic. He received 500 mL of normal saline prior to transfer. On arrival to the PICU he is found to be lethargic, hypothermic, hypotensive, and tachycardiac.

- Should this patient receive additional IV fluids?
- Should this patient be intubated?
- What antibiotics are indicated in this patient?
- What are the risk factors for this patient?

Shock and respiratory failure in the pediatric oncology patient are the most common reasons for admission to the pediatric intensive care unit. Although the oncology patient's clinical presentation of septic shock may be similar to that of noncancer patients (see **Chapter 7**), the critically ill oncology patient presents additional challenges to the healthcare provider. These patients typically present with fever, neutropenia, septic shock, and varying degrees of preexisting end-organ dysfunction.

B. Treatment

The general principles for the management and diagnosis of septic shock are covered in **Chapter 7**. The ultimate therapeutic goal in septic shock is to restore and maintain optimal organ perfusion. Acceptable intermediate goals include restoration of the patient's mental status and urine output (1 mL/kg/h). Typical fluid requirements range from 40 to 200 mL/kg during the initial phase of resuscitation. Aggressive fluid management (60 mL/kg in the first hour); broad-spectrum antimicrobial coverage that includes gram-positive, gram-negative, antifungal, and antiviral medications (depending on the clinical presentation); early use of inotropic and vasopressor support; and positive pressure ventilation maximize the potential for a positive outcome. Early implementation of renal replacement therapy is indicated in the fluid-overloaded patient with renal insufficiency. The practitioner should be attentive to patients presenting in shock but not responding to conventional resuscitative measures. A significant contributing factor to the shock state in these patients may be a cardiogenic component resulting from chemotherapy-related (anthracyclines, high-dose cyclophosphamide, 5-fluorouracil) or radiation-related cardiomyopathy. The use of corticosteroids is indicated in patients with vasopressor-resistant

> !
>
> *Vasopressor Support in Sepsis*
>
> - *Dopamine 5–10 mcg /kg/min*
> - *Norepinephrine 0.05–0.1 µg /kg/min*
> - *Epinephrine 0.05–0.1 µg /kg/min*
> - *Hydrocortisone 2 mg/kg*
>
> !

shock, purpura fulminans, or suspected or proven adrenocortical insufficiency. The initial recommended dose is 2 mg/kg of hydrocortisone. Early transfer to a pediatric intensive care unit for inotropic and vasopressor support and invasive cardiopulmonary monitoring is indicated in patients who do not respond to fluid resuscitation.

The care of these patients should be carefully directed to avoid end-organ failure, as they have substantially greater mortality from multiple-organ-system failure than do noncancer pediatric patients.

C. Prognosis

Although the survival rates for pediatric cancer patients with septic shock are lower than the survival rates for noncancer pediatric patients, recent data support an aggressive approach in the care of these patients.

IV. WATER AND ELECTROLYTE PROBLEMS

Water and electrolyte disorders (see **Chapter 9**) are commonplace in the pediatric oncology patient. These disorders are usually the result of the primary tumor's impact on the kidney and/or the urinary tract, or secondary to toxic effects of chemotherapy on the kidney.

A. Tumor Lysis Syndrome

Case Study

A 12-year-old, previously healthy female presents to the emergency department with fever, tachypnea, oliguria, petechia, and generalized edema. Her initial complete blood count (CBC) shows a WBC count of 250,000 mm^3, platelets at 32,000/mm^3, hemoglobin at 7.2 g/dL, lactate dehydrogenase (LDH) at 3000 international units/L, uric acid at 12 mg/dL, potassium at 6.2 mmol/L, phosphorus at 9 mg/dL (2.9 mmol/L), and calcium at 6 mg/dL (1.5 mmol/L).

- What are this patients major risks?
- What is the most important treatment strategy?
- Should you call for help?

Tumor lysis syndrome (TLS) is characterized by hyperuricemia, hyperkalemia, hyperphosphatemia, and hypocalcemia. It most often develops approximately 12 to 72 hours after the initiation of chemotherapy but may also occur after administration of steroids, hormones, or radiation therapy.

Tumor lysis syndrome occurs most frequently in patients with a large tumor burden (Burkitt lymphoma, lymphoblastic lymphoma, and leukemia) or in those in whom a tumor is widely disseminated, rapidly proliferating, or highly sensitive to chemotherapy. The incidence of TLS is unknown. Patients with leukemia or Burkitt lymphoma with elevated LDH (>500 units/L) have the highest risk of developing TLS or anuria. Laboratory evidence of TLS is far more frequent than the actual symptomatic clinical syndrome.

1. Symptoms

Tumor lysis syndrome affects children of all ages. Symptoms commonly found in patients with TLS include anorexia, malaise, weakness, vomiting, hiccups, paresthesia, tetany, carpopedal spasm, and seizures.

2. Pathophysiology

The high cell turnover found in many acute leukemias and lymphomas results in an increase in the by-products of cellular breakdown, which is dramatically accentuated by chemotherapy. This leads to a dramatic rise in plasma levels of cellular by-products, such as uric acid, urea nitrogen, phosphorus, and potassium, with rapid saturation of renal homeostatic mechanisms and ensuing hyperkalemia, hyperuricemia, and hyperphosphatemia. As a result of calcium phosphate precipitation in the microvasculature, phosphorus elevation leads to hypocalcemia. The glomerular filtration rate then declines and progresses to renal failure as a result of the precipitation of calcium phosphate and uric acid crystals in the renal tubules. The risk of acute renal failure increases if the primary tumor infiltrates or obstructs the normal flow of urine. Other risk factors for acute renal failure include preexisting renal pathology and dehydration.

3. Treatment

The key to the management of TLS is early diagnosis of the primary condition, recognition of the risk factors, and aggressive management. In patients with high risk of TLS, cytoreductive chemotherapy should be delayed until preventive treatment measures are initiated. A summary of TLS treatment is presented in **Table 19-2**. Essential treatment measures are as follows:

- **Monitoring.** Patients with TLS should be monitored for electrocardiographic changes associated with hyperkalemia (prolonged PR, flattened P, widened QRS, peaked T wave) and/or hypocalcemia (prolonged QT interval).

- **Hydration.** Vigorous IV hydration should begin at least 24 hours before the initiation of chemotherapy. Infusion rates are usually 2 to 4 times maintenance. Urine alkalinization is recommended. The goal is to promote uric acid solubility and excretion by increasing the urinary pH to 7 to 7.5. Recommended solutions are 5% dextrose in 0.25% normal saline with 60 to 100 mmol of sodium bicarbonate/L.

Table 19-2. Treatment of Tumor Lysis Syndrome

- Hydrate with 5% dextrose in 0.25% normal saline + 60-100 mmol sodium bicarbonate/L at 2-4 times maintenance. Monitor urine output.
- Control uric acid:
    - Urate oxidase (rasburicase): 0.2 mg/kg once daily in a 30-minute IV infusion for 5 days. Contraindicated in patients with glucose-6-phosphate dehydrogenase (G6PD) deficiency.
    - Allopurinol: 10 mg/kg/day PO 24-48 hours prior to initiation of chemotherapy.
- Keep urine pH 7-7.5. Maintain specific gravity ~1.010.
- Restrict potassium and phosphorus. Monitor hyperkalemic patients with a cardiopulmonary monitor.
- Replace calcium in symptomatic patients only.
- Consider early renal replacement therapy in patients with refractory hyperkalemia or with rapid decline in renal function.

- **Hyperkalemia and Hyperphosphatemia.** Potassium and phosphorus should be restricted.

- **Urine Output.** Urine flow should be maintained at about 2 to 4 mL/kg/h. Diuretic use is discouraged in the volume-depleted patient. Osmotic diuretics (mannitol) and/or furosemide may be used in normovolemic or fluid-overloaded patients with poor urine output.

- **Uric-Acid Control.** Uric-acid control may be obtained with recombinant urate oxidase (rasburicase) or with a xanthine oxidase inhibitor (allopurinol). The usual dose of rasburicase in children is 0.15 to 0.2 mg/kg IV given over 30 minutes, once per day for 5 days. This produces a sharp and sustained drop in uric acid levels. Urate oxidase infusions are contraindicated in patients with glucose-6-phosphate dehydrogenase (G6PD) deficiency. Allopurinol reduces the conversion of nucleic acids to uric acid but does not affect existing uric-acid levels. The initial oral dose is 10 mg/kg/day, starting 24 to 48 hours prior to initiation of chemotherapy. A recent study showed a more rapid reduction of uric acid and lower plasma levels in a group of children randomized to rasburicase when compared to the group treated with allopurinol.

- **Management of Severe Electrolyte Disturbances.** Patients with potassium levels >6.5 mmol/L or with electrocardiographic signs of hyperkalemia should receive insulin, glucose, bicarbonate, and calcium (see **Chapter 9**). Diuretics should be used with caution in dehydrated patients. Kayexalate, taken orally at 1 g/kg, may be helpful in preventing potassium rebound after the transient effect of acute hyperkalemia treatment. Renal replacement therapy (hemodialysis, continuous venovenous hemofiltration) should be considered early in patients with refractory hyperkalemia or in patients with rapid decline in renal function. Calcium replacement during TLS is indicated only in patients with neuromuscular irritability secondary to hypocalcemia, including seizures, arrhythmias, or positive Chvostek or Trousseau signs. Calcium replacement in nonsymptomatic hypocalcemic patients may aggravate calcium phosphate precipitation in the renal tubules. Hyperphosphatemia is managed with oral phosphate binders such as sevelamer hydrochloride, calcium carbonate, calcium acetate, or aluminum hydroxide.

V. NEUROLOGIC EMERGENCIES

A. Hyperleukocytosis and Stroke

1. Definition

Hyperleukocytosis is defined as a WBC of ≥100,000/mm^3 in the peripheral blood.

2. Risk Factors

Hyperleukocytosis occurs in children with leukemia and myeloproliferative disorders. Children with hyperleukocytosis are at increased risk for stroke due to leukostasis (sludging of leukemic cells in capillary vessels). Children with acute myeloid leukemia (AML) are at the greatest risk, followed by children with acute lymphoblastic leukemia (ALL) and children with chronic myelogenous leukemia (CML). Patients with hyperleukocytosis are at risk for tumor lysis syndrome, cerebral stroke (ischemia, hemorrhage, edema), and pulmonary stasis.

3. Clinical Findings

Clinically significant hyperleukocytosis occurs with WBC of >200,000/mm^3 in AML and in excess of 300,000/mm^3 in ALL and chronic myelocytic leukemia. Most patients are asymptomatic at presentation. Some patients, however, may present with subtle signs, such as headaches and blurred vision. In some instances the presentation is more dramatic and includes full-blown symptoms of cerebral stroke (changes in mental status, seizures, and increased intracranial pressure) or pulmonary leukostasis (hypoxia, cyanosis, and acidosis).

Children with hyperleukocytosis often develop a consumptive coagulopathy, likely through activation of the extrinsic pathway. The platelet count, PT (prothrombin time), aPTT (activated partial thromboplastin time), and fibrinogen should be monitored frequently. If a coagulopathy is confirmed, it must be treated aggressively. Computed tomographic or magnetic resonance imaging (MRI) with and without contrast is useful in evaluating the nature and extent of a stroke.

4. Treatment

The management of stroke is supportive. Treating the underlying malignancy with cytotoxic therapy may prevent additional strokes. The platelet count should be maintained at >50,000/mm^3. Packed red blood cell (PRBC) transfusions are discouraged in patients with asymptomatic anemia because of the risk of worsening hyperviscosity. Leukopheresis or exchange blood transfusion is the treatment of choice along with hydration, urine alkalinization, and administration of allopurinol or rasburicase (see discussion in Part IV, Section A.3).

B. Spinal Cord Compression

1. Pathophysiology

Case Study

A 15-year-old high school basketball player presents to the emergency department with a 1-month history of progressive back pain radiated to the right lower extremity, initially relieved by ibuprofen. The patient now complains of right lower-extremity weakness and paresthesias. On physical examination, there is tenderness to percussion on the back and decreased strength and hyporeflexia on the right lower extremity.

- What tests would be useful to evaluate the severity of this patient's condition?

- What pharmacologic treatment should initiated?

- Should you call for help?

Spinal cord compression most frequently results from metastatic spread (85%). The most common metastatic tumors involving the spinal cord are sarcomas (Ewing sarcoma, osteosarcoma), neuroblastomas, lymphomas, germ cell tumors, and metastatic central nervous system neoplasms. Tumors typically infiltrate by local extension into the epidural space through the intervertebral foramina from nearby structures, such as the ribs (sarcomas) and paravertebral adenopathy (lymphomas), or by hematogenous spread. Most primary spinal cord tumors are astrocytomas or ependymomas. Tumor spread into the epidural space may cause injury to the spinal cord by direct mechanical distortion or by vascular compromise with ischemia and edema or infarction.

2. Symptoms

Pain, either local or radicular, is the most frequently encountered presenting sign of spinal cord compression in children (80%). The onset of pain is often insidious and follows a gradually progressive course (weeks to months). However, once symptoms other than pain appear, progression may be rapid. In contrast to back pain from other causes, pain from vertebral metastasis may worsen with a recumbent position. Local vertebral tenderness to percussion often is present. Weakness and sensory loss are also common symptoms. Autonomic dysfunction (bladder or bowel incontinence) is a late sign of epidural compression. Lesions above T10 produce hyperreflexia and Babinski, whereas lesions below T10 that compress the conus or cauda equina produce hyporeflexia.

The duration, severity, and rapidity of onset of neurologic dysfunction are strong predictors of whether function can be maintained or restored.

3. Diagnosis

For children with suspected spinal cord involvement, MRI with gadolinium enhancement of the entire spine is the recommended diagnostic tool. Craniospinal T1-weighted and T2-weighted MRI allows demonstration of epidural involvement, intraparenchymal spread, and compression of nerve roots. Conventional radiographs may help reveal bone destruction but do not provide information about the spinal cord structure. Lumbar puncture is relatively contraindicated in spinal cord tumors except in leptomeningeal disease (diffuse seeding of the leptomeninges by tumor metastases).

4. Treatment

The prognosis for recovery in patients with neurologic dysfunction is related to the severity and duration of symptoms at the time of diagnosis. Early diagnosis and treatment are crucial. Non-oncologic diagnoses must be excluded (tuberculosis, osteomyelitis). The treatment of a child with cancer with confirmed spinal cord compression should include high-dose steroids (dexamethasone 1-2 mg/kg), emergent laminectomy, and posterior decompression, followed by radiation and chemotherapy as indicated. Prompt referral to a pediatric neurosurgeon and a pediatric oncologist is recommended.

!

Spinal Cord Compression Diagnosis and Treatment

- *Emergent MRI with gadolinium*
- *Dexamethasone 1-2 mg/kg IV*
- *Emergent laminectomy and posterior decompression*
- *Radiation and chemotherapy*

!

Key Points

Oncologic Emergencies and Complications

- Early admission to the PICU should be considered for pediatric oncology patients who arrive in the emergency department.
- Preexisting organ dysfunction from chemotherapy or its complications is not uncommon in pediatric oncology patients.
- Fever in neutropenic patients should be addressed aggressively with early use of broad-spectrum antimicrobials, colony-stimulating factors, and a methodical search for the infectious source.
- Resistant bacterial or fungal infections should be considered in patients with a history of longstanding fever and infections.
- Respiratory distress in the pediatric cancer patient may reflect bacterial, fungal, or viral infection or toxicity.
- High-resolution CT should be utilized in patients with respiratory insufficiency irrespective of the plain radiographic findings. Bronchoalveolar lavage should be considered early to clarify etiology.
- Early institution of a lung-protective strategy, including the use of high-frequency oscillatory ventilation, may improve the outcome in patients with respiratory failure.
- For patients with shock who do not respond to conventional fluid challenges, consider early evaluation for cardiac dysfunction.
- The possibility of previous high-dose steroid use and the risk of adrenal insufficiency should be taken into consideration.
- Tumor lysis syndrome is characterized by hyperuricemia, hyperkalemia, and hyperphosphatemia.
- Tumor lysis syndrome may result in renal failure and potentially fatal cardiac arrhythmias. Frequent laboratory studies, aggressive hydration, and alkalinization are helpful in reducing these risks.
- Hyperleukocytosis can cause coagulopathy and hyperviscosity, leading to lung injury and stroke. Prompt initiation of cancer therapy is recommended.
- Emergence of leg weakness, paresthesias in the lower extremities, and/or bowel or bladder dysfunction in children with a history of cancer are symptoms suggestive of spinal cord compression.

Suggested Readings

1. Carcillo JA, Fields AI. Clinical practice parameters for hemodynamic support of pediatric and neonatal patients in septic shock. *Crit Care Med.* 2002;30:1365-1378.

2. Fiser RT, West NK, Bush AJ, et al. Outcome of severe sepsis in pediatric oncology patients. *Pediatr Crit Care Med.* 2005;6:531-536.

3. Hagen SA, Craig DM, Martin PL, et al. Mechanically ventilated pediatric stem cell transplant recipients: effect of cord blood transplant and organ dysfunction on outcome. *Pediatr Crit Care Med.* 2003;4:206-213.

4. Hughes WT, Armstrong D, Bodey GP, et al. 2002 guidelines for the use of antimicrobial agents in neutropenic patients with cancer. *Clin Infect Dis.* 2002;34:730-751.

5. Jacobe SJ, Hassan A, Veys P, et al. Outcome of children requiring admission to an intensive care unit after bone marrow transplantation. *Crit Care Med.* 2003;31:1299-1305.

6. Mejia R, Cortes J, Brown D, et al. Oncologic Emergencies and Complications. In: Rogers MC, ed. *Rogers Textbook of Pediatric Intensive Care.* Philadelphia, PA: Lippincott Williams & Wilkins; 2008:1710-1724.

7. Porcu P, Cripe LD, Ng EW, et al. Hyperleukocytic leukemias and leukostasis: a review of pathophysiology, clinical presentation and management. *Leuk Lymphoma.* 2000;39:1-18.

8. Rheingold SR, Lange BJ. Oncologic emergencies. In Fleisher GR, Ludwig S, Henretig FM, Ruddy RM, Silverman BK. *Textbook of Pediatric Emergency Medicine.* 5th ed. Philadelphia, PA: Lippincott Williams & Wilkins; 2005:1202-1230.

9. Walsh TJ, Teppler H, Donowitz GR, et al. Caspofungin versus liposomal amphotericin B for empirical antifungal therapy in patients with persistent fever and neutropenia. *N Engl J Med.* 2004;351:1391-1402.

10. Watson RS, Carcillo JA. Scope and epidemiology of pediatric sepsis. *Pediatr Crit Care* Med. 2005;6:S3-S5.

Chapter 20:

ACUTE RENAL FAILURE

Objectives

- Describe the incidence and etiology of acute renal failure.
- Recognize risk factors to implement preventive strategies.
- Review the evaluation and treatment of acute renal failure.
- Identify common fluid and electrolyte abnormalities.
- Compare renal replacement therapies.

Case Study

A 3-year-old boy is admitted with a 4-day history of abdominal pain and bloody diarrhea. He becomes listlessness and oliguric the day before admission. On physical examination the child is tachycardic (150 beats/min), pale and some petechiae are evident in abdomen and extremities.

- What part of this patient's history could be of help for making a diagnosis?

- What findings of the physical examination and laboratory tests should be relevant?

I. INTRODUCTION

The rapid drop in glomerular filtration rate (GFR) and the inability of the kidney to regulate fluids, plasma electrolytes, and acid-base homeostasis are the hallmarks of acute renal failure (ARF).

The increased survival of critical illnesses and the incorporation of new therapeutic techniques and drugs, such as immunosuppressive agents, have modified the epidemiology of ARF. The causes of ARF may differ from one geographic area to another. For example, incidences of hemolytic uremic syndrome (HUS) vary between countries with differing levels of social development. In the US adult population, the incidence of ARF is 21 per 100,000, of which 21% are prerenal and 45% are due to acute tubular necrosis. There are no large-scale US studies of the incidence of ARF in children, though an incidence of 0.8 per 100,000 has been estimated at some tertiary centers. The incidence of ARF in neonatal intensive care units ranges between 8% and 24% of admissions, whereas in pediatric intensive care units (PICUs) it ranges between 2.5% and 4.5%. In adult ICUs, the figures cited are between 7% and 25%.

II. DEFINITION

An acute decrease of the urinary volume (urinary output <0.5-1 mL/kg/h) usually raises suspicion of ARF. Oliguria may be the result of a physiologic homeostatic response in response to a drop in renal blood flow secondary to hypovolemia or hypotension (prerenal failure). Oliguria can also be the result of an obstruction of the urinary excretory pathways (postrenal failure). These mechanisms and others result in renal failure. A sharp rise in serum creatinine concentration by more than 50% of its basal value, together with a rise of blood urea nitrogen (BUN), are proof of ARF. In some circumstances, there may be a rise of creatinine and BUN in the presence of a normal urinary volume (non-oliguric ARF). Non-oliguric renal failure is the most common type of renal failure in neonates (60%), followed by oliguric failure (25%) and anuria (15%).

> **!** *An increase in creatinine equal to or above 0.5 mg/dL in 24 hours indicates renal failure.*

To summarize, the diagnosis of ARF is based on two criteria: oliguria and elevation of the serum creatinine level above baseline. Oliguria, though nonspecific, is the earliest and most sensitive indicator. The level of creatinine is influenced by the patient's volume of distribution, liver function, muscle mass, and catabolism. Back-leaking and tubular secretion of creatinine rise as the glomerular filtrate drops.

ARF is defined as a serum creatinine level twice the basal value. In full-term newborns, the creatinine level is similar to that of the mother until day 7, whereas in premature infants younger than 32 weeks, serum creatinine is higher. When the basal creatinine is unknown, ARF in the PICU is defined as a serum creatinine level twice the upper limit for age and sex.

III. ETIOLOGY

It is necessary to differentiate ARF due to preexisting renal disease from ARF secondary to other conditions, such as sepsis and shock, or as an effect of multiorgan failure or the action of nephrotoxins.

The most frequent causes of primary renal failure in children are HUS, rapidly progressive glomerulonephritis, and acute interstitial nephritis. Occasionally, the cause is an undiagnosed chronic renal disease, such as renal dysplasias or cystic disease.

In the neonate, bilateral renal vein thrombosis associated with umbilical vein catheter and severe dehydration can cause ARF. It can also arise in a child with a decompensated nephrotic syndrome. The most frequent causes of ARF in neonates, however, are severe perinatal asphyxia and sepsis and, where applicable, cardiac surgery.

> !
>
> *Prerenal failure is a high-risk condition that must be identified and corrected promptly to avoid structural damage to the kidney.*
>
> !

In children, ARF most commonly results from comorbid conditions. These can include hematologic and oncologic diseases, urologic conditions, and hepatic insufficiency. ARF may also occur following cardiovascular surgery or liver transplantation. The most frequent causes, however, are ischemia and sepsis. The use of antibiotics, antimycotics, chemotherapy, nonsteroidal antiinflammatory drugs, and angiotensin-converting enzyme inhibitors also contribute to ARF. Ischemia is a frequent cause in young children, whereas nephrotoxic causes predominate in school-age children and adolescents. ARF, when it occurs in patients with multiorgan failure, usually has multiple etiologies that include ischemia, sepsis, inflammatory mediators, and nephrotoxic drug effects.

Hypovolemia or a decrease in effective arterial volume restricts renal perfusion and adversely affects renal function. Causes of hypovolemia include: hemorrhage, intestinal obstruction, severe burns, decompensated nephrotic syndrome, and trauma. It can also arise as a result of polyuria, which may be caused by osmotic diuresis in diabetic ketoacidosis, the different forms of diabetes insipidus, a salt-wasting syndrome, or mineralocorticoid deficiency. A fall in effective arterial volume is also found in heart failure and any situation that involves a decrease in cardiac output.

HUS consists of microangiopathic hemolytic anemia and thrombocytopenia associated with oliguria or anuria preceded by bloody diarrhea. The cause is frequently an intestinal infection by a verotoxin-producing strain of Escherichia coli. HUS may have a multisystemic course that involves the nervous system, the colonic wall, the pancreas, or the myocardium. According to some reports, HUS is responsible for one-third of all ARF cases presented to PICUs.

Urinary tract obstruction, like posterior urethral valves or bilateral ureter obstruction, can cause kidney damage and loss of function. Causes of ARF are summarized in **Table 20-1.**

Table 20-1. Causes of ARF

Prerenal Failure

Intravascular volume depletion
- Hemorrhage/bleeding
- Severe dehydration
- Gastrointestinal losses
- Third space losses (burns, trauma, capillary leak syndrome)
- Urinary losses (central or nephrogenic diabetes insipidus, osmotic diuresis, salt-wasting, diuretics)

Decreased effective intravascular blood volume
- Congestive heart failure
- Low cardiac output
- Tamponade or pericarditis
- Liver failure

Renal Failure

Acute tubular necrosis
- Hypoxic ischemic: sepsis and septic shock
- Drug related: aminoglycosides, amphotericin B, cisplatin, nonsteroidal antiinflammatory, angiotensin II receptor antagonist, radiocontrast agents, fluorinated anesthetics
- Endogenous toxins: rhabdomyolysis, hemolysis, tumor lysis syndrome

HUS

Acute glomerulonephritis

Acute interstitial nephritis: drug-induced or idiopathic

Infection/pyelonephritis

Vascular injury: cortical bilateral necrosis, renal or arterial thrombosis

Postrenal

Urethral obstruction: urinary catheter obstruction, stone, blood clots, posterior urethral valves

Bladder obstruction: neurogenic bladder, stone, tumor

Bilateral urethral obstruction: tumor mass

Modified from Barletta GM, Bunchrman T. Acute renal failure in children and infants. *Curr Opin Crit Care.* 2004; 10:499-504.

IV. RISK FACTORS

There is strong evidence that suggests an association between sepsis and ARF. Hypovolemia, is a significant risk factor. Liver failure can cause a hepatorenal syndrome. Although a cause-effect relationship has not been established, patients on mechanical ventilation appear to be at an increased risk of developing ARF. Hypotension and shock are often implicated in the development of ARF, though usually in the presence of other predisposing factors. Rhabdomyolysis can generate ARF, though it has not been clearly established at what level of creatine kinase and myoglobin this occurs. Myoglobin in the presence of hypovolemia or ischemia is particularly nephrotoxic.

In the postoperative course of cardiovascular surgery, the underlying cardiac pathology, the type of surgery performed, and the duration of cardiopulmonary bypass are all factors that may increase the risk for ARF. For transplant recipients, risk factors include the duration of the surgery and the amount of blood lost. The type of medication utilized (particularly tacrolimus and cyclosporin) may also contribute.

The risk associated with contrast media has been reduced with the employment of nonionic isosmolar substances. The total amount of contrast administered is directly proportional to the risk involved in the presence of other predisposing risk factors. Drugs most commonly associated with nephrotoxicity include aminoglycosides, vancomycin, amphotericin B, intravenous (IV) immunoglobulin, acyclovir, and immunosuppressive agents. Contrast media can produce ARF, however the risk has been reduced with the employment of nonionic isosmolar substances.

In patients with low effective arterial volume in whom filtration is maintained at the expense of vasoconstriction of the efferent arteriole, vasodilators, like nifedipine or angiotension converting enzyme inhibitors, may cause a sharp drop in filtration.

Tumor lysis syndrome, especially occurring in children with lymphoma (who may develop it before beginning therapy), can also precipitate ARF (**See Chapter 19**).

In a prospective analysis of children admitted to intensive therapy, Bailey and colleagues identified multiple risk factors associated with ARF, including thrombocytopenia, hypoxemia, hypotension, disturbances of coagulation, and an age greater than 12 years old. Thrombocytopenia and coagulation disturbances reflect the underlying diseases of an oncologic and hematologic nature or the presence of HUS, rather than being individual risk factors. Baseline risks, acute clinical conditions, and diagnostic/therapeutic agents associated with the development of in-hospital ARF are shown in **Table 20-2.**

Table 20-2. Risk Factors for Acute Renal Failure

Baseline Risks	Acute Clinical Conditions	Nephrotoxic Agents
Chronic kidney disease	Sepsis	Antimicrobial agents
Heart failure	Hypotension	Chemotherapeutic drugs
Congenital heart disease	Hypovolemia	Immunosuppressive agents
Liver failure	Rhabdomyolysis	Nonsteroidal antiinflammatory drugs
Hypoalbuminemia	Nonrenal solid organ transplantation	Contrast media
	Abdominal compartment syndrome	
	Mechanical ventilation	

Modified from Leblanc M, Kellum J, Gibney N, et al. Risk factors for acute renal failure: inherent and modificable risks. *Curr Opin Crit Care.* 2005; 11:533-536.

V. CLASSIFICATION OF ARF

Diverse factors that affect the intravascular volume or the arterial effective volume can lead to failure of renal function and can be rapidly corrected by fluid resuscitation and/or restoration of the mean arterial pressure. The most frequent situations linked to prerenal failure are sepsis and septic shock. There are, however, other causes, such as low cardiac output, trauma, hypovolemia, hepatorenal syndrome, or abdominal compartment syndrome that may also aggravate prerenal failure. All of these causes, if not promptly resolved or if particularly intense, may lead to acute tubular necrosis or, in extreme cases, bilateral cortical necrosis.

> ! *Traditional indicators used to differentiate prerenal from renal failure are scarcely useful in the critically ill patient.* !

Drug-induced nephrotoxic injury is a significant cause of renal parenchymal failure in the PICU. It may improve after stopping the responsible agent. Structural changes involving the glomeruli and tubules can be seen in biopsy specimens. A careful medical history and a meticulous physical examination, laboratory studies, and imaging studies should be completed. Renal biopsy may be indicated in other conditions, such as when glomerular lesions needing immunosuppressant therapy are suspected.

Postrenal failure is the least frequent in the pediatric population and can be observed in obstructive uropathies, especially during the first year of life. Tumor lysis syndrome may provoke an obstructive lesion associated with calcium phosphate or uric acid precipitation.

Urinary parameters and fractional excretions can contribute to differentiate prerenal from renal failure (**Table 20-3**); however their use is limited to initial stages of renal failure before the use of diuretics or vasoactive drugs.

Table 20-3. Urinary Parameters for the Differential Diagnosis Between Prerenal and Renal ARF*

Urinary Indices	Prerenal	Renal
Urinalysis	Hyaline casts	Abnormal
Specific gravity	1.020	1.010
U osm (mOsm/kg H_2O)	>500	<300
U Na (mmol/L)	<20	>40*
Fractional excretion		
Sodium (%)	<1	>2*
Urea (%)	<0.35	>0.35
Uric acid (%)	<7	>20
BUN/creatinine	>20	<20

*Not useful when the patient has received furosemide in the last 12 hours or is receiving dopamine.

VI. DIAGNOSIS

A. Clinical Diagnosis

ARF may occur in some patients with clinical conditions leading to hypovolemia, such as dehydration, trauma, sepsis, or exposure to nephrotoxins. The presence of peripheral edema and hypervolemia (heart failure) is suggestive of initial renal injury. The presence of cutaneous signs, such as petechia or purpura, may suggest a diagnosis of HUS.

The presence of anuria is indicative of complete obstructive lesion, vascular lesion, rapidly progressive glomerulonephritis, or bilateral cortical necrosis. Anuria with bladder distention is suggestive of an obstructive uropathy.

B. Laboratory Diagnosis

The upper normal creatinine values vary with age. Both creatinine and BUN values can be higher or lower depending on specific clinical conditions (**Figure 20-1**). Normal values of creatinine, BUN, and diagnostic criteria for oliguria are found in **Table 20-4.** Other metabolic alterations frequently seen in patients with ARF include:

- Metabolic acidosis with wide anion gap due to the presence of sulphates and phosphates
- Hyperkalemia
- Hyponatremia
- Hyperphosphatemia and hypocalcemia

Figure 1. Clinical Situations That Influence BUN and Creatinine Values

↑ **BUN** ↓

↑ BUN:
- Hypercatabolic states
- Sepsis
- Starvation
- GI bleeding
- Corticosteroids
- High protein diet
- Dehydration
- Renal hypoperfusion

↓ BUN:
- Malnutrition
- Low protein diet
- Liver failure
- Nephrotic syndrome
- Hypometabolism

↑ **Creatinine** ↓

↑ Creatinine:
- Rhabdomyolysis
- Cimetidine
- TLS
- Dehydratation

↓ Creatinine:
- Liver failure
- Loss of muscle mass
- Hyperlipemia

GI, gastrointestinal; TLS, tumor lysis syndrome

Table 20-4. Normal Values of Creatinine, BUN, and Oliguria Diagnosis Criteria

Value	Neonate	Infant	Child	Adolescent
BUN, mg/dL	3-12	5-18	7-18	7-18
Creatinine, mg/dL	0.3-1.0	0.2-0.5	0.3-0.7	0.5-1.0
Oliguria	<1 mL/kg/h	<1 mL/kg/h	<0.5 mL/kg/h	< 300 mL/d

The presence of proteinuria, hematuria, or casts in a urinalysis is suggestive of a glomerular lesion, whereas the presence of eosinophils suggests interstitial nephritis.

C. Diagnostic Imaging

Renal ultrasound may help rule out obstructive uropathy or chronic lesions and show the kidney's size and echogenicity. A Doppler ultrasound may be helpful to rule out renal vascular lesions. Scintirenography study with technetium diethylene triamine pentaacetic acid scan (TcDTPA) is useful for calculating the glomerular filtration rate of each kidney (**Table 20-5**). The initial phase reflects renal perfusion. Activity measured after the first few minutes shows functional mass. TcDTPA is eliminated through the urine and may help evaluate the renal excretory system. Scintirenography study may be indicated in established renal disease or during the recovery phase of ARF.

Table 20-5. Renal Imaging

US: size and shape of both kidneys
- Suspicion of urinary tract obstruction
- (hydronephrosis, renal calculi, bladder distension, and thickness)
- Suspicion of occlusion of renal vessels
- Suspicion of chronic renal disease
- Suspicion of unilateral kidney absence

Radionuclide scanning: TcDTPA (some GF rate is required)
- Renal perfusion and renal mass function (glomerular filtration)
- Visualization of the urinary collecting system
- Visualization of small cortical lesions

TcDMSA: visualization of renal structure
(60-70% is retained within the renal cortex)

Doppler US: assesses renal blood flow velocity patterns and absence or presence of diastolic flow

US, ultrasound; GF, glomerular filtration; TcDMSA, technetium labeled dimercaptosuccinic acid

VII. MANAGEMENT OF ARF

Children with ARF should be managed in a center that has the capability to offer renal replacement therapies, including peritoneal dialysis, hemodialysis, and continuous venovenous replacement therapies. If these therapies are unavailable, children should be stabilized and transferred to a center where renal support treatment is offered. Dialysis can rapidly restore fluid and electrolyte homeostasis.

> ! *The objectives of the management of children with ARF are to maintain fluid, electrolyte, and metabolic homeostasis, prevent progression of the renal failure, treat the underlying cause of ARF, and provide adequate nutritional support.* !

A. Prevention of Renal Injury

> ! *Maintenance of an adequate organ (renal) perfusion is the basis of the preventive strategy.* !

Prevention of renal injury consists of anticipating and avoiding potential renal injury. Preventive strategies should be included in the management of all critically ill patients before the onset of ARF or once renal failure is established in order to avoid postinjury progression.

1. Renal Blood Flow

Primary prevention methods consist of ensuring adequate renal blood flow and avoiding nephrotoxicity. Early recognition and adequate management of hemodynamic instability or risk factors that may lead to hemodynamic decompensation are key elements for ensuring maintenance of renal blood flow. Aggressive fluid resuscitation may result in a reduction of end organ failure, including ARF. The use of vasopressor agents is discussed in **Chapter 7.** Dopamine and norepinephrine are the preferred first-line alpha-adrenergic agents in fluid refractory warm shock. There is evidence that suggests that reversing hypotension with norepinephrine after adequate fluid resuscitation may improve renal blood flow. There is, however, evidence against the use of low-dose dopamine for the prevention of ARF. Loop diuretics or osmotic agents, such as mannitol, have shown to be no better than hydration alone for the prevention of renal injury.

Infusion of normal saline solution starting at 20 mL/kg or more should be given to patients with suspected prerenal ARF in order to improve or limit renal injury and avoid the progression from a prerenal situation to parenchymal injury. Care should be taken to detect and avoid fluid overload. Frequent clinical evaluation, close monitoring of vital signs, and meticulous measurement of the urinary output will help with the early recognition of signs of improvement or fluid overload (tachypnea, crackles, or hepatic congestion) after volume administration. Signs of fluid overload are an indication to stop fluid administration. Close monitoring of the central venous pressure is useful in guiding the amount of fluid to be administered without pushing the central venous pressure beyond 6 to 8 mm Hg. Patients that respond to volume administration should be given adequate maintenance fluids.

2. Nephrotoxic Medications and ARF

Patients at risk should be carefully hydrated prior to the administration of potential nephrotoxins (eg, cancer chemotherapy agents, aminoglycosides, immunosuppressants, and others). Patients at risk for tumor lysis syndrome should be carefully hydrated (see **Chapter 19**). Nephrotoxic drugs should be avoided or adjusted to creatinine clearance. Drugs with renal elimination should be given at lower doses or longer intervals in accordance with the degree of renal function. Creatinine clearance can be difficult to calculate in patients receiving diuretics or electrolyte infusions. In these situations, the glomerular filtration rate (GFR) may be calculated with the following formula:

$$\text{GFR} = \text{length (cm)} \times (K/\text{Pcr})$$

Pcr = plasma creatinine; K is constant for different age groups; younger than 1 year, K = 0.45; 1 to13 years, K = 0.55; adolescent male, K = 0.7; adolescent female, K = 0.55. This formula is not fully accurate; however, it is useful as a guide for drug dosage in relation to the creatinine clearance during ARF.

B. Management of Fluid and Electrolytes

Strict monitoring of input and output is mandatory for all patients with ARF. Indwelling urinary catheters (ie, Foley catheters) are not necessary in stable patients and should be avoided in order to reduce the risk of infection. Urinary catheters are indicated in young children with gastroenteritis and with suspected oliguria or anuria. Daily or twice daily weight measurements should be obtained in all patients with ARF.

1. Fluid Management

The objective in prerenal ARF is to achieve normovolemia. Fluid calculations in dehydrated patients should include the previous deficit, insensible losses, and ongoing losses. In euvolemic patients, fluid should be calculated to replace insensible and ongoing losses.

Fluid intake restriction is indicated in patients with fluid overload while replenishing insensible water losses (1 mL/kg/h). Replacement of partial urine losses may be considered, depending on the clinical situation. A trial of furosemide (1-4 mg/kg, to obtain 10 mL/kg urine in the following 4 hours) can be performed in patients with oliguria and fluid overload, in an attempt to stimulate urinary output and improve signs of fluid overload. Severe fluid overload is an indication for dialysis.

2. Management of Sodium

Hyponatremia is a frequent finding during ARF. Hyponatremia is usually dilutional. Less frequently, hyponatremia is caused by sodium loss during ARF with adequate urinary output. Fluid restriction is indicated in oliguric patients with dilutional hyponatremia. If adequate restriction is achieved, sodium levels should improve progressively. In patients with anuria maintenance, sodium should not be given. Correction with a 3% saline solution should be considered in patients with serum sodium <120 mEq/L or if clinical signs of hyponatremia are present. Correction with a 3% saline solution should be considered in patients with serum sodium <120 mEq/L or if clinical signs of hyponatremia are present, but only as a transient measure while dialysis is being prepared. Infusion of hypertonic saline solutions should be adjusted to raise the sodium level by no more than 0.5-1.0 mmol/kg/h. The amount of sodium necessary to achieve a desired sodium level (120-125 mmol/ L) in symptomatic patients is as follows:

$$\text{mmol of Na+ to administer} = (\text{Desired Na}^+ - \text{Measured Na}^+) \times \text{weight in Kg} \times 0.6$$

An infusion of 1 mmol/kg/h will raise the sodium by about 1 mmol/L/h. In the less common cases of hyponatremia secondary to sodium losses, sodium replacement may be indicated relative to the amount lost.

3. Management of Potassium

Hyperkalemia is a frequent finding during ARF. It can be fatal due to cardiac conduction abnormalities. It is secondary to decreased elimination, while endogenous production continues from tissue degradation, soft tissue injury, or hemolysis. Potassium restriction should always be indicated in patients with ARF.

Hypocalcemia and hyponatremia may exacerbate cardiac toxicity. Dialysis is the proper treatment for hyperkalemia secondary to ARF with potassium values of >7 mmol/L. Medical management, as described in **Chapter 10**, should be started with a potassium level ≥5.5 mmol/L. Patients with mild elevations of potassium (up to 6.5 mEq/L) and without ECG abnormalities can be managed medically. However, if renal function does not improve promptly, dialysis should be considered.

4. Management of Phosphorus and Calcium

Hyperphosphatemia can be managed with chelating agents that bind calcium in the gut (calcium carbonate 300-400 mg/kg/day), therefore preventing absorption. However, in cases of severe hyperphosphatemia, (phosphorus >10 mEq/L) dialysis should be started. Hypocalcemia should only be corrected in symptomatic patients only.

> **!**
>
> *In the presence of hypocalcemia with hyperphosphatemia, management should be aimed at reducing the phosphorus rather than increasing the levels calcium.*
>
> **!**

5. Management of Metabolic Acidosis

Metabolic acidosis is secondary to an inadequate excretion of hydrogen ions and ammonia. Severe acidosis can increase myocardial irritability, affect peripheral vascular resistance, enzyme activity, and energy production. Treatment of acidosis should be aimed at improving associated causes of acidosis, which include poor cardiac output, exogenous acid administration (eg, hyperchloremia secondary to sodium chloride administration), or respiratory acidosis. Mild-to-moderate metabolic acidosis with a pH >7.20 can be treated with oral bicarbonate supplements. Severe metabolic acidosis with pH <7.20 or metabolic acidosis in the presence of hyperkalemia should be corrected intravenously. Intravenous sodium bicarbonate should be given slowly in patients with anuria or oligoanuria, because they may not tolerate a rapid volume expansion. The formula for bicarbonate correction is as follows:

$$\text{mmol of sodium bicarbonate to administer} = \text{base deficit} \times \text{weight in kg} \times 0.3$$

Half the correction should be given in 1 hour, and the remainder over 3 hours.

C. Renal Replacement Therapies

Indications for renal replacement therapies include the following:

Fluid overload
Pulmonary edema
Congestive heart failure
Persistent anuria or oliguria
Refractory hypertension
Critically ill patient with oliguria and high fluid requirements (eg, parenteral nutrition, antibiotics, sedation, inotropes)
Critically ill patient with oliguria needing negative fluid balance

Electrolyte or acid-base disorders
Hyponatremia or hypernatremia
Hyperkalemia with potassium >7 mEq/L
Persistent acidosis

Toxin removal
Urea
Uric acid
Exogenous toxins

1. Peritoneal Dialysis

Children have a peritoneum with a greater surface area proportional to body mass. This makes peritoneal dialysis more effective in this age group. Access to the peritoneum is easier in the pediatric population, especially in small children where vascular access for other dialytic techniques can be a problem. Peritoneal dialysis is well tolerated, even in hemodynamically unstable patients.

Absolute contraindications for peritoneal dialysis are loss of peritoneal membrane surface, diminution of the abdominal continent (omphalocele or diaphragmatic hernia), extensive adhesions, ventriculoperitoneal shunt, and causes of peritoneal instability, such as peritonitis. Relative contraindications include recent abdominal surgery, large polycystic kidneys, cirrhosis with ascites, gastrostomy, or colostomy.

Rigid catheters placed at the bedside or flexible catheters placed by the surgeon can both be used in peritoneal dialysis. The latter are being used more frequently, because they are associated with fewer complications and last longer.

a. Prescription of Peritoneal Dialysis

Peritoneal dialysis can be done with automated machines or manually. When performing manual peritoneal dialysis, using sets with closed drainage systems helps to reduce the incidence of peritoneal contamination. The dialysis solution should be appropriately warmed.

During a peritoneal dialysis session, the following points should be specified:

- Composition of the dialysis solution
- Dialysis fill volumes
- Time of permanence of fluid during each cycle (dwell time)
- Number of cycles
- Addition of electrolytes or medication (potassium, heparin or antibiotics)

b. Choice of Dialysis Solution

Peritoneal dialysis solutions glucose concentrations vary from 1% glucose to 4.25% glucose. In general, initiation of dialysis is done with the lowest concentration of glucose solution possible for the patient. Concentrations of glucose can be increased gradually to obtain the expected ultrafiltrate. With glucose concentrations greater than 3%, rapid ultrafiltration or hyperglycemia must be carefully monitored.

c. Dialysis Fill Volume

On the first day of peritoneal dialysis, cycle fill volumes should be lower, approximately 20 mL/kg. On subsequent days, volume can be progressively increased up to 40 to 45 mL/kg, but should not exceed 1,200 mL total.

d. Dwell Time

Dwell time varies between 20 to 60 minutes, depending on the objective. Shorter time periods are used for fluid removal, while longer periods are used for solute clearance.

e. Dialysis Solution Additives

Potassium chloride is added when serum potassium is lower than 3.5 mmol/L. Usual doses are 3 to 3.5 mmol/L of dialysis solution. Heparin should be added (250 U/L) to the dialysis solution if the fluid obtained from peritoneum has blood or fibrin. An antibiotic should be added to the dialysis solution in patients with peritonitis due to peritoneal dialysis.

f. Complications of Acute Peritoneal Dialysis

The most frequent complication is mechanical blockage, which is usually caused by omental obstruction or fibrin accumulation. Changing the position of the patient or increasing the volume of the dialysis solution may be helpful in patients with omental obstruction. Fibrin accumulation can be prevented by flushing the catheter or by administering heparin. Sometimes, obstruction of the catheter with fibrin can be resolved with the use of fibrinolytics. Other complications include pain, intraperitoneal bleeding, leakage around the catheter, local infection, peritonitis, restriction of lung volumes, hydrothorax, and vascular volume contraction. Possible metabolic complications, such as hyperglycemia, hypokalemia, hypernatremia, metabolic alkalosis, or protein losses, also should be monitored.

2. Extracorporeal Renal Replacement Techniques

These therapies involve the circulation of blood through an extracorporeal filter with the objective of eliminating solutes or fluid. It can be classified in intermittent or continuous and arteriovenous or venovenous techniques. The discussion of these techniques is beyond the scope of this textbook and will not be covered.

D. Nutritional Support

Children with ARF have an increased rate of catabolism and are at risk of malnutrition. Adequate nutrition is essential for the treatment of ARF. Providing sufficient nutrition may be difficult, however, because of restrictions on the amount of fluid that may be administered.

Concentrated enteral or parenteral nutrition should be used to achieve these goals. The enteral route is always preferred. Lipids and concentrated glucose solutions should be used in order to improve caloric concentration. Essential amino acids can be used to decrease urea production. In some situations, dialysis techniques may be used to increase the amount of fluid that can be administered and to decrease nutritional limitations.

!

Nutritional plans should aim at achieving adequate caloric intake (45- 55 Kcal/kg/day), fluid restriction, limited protein intake (0.5-1 g/kg/day), and reduced or absent potassium intake.

!

E. Management of Anemia

!

Blood transfusion may increase the serum potassium concentration and may worsen arterial hypertension, cardiac failure, and acute pulmonary edema.

!

Anemia in children with ARF is usually mild and secondary to hemodilution. Anemia can also be secondary to hemolysis in situations such as HUS and systemic lupus erythematous, or it can be caused by blood loss secondary to gastrointestinal bleeding or multiple blood extractions. Transfusion of packed red blood cells is recommended if the hemoglobin value is lower than 7 g/dL.

F. Management of Hypertension

Hypertension is usually secondary to volume overload in patients with oliguria. Dialysis is indicated in hypervolemic, hypertensive patients failing to respond to fluid restriction and diuretics. Patients with severe hypertension and encephalopathy or cardiomyopathy should be treated aggressively (**Table 20-6**). Less severe hypertension can be treated with nifedipine 0.25 to 0.5 mg/kg dose up to 10 mg/dose. Doses of antihypertensive agents may need to be adjusted to the glomerular filtration rate.

Table 20-6. Medications in Hypertensive Emergencies

Medication	Loading Dose	Maintenance	Maximum Dose	Route
Labetalol	0.2-1.0 mg/kg (max 20 mg)	0.4-1.0 mg/kg/h	3 mg/kg/h	IV
Nicardipine	None	0.5-5.0 µg/kg/h	5 µg/kg/h	IV
Nitroprusside sodium (monitor thiocyanate levels)	None	0.3 µg/kg/min	10 µg/kg/min	IV
Hydralazine	0.2 mg/kg	5-20 mg every 4 h	20 mg	IV

VIII. OUTCOMES

Outcomes of ARF vary widely in the pediatric population. Prospective, multicenter outcome studies of ARF in critically ill children are insufficient. Expected survival rates depend on the absence of complications, such as multiorgan failure or sepsis. Recovery of normal renal function can take weeks to months. A percentage of children will progress to chronic renal failure.

Key Points

Acute Renal Failure

- Oliguria is the most frequent clinical manifestation of ARF.
- Increases in serum creatinine concentration by more than 50% of basal value, together with a rise of the BUN, are suggestive of ARF.
- Sepsis and hypovolemia are significant risk factors for developing ARF.
- Nephrotoxic medications to avoid in ARF include vancomycin, aminoglycosides, amphotericin B, IV immunoglobulin, acyclovir, or immunosuppressants.
- Traditional indicators used to differentiate prerenal from renal failure may support the diagnosis during the initial phase before the patient has received diuretics or vasoactive drugs. They are usually not useful in the critically ill child who needs multiple pharmacologic therapies.
- Metabolic acidosis, hyperkalemia, and hyponatremia are frequent metabolic conditions found in patients with ARF.
- Preventive strategies to avoid primary or secondary renal injury consist mainly of ensuring adequate renal blood flow and avoiding nephrotoxicity.
- Patients should be monitored for signs of fluid overload.
- Strict fluid balance and daily weight records are essential.
- Hyponatremia is usually dilutional and should be treated with fluid restriction or with dialysis. Hyperkalemia ≥7 mEq/L is an indication for dialysis.
- Broad indications for renal replacement therapies include fluid overload, electrolyte or acid base disorders, and toxin removal.
- An ideal nutrition plan should offer adequate caloric intake with fluid restriction, limit protein intake, and reduce or eliminate potassium intake.

Suggested Readings

1. Andreoli S. Acute renal failure. *Curr Opin Pediatr.* 2002; 14:183-188.

2. Bailey D, Phan V, Litalien C, et al. Risk factors of acute renal failure in critically ill children: A prospective descriptive epidemiological study. *Pediatr Crit Care Med.* 2007; 8: 29-35.

3. Barletta GM, Bunchrman T. Acute renal failure in children and infants. *Curr Opin Crit Care.* 2004; 10:499-504.

4. Bellomo R. Defining, quantifying, and classifying acute renal failure. *Crit Care Clin.* 2005; 21:223-237.

5. Kellum J, Leblanc M, Gibney N, et al. Primary prevention of acute renal failure in the critically ill. *Curr Opin Crit Care.* 2005; 11:537-41.

6. Lameire N, Hoste E. Reflections on the definition, classification, and diagnostic evaluation of acute renal failure. *Curr Opin Crit Care.* 2004; 10:468-475.

7. Leblanc M, Kellum J, Gibney N, et al. Risk factors for acute renal failure: Inherent and modifiable risks. *Curr Opin Crit Care.* 2005; 11:533-536.

8. Stickle S, Brewer E, Goldstein S. Pediatric ARF epidemiology at a tertiary care center from 1999 to 2001. *Am J Kidney Dis.* 2005; 45:96-101.

9. Strazdins V, Watson A, Harvey B. Renal replacement therapy for acute renal failure in children: European guidelines. *Pediatr Nephrol.* 2004; 19:199-207.

10. Uchino S, Kellum J, Bellomo R, et al. Acute renal failure in critically ill patients: A multinational, multicenter study. *JAMA.* 2005; 294:813-818.

Chapter 21:

Postoperative Management

Objectives

- Discuss the anesthetic factors and their relation to the postoperative period.
- Identify particular pediatric age groups at increased risk.
- Describe a stratified approach to postoperative pain management.
- Identify and recognize the potential postoperative complications.
- Summarize the management of fluid, electrolyte, and nutritional support.
- Recognize and manage malignant hyperthermia.

Case Study

A 4-year-old female was admitted with signs of septic shock and an acute abdomen. She has a known history of asthma that is well controlled with beclomethasone metered dose inhaler. She undergoes an exploratory laparotomy with surgical findings consistent with ruptured acute appendicitis and intra-abdominal abscess. She was given a caudal block by the anesthesiologist. Soon after arrival to the ward she is noted to be febrile (39.5° C [103.1°F}), agitated with inspiratory stridor. Prior to your arrival to her bedside she was given intravenous morphine sulfate 0.1 mg/kg.

- What would you want to know about her preoperative and intraoperative course?

- What is the most likely etiology of her stridor and how would you manage it?

- What are the potential complications of administering morphine in this situation?

- What would be the best approach to her pain management?

- How would you manage her hydration in the first 24 hours postoperatively?

I. INTRODUCTION

The postoperative management of the pediatric patient is a continuum of the perioperative management of the surgical patient. Often, the status and stabilization of the patient prior to surgery and their anesthetic management determines their physiologic status and disposition in the postoperative period. Key concepts include fluid and electrolyte therapy, pediatric analgesia, and cardiopulmonary evaluation and management. This chapter attempts to integrate these principles and relate them specifically to the postoperative management of the pediatric patient.

II. PREOPERATIVE AND ANESTHETIC CONSIDERATIONS

With the advent of modern anesthetic techniques and specialty training in pediatric anesthesiology, anesthetic-related mortality in children is approximately 1:100,000. This risk significantly rises in very young children and patients with preexisting conditions. The overall risk for infants is 1:40,000, with the risk of complication being 4.3:1,000. Preoperative severity of illness remains a significant risk factor, therefore, in 1941, the American Society of Anesthesiologists (ASA) developed the physical status classification to estimate severity of illness of patients prior to receiving sedation or anesthesia (**Table 21-1**). This system does not predict risk but allows the anesthesiologist to tailor the anesthetic to the patient's underlying condition. Therefore, the higher the ASA class, the greater the likelihood that the patient will have a complicated postoperative course and require intensive management and monitoring.

Table 21-1. ASA Physical Status Classification*

Class	Definition
P 1	Normal healthy patient
P 2	Patient with mild systemic disease
P 3	Patient with severe systemic disease
P 4	Patient with severe systemic disease that is a constant threat to life
P 5	Moribund patient who is not expected to survive without the operation
P 6	A declared brain-dead patient whose organs are being removed for donor purposes

*ASA Relative Value Guide 2008. Available at www.asahq.org/clinical/physicalstatus.htm.

The preoperative patient history is essential to identify patients with underlying conditions at potential risk for intraoperative, as well as postoperative complications. This history must be obtained to guarantee appropriate management of the pediatric patient in the postoperative period and is essential to be included in the sign-out process. Examples include prior medications, allergies, chronic medical conditions (ie, asthma, epilepsy), and reactions to any prior anesthetic agents or procedures. Pertinent information about the intraoperative course should be relayed to the medical team providing postoperative care. This would include the anesthetic agents used, the amount of opioids administered, blood loss, fluids administered, difficulty in airway and ventilatory management, and the occurrence of any untoward events.

> !
>
> *A prolonged and complicated postoperative recovery is directly dependant on preexisting conditions, severity of illness, and the duration of anesthesia.*
>
> !

III. RESPIRATORY CONSIDERATIONS

A. Postoperative Apnea

Postoperative apnea is defined as the cessation of respirations for 15 seconds or more or the cessation of breathing for less than 15 seconds when associated with bradycardia. Premature infants are at increased risk for apnea (central and obstructive) within the first 24 to 48 hours after surgery and anesthesia. It will usually present in the first 2 to12 hours postoperatively. This may be due to immaturity of the respiratory center in the brainstem and easy fatigability of the neonatal diaphragm due to decreased musculature development. In neonates, apnea is a stress response and may be associated with inadequate anesthesia and analgesia.

> !
>
> *The risk of apnea in preterm infants is inversely proportional to the postconceptual age at time of surgery.*
>
> !

It is generally agreed that both premature and full-term infants are at risk for apnea if they are younger than 44 weeks postconceptual age.

The age at which this risk disappears continues to be controversial. Anesthesia should be avoided in the full-term infant less than 44 weeks postconceptual age, unless emergent surgery is required. Full-term infants less than 1-month-old and premature infants less than 60 weeks postconceptual age should be considered at risk for apnea after general anesthesia and require inpatient monitoring and observation for 24 hours postsurgery.

Anemia is an independent risk factor that increases the chances of postoperative apnea in the neonatal population. It is recommended that infants with a hematocrit of less than 30% should have their elective surgery postponed and be given oral hematinics until their hematocrit is greater than 30%. If surgery cannot be delayed, then these patients will require postoperative inpatient observation and monitoring. Children with a known history of obstructive sleep apnea and infants being treated for apnea of prematurity should also be observed postoperatively.

B. Respiratory Depression

Respiratory depression in the immediate postoperative period is usually caused by opioids, residual anesthetic effect, or inadequate neuromuscular blockade reversal. Severe chest or abdominal pain may also cause respiratory splinting with resultant hypoventilation and delay the elimination of any inhaled anesthetic agents. If excessive opioid effect is suspected, then reversal with naloxone is warranted. The half-life of naloxone is relatively short compared with most opiates, and the patient should be monitored for recurrence of respiratory depression.

> !
>
> *Respiratory depression is associated with prolonged or delayed emergence from anesthesia.*

C. Upper Airway Obstruction

> !
>
> *Decreased pharyngeal tone frequently results in upper airway obstruction in the postanesthetic period.*

Upper airway obstruction is frequently encountered while the child is still somewhat sedated after anesthesia. Protective reflexes are intact, but pharyngeal hypotonia with posterior displacement of the tongue may occur.

This results in inspiratory obstruction with the patient exhibiting paradoxical respiration or seesaw-type breathing (the chest caves in while the abdomen rises). If this respiratory pattern is seen, it should be quickly recognized as providing ineffective ventilation. Usually, providing chin lift or jaw thrust will arouse the patient and open the airway. Sometimes the use of a nasal airway adjunct is necessary. In all these situations, the healthcare provider should be prepared to provide a definitive airway and support oxygenation and ventilation.

1. Postextubation Stridor

Postextubation stridor occurs in 1% to 2% of all postoperative pediatric patients. Etiologies include the following: subglottic edema arising from the use of oversized endotracheal tubes, traumatic or repeated attempts at intubation, coughing or bucking with the endotracheal tube in place, or a change in positioning of the endotracheal tube.

> !
>
> *Postextubation stridor is most often seen in the 3-month-old to 4-year-old age group.*

The use of uncuffed, atraumatic, nonirritant endotracheal tubes and the use of appropriately sized endotracheal tubes with a leak below 30 cm H_2O decreases the risk of airway trauma. Mild stridor generally can be managed by providing a cool mist, however, if the patient has evidence of significant stridor and work of breathing, administration of racemic epinephrine nebulizer therapy (0.25 mL to 0.5 mL of 2.25% solution in 2 mL to 3 mL of normal saline solution) may be effective. The patient will require observation to monitor for any rebound edema with consideration for administration of concomitant administration of corticosteroids (dexamethasone 0.5 mg/kg IV/IM) for persistent or severe stridor.

2. Other Causes of Upper Airway Obstruction

Other reasons for upper airway obstruction may include laryngomalacia, soft tissue swelling of oropharyngeal structures (eg, tongue), uncontrollable bleeding from the nasopharynx, oropharynx or hypopharynx, or posterior pharyngeal narrowing after cleft palate repair. Usually, these patients will improve with upright positioning, adequate analgesia, suctioning and clearing of secretions, and control of any active bleeding.

D. Lower Airway Disease

Lower airway disease should be suspected when a child is exhibiting tachypnea, diminished bilateral breath sounds, retractions, and expiratory wheezing. The most common etiologies are bronchospasm, secretions, or aspiration. Atelectasis can occur in the first 48 hours postoperatively and is usually caused by retained secretions due to hypoventilation secondary to pain. Coughing and clearing of secretions can often be accomplished with the aid of incentive spirometry in the children older than 6 years old or encouraging younger children to blow bubbles. This is often effective in the prevention of atelectasis and providing effective pulmonary toilet. In the presence of bronchospasm, the patient may require bronchodilator nebulizer or metered-dose inhaler therapy in addition to the use of corticosteroids.

E. Pulmonary Edema

Pulmonary edema is usually rare in otherwise healthy patients, unless the patient is known to have congestive heart failure or received an excessive amount of intravenous (IV) fluids intraoperatively. Postobstructive pulmonary edema occurs after the acute relief of chronic severe upper airway obstruction or after postextubation obstruction, such as laryngospasm, in which the patient was making vigorous inspiratory efforts against a closed glottis. It is frequently seen in children following a tonsillectomy and adenoidectomy for obstructive sleep apnea.

> **!** *Patients with a history of obstructive sleep apnea are at increased risk to develop postobstructive pulmonary edema.*

Management is supportive with mild cases requiring oxygen and possibly one dose of IV diuretic (furosemide 1 mg/kg IV). Patients in severe respiratory distress will require intubation and provision of adequate positive end-expiratory pressure. Usually, the pulmonary edema in these cases rapidly resolves with appropriate management.

IV. HEMODYNAMIC CONSIDERATIONS

A. Dysrhythmias

Children tend to be quite healthy and abnormal electrocardiogram results and arrhythmias are uncommon postoperatively, unless there is an underlying cardiac pathology or electrolyte disturbance. Abnormalities of heart rate tend to be the most frequent dysrhythmias seen, and sinus tachycardia is the most common.

> !
>
> *Sinus tachycardia is the most frequent dysrhythmia seen postoperatively and is usually due pain and hypovolemia.*
>
> !

Sinus tachycardia rarely needs specific therapy, but its underlying etiology must be determined. Tachycardia may be an early indicator of compensated shock, with the most common cause in the postoperative patient being hypovolemia. On physical examination, there may be associated cool extremities, decreased urine output, and hypotension indicative of decompensated shock. One should promptly initiate fluid resuscitation. Other factors that may result in sinus tachycardia include emergence delirium, pain, anemia, anxiety, hyperthermia, hypercarbia, and the presence of parasympathomimetic agents, such as atropine and glycopyrrolate.

> !
>
> *The most common causes of bradycardia is hypoxia and increased parasympathetic tone.*
>
> !

Bradycardia in infants requires immediate attention, because this age group is heart rate dependent for their cardiac output. The most life-threatening cause of bradycardia is hypoxia, and, thus, administering oxygen and providing assisted ventilation is paramount in the initial management. Tracheal suctioning, nasogastric tube insertion, or the application of ophthalmic pressure can result in increased parasympathetic tone and is a common cause of bradycardia in this age group.

In neurologically injured or impaired patients, bradycardia may be a sign of increased intracranial pressure, and, when associated with hypertension and decreased ventilatory rate, it is a sign of impending cerebral herniation and is a medical emergency. In this situation, the patient should be emergently hyperventilated and administered IV osmotic therapy with either mannitol or 3% hypertonic saline solution.

B. Abnormal Blood Pressure

Hypertension in children rarely has a pathologic etiology and, like tachycardia, usually does not require specific therapy, but the underlying cause needs to be determined. Hypertension with associated tachycardia is usually due to increased agitation, anxiety and/or pain. When accompanied with normal or decreased heart rate, this may be a sign of hypothermia or increased intracranial pressure. In all these situations, antihypertensive medication is not indicated. Antihypertensive therapy is indicated in patients who are known to have chronic renal disease with preexisting hypertension.

Hypotension in the postoperative patient should be considered a medical emergency. This may be seen in the patient who is initially cold with vasoconstriction and is then rapidly rewarmed. However, the most common cause of hypotension is volume depletion. In all of these situations, volume therapy needs to be initiated as soon as possible. If the patient does not respond in the expected fashion, then one must consider that the patient may be in shock due to sepsis or cardiac dysfunction. In these situations, vasopressor and/or inotropic support needs to be considered, and the patient should be managed in a monitored setting that can provide for arterial and central venous monitoring.

V. NEUROLOGIC CONSIDERATIONS

A. Altered Consciousness

Altered consciousness poses a diagnostic dilemma for the anesthesiologist and the medical team managing the patient postoperatively. This is a common reason for unanticipated admission of children to the pediatric intensive care unit (PICU) from the recovery room. The causes for this can usually be directly traced to prolonged anesthetic effect along with other less common etiologies (**Table 21-2**).

Table 21-2. Causes of Altered Consciousness in the Postoperative Period

Prolonged anesthesia or delayed emergence due to residual anesthetic effect
Prolonged neuromuscular blockade
Metabolic and electrolyte imbalances
Hypoglycemia
Diabetic ketoacidosis
Hypokalemia → severe muscular weakness
Hypernatremia and hyponatremia
Hypercarbia secondary to hypoventilation
Narcosis with markedly elevated CO_2 levels
Neurologic events
Postictal
Embolic event
Hypoxic ischemic injury
Intracranial mass lesion and raised intracranial pressure or herniation

1. Residual Anesthetic Effect

The most common anesthetic agents used in the operating room are inhalational anesthetic agents. The elimination of inhalational anesthetic gases is dependent on minute ventilation, cardiac output, drug solubility, and the depth and duration of anesthesia. Therefore, ventilation and cardiac output must be optimized, and very often the patient will require prolonged recovery room stay and may possibly require observation in a step down unit or PICU. As previously discussed, the effect of excessive opioid administration is a cause of respiratory depression, and this must be evaluated in the patient who fails to awaken. A trial of naloxone can be given; however, it should be used judiciously, because it not only reverses the depressive effects but also the analgesia, resulting in a child who is in pain, agitated, hypertensive, and exhibiting uncontrollable behavior. It is prudent to continue to actively manage the airway and ventilate the patient until the residual anesthetic or excessive opioid effects abate without the acute removal of analgesia. This can be safely done in an ICU setting. If there is no improvement in the patient's sensorium, then other etiologies must be sought.

> !
>
> *It is preferable to actively manage the airway and ventilate the patient until the residual anesthetic effect wears off without acute reversal of analgesia.*
>
> !

2. Prolonged Neuromuscular Blockade

Neuromuscular blocking agents are commonly used in general anesthesia during induction and endotracheal intubation. Neuromuscular blocking agents can be divided into two types: depolarizing and nondepolarizing. Succinylcholine is a depolarizing neuromuscular blocking agent, and its routine use by pediatric anesthesiologists has fallen out of practice due to its side effect profile. Succinylcholine noncompetitively binds to the acetylcholine (ACh) receptors of the motor endplate, resulting in depolarization and, initially, muscle fasciculation. It then diffuses from the receptor and is metabolized by hepatic and plasma pseudocholinesterase. Prolonged blockade after administration of succinylcholine is most commonly caused by an abnormal genetic variant of pseudocholinesterase. The patient is managed with supportive ventilation until the effects of neuromuscular blockade (NMB) have dissipated. Other causes of prolonged depolarizing NMB are pregnancy, hepatic dysfunction, and hypermagnesemia.

Nondepolarizing neuromuscular blockers such as pancuronium, rocuronium, vecuronium, atracurium, cisatracurium, and mivacarium are commonly used during the anesthetization of pediatric patients. These drugs competitively inhibit ACh receptors causing muscular paralysis without depolarization. This type of agent can be reversed or antagonized by administering an inhibitor of acetylcholinesterase, resulting in elevated synaptic concentrations of ACh, which then competitively displaces the neuromuscular blocking agent from the receptor. Nondepolarizing NMB reversal drugs commonly used are neostigmine (0.07 mg/kg IV), edrophonium (1 mg/kg IV), and pyridostigmine (0.2 mg/kg IV). Due to the muscarinic effects of these reversal agents, atropine (0.02 mg/kg IV) or glycopyrrolate (0.01 mg/kg IV) should be concomitantly given. The common causes of failure to reverse nondepolarizing agents are given in **Table 21-3.**

Table 21-3. Failure of Reversal or Recurring Blockade by Nondepolarizing Agents

Respiratory acidosis
Hypokalemia
Hypermagnesemia
Hypothermia
Drug interactions
Antibiotics: aminoglycosides, tetracyclines, polymyxins, lincomycins
High-dose corticosteroids
Calcium-channel blockers
Local anesthetics (quinidine)
Alkylating cytotoxic agents
Myasthenia gravis
Muscular dystrophies and myotonia

Patients with prolonged NMB will not be able to breathe or move but will retain autonomic and ocular reactivity. Patients with persistent NMB can be evaluated using a peripheral nerve stimulator with the administration of a train of four electrical impulses, while observing for corresponding twitches. Usually, the fourth twitch is abolished when greater than 75% of the ACh receptors on the motor endplate are blocked. In adults, when less than 75% of the receptors are blocked, the patient can still effectively breathe. Children, on the other hand, have decreased functional residual capacity and a higher incidence of postextubation airway obstruction. Thus, other indications of the reversal of NMB include their ability to lift their head for more than 5 seconds, exhibit hand grip, and sustain a leg raise.

B. Emergence Delirium

Less than 3% of children will experience emergence delirium, which is most commonly seen in children 3 to 9 years of age. These patients become extremely restless, combative, disoriented, and may scream and cry within the first few hours postoperatively. Other causes for this are hypoxia, hypoglycemia, and severe pain, all of which must be considered. These patients pose a risk of harming themselves and often will require restraints and comforting. Sometimes sedation with benzodiazepines is required; however, delirium may reoccur after the sedative effects have worn off.

> ! *The agents often implicated with emergence delirium are barbiturates, inhaled anesthetics, and ketamine.* !

VI. PAIN MANAGEMENT

Approximately 40% to 75% of children will experience significant pain in the first 24 hours after surgery. In the not so recent past, children were denied pain relief as it was felt that they did not have the ability to experience pain or tolerate potent analgesia, and this practice resulted in inadequate procedural pain management. There is no reason for a child to experience pain, as we now have an armamentarium of medications and techniques available to us. This requires a multidisciplinary approach, which includes the involvement of the child, parents, bedside nurse, physician team (anesthesiologist, surgeon, primary care physician), and child life specialist. The strategies used are determined by the procedure performed, anesthetic technique used, expected duration of the recovery period, and anticipated severity of postoperative pain. It becomes obvious that pain management must be integrated throughout the preoperative, intraoperative, and postoperative periods.

A. Physiology

Newborns will often cry after noxious stimuli for short periods and then fall asleep without the use of any analgesics. Newborns lack myelin in the thalamocortical tracts and have higher plasma and cerebrospinal fluid concentrations of endogenous opioids compared with older children. This led to the presumption that infants experience minimal perception of pain and that analgesics were not necessary in this population. This has had the effect of propagating the misperception that children as a group do not require as much analgesia as adults. Nothing could be further than the truth. It has been clearly shown that children of all ages experience pain.

> ! *Newborns experience pain in a manner similar to adults.* !

At birth, peripheral nociceptors are fully developed and functional, reflexive expressive pathways are structurally and functionally immature, and central pain perception is not well understood. Therefore, the response of infants and young children to pain is variable and often unpredictable. In neonates, there are fewer µ1-opioid receptors (analgesia) relative to µ2-opioid receptors (respiratory depression). In premature infants, the volume of distribution of some opioids is larger and elimination half-life prolonged. This may explain the increased sensitivity of the neonatal population to the respiratory depressive effects of opioids compared with older children and adults.

B. Pain Assessment

Pain assessment in children can be quite difficult. This is particularly true in preverbal and developmentally delayed children. Often, their response to pain is age-specific and difficult to distinguish from agitation and anxiety. Many children respond to pain by withdrawing from their surroundings and do not volunteer information out of fear of further painful interventions. This can often be misinterpreted by the medical staff that the patient is not experiencing pain. In an attempt to objectively assess pain in this population, validated, developmentally appropriate tools have been developed and applied. Analog scales are used with pictures of faces in various degrees of pain and distress ranked from 0 to 10. These are often used in the assessment of pain in preverbal children. Other analog scales encompassing visual/verbal scales and age and developmentally specific pain-associated behaviors have been developed. Ultimately, what is most important is the consistent application of a pain assessment tool that is tailored toward the appropriate population.

C. Analgesics

> !
>
> *The combination of analgesic agents should be tailored to the individual child's severity of pain and circumstances.*
>
> !

A variety of analgesic drugs can be used in the postoperative pain management of children. This includes nonopioids, nonsteroidal antiinflammatory drugs (NSAIDS), opioids, and regional analgesia.

These modalities can be used singularly or in combination, and should be tailored to the individual patient's circumstances and pain level. The stratified approach to the use of analgesics in pain management is often used based on the severity of pain being experienced (**Figure 21-1**). In this approach, nonopioids, including acetaminophen and NSAIDS (eg, ibuprofen), can be used for mild pain. Lower potency opioids (codeine, hydrocodone and oxycodone) are often used in combination with nonopioids for moderate pain, while for severe pain IV opioids (morphine, fentanyl, hydromorphone, methadone) are utilized in combination with potent IV NSAIDS (ketorolac 0.5 mg/kg IV/IM every 6 h). This closely follows the Analgesic Ladder model of pain management developed by the World Health Organization (**Figure 21-1**).

Figure 21-1. Stratified Approach to Analgesic Management

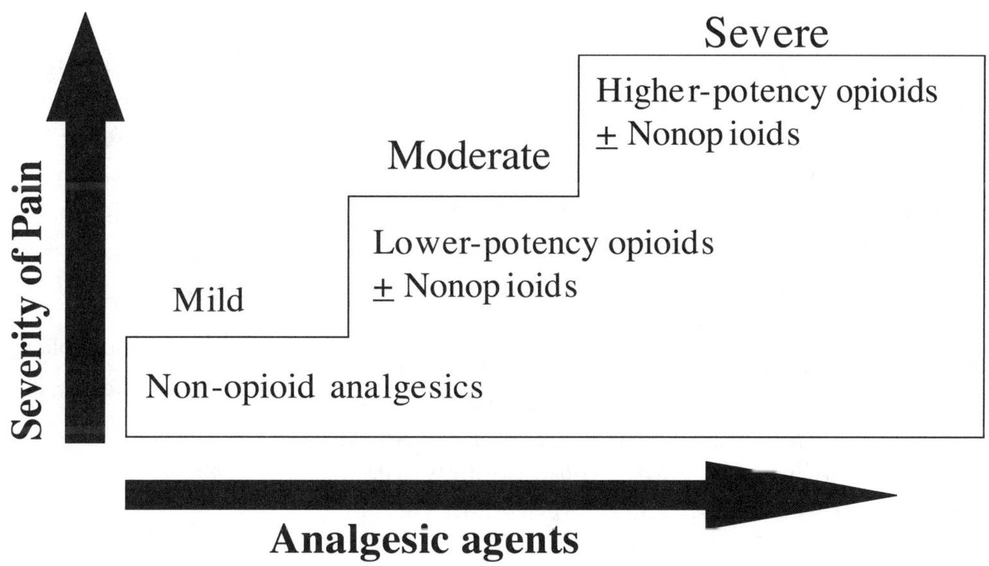

D. Patient Controlled Analgesia

Typically, opioids are administered to patients after they complain or are noted to experience pain. This leads to a vicious cycle of pain followed by delayed administration of an analgesic by the healthcare provider, with the resultant risk of persistent pain or increased sedation. This places the patient at risk for the side effects of opioids with inadequate pain relief. Patient-controlled analgesia (PCA) administration allows us to break this vicious cycle. The goal is twofold; maintain therapeutic levels of opioids to ensure adequate analgesia and have a system that is rapidly responsive to the patient's analgesic needs. The PCA regimen usually employed uses an opioid that can be dosed on demand, continuously, or both (**Table 21-4**).

Table 21-4. PCA Dosing Regimen

Opioid Drug	Demand Dose	Lock-out Interval (min)	Basal Infusion	One Hour Limit
Morphine	0.02 mg/kg (adult dose: 1 mg)	10	0-0.02 mg/kg/h (adult dose: 2 mg/h)	1 mg/kg
Fentanyl	0.5 µg/kg (adult dose: 50-100 µg)	10	0-0.5 µg/kg/h (adult dose: 50-100 µg/h)	2.5 µg/kg
Hydromorphone	4 µg/kg (adult dose: 200 µg)	10	0-4 µg/kg/h (adult dose: 200 µg/h)	20 µg/kg

Adapted from Landsman IR, Vustar M, Hays SR. Pediatric anesthesia. In: Grosfeld JL, O'Neill JA, Fonkalsrud EW, eds. *Pediatric Surgery*. 6th ed. St Louis, MO: Mosby; 2006: 242-243.

A microprocessor linked to an infusion pump with a push-button to deliver the programmed regimen is at the heart of this modality of pain management. With the advent of smart technology, end-tidal CO_2 monitoring and pulse oximetry provides feedback to the microprocessor in the PCA pump, cutting off the administration of the opioids and alerting the nurse in the event that signs of respiratory depression arise. Continuous infusions should only be administered in patient care units where there is close cardiorespiratory monitoring. It has been speculated that continuous infusions may facilitate a normal sleeping pattern in the postoperative patient who is awoken by the experience of pain and must then push the button to self-administer a demand opioid dose. There is, however, no evidence to support this assumption. In older children and adolescents, use of demand dosing is often used, because these patients are developmentally able to follow instructions and possess adequate hand strength and dexterity.

> **!** *If a child can play video games, they can operate their PCA pump.*

This ensures a margin of safety, while providing adequate analgesia and minimizing side effects. The practice of opioid proxy administration with the PCA demand button by parents or nurses (when they think the patient is experiencing pain) is strongly discouraged. This has shown to increase the incidence of opioid overdosing and untoward events, especially in poorly monitored patient care environments.

E. Regional Anesthesia

Regional anesthesia is the use of local anesthetics and/or opioids in an attempt to block the afferent pathways from nocioceptors to the central nervous system. These techniques include local analgesic infiltration, peripheral nerve blocks, nerve-plexus blocks, or epidural/intrathecal nerve blocks. The anesthetic agent is administered as a single injection or by continuous infusion as in neuraxial blocks. Neuraxial blocks involve the injection of local anesthetics and/or opioids using spinal or epidural approaches.

Regional anesthesia can be advantageous in patients who exhibit increased sensitivity to the side effects of opioids, which often occurs in neonates and young children. There is a lower risk of adverse effects, such as nausea, vomiting, sedation, and respiratory depression that is frequently encountered with parenteraly administered opioids. The use of long-acting local anesthetics can reduce the need for high potency opioids and provide hours of pain relief in the immediate postoperative period when the severity of pain is usually at its greatest.

1. Caudal Block

The most common block used in children is the caudal block. In this technique, the epidural space is accessed via the sacral hiatus, and a single injection of 1 mL/kg of local anesthetic is administered. Its success rate is high with a low rate of complication. It usually provides analgesia below the umbilicus, and, with the use of only a local anesthetic, the patient is pain-free for several hours. In general, children do not exhibit hemodynamic instability or urinary retention. The addition of opioids will prolong analgesia but increase the risk of side effects. This technique usually works well when severe pain is only anticipated for the first 24 hours postoperatively.

2. Epidural Anesthesia

Patients requiring a longer duration of analgesia may have an epidural catheter inserted, and either intermittent injection or continuous infusion of anesthetic can be administered. The level of anesthesia being provided depends upon the position of the catheter tip relative to the site of pain and the opioid used. The combined effect of local anesthetics and opioids is synergistic, thus allowing lower doses of each agent required to provide adequate analgesia. The most common complication encountered is respiratory depression, because the level of anesthesia is too high or, more frequently, because IV or intramuscular opioids are used to supplement the epidural opioid.

> **!** *Exercise caution with the use of supplemental IV opioids with either the caudal block or epidural anesthesia due to the increased risk of respiratory depression.*

Patients with an indwelling epidural catheter should be closely monitored to observe for respiratory depression and neurologic complications.

VII. FLUID AND ELECTROLYTE CONSIDERATIONS

Total body water averages 60% of body weight in men, 50% in young women, and 75% to 80% of body weight in the infant. By the age of 1 year, total body water is 65% of body weight. Approximately two thirds is located in the intracellular compartment and the remainig third extracellular. Small infants can have extraordinary insensible fluid losses, especially if under radiant warmers or requiring phototherapy. Under these conditions, fluid requirements are increased 10% to 20%. It is important to note that pulmonary insensible water loss is negligible when patients are mechanically ventilated due to humidity in the circuits.

Volume deficit is the most common fluid problem in the surgical pediatric patient. It is usually due to ongoing loss of GI fluids (vomiting, nasogastric tubes, and surgical drains), cerebrospinal fluid loss through external ventricular drains, and sequestration of fluids (peritonitis, ileus, burns). The clinical findings will depend on the severity of vascular volume depletion and may consist of irritability that progresses to apathy and lethargy, increased heart rate, mottled and cold extremities, and decreased urinary output. Hypotension is a late finding in shock. Laboratory evaluation will usually show increased blood urea nitrogen with or without elevation in creatinine and hemoconcentration with an inappropriately elevated hematocrit. In severe volume depletion with significant compromise in oxygen delivery, there will be a metabolic acidosis and increased blood lactate.

!

Measurements of urinary output trends are helpful in detecting a low intravascular volume status and in assessing the response to ongoing interventions.

!

Children with anticipated perioperative large volume shifts or losses and large volume fluid resuscitation should be monitored invasively with continuous measurement of central venous pressure and arterial pressure. An indwelling urinary catheter should be utilized.

After the acute correction of shock, fluid management should provide for the correction of the remaining deficit, maintenance fluid, and replacement of ongoing losses. In the critically ill postoperative patient, it is safe to assume that any ongoing losses are more likely to be isotonic than hypotonic in composition. It is also safe to assume that in the stressed postoperative patient, there are going to be hemodynamic and nonhemodynamic stimuli for the release of antidiuretic hormone. In this setting, it is prudent to use isotonic fluids in the early postoperative period to decrease the risk of hyponatremia and potential neurologic complications. Frequently assess the patient for adequacy of hydration and circulation, determine serum electrolytes every 6 to 8 hours, and adjust electrolyte delivery in the fluids accordingly.

!

Ongoing fluid loss secondary to third spacing is usually isotonic in composition.

!

The neurosurgical or head-injured patient that develops the syndrome of inappropriate secretion of antidiuretic hormone poses a special circumstance. These patients are usually euvolemic or have a mild excess of total body water with varying degrees of hyponatremia. These patients are managed with the provision of maintenance sodium and fluid restriction to 50% of maintenance. The goal is to increase serum sodium at a rate of less than 1 mEq/h.

VIII. POSTOPERATIVE NAUSEA AND VOMITING

> *The causes of PONV include the stress and trauma of surgery combined with the emetic effect of the anesthetic agents, pain, and the side effects associated with the use of opioid analgesics.*

One of the most distressing aspects of the postoperative period for patients, parents, and nurses alike is the nausea and vomiting associated with the anesthetic. Postoperative nausea and vomiting (PONV) can occur within the first 1 to 2 hours after surgery and for to several hours afterward. Up to 50% of children will experience PONV, depending on the anesthetic used and the procedure performed. Patients at high risk who have received inhaled anesthetics have an 80% incidence of PONV.

Preoperative fasting does not prevent PONV, but it has been shown that hydration and glucose supplementation will ameliorate it. The use of ondansetron (0.15 mg/kg/dose IV every 4 to 6 hours) and other serotonin antagonists are the mainstay of pharmacologic management of PONV (**Table 21-5**). Ondansetron is very efficacious when used prophylactically and in the management of active vomiting and should be used in high-risk patients (eg, strabismus surgery).

Table 21-5. Measures to Reduce Incidence of PONV

Prophylactic use of antiemetics preceding, during, or after anesthesia
Droperidol is effective prophylactically and as treatment of ongoing vomiting; use with caution due to rare incidence of prolonged QT interval and ventricular arrhythmias
Metoclopromide is used prophylactically
Ondansetron and other serotonin antagonists are very efficacious
Induction or maintenance of anesthesia with propofol versus inhaled anesthetics
Use of nonopioid analgesics (eg, acetomenophen, ketorolac)

IX. NUTRITIONAL CONSIDERATIONS

Acute malnutrition is frequently encountered in the postoperative pediatric patient. In this setting, malnutrition is multifactorial and may be caused by prolonged bowel dysfunction or food intolerance after surgery, increased catabolism, lack of aggressive intervention, or missed opportunities to increase nutritional support. To complicate the picture further, many children have chronic malnutrition due to a preexisting chronic condition.

> !
>
> *The unique challenge in the pediatric patient is the provision of nutrition to help meet the increased demands of critical illness and healing and also meet the demands of normal growth and development.*
>
> !

A. Nutrition Assessment

On admission, all patients at risk should be assessed by obtaining base measures, such as weight, height, and head circumference. Children less than 2 years old should be plotted on normative growth charts. Comparison can be made with previous measures from the clinics or prior admissions, if available. Body mass index can de determined in older children. Also, base measures of specific visceral proteins such as albumin, transferrin, pre-albumin and retinol-binding protein can de determined. These proteins have a rapid turnover. However, during periods of increased catabolism, their synthesis is decreased. Increasing levels are indicative of resolving stress and/or adequate nutrition. Pre-albumin and retinol-binding protein, due to their short half-life (2 days and 12 hours, respectively), are better suited to reflect quick change in the patient's metabolic state.

B. Stress Response

During acute physiologic stress, there is activation of the hypothalamic-pituitary axis, activation of the sympathetic nervous system, increased cytokines, increased counter-regulatory hormones, increase in endogenous catecholamines, and insulin resistance. Elevated cortisol induces muscle breakdown and promotes gluconeogenesis (conversion of non-carbohydrate energy sources into glucose). The increased levels of catecholamines stimulate glycogen breakdown in the liver and skeletal muscle and mobilization of free fatty acids, all which fuels the hypercatabolic state.

C. Nutritional Support

The breakdown of lean body tissue is central during the stress response. Therefore, the goals are to limit protein breakdown during the acute phase of illness by provision of amino acids and adequate nonprotein calories (**Table 21-6**).

Table 21-6. Nutritional Requirements (Energy and Protein)

Age (years)	Energy (Kcal/kg/day)	Protein (gm/kg/day)
< 1	50-80	2.0-2.5
1-7	45-65	1.5-2.0
> 7	30-60	1.5-2.0

Carbohydrates in the form of glucose provide 4 kcal/gram of energy. Children require a glucose infusion rate of 5 to 8 mg/kg/min to meet metabolic demand. The threshold for ketosis is a glucose infusion rate of less than 2 mg/kg/min but may be higher in the context of the stress response due to the state of insulin resistance. Overfeeding with glucose delivery rates of more than 10 mg/kg/min should be avoided, because it promotes lipogenesis and increased CO_2 production. If hyperglycemia develops despite an adequate glucose delivery, insulin supplementation (starting infusion of regular insulin at 0.05 U/kg/h to 0.1 U/kg/h) may be indicated to facilitate cellular uptake. When reintroducing enteral nutrition, a lactose-free formulation may be better tolerated.

Fats provide 9 kcal/gram of energy. In patients unable to tolerate enteral feedings, fat can be administered parenterally as a 20% emulsion. As little as 0.5 g/kg/day is enough to provide essential fatty acids (linoleic and linolenic acids), which can be increased by 1 g/kg/day to a limit of 3 g/kg/day. Triglyceride levels are best determined at least 4 hours after discontinuing a lipid infusion. Hypertriglyceridemia is frequently due to an excess caloric load from carbohydrates. When the enteral route is used, medium-chain triglycerides offered in some formulas are able to directly enter the portal system, facilitating digestion.

The breakdown of protein produces 4 kcal/gram of energy. Although unable to prevent the catabolism of proteins during the stress response, amino acids should be provided in an amount sufficient to prevent deficiency of essential amino acids and to facilitate the synthesis of new protein. Maintaining this balance between breakdown and synthesis may require protein intake of 2 to 3 g/kg/day.

D. Route of Administration

The use of IV delivery devices and central venous catheterization allows the administration of parenteral nutrition to surgical patients who would otherwise suffer the consequences of malnutrition (poor wound healing, infections, even death).

Feeding via the native gastrointestinal tract is always preferred and provides many benefits, especially in critically ill children (**Table 21-7**).

Table 21-7. Advantages of Enteral Feeding

Advantages of Enteral Feeding
Stimulates the release of gut trophic factors
Maintains enerocyte mass better
Preserves gut motility
Improves mesenteric blood flow
Decreases incidence of nosocomial infections
Cuts down on costs

Delayed gastric emptying is common in critical illness. If attempts to feed into the stomach fail or if the risks of aspiration are high, transpyloric tube feeding is usually successful. There may be the added advantage that transpyloric feeding can be continued around the period of planned extubation, providing uninterrupted nutrition. Parenteral nutrition continues to play an important role in the support of patients with hemodynamic instability at risk for bowel ischemia and in patients with congenital or acquired abnormalities of the gut, such as necrotizing enterocolitis, bowel atresias, mecononium ileus, dysmotility syndromes, and short-gut syndrome. Complications of prolonged parenteral nutrition are numerous and every effort should be made to provide some nutrition by the enteral route (**Table 21-8**).

> **!** *"If the gut works, then use it."* **!**

Table 21-8. Complications of Parenteral Nutrition

Catheter-related infections

Electrolyte disturbances

Hepatic

- Fatty liver
- Cholestasis
- Hepatic fibrosis
- Biliary cirrhosis (parenteral nutrition associated liver disease)

X. HEMATOLOGIC CONSIDERATIONS

Intraoperative blood loss is carefully monitored by both the surgeon and the anesthesiologist. Most often, the rate of blood loss is gradual and surgically controlled. Patients usually do not require blood products, unless there has been significant blood loss or their initial hematocrit was low. Large volumes of blood products required intraoperatively and ongoing bleeding can have a major impact on the patient's status in the postoperative period. The rate of fall of the patient's hemoglobin and hematocrit can be used as an estimation of the extent of the patient's blood loss when that loss has been gradual. This cannot be used, however, when active bleeding is vigorous, in which case, hemodynamic instability is a closer reflection of blood volume depletion. Direct measurement of blood losses as observed from the amount collected from indwelling drains (eg, thoracostomy tubes) is also used to estimate the extent of ongoing blood loss. Occult bleeding occurring in closed compartments, such as the intra-abdominal compartment and thigh, is an exception to this practice.

The optimal fluid to replace blood loss until the lowest acceptable hemoglobin is reached remains controversial; some professionals prefer isotonic crystalloid solutions, others colloids. Typically, the amount of isotonic crystalloid solution (lactated Ringers solution or 0.9% normal saline solution) that is infused should equal 2 to 3 times the volume of the estimated blood loss. The trigger for initiation of packed red blood cell (PRBC) transfusion is a hemoglobin of 7 mg/dL or less in the older child and 10 mg/dL or greater in the neonate.

> !
>
> *The goal of blood replacement therapy is to maintain euvolemia, optimize arterial oxygen content, and maintain clotting factor and component levels.*
>
> !

The etiology of postoperative bleeding must be determined and corrected, especially if such bleeding is ongoing and/or brisk. The most common cause for bleeding is usually poor surgical hemostasis. The other major reason is coagulopathy due to hemodilution of clotting factors and/or platelets, massive PRBC transfusion, or other underlying conditions, including sepsis and disseminated intravascular coagulopathy. In blood product administration, start administering fresh frozen plasma when the estimated blood loss approaches one blood volume. An equal amount of fresh frozen plasma and PRBCs should be transfused. The need for platelets is variable. A platelet count of greater than 20,000/mm^3 may be acceptable in patients where there is no ongoing bleeding, but when there is evidence of active bleeding, a platelet count of greater than 100,000/mm^3 is desirable. Two units of platelets per 10 kg will raise the platelet count by 10,000 to 15,000/mm^3.

PRBCs and fresh frozen plasma contain citrate that chelates calcium and can cause a fall in the serum ionized calcium level. The mobilization of calcium and the hepatic metabolism of citrate are usually rapid enough in older children and adults to prevent a significant fall in the ionized calcium. Neonates have inadequate calcium stores and are susceptible to acute hypocalcemia and its attendant hypotension and require IV calcium replacement (calcium chloride 10-20 mg/kg or calcium gluconate 50-100 mg/kg). Calcium may also be required if massive amounts of blood products have been transfused. Large transfusions of cold blood products will precipitate hypothermia and should be warmed prior to their administration.

XI. THERMAL REGULATION

As part of the intraoperative management, the anesthesiologist optimizes body temperature control with the primary goal being normothermia. Some patients are more prone to develop hypothermia or hyperthermia during anesthesia. This is a major concern in infants, patients having prolonged procedures, in instances that require large areas of surgical site exposure, when radiant warmers or thermal blankets are used, and after the administration of large volumes of unwarmed IV fluids or blood products.

A. Hypothermia

Shivering is a very common occurrence in the immediate postoperative period with the patient often complaining of feeling extremely cold. The use of warm blankets may remedy this chill and tends to be comforting and subjectively appears to reduce shivering. Hypothermia, on the other hand, can be a cause of shivering and must be ruled out.

> !
>
> *Infants and small children are at increased risk for hypothermia due to their larger body surface area to mass ratio, higher metabolic rates, and decreased fat stores.*

Hypothermia, if not promptly attended to, can lead to life-threatening situations, especially in neonates (**Table 21-9**). During the rewarming, one must be cautious to avoid cutaneous hyperthermia and burns (especially with improper use of radiant warmers).

Table 21-9. Deleterious Effects of Hypothermia

Deleterious Effects of Hypothermia
Respiratory acidosis
Apnea
Hypotension
Bradycardia
Prolongation of neuromuscular blockade
Prolongation of the effects of narcotics

B. Fever

Fever in the first 24 hours postoperatively is relatively common. This is often due to the release of pyrogens from surgically traumatized tissue. However, if fever persists beyond this period, then one must rule out infection, which in all likelihood was present or occult prior to surgery. Excessive ambient environmental heat with no opportunity for heat loss, which is seen when infants are bundled and warming devices have been used, may be another cause of hyperthermia. Dehydration secondary to inadequate fluid replacement also predisposes the patient to temperature elevation. In all these cases, fever results in increased metabolic demand with resultant tachycardia, tachypnea and carbon dioxide production, and induces increased stress on the patient. If, within hours of having received an inhalational anesthetic, the patient's temperature is in excess of 39°C (102.2°F), especially if succinylcholine was used, then malignant hyperthermia should be considered.

> !
>
> *Malignant hyperthermia should be suspected if the patient received succinylcholine and the temperature is greater than 39°C (102.2°F).*

C. Malignant Hyperthermia

Malignant hyperthermia (MH) is a familial disorder of muscle hypermetabolism that may complicate the anesthesia or postanesthesia course and require further management in the PICU. The prevalence of MH during general anesthesia varies from 1:15,000 in children to 1:50,000 in adults. Malignant hyperthermia results from a genetic defect in one of the receptors that control the release and reuptake of sarcoplasmic calcium in skeletal muscle. Children with underlying myopathy are at increased risk. Agents inciting MH include inhalational anesthetics agents and depolarizing muscle relaxants, such as succinylcholine. Exaggerated jaw rigidity (masseter spasms) after succinylcholine and excess carbon dioxide production are often the earliest signs; skeletal muscle rigidity, tachycardia, and hyperthermia then ensue. This hypermetabolic state leads to ATP depletion and anaerobic metabolism with lactic acidemia and metabolic acidosis. If not controlled, the intense muscle activity leads to rhabdomyolysis, hyperkalemia, and eventual multiple organ system failure.

Treatment consists of avoidance or removal of triggering agents, muscle relaxation with dantrolene sodium, and supportive care. Dantrolene causes complete and sustained relaxation of skeletal muscle by inhibiting intracellular calcium release in the myocyte by direct action on calcium release channels. Dosing of dantrolene is 1 to 3 mg/kg IV, repeated every 15 minutes, as needed, to a maximum dose of 10 mg/kg in the setting of acute MH. Recurrence is prevented by administration of dantrolene 1 mg/kg IV every 6 hours for 24 to 48 hours postoperatively. Supportive care involves airway protection by orotracheal intubation and mechanical ventilation if large doses of dantrolene are needed to control acute MH, active cooling to less than 38°C but avoidance of hypothermia, and correction of acidosis and hyperkalemia. In the presence of rhabdomyolysis and myoglobinuria, it is important to maintain a brisk urine output with IV hydration and osmotic diuretics, such as mannitol. As with other hyperthermia syndromes, coagulopathy, pulmonary edema, and cerebral edema can be potential complications. When suspicion of malignant hyperthermia has been raised by well-documented clinical events or strong family history, genetic evaluation and muscle testing could secure a diagnosis and indicate appropriate precautions for both the index patient and relatives of all ages.

Key Points

POSTOPERATIVE MANAGEMENT

- The postoperative management of the pediatric patient is part of the continuum of care in the perioperative management of the surgical patient.
- A prolonged and complicated postoperative recovery is directly dependent on preexisting conditions, severity of illness, and the duration of anesthesia.
- A stratified approach to the use of analgesics in pain management is used based on the severity of pain and incorporating behavioral modification, nonopioids, opioids, and regional anesthesia.
- Full-term infants less than 1 month old and premature infants less than 60 weeks postconceptual age should be considered at risk for apnea after general anesthesia and require inpatient monitoring and observation for 24 hours postsurgery.
- Naloxone should be used if respiratory or central nervous system depression is suspected to be due to excessive opioids. However, it should be used judiciously, because it not only reverses the depressive effects but also the analgesia, resulting in a child who is in pain, agitated, hypertensive, and behaviorally uncontrollable.
- Emergence delirium is usually treated with benzodiazepines, but other causes, such as hypoxia, hypoglycemia, and severe pain, must be ruled out.
- Volume deficit is the most common fluid problem in the surgical pediatric patient and is usually due to ongoing loss of gastrointestinal fluids, cerebrospinal fluid loss through external ventricular drains, and third-spacing of fluids.
- In the critically ill postoperative patient, it is safe to assume that any ongoing losses are more likely to be isotonic than hypotonic in composition.
- Prophylactic use of antiemetics preceding, during, and after anesthesia should be used to prevent and treat PONV.
- Early institution of nutrition shortens the postoperative period and speeds recovery, and the enteral route is preferred.
- If, within hours of having received an inhalational anesthetic, the patient's temperature is in excess of 39°C (102.2°F), and especially if succinylcholine was used, then malignant hyperthermia should be considered.

Suggested Readings

1. Binda RE, Mestad PH, Perryman KM. Anesthetic considerations. In: Ashcraft KW, Holcomb GW, Murphy JP, eds. *Pediatric Surgery.* 4th ed. Philiadelphia, PA: Saunders; 2005:29-37.

2. Brandon BW. Malignant Hyperthermia. In: Fuhrman BP, Zimmerman JJ, eds. *Pediatric Critical Care.* 3rd ed. St Louis, MO: Mosby; 2006:1780-1791.

3. Kaus SJ, Rockoff MA. Malignant hyperthermia. *Pediatr Clin North Am.* 1994; 41(1):221-237.

4. Landsman IR, Vustar M, Hays SR. Pediatric anesthesia. In: Grosfeld JL, O'Neill JA, Fonkalsrud EW, eds. *Pediatric Surgery.* 6th ed. St Louis, MO: Mosby; 2006: 221-249.

5. Lyons KA, Brilli RJ, Wieman RA, et al. Continuation of transpyloric feeding during weaning of mechanical ventilation and tracheal extubation in children: a randomized controlled trial. *J Parenter Enteral Nutr.* 2002; 26(3):209.

6. Rusyniak DE, Sprague JE. Hyperthermic syndromes induced by toxins. *Clin Lab Med.* 2006; 26(1):165-184, ix.

7. Steinhorn DM, Russo LT. Nutrition issues in critically ill children. In: Fink MP, Abraham E, Vincent JL, Kochanek P, eds. *Textbook of Critical Care.* 5th ed. Philadelphia, PA: Saunders; 2005:951-959.

8. Valley RD. Postanesthesia care issues. In: Bagwell JM, ed. *Clinical Pediatric Anesthesia.* Philidelphia, PA: Lippincott Williams & Wilkins; 1997:461-475.

9. Wetzel RC. Anesthesia and perioperative care. In: Behrman RE, Kliegman RM, Jenson HB, eds. *Nelson Textbook of Pediatrics.* 17th ed. Philiadelphia, PA: Saunders; 2003: 342-357.

10. Yaster M, Bean JD, Schulman SR, et al. Pain, sedation and postoperative anesthetic management in the pediatric intensive care unit. In: Rogers MC, Nichols DG, Ackerman AD, et al, eds. *Textbook of Pediatric Intensive Care.* 3rd ed. Philidelphia, PA: Lippincott Williams & Wilkins; 1997:1547-1593.

Chapter 22:

Sedation, Analgesia, and Neuromuscular Blockade

Objectives

- Identify the indications, risks, and monitoring needs for patients undergoing elective procedural sedation.
- Explain the various benefits and side-effects of commonly used sedating agents.
- Describe the differences between mild, moderate, and deep sedation.
- State the benefits of the appropriate use of therapeutic analgesia in critically ill patients.
- Know the reversal agents for benzodiazepines and opioid agents.
- Describe the indications and potential risks of neuromuscular blocking agents.

Case Study

A 3 year-old girl presents with a heart rate of 170, a mottled appearance, a systolic blood pressure of 70 mm Hg, hypothermia, and moderate respiratory distress several days after being diagnosed with influenza. She is placed on oxygen via face mask, and fluid resuscitation is begun with isotonic saline as preparations are made for intubation.

- Which medications should be used to intubate the child?

- What can be used to provide analgesia and sedation before transfer to the PICU?

-Which medicines are best avoided in the presence of shock?

I. INTRODUCTION

Analgesia and sedation are integral in the care of critically ill children. Indeed, it has been recognized for many years that inadequate analgesia and sedation during or following painful procedures may have long-lasting effects on a child's stress response, thus adversely affecting the physiologic, neurodevelopmental, and psychological outcomes. Additionally, the placement and maintenance of invasive monitoring and therapeutic devices for acute stabilization and management of critically ill children would be extremely difficult, if not impossible, without these agents. Thus, the primary goal of analgesia and sedation is to facilitate optimal patient care.

> **!**
>
> *Basic principles must be applied by the prudent clinician caring for any patient requiring sedation. Untoward and even fatal complications may accompany any sedation.*
>
> **!**

Although this discussion centers on the use of sedatives, analgesics, and neuromuscular blockade in the setting of pediatric critical illness, basic principles must be applied by the prudent clinician caring for any patient requiring sedation. Untoward and even fatal complications may accompany any sedation.

The "Guidelines for Monitoring and Management of Pediatric Patients During and After Sedation for Diagnostic and Therapeutic Procedures: An Update," recently published by the American Academy of Pediatrics (AAP) and the American Academy of Pediatric Dentistry (AAPD), emphasizes the following:

- No sedative medication should ever be administered without medical supervision.
- A careful pre-sedation evaluation should be completed to ensure the identification of conditions that could increase risk.
- Appropriate fasting should be ensured for elective procedures; a risk/benefit assessment should be performed prior to medicating children who require unplanned sedations for emergencies.
- Focused physical examinations with an emphasis on the pediatric airway should be performed.
- Practitioners should have a solid knowledge of the pharmacology and potential interactions of the drugs utilized.
- Age- and size-specific airway equipment should be checked and immediately available prior to the administration of any agent.
- Emergency drugs for agent reversal and cardiopulmonary support must be immediately available.
- Adequate staffing is imperative. One person's sole responsibility should be to monitor the sedated child's vital signs.

- Appropriate monitoring must be maintained, including, at a minimum, continuous pulse oximetry for all patients requiring moderate or deeper levels of sedation.
- The patient must have recovered to the pre-sedation level of consciousness before discharge to a lower level of care is contemplated.

Several excellent recent publications address the safe and effective use of opioids and sedating agents in the emergency department and intensive care units. The Joint Commission (formerly the Joint Commission on Accreditation of Healthcare Organizations) mandates that the standard of care for sedated children be uniform throughout an institution. Institutional guidelines should be based on the recommendations of the AAP and the American Society of Anesthesiologists (ASA). (See **Appendix 13**).

II. LEVELS OF SEDATION AND RISK FACTORS

Procedural sedation occurs along a continuum ranging from minimal sedation or anxiolysis to general anesthesia. Patients, particularly children, are apt to transition from the desired depth to unintended, deeper planes. It is therefore imperative to have the ability to quickly recognize this phenomenon so that appropriate rescue measures can be implemented in a timely manner.

A. Levels of Sedation

1. Mild Sedation

Mild sedation is a drug-induced state during which patients respond normally to verbal commands. Although cognitive function and coordination may be impaired, ventilatory and cardiovascular function should remain unaffected.

2. Moderate Sedation

Moderate sedation (formerly known as conscious sedation) is a drug-induced depression of consciousness during which patients respond purposefully to verbal commands alone or to those accompanied by light tactile stimulation. No intervention is required to maintain a patent airway, and spontaneous ventilation is adequate. Cardiovascular function is usually maintained.

3. Deep Sedation

Deep sedation is a drug-induced depression of consciousness during which patients cannot be easily aroused but respond purposefully to repeated or painful stimulation. The ability to independently maintain ventilatory function may be impaired. Patients may require assistance in maintaining a patent airway, and spontaneous ventilation may be inadequate. Cardiovascular function is usually maintained.

4. General Anesthesia

General anesthesia is a medically controlled state of unconsciousness frequently accompanied by a loss of protective reflexes, including the abilities to maintain a patent airway independently and to respond purposefully to physical stimulation or verbal command.

B. American Society of Anesthesiologists Physical Status Classification System

The ASA physical status classifications are utilized during pre-sedation and pre-anesthetic evaluation. In ASA class P1 are previously healthy patients. Class P2 includes patients with mild, adequately controlled chronic disorders, such as asthma or a history of seizures. Children who fall within class P3 have disorders that may pose a threat to life, such as malignancies, morbid obesity, and chronic end-organ dysfunction. Because ASA class P4 implies the presence of acute conditions that pose a constant threat to life, children in this group should receive planned sedation only from appropriately trained anesthesiologists and intensivists. Sedation for intubation and other invasive procedures should proceed with extreme caution in emergent situations.

C. Risk Factors

Factors that increase the risk of complications during sedation include early infancy (less than 6 months of age), a history of prematurity, lack of provider experience, and ASA classification of P3 or greater. The role of fasting is undetermined at this time, but following ASA fasting guidelines appears prudent with elective sedations. Airway protective strategies, such as cricoid pressure during intubation and the use of appropriate tidal volumes during bag-mask ventilation, may prevent aspiration in patients at risk for delayed gastric emptying or those known to have a full stomach.

Factors that increase risk and are discernible on history or physical examination include but are not limited to chromosomal abnormalities, facial dysmorphisms, a uvula that is not readily visible without phonation (also known as Mallampati classes III and IV), large tonsils, known airway abnormalities or cardiac disease, suspicion of mediastinal mass, obesity, loose teeth, and dental appliances. The incidence of complications increases when multiple drugs are used in the initial stages. It is best to have a sound knowledge of 2 or 3 agents from each drug class.

III. ANALGESIA, SEDATION AND NEUROMUSCULAR BLOCKADE

A. Sedative Drugs

1. Benzodiazepines

Benzodiazepines are very useful anxiolytics, amnestics, and anticonvulsants. They appear to promote cellular hyperpolarization through interactions between the inhibitory neurotransmitter γ-aminobutyric acid (GABA) and the $GABA_A$ receptor, a membrane chloride channel.

Benzodiazepines, even at pharmacologic dosages, may decrease the ventilatory response to carbon dioxide. This effect becomes much more evident from the clinical standpoint when benzodiazepines are used in conjunction with opioids or any other central depressant, such as a barbiturate. Apnea and severe hypoventilation are extremely common in settings such as status epilepticus when these drugs are used in combination. Thus, age- and size-appropriate equipment should be readily available for rescue when these drugs are used. All patients receiving sedation should receive oxygen.

Significant cardiovascular effects may be noted at pharmacologic dosages, particularly in the presence of hypovolemia or when other agents that decrease systemic vascular resistance, such as opioids, are utilized. Life-threatening hypotension may occur if large, single boluses are used instead of carefully titrated doses over several minutes to allow maximal effect between aliquots. From a neurologic standpoint, these drugs are effective anticonvulsants and decrease both cerebral oxygen consumption and skeletal muscle tone. It should be noted, however, that they have no intrinsic analgesic effect.

The benzodiazepine most commonly used in clinical practice is midazolam. Although the dosages commonly cited in pediatric sources are 0.05 to 0.1 mg/kg, it is prudent to use aliquots no larger than 1 to 2 milligrams in children to prevent hemodynamic instability. Duration of action for a single intravenous dose of midazolam ranges from 30 to 60 minutes, with marked individual variability.

Lorazepam and diazepam are painful when injected intramuscularly and are not usually administered as continuous infusions due to their propylene glycol content. Intermittent dosing may be considered when a longer duration of action is desired than that attained with midazolam.

2. Barbiturates

The use of barbiturates is diminishing in the sedation of acutely ill children. Respiratory depression may be noted, particularly when these agents are used in combination with benzodiazepines. Barbiturates can cause profound hypotension by decreasing systemic vascular resistance as well as myocardial contractility. Hypotension can occur very rapidly and is often more pronounced in patients that are hypovolemic. The lack of any reversal agent makes barbiturates less desirable than benzodiazepines for use as sedating agents.

Despite these pitfalls, phenobarbital remains a useful drug for the management of acute seizures and status epilepticus. Pentobarbital may be employed to decrease cerebral oxygen consumption and intracranial pressure in children with severe brain injuries. It is also useful in the management of intractable status epilepticus.

Phenobarbital is usually started with a 20 mg/kg loading dose, followed by intermittent dosing. Pentobarbital is generally introduced in aliquots of 1 to 2 mg/kg (no more than 5 mg/kg total over 30 to 60 minutes), followed by a continuous infusion starting at 1 mg/kg/hour. In patients on continuous infusions, meticulous hemodynamic monitoring and serial measurements of pentobarbital serum concentration are essential given the effects of the drug on myocardial contractility and systemic vascular resistance. Additional concerns are leukocyte dysfunction and the potential for ileus with abdominal hypertension.

3. Other Sedative Drugs

a. Propofol

Propofol has a mechanism of action somewhat similar to benzodiazepines in that it exerts its clinical effects through interactions with GABA A receptors. An easily titratable level of sedation is reliably obtained. Amnesia is characteristic of this agent. Thus, it is an extremely valuable drug in the setting of planned procedural sedation in hemodynamically competent children. Because it lacks analgesic effect, it should be used in conjunction with an opioid if the procedure contains painful elements. Warming the emulsion to body temperature, admixing it with plain 1% lidocaine (usually 1 mL 1% lidocaine mixed with the first 10 mL propofol to be used for the induction), performing a modified Bier block with lidocaine, using large veins, or administering fentanyl several minutes before injecting the propofol may decrease the pain on injection that is observed in younger children.

The role of propofol in the management of the critically ill child is limited because it commonly leads to respiratory depression and has negative inotropic and chronotropic effects. Use of this agent in hypovolemic patients or those with decreased myocardial performance may precipitate a cardiopulmonary arrest, particularly if doses larger than 1 mg/kg are used during the induction. A highly lethal propofol infusion syndrome has been observed in children, and there have been recent adult reports as well. Thus, it is not a suitable agent for children requiring acute stabilization and transport and is best used only in the setting of an ICU for clearly defined indications and limited periods of time, typically no longer than 12 to 24 hours.

b. Ketamine

Ketamine is the only drug that truly creates a dissociated state and is one of the most useful drugs available for emergency care. Ketamine produces intense analgesia, amnesia, and a cataleptic-like state that facilitates emergent procedures. Airway reflexes are typically maintained, although apnea with fatal consequences has been reported. Laryngospasm may occur in the presence of airway secretions or if painful procedures are initiated before the child is adequately sedated. Children with depleted catecholamine stores, particularly during a prolonged illness, have developed cardiovascular collapse during induction with ketamine. However, it is generally a very safe drug to use in the acutely ill child. Systemic vascular resistance is usually well maintained and balances any increase in pulmonary vascular resistance or myocardial depression. Ketamine is the drug of choice for intubating patients with acute severe asthma or septic shock. Although it may have intrinsic neuroprotective effects, most practitioners avoid using it when increased intracranial pressure is suspected.

Children receiving ketamine should be premedicated with atropine, or at the very least glycopyrrolate, to offset the sialorrhea that is frequently observed. Noxious stimuli should be avoided until the child is clearly sedated to prevent laryngospasm. An appropriate dose of a benzodiazepine may be administered to decrease the frequency and severity of emergence phenomena.

> *Ketamine is the drug of choice for intubating patients with acute severe asthma or septic shock.*

c. Etomidate

Etomidate is structurally unrelated to other anesthetic agents and acts by depressing the reticular activating system and potentiating inhibitory neurotransmitters. Although it is devoid of an intrinsic analgesic effect, it is used for emergent intubation in situations where impaired cardiovascular performance or increased intracranial pressure are clinically evident. Because even a single dose has been associated with an increased risk of mortality and adrenal suppression, this agent should be used to attain adequate conditions for emergent intubation only in the presence of compelling circumstances contraindicating the use of other drug combinations. The typical dose under these circumstances is 0.3 mg/kg.

d. Dexmedetomidine

Dexmedetomidine is a selective α_2-agonist with potent sedative and analgesic effects. The role of this drug appears to be expanding in pediatric medicine. Attractive features include a low incidence of clinically significant respiratory depression and the apparent lack of tachyphylaxis. However, hypertension and hypotension have been observed during induction, and occasionally during infusions. Bradycardia may be marked, especially in the presence of other negative chronotropic drugs such as propofol, succinylcholine, digoxin, and pyridostigmine. Its use should be restricted to hemodynamically stable patients who are closely monitored in an ICU.

B. Opioids

Morphine and fentanyl are the most commonly used opioid analgesics. Morphine and other clinically important opioids act by binding to opioid receptors located on neuronal cells. Conformational changes in receptor proteins in turn activate other proteins, eventually decreasing intracellular cyclic adenosine monophosphate levels and hyperpolarizing the neuronal membrane.

1. Fentanyl

Fentanyl is a synthetic opioid analgesic commonly utilized during the stabilization of patients with significant hemodynamic compromise or severe bronchospasm because the related histamine release is much less significant than that observed with morphine. Fentanyl also is useful for procedural analgesia because it has a more rapid onset and a shorter duration of action than morphine. It is important to recognize, however, that very significant respiratory depression and hypotension can occur in patients who receive fentanyl and benzodiazepines simultaneously. Patients should receive adequate fluid resuscitation prior to the administration of opioids and benzodiazepines. Equipment required for airway control must be readily available when these medications are utilized.

> **!**
>
> *Very significant respiratory depression and hypotension can occur in patients who receive fentanyl and benzodiazepines simultaneously.*
>
> **!**

Additionally, it should be noted that rapid infusions of greater than 2 µg/kg of fentanyl can precipitate chest wall rigidity, which may require neuromuscular blockade for reversal. All patients requiring bag-mask or mechanical ventilation should be watched closely for hypotension.

2. Morphine

Morphine is an acceptable choice in hemodynamically stable patients who do not have a history of reactive airway disease. The duration of analgesia is much longer than that of fentanyl; therefore, it is more useful for patients with ongoing pain. Morphine's duration of action is 2 to 4 hours rather than the 30 to 60 minutes observed with fentanyl. Dysphoria is occasionally observed, and pruritus may occur as well. Active metabolites include morphine-6-glucuronide, which has intrinsic analgesic effects, and morphine-3-glucuronide, which has excitatory and possibly anti-analgesic effects. This should be kept in mind when this agent is utilized in patients with underlying hepatic or renal dysfunction because the duration of action and the balance of products of metabolism may not be predictable.

3. Use of Opioids and Benzodiazepines in Ventilated Patients

Adequate relief of the pain, discomfort, and anxiety provoked by medical or surgical disease is an essential component of critical care. The relationship between oxygen consumption and delivery is optimized by prudent analgesia and sedation. Neuromuscular blockade is rarely necessary to facilitate ventilator synchrony in the presence of adequate sedation, when the discomfort the child is likely to experience is limited to mechanical ventilation and the attendant invasive devices. A reasonable starting point is 1 to 2 µg/kg/h of fentanyl to control pain and discomfort with 0.05 to 0.1 mg/kg/h of midazolam to induce amnesia and sedation. Higher doses of fentanyl may be required when children are recovering from painful procedures or appear to have pain unresponsive to the initial doses.

Neonates and young infants can sometimes be managed with intermittent dosing of analgesia and sedation medications, particularly if they do not have a surgical or painful disease process. Older patients usually require maintenance infusions. It is helpful to remember that although opioids are excellent analgesics, they are not necessarily good sedatives; similarly, benzodiazepines do not have any analgesic effect. For that reason, it is important to consider whether pain or anxiety is the predominant symptom to be controlled. Daily interruption of continuous sedating medication has been found to improve outcomes in intubated adult patients and should be considered for pediatric patients.

Once the child has improved from the hemodynamic standpoint, it is worthwhile to consider whether a longer acting opioid such as morphine can be substituted for fentanyl. Morphine infusions or intermittent doses are less likely than fentanyl infusions to induce the phenomenon of pharmacologic tolerance. Moreover, morphine has active metabolites that have analgesic properties, and it may have some additional benefits in terms of fluid allotment and expense. A longer acting enteral agent such as methadone can be considered once a child has resolved any physiologic instability and is approaching extubation.

Supplemental analgesia and sedation are necessary for painful procedures. Local anesthetic infiltration for procedures such as placement of invasive lines or thoracostomy tubes should always be utilized, particularly in the presence of neuromuscular blockade.

Opioid and benzodiazepine requirements should be reviewed on a daily basis, especially when clinical assessment is complicated by concurrent use of neuromuscular blocking agents. It may be necessary to increase the dosage about every 3 days. One may find, however, that as a child's clinical condition improves it is sometimes possible to begin tapering the infusions to enable interactive ventilator strategies.

Tolerance to opioids is dependent on several factors, including duration of administration, developmental differences between neonates, infants and older children, and the use of synthetic rather than naturally occurring opioids. Some medications, such as methadone, may have a lower tolerance and dependence potential when compared to morphine. Concerns of tolerance, dependence and addiction should be addressed with appropriate specialists, so that pain can be appropriately treated in all cases.

4. Minimizing the Use of Opioids and Benzodiazepines

The management of pain should be clearly separated from strategies to control anxiety and undesirable behaviors, particularly in patients requiring prolonged stay in the pediatric intensive care unit (PICU) with repeated trips to the operating room. Some surgical pain may be obviated with the use of preemptive analgesia, epidural techniques, nerve blocks, and incisional infiltration. Propofol and dexmedetomidine may be useful in carefully selected patients during brief periods. Examples include the child recovering from an airway procedure who is agitated and a few hours away from extubation and patients who are rapidly recovering from head injury.

Pain control in the acute postoperative phase may be safely achieved with fentanyl or morphine. Other opioids may be useful in selected cases. Patient-controlled devices may be appropriate for some children. Other drugs, such as appropriately dosed, scheduled acetaminophen, may be very effective in augmenting the analgesia achieved with opioids. Some patients, particularly those recovering from orthopedic procedures, may benefit from a limited course of nonsteroidal agents, such as ketorolac. The use of low-dose ketamine (ie, 0.2-0.3 mg/kg/h) in addition to a morphine infusion may delay the need to escalate opioid infusions. Several recent reports highlight the utility of this drug in certain settings. One example is in children with extensive burns requiring repeated painful procedures.

Chloral hydrate may be useful in younger children who have infrequent episodes of breakthrough agitation, but it is a mucosal irritant, may produce habituation with withdrawal, and has significant drug interactions. Pentobarbital should be used cautiously because it can cause myocardial depression in some patients and may likewise produce withdrawal symptoms if stopped suddenly after prolonged exposure.

Severe behavioral symptoms in cognitively impaired patients or in patients who appear to be confused may respond to the use of haloperidol or risperidone in small doses. These drugs may be very effective in calming disruptive behavior but should be avoided in patients with underlying prolonged QT syndrome, hemodynamic instability, and seizure disorders. Although they are generally well tolerated, they may cause dystonia, which usually responds to diphenhydramine. Neuroleptic malignant syndrome may occur in very rare instances.

Experience with clonidine in pediatric patients to enhance sedation or manage withdrawal symptoms is limited. However, it may be particularly useful in the management of children who are also hypertensive. Use of the transdermal patch is complicated by the fact that the lowest commercially available dose is 0.1 milligram. Rebound hypertension and signs and symptoms of withdrawal may be precipitated if clonidine, and perhaps dexmedetomidine, is discontinued abruptly after prolonged exposure.

All patients receiving opioid and benzodiazepine medications are at increased risk of exposure keratitis, atelectasis, constipation or even ileus, decubiti, deconditioning, and foot drop. These and other complications of immobility or decreased activity may be minimized with early initiation of ocular lubrication, pulmonary toilet, enteral nutrition, a bowel program, physical therapy, and appropriate splinting.

Opioid- and benzodiazepine-withdrawal syndromes should be anticipated in all patients requiring 5 or more days of therapy, particularly when synthetic opioids have been administered as a continuous infusion. A long-acting agent, such as lorazepam, can be started 1 to 2 days prior to anticipated extubation to prevent withdrawal to benzodiazepines; the midazolam infusion can be tapered and stopped gradually once the child is close to extubation. Likewise, methadone can be started at a dosage that approximates the opioid equivalent (while also accounting for pharmacokinetic differences between the 2 agents). It may be initially dosed at intervals of 6 hours for approximately 1 day and subsequently decreased to longer intervals. Smaller dosages are often effective, with careful titration and consultation with a pediatric intensivist or pain specialist. Although methadone is given in three to four divided doses the first day, the dosing interval is gradually increased and the total daily dose is tapered to avoid drug accumulation.

Lorazepam and methadone are usually tapered on an individualized basis over several days to weeks, depending on the duration of previous treatment with benzodiazepines and opioids, with the goal of preventing physiologically significant complications of withdrawal, such as agitation, seizures, tachycardia, hypertension, diarrhea, and vomiting. Recovery from critical illness and its associated psychological derangements is also expedited by appropriately tapering these agents.

5. Reversal of Opioids and Benzodiazepines

Respiratory depression complicating exposure to any agent - including benzodiazepines and opioids - centers on appropriate support of the airway and assisted ventilation, as required. The use of flumazenil for suspected benzodiazepine ingestion has generally fallen out of favor due to the propensity of this agent to precipitate seizures.

Naloxone, on the other hand, is useful for accidental and intentional opioid overdoses. The recommended pediatric dose for rapid, full reversal of opioid-induced respiratory depression is 0.1 mg/kg, up to 2 mg per dose, preferably given IV although other routes such as the intramuscular and intratracheal routes may be used. Repeat doses, or even a continuous infusion, may be required for re-sedation or recurrent respiratory depression, as the offending opioid may have a longer half life than naloxone. Meticulous attention to the airway, breathing pattern, and circulation is essential.

The administration of full reversal doses of naloxone may precipitate pain in the opioid-naive patient, and withdrawal syndrome in patients with more chronic exposure. Tachycardia and hypertension, which may be poorly tolerated by children recovering from cardiac surgery, may be observed. Agitation and violent behavior may also complicate the administration of naloxone. Thus, it should be used cautiously in these settings. One approach is to administer small aliquots, carefully titrated to the desired effect.

6. Nonpharmacologic Strategies to Control Agitation

The PICU environment may be very upsetting to patients and their families. Units that allow privacy, continuous access to a supportive parent, and controlled sound and lighting may decrease anxiety in young patients. Likewise, promotion of a circadian rhythm by encouraging exposure to sunlight during the day and quiet, dark conditions at night may minimize the need to escalate drug therapy. Child life specialists can be very helpful in distracting and entertaining patients in ways that permit reduced doses or brief daytime holidays from opioid and sedative infusions.

C. Neuromuscular Blocking Agents

Neuromuscular blocking agents (commonly called muscle relaxants) are frequently used in the ICU to produce skeletal muscle paralysis. These drugs are devoid of any intrinsic analgesic or sedative effects because they exert their actions exclusively at the synaptic cleft of the neuromuscular junction with a depolarizing or non-depolarizing mechanism.

> !
>
> *These drugs are lethal if used improperly and should be used only by adequately equipped practitioners with excellent airway skills. Assistance should be summoned as soon as an airway emergency is detected.*
>
> !

Adequate intubating conditions are often difficult to obtain without the use of neuromuscular blocking agents. The choice of a particular drug depends on specific patient characteristics and the practitioner's preferences. These drugs are lethal if used improperly and should be used only by adequately equipped practitioners with excellent airway skills. Assistance should be summoned as soon as an airway emergency is detected. Unexpected airway difficulties must be managed in accordance with the published ASA algorithm as soon as they are recognized. Bag-mask ventilation with 100% oxygen is preferable to multiple intubation attempts, which may result in loss of airway landmarks and subsequent cardiopulmonary arrest.

1. Succinylcholine

Succinylcholine binds to the cholinergic receptor at the myoneural junction, causing depolarization. It is very popular in some centers, particularly for rapid-sequence intubation techniques, due to its quick onset and duration of action. Intubating conditions may be adequate within a minute of injection, and neuromuscular function may begin to return within 4 to 6 minutes. Nonetheless, succinylcholine carries intrinsic risks that must be carefully considered before it is used. Because succinylcholine acts on muscarinic receptors and autonomic ganglia, it may cause significant bradycardia, which may be poorly tolerated in patients with myocardial dysfunction and in younger children. Thus, it should always be preceded by the use of atropine, particularly if a second dose of the drug will be required. Tachycardia is *not* a contraindication to atropine use; any additional rise in heart rate will be small, transient, and less risky than an episode of bradycardia during intubation or instrumentation.

> !
>
> *Significant hyperkalemia resulting in cardiac arrest has occurred in patients given succinylcholine.*
>
> !

Significant hyperkalemia resulting in cardiac arrest has occurred in patients given succinylcholine during recovery from burns or crush injuries, in patients who have been bedridden, have underlying renal dysfunction, any kind of myopathy, or intraabdominal processes, to name only a few of the risk factors. Cardiac arrest following succinylcholine administration requires specific interventions to address the hyperkalemia, including calcium chloride (10 mg/kg), bicarbonate, and glucose-insulin infusions in addition to the American Heart Association Pediatric Advanced Life Support (PALS) and Advanced Cardiac Life Support (ACLS) protocols.

Succinylcholine releases histamine and may precipitate malignant hyperthermia. The diffuse muscle pain reported in a high percentage of patients awakening soon after the administration of this drug is less serious but troublesome. A small defasciculating dose of a non-depolarizing agent can be used to prevent myalgia, increased masticator muscle tone, and increased intracranial and intraocular pressure. Like ketamine, succinylcholine may be given intramuscularly in emergent situations before vascular access has been secured. The typical dosage for intramuscular administration is 3 mg/kg, compared to 1 mg/kg when it is injected via a peripheral or central venous catheter.

A wide variety of non-depolarizing neuromuscular agents is currently available. All of these agents share a common mechanism of action that involves competition with acetylcholine for cholinergic receptors at the myoneural junction, but they differ in terms of metabolism and duration of action. The use of any non-depolarizing neuromuscular agents carries with it the small but real risks of hypersensitivity, histamine-related bronchospasm, and true anaphylaxis.

2. Rocuronium

Rocuronium has an onset of action that approximates that of succinylcholine when a dose of 1 mg/kg is administered intravenously. Return of neuromuscular function is also quite rapid, often within 15 to 20 minutes. This makes rocuronium an attractive agent for brief procedures. One potential disadvantage, however, is that due to its brief duration of action, patients may become quite active in an unexpected fashion, risking loss of invasive medical devices, ventilator dyssynchrony with high airway pressures, and associated negative outcomes.

3. Vecuronium

Vecuronium shares the steroidal structure of rocuronium and is also commonly used for acute airway management at doses of 0.1 mg/kg intravenously. Duration of action is longer, typically in excess of 30 minutes. Vecuronium and rocuronium may be less likely to precipitate bronchospasm than atracurium. These drugs do not typically cause the tachycardia associated with pancuronium and are practical for long-term infusion in patients who do not have renal or hepatic insufficiency and do not require corticosteroids.

4. Atracurium and Cis-atracurium

Atracurium and cis-atracurium may have a relatively higher propensity to cause histamine release with consequent hypotension and bronchospasm, thus making them unsuitable for acute airway management. They differ structurally from the steroidal agents vecuronium and rocuronium in that they are benzylisoquinolines. Given the relatively large infusion volumes that are required, they are best used in the PICU for specific indications. The elimination of these drugs is independent of hepatic and renal function because they undergo a unique metabolism termed Hoffman degradation, making them useful in patients with multiorgan dysfunction in whom prolonged neuromuscular blockade may be a concern with other agents.

Cis-atracurium is used more commonly than atracurium because the latter is associated with formation of the toxic metabolite laudanoside in much greater quantities than the former. It is the drug of choice when neuromuscular blockade is required for extended periods of time, particularly if corticosteroids are required in the treatment of a child's underlying medical condition.

Prolonged neuromuscular blockade may contribute to the myopathy of critical illness, particularly in the presence of hypothermia; electrolyte abnormalities, including hypokalemia, hypophosphatemia, and hypermagnesemia; and metabolic disturbances such as hyperglycemia. Many drugs commonly used in critical care patients, such as corticosteroids and aminoglycosides, may significantly increase the duration of action of neuromuscular blocking agents.

Other problems that should be viewed as potentially avoidable secondary injuries include ileus, exposure keratitis, decubiti, deconditioning, and foot drop. Many PICUs have protocols in place that include daily neuromuscular blockade holidays, early initiation of enteral nutrition, bowel programs, ocular lubrication, range of motion exercises, and splinting to minimize the risk of secondary injury in children requiring pharmacological paralysis. Titrating the blockade to allow some patient movement while preventing dislodgement of medical devices may be preferable to the use of peripheral nerve stimulators, which can be painful.

Key Points

SEDATION, ANALGESIA, AND NEUROMUSCULAR BLOCKADE

- Adequate preparation is key
- All patients requiring sedation should receive oxygen
- Respiratory depression is best managed with supportive measures, including assisted ventilation for as long as necessary.
- Opioids are poor sedatives, and sedatives lack analgesic effects.
- Improper use of sedatives, analgesics, and neuromuscular blocking agents may be deadly.

Suggested Readings

1. Cook DR. Neuromuscular blocking agents. In: Fuhrman BP, Zimmerman J, eds. *Pediatric Critical Care*. Philadelphia, PA: Mosby Elsevier; 2006:1729-1747.

2. Cote CJ, Wilson S, Work Group on Sedation. Guidelines for monitoring and management of pediatric patients during and after sedation for diagnostic and therapeutic procedures: an update. *Pediatrics*. 2006;118(6):2587-2602.

3. Cravero JP, Blike GT. Pediatric sedation. *Curr Opin Anaesthesiol*. 2004;17(3):247-251.

4. Doyle L, Colletti JE. Pediatric procedural sedation and analgesia. *Pediatr Clin North Am*. 2006;53(2):279-292.

5. Heard CMB, Fletcher JE. Sedation and analgesia. In: Fuhrman BP and Zimmerman J, eds. *Pediatric Critical Care*. Philadelphia, PA: Mosby Elsevier; 2006:1748-1792.

6. Johnson YJ, Finkel JC. Sedation for procedures and mechanical ventilation in children with critical illness. In: Slonim AD, Pollack MM, eds. *Pediatric Critical Care Medicine*. Philadelphia, PA: Lippincott Williams & Wilkins; 2006:804-809.

7. Tobias JD. Dexmedetomidine: applications in pediatric critical care and pediatric anesthesiology. *Pediatr Crit Care Med*. 2007;8(2):115-131.

8. Twite MD, Rashid A, Zuk J, et al. Sedation, analgesia, and neuromuscular blockade in the pediatric intensive care unit: survey of fellowship training programs. *Pediatr Crit Care Med*. 2004;5:521-532.

Chapter 23:

TUBES, LINES AND SHUNTS

Objectives

- Describe the distinguishing characteristics of various tubes, catheters, shunts, and wires.
- Compare the various age-specific catheter and tube sizes that may be utilized.
- Recognize circumstances that may indicate the need for implementation of various technologies.
- Distinguish potential complications associated with the use of individual technologies.

Case Study

A 3-month-old with a history of prematurity status post, tracheostomy tube, nasoduodenal tube, and Broviac® catheter placement shortly after birth is brought to the emergency department by his parents after the feeding tube is dislodged and for evaluation of redness and green-colored drainage at the central venous catheter insertion site. The child is tachypneic with increased work of breathing, irritable, and febrile.

- What are the priorities of assessment and management?

- How would you evaluate the proper placement of the nasoduodenal tube?

- What additional studies would you like to perform during this patient's evaluation?

I. INTRODUCTION

Advances in medical science and technology have allowed children with complex medical conditions and special health care needs to live longer lives. The advances in technology have also made it possible for these technology dependant children to remain outside of the hospital setting and live in the community, while continuing to receive complex care. Children with chronic health conditions account for a substantial share of severe acute illness in a region. Because they have underlying conditions and reliance upon technology, they are at significant risk for complications associated with the medical devices, including malfunction, infection, dislodgement, and exacerbation of their underlying illnesses. The various tubes, catheters, and wires are not exclusively utilized in the care of the chronically ill child, but may also need to be implemented in the care of a child with critical illness.

II. TUBES

A. General Information

There are several different types of tubes that may be used in the care of critically ill children. These tubes fall into several different categories. They include gastrointestinal tubes and thoracostomy tubes. Each of the various tube types have a range of sizes that may be utilized. The specific size is determined by the pediatric patient's age, weight, and anatomical size.

B. Gastrointestinal Tubes

A variety of gastrointestinal tubes are used in medical practice. These tubes are usually made of polyurethane or silicone. Tubes have single or double lumens, are weighted or non-weighted, and are vented or non-vented. The name of the tube generally refers to the anatomical site of insertion and intended use. Typically, gastrointestinal tubes are used to access the stomach for decompression (air), removal of gastric contents (blood, secretions, ingested drugs, or toxins), or to instill products (medications, feedings, lavage fluids, or warmed lavage fluids to correct hypothermia). The diameter of a gastrointestinal tube is measured in French (F) units with each French unit equal to 0.33 millimeters. The size range that may be utilized in pediatrics is from 5 F to 14 F or larger (**Table 23-1**).

Table 23-1. Nasogastric Tubes: Typical Weights and Tube Sizes for Age

Age	Weight (kg)	NG-tube Size (F)
0 – 6 months	3.5 – 7	5 – 10
1 year	10	10
2 years	12	10
3 years	14	10 – 12
5 years	18	12
6 years	21	12
8 years	27	14
12 years	varies	14 – 16

1. Orogastric and Nasogastric Tubes

Orogastric (OG) or nasogastric (NG) tubes are used for both diagnostic and therapeutic purposes. They are frequently indicated for stomach decompression when a child is on invasive or noninvasive mechanical ventilatory support and for evacuation of gastric contents after an overdose, hemorrhage, or an ileus (**Figure 23-1**).

Figure 23-1. Nasogastric Tube

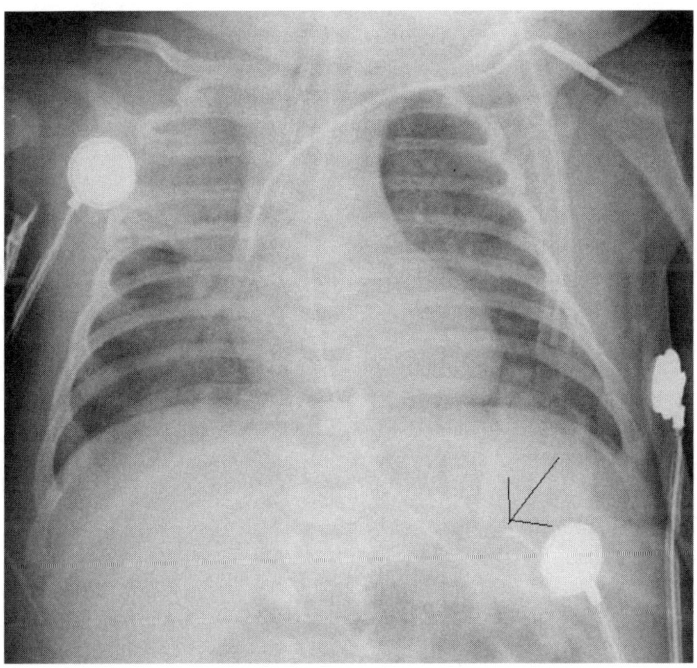

OG intubation is performed by passing a tube through the oral cavity, while in NG intubation the tube is passed through a nostril. In both instances, the tube is advanced through the oropharynx and esophagus and into the stomach. Orogastric intubation is specifically recommended for patients with suspected or confirmed anterior fossa skull fracture or maxillofacial injury. These patients are at high risk for inadvertent placement of the tube into the brain via the cribriform plate or ethmoid bone when the tube is attempted to be placed nasally.

!

Nasogastric intubation is contraindicated in suspected or confirmed anterior fossa skull fracture or maxillofacial injury.

!

The Salem sump is a vented, non-weighted, double lumen tube commonly utilized in patients requiring suction. The second lumen of the sump tube is the air vent, which allows air to continually irrigate the distal tip of the tube. This continual air irrigation decreases the likelihood of tube adherence to the gastric mucosa, resulting in gastric irritation. The Salem sump is not the optimal tube to utilize for feeding because of the stiffness of tubing material. It is more commonly used for decompression, lavage, or medication administration.

2. Feeding Tubes

A feeding tube is a medical device used to provide enteral feeding or tube feeding to patients who are unable to obtain sufficient nutrition by swallowing. Placement may be temporary for the treatment of acute conditions or, in the case of chronic conditions, lifelong. Small bore, weighted or non-weighted, single-lumen tubes are preferred for enteral feedings. Both weighted and non-weighted small-bore nasogastric tubes are available. They may or may not have a stylet guidewire in the packaging. If packaged with the tube, the guidewire is already in the lumen to assist in placement of the tube. After successful placement, the guidewire is removed and discarded.

Figure 23-2. Nasogastric Tube (NGT)

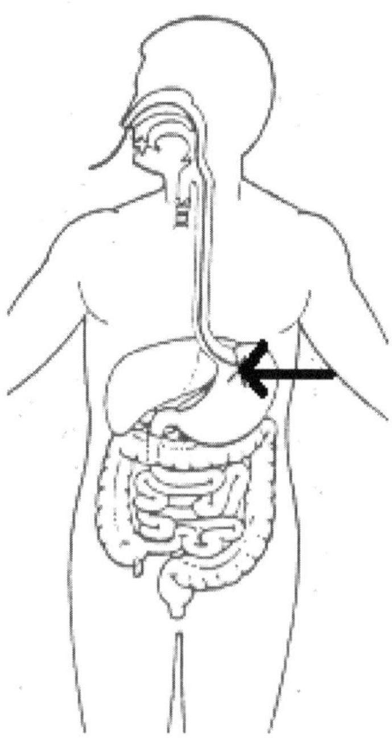

The small-bore feeding tubes are preferable to larger-bore nasogastric tubes over the course of time, because the risk of complications (tissue necrosis at the nares and sinusitis) is lower. Small-bore feeding tubes are not designed for drainage of gastric contents. The tube can be used for administration of nutrients, fluid, and medications. These tubes may be utilized for the short-term or long-term, depending upon the child's needs, prognosis, and family preference. The nonsurgical placement of these tubes includes NG, nasoduodenal (ND), and nasojejunal (NJ). The placement of the distal tip of the tube will dictate what type of feeding regime the child must receive. Nasogastric placement allows for both bolus and continuous feeding regimens to be implemented. Nasoduodenal or NJ tube placement will allow only infusion of continuous feedings and will not permit bolus feedings because of the inability of the duodenum or jejunum to appropriately tolerate absorption of nutrients in large volumes (**Figures 23-2, 23-3, and 23-4**).

Figure 23-3. Nasoduodenal Tube (NDT)

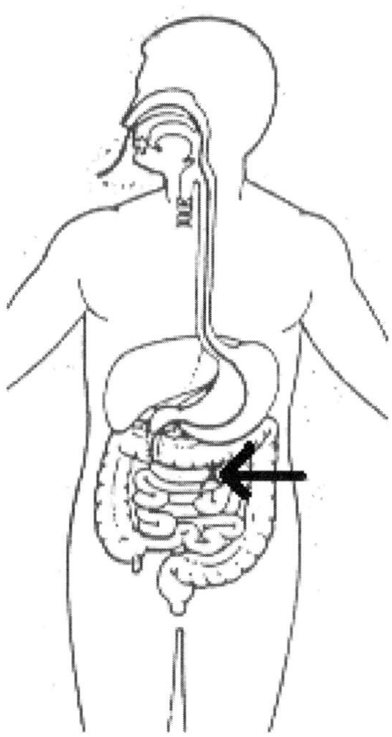

Figure 23-4. Nasojejunal tube (NJT)

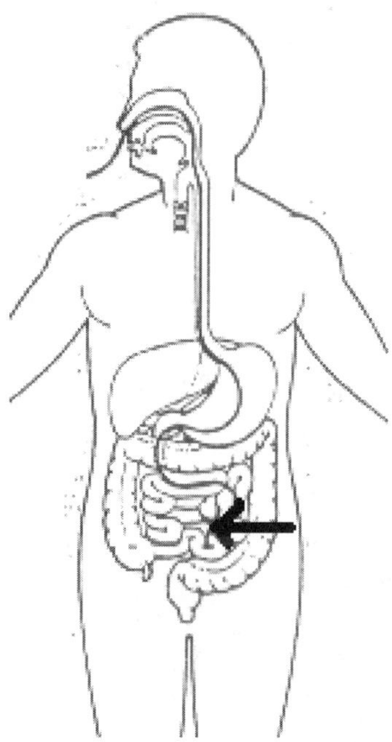

3. Complications

The most frequent complications associated with intubation of the gastrointestinal system are listed in **Table 23-2.** If equipment failure is suspected, remove all connecting materials and flush the feeding tube with 5 to 10 mL of water or air. If the tube flushes easily, it is likely that the equipment has malfunctioned. If unable to flush the tube, it is probably obstructed and needs to be exchanged.

Table 23-2 Frequent Complications Associated With Small-Bore Feeding Tube Placement

Coughing or dyspnea, indicating bronchial placement
Pneumothorax from inadvertent pleural placement
Tube coiled in esophagus or posterior pharynx
Esophageal tear related to trauma of tube placement
Tube dislodged or removed by patient
Aspiration of stomach contents despite appropriate placement
Clogging of enteral tube with enteral formula or medication fragments
Skin irritation or breakdown at insertion site

C. Gastrostomy Tubes

There is a large population of children with surgically placed enteral access tubes. These surgically placed feeding tubes include gastric tubes and jejuonostomy tubes. The tubes can also be used in reverse to decompress or drain stomach contents. Occasionally, there may be a need to insert an NG or OG tube to facilitate decompression of the stomach in addition to the gastrostomy tube.

Gastrostomy or gastric feeding tubes (G-tubes) (**Figure 23-5 and 23-6**) are the most common and can be placed in a number of ways. The Stamm gastrostomy requires laparotomy and results in a tube that is placed within the stomach.

Figure 23-5. Gastrostomy Tube

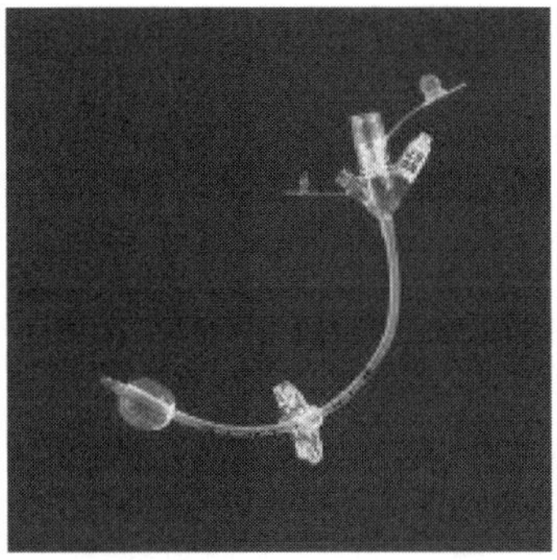

Figure 23-6. Gastrostomy Tube

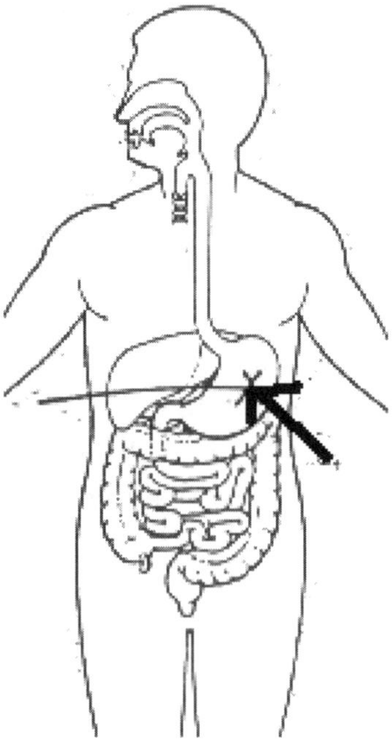

Percutaneous endoscopic gastrostomy (PEG) tubes avoid the need for laparotomy and, instead, depend on the traction exerted on the tube as it is anchored to the skin to maintain contact between the gastric opening and the anterior abdominal wall. PEG tubes often are tubes with rigid crossbars in the stomach, which precludes traction removal and requires another endoscopy for removal. Unlike in the adult population, these tubes cannot simply be cut and allowed to pass through the GI tract of a young child. They have been associated with small bowel obstruction and cases of esophageal erosion and perforation, because the device may “reflux” into the esophagus where it becomes lodged. Other potential complications include loss of contact between the stomach and abdominal wall resulting in intra-peritoneal soilage and injury to other viscera in the process of placement.

The tubes used for laparoscopic G-tubes are either primary MIC-key buttons or other balloon catheters. Laparoscopy-assisted G-tubes are anchored in a manner similar to the PEG. This procedure, however, avoids laparotomy, while minimizing the risk of injury to adjacent organs, such as the colon, in the process of placing the G-tube. The types of catheters used in each instance may be different. Operative G-tubes are generally Malecot or Pezzer catheters, which are simply removed by traction (**Figure 23-7**).

Figure 23-7. Mic-Key button

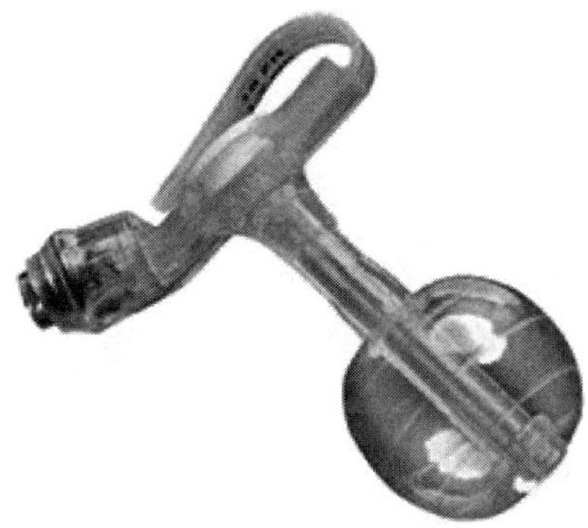

1. Complications

> ! *A Foley catheter needs to be placed promptly into the gastrocutaneous tract to maintain patency of the tract for patients with dislodged G-tubes.* !

Avoid excessive force when replacing G-tubes, because this may push the stomach away from the anterior abdominal wall and result in a gastric leak into the peritoneal cavity. If there is any difficulty in replacing the gastrostomy tube or the gastrostomy was created within the past month, a contrast study should be obtained to verify correct placement of the tube.

Judging by the thickness of the child’s abdomen, place the Foley catheter into the stomach wall a length sufficient to avoid inflating the balloon in the subcutaneous tract, approximately a 2 cm distance. To avoid the opposite extreme, take care not to push the Foley catheter so far that it passes through the pylorus and is inflated in the duodenum. This will result in gastric outlet obstruction and also has the potential for rupturing the duodenum. The pylorus is frequently within 5 to 7.5 cm of the site where the tube enters the stomach.

This also is the basis for evaluating feeding difficulties in a child with a Foley catheter used as a feeding tube. If not properly secured to the skin, the stomach will propel the balloon forward and through the pylorus as if it were a bolus of food, resulting in a very proximal small bowel obstruction (emesis may or may not be bilious, usually there is gastric, but no diffuse abdominal distension). These children usually present with excessive leakage around the G-tube site. The diagnosis is determined by examining how much tubing is protruding from the site. The problem is resolved by deflating the balloon, pulling the catheter out, replacing it to the proper depth (inserted approximately 2-4 cm), then securing it appropriately with tape. The best solution is a button G-tube, because this cannot be sucked into the stomach.

D. Jejunostomy Tubes

!

Small-bore feeding tubes are prone to clogging, particularly with certain medications and if not flushed as directed.

!

A jejuonostomy tube is similar to a gastric tube, though it generally has a finer bore and smaller diameter and is surgically inserted into the jejunum rather than the stomach. Jejunostomy tubes are indicated in medical conditions that require bypassing the upper gastrointestinal tract. These tubes may be used as soon as 12 hours after surgery.

Commercially prepared formulas are generally used for feeding through these tubes to provide nutrition and to avoid clogging when used with a pump or drip feedings (**Figure 23-8**).

Figure 23-8. Jejunostomy Tube (J-tube)

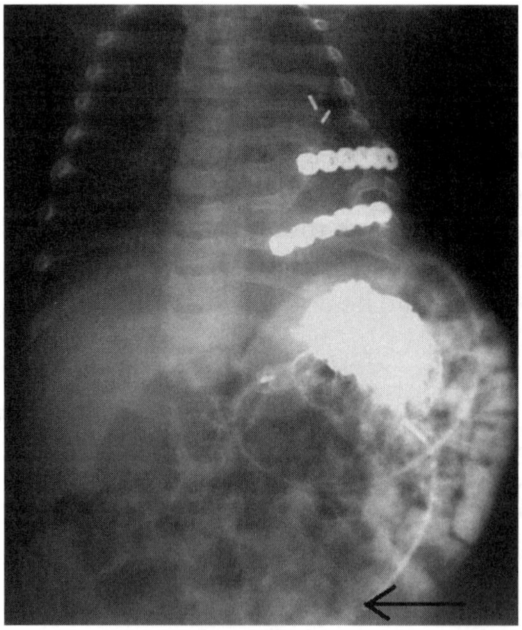

E. Thoracostomy Tubes

A tube thoracostomy, chest tube, or chest drain is a flexible plastic tube that is inserted through the side of the chest into the pleural space. It is used to remove air (pneumothorax), fluid (pleural effusion, blood, chyle), or pus (empyema) from the intrathoracic space. Needle thoracostomy may be accomplished more quickly than chest tube insertion; therefore, depending upon the child's clinical condition and the urgency of the circumstances, needle thoracostomy may precede the use of tube thoracostomy.

Chest tubes are sterile, flexible nonthrombogenic catheters made of vinyl or silicone and of varying French sizes and lengths. The size of the tube utilized is dictated by the anatomy of the patient and the reason for placement (**Table 23-3**). The insertion site selected for chest tube insertion is determined by the indication for the tube. If draining air, the tube is placed near the apex of the lung; if draining fluid, the tube is directed toward the base of the lung.

Table 23-3. Chest Tube Size

Age	50th percentile weight (kg)	Tube size (French)
New born	3-5	10-12
Infant	6-9	10-12
Toddler	10-11	16-20
Young child	12-14	20-24
Child	15-22	20-32
Older child	24-30	28-32

1. Complications

Complications of tube thoracostomy may occur during penetration of the pleural cavity, during placement of the tube, or after tube placement. Complications that can occur include damage to the thoracic nerve and damage to intercostal arteries. Excessive bleeding may also occur during penetration of the pleural cavity. During insertion of the tube, there may be bleeding secondary to vessel damage and damage to intrathoracic and abdominal organs. Organs that may be perforated by the tube during insertion include the lung, heart, diaphragm, liver, stomach, and spleen. Other complications appear to be directly related to tube location after placement. A tube that is not inserted far enough may cause an air leak and subcutaneous emphysema if any of the side drainage holes are outside the pleural space. A tube inserted too far will press against the parietal pleura or thoracic structures, resulting in pain and further tissue injury.

Complications may also occur after the tube is placed. A tube may become dislodged or disconnected. Pain at the insertion site may cause the child to splint, leading to atelectasis. The skin at the insertion site may also become irritated, erythematous, or excoriated, particularly if the occlusive dressing becomes saturated or requires frequent changing. See **Appendix 11.**

> !
>
> *Radiologic confirmation is necessary to verify correct tube placement.*
>
> !

III. CATHETERS

A. Introduction

A catheter is a tube that can be inserted into a body cavity, duct, or vessel. Catheters allow drainage or injection of fluids and access by surgical instruments. The process of inserting a catheter is called catheterization. Placement of a catheter into a particular part of the body may allow for the following:

- Draining urine from the urinary bladder, in which a catheter is inserted through the urethra or the suprapubic region into the bladder
- Drainage of cerebral spinal fluid into a body cavity
- Administration of intravenous fluids, medications, or parenteral nutrition
- Direct measurement of pressure in an artery or vein

B. Urinary catheters

In urinary catheterization, a plastic urinary tube urinary catheter (eg, Foley catheter) is either inserted into the patient's urinary tract via the urethra into their bladder or via suprapubic catheterization. If the catheter is to remain indwelling for an indefinite period of time, a balloon located at the end of the catheter is usually inflated with sterile water to prevent the catheter from inadvertently slipping out. In this manner, the patient's urine is collected, measured, and then contained for various medical purposes and tests. Catheters come in a large variety of sizes, materials (latex, silicone, polyvinyl chloride, or Teflon®), and types (Foley catheter, straight catheter, or coude tip catheter). The smallest size is usually recommended when placing a catheter in the urethra, although a larger size is sometimes needed to control leakage of urine around the catheter (**Table 23-4**). A large size may also be necessary when the urine is thick, bloody, or contains large amount of sediment or clots. Individuals with specific medical conditions (spina bifida or urogenital abnormalities, patients who have undergone repeated or prolonged surgeries or mucous membrane exposure to latex devices, especially early in life, atopic history or history of food allergy) are at a high risk for latex allergies

> !
>
> *Inquire about latex allergy history when treating a chronically ill child.*
>
> !

or may have developed allergies or sensitivities to latex after long-term latex catheter use. In such cases, silicone or Teflon® types should be used.

Table 23-4. Urinary Catheter Sizes

Age	50th percentile weight (kg)	Tube size (French)
Newborn	3-5	5-8
Infant	6-9	5-8
Toddler	10-11	8-10
Young child	12-14	10
Child	15-22	10-12
Older child	24-30	12-14

Intermittent catheterization may be used to collect urine specimens for laboratory testing. Patients with neurologic injuries, especially spinal cord injuries, may require clean intermittent catheterization for the long-term.

A urine collection system is attached to the catheter in circumstances that require the urinary catheter to remain indwelling. The connection of a collecting system maintains a sterile environment.

C. Intraventricular Cerebral Spinal Fluid Shunt

Cerebral spinal fluid (CSF) shunts are catheters that drain cerebral spinal fluid typically from the ventricles of the brain to another area of the body where the fluid can be absorbed. It involves surgical placement of a ventricular catheter made of silastic tubing, into the cerebral ventricles to shunt the CSF. There are a variety of medical conditions that may necessitate the placement of a CSF shunt. The most common is hydrocephalus, which occurs when the lateral ventricles become dilated with excess CSF. Hydrocephalus results from an imbalance between the production and absorption of CSF. This can be an imbalance resulting from a blockage in the normal flow of CSF, a reduction in reabsorption, or excess production of CSF.

The CSF shunt is frequently placed in a lateral ventricle of the brain to drain the CSF. The shunt drain is connected into a subcutaneous reservoir, which is usually placed under the skin of the scalp, outside the skull. This reservoir may contain a one-way valve with high, medium, or low pressure and a pumping mechanism. The reservoir is connected to a conduit, which is tunnelled under the skin to the abdomen or chest. Most shunt catheters drain the fluid into the peritoneal cavity (ventriculo-peritoneal shunt), but alternative sites include the right atrium (ventriculo-atrium shunt), pleural cavity (ventriculo-pleural shunt), gallbladder, and, in rare circumstances, the bladder (**Figures 23-9, 23-10, 23-11**).

Figure 23-9. Ventriculoperitoneal Shunt – Skull image

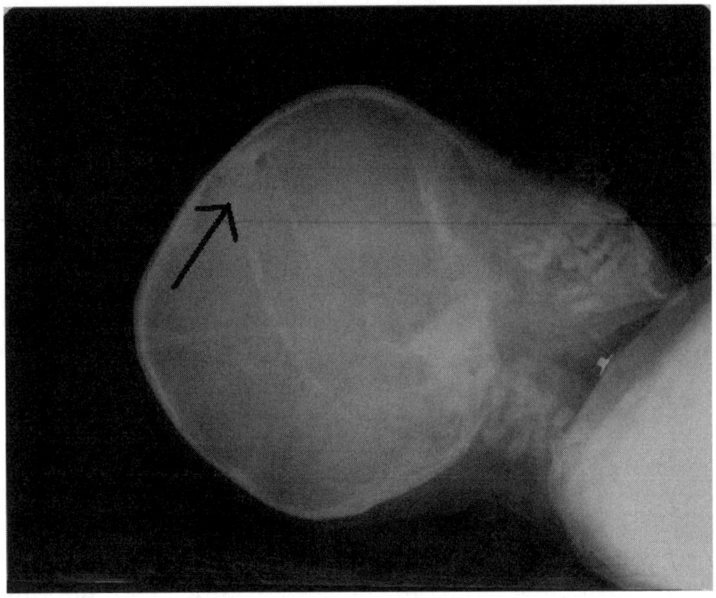

1. Complications

The most common causes of shunt catheter complications are shunt failure and shunt infections. Shunt failure is typically related to malfunction of the system or obstruction of the catheter tubing. Shunt failure can also be related to the shunt becoming dislodged, damaged, or displaced. The shunt may crack, disconnect, or become damaged if there is a traumatic incident or the child may outgrow the length of catheter tubing that was surgically placed and the stretching of the catheter may cause it to snap or disconnect. The child may begin to exhibit or complain of signs and symptoms of increased intracranial pressure as the CSF accumulates in the ventricles when the shunt is not functioning properly.

The shunt may become obstructed because of blood or protein clots forming inside the catheter, resulting in catheter obstruction, CSF accumulation, and increased intracranial pressure.

Often, the early signs of shunt obstruction are nonspecific. If the shunt is suspected to be malfunctioning, a shunt series that includes plain films of the skull, chest, and abdomen should be ordered. This radiographic imaging should be examined to determine if the continuity of the shunt is intact. In addition, a computerized tomographic (CT) image of the head may need to be obtained to examine the brain for the presence of hydrocephalus. The shunt failure rate is relatively high, and it is not uncommon for patients to require multiple shunt revisions within their lifetime.

!

Signs and symptoms of CSF shunt obstruction include headache, nausea or vomiting, irritability, bulging fontanel in infants, bradycardia, hypertension, change in pupillary size, ataxia, listlessness, apnea, change in mental status, and seizures.

!

Figure 23-10. Ventriculoperitoneal Shunt – Chest image

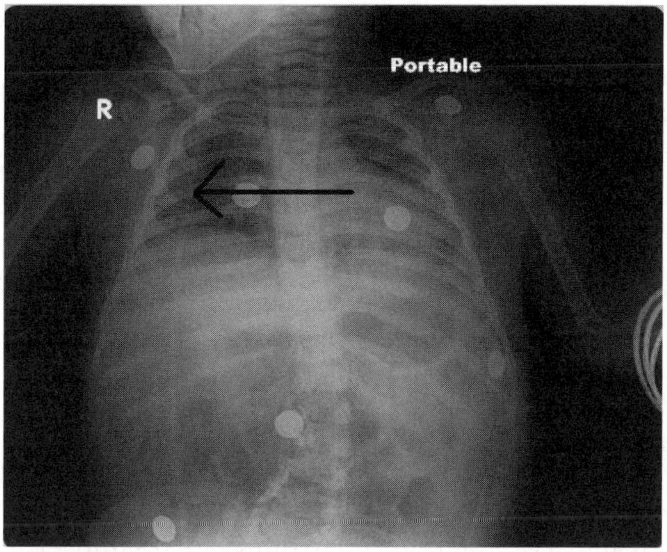

Figure 23-11. Ventriculoperitoneal Shunt – Abdomen image

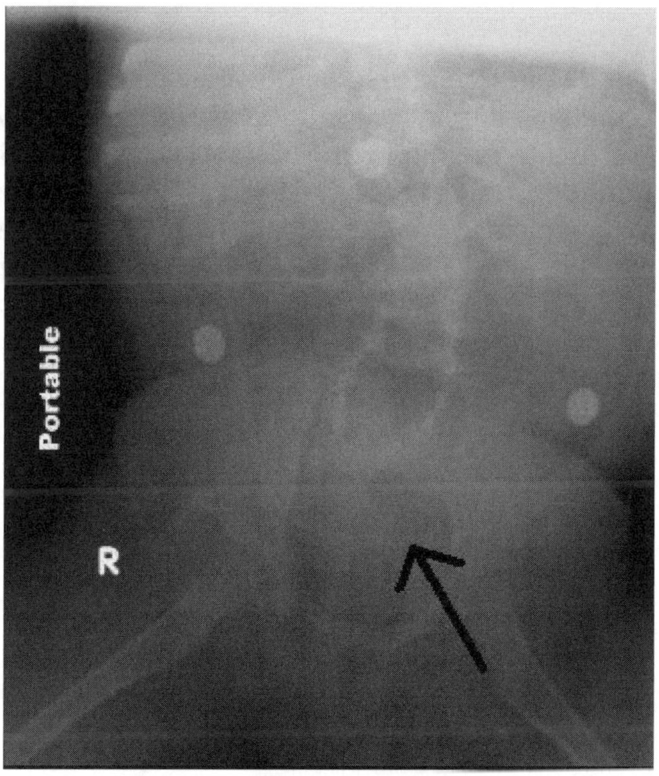

CSF shunts may also become infected. Children with potential shunt infections require the sampling of CSF from the shunt and antibiotic therapy. Shunt infection and obstruction, dislodged, damaged, or displaced shunts may require emergent surgical intervention. The child should be promptly transported to a facility that can provide definitive care, including surgical intervention and replacement of the shunt.

Signs and symptoms of shunt infection include fever, erythema, or tenderness at the shunt site, meningeal signs, vomiting, signs and symptoms of shunt malfunction, abdominal pain, and peritonitis.

The distal portion of the shunt may also have complications. The distal portion of the shunt may cause erosion or perforation of the stomach or intestines, resulting in symptoms of perforation or peritonitis. Adhesions may cause the distal portion of the shunt to be stretched, which may result in cracking, fracture, or obstruction. A pseudocyst may also develop when the omentum wraps around the abdominal end of the catheter, creating a sac or cyst into which the CSF drains. When sufficient fluid flows into this sac or closed space, abdominal pain and shunt obstruction can develop.

D. Indwelling Venous Access Catheters

Indwelling venous access catheters are used to deliver fluids, parenteral nutrition, medication, and blood products directly into a central vein and to draw blood samples. There are a variety of catheters available for long-term use. The type of catheter used is determined by the patient's needs and the preference of the health care team.

1. Tunneled Lines

Indwelling venous access devices are classified by how they are placed in the patient. Some catheters exit the skin directly above the vascular site after being tunnelled beneath the subcutaneous tissue of the chest, neck, groin, or arm and are inserted into a large central vein. These catheters are typically Broviac®, Shiley dialysis catheter, Hickman®, and Permacath® (**Figure 23-12**). These catheters are most often used for the administration of chemotherapy, medications, parenteral nutrition, and the Shiley catheter is most commonly used for the purpose of dialysis or apheresis. These catheters may remain in place for extended periods of time until they are no longer necessary or malfunction.

Figure 23-12. Broviac Catheter

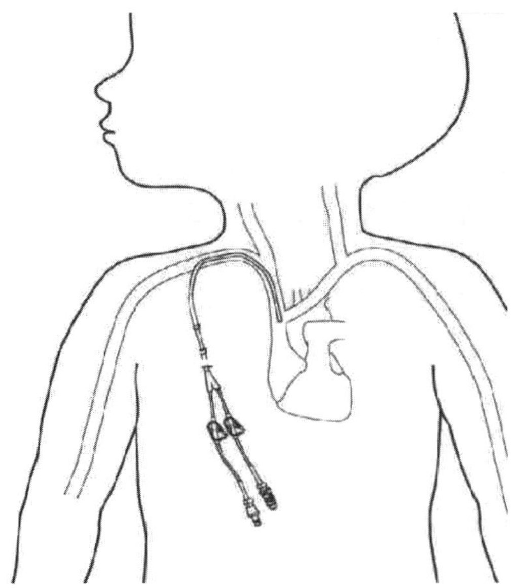

The insertion of these catheters is typically done under sedation or general anesthesia by a radiologist or surgeon. The catheter may have single, double, or triple lumens. The catheter is secured by means of a Dacron cuff just under the skin at the exit site, which prevents catheter dislodgement and forms a barrier for infection. The lumens are secured at the exit site with an occlusive dressing. External catheter lumens are typically flushed on a scheduled basis with an anticoagulant solution to prevent blood clots from forming inside the catheter (**Table 23-5**).

Table 23-5. Heparin Flush Table

Intravenous Catheter and Central Line Catheter	Peripheral IV Catheter	Central Line Catheter	Percutaneous Inserted Central Line Catheter (PICC)	Tunneled Central Line Catheters Catheter	Implanted Port
Description	Range in size from 24G to 16G. Always use a T or Y connector	Any venous catheter in which the tip of the catheter is lying in or past the SVC; placed percutaneously	Peripherally inserted central catheter; can be either open ended PICC or Groshong® PICC	Central venous catheters that are tunneled through subcutaneous tissue	Surgically implanted port (Port-a-Cath®, Pas-Port®, Infus-a-Port®, Medi-Port® have a flat septum; Groshong® port has a domed septum)
Site care (all IV tubing and caps are changed every 96 h)* (TPN/lipid tubing is changed every 24 h with solution changes)	q96h with site rotation and PRN*	Once a week if transparent dressing; q48h if gauze used and PRN. Use central line dressing kit. Do not use ChloraPrep® on infants <2 mo. NICU use povidone-iodine x3, then rinse with sterile saline solution, apply dressing. Non-NICU infants <2 mo. use alcohol x3, apply dressing. All others 2 mo or older, use ChloraPrep® x1, apply dressing.	Initial gauze dressing removed in 24 h, then once a week if transparent dressing q48 if gauze used and PRN. Use central line dressing kit. Do not use ChloraPrep® on infants <2 mo, use alcohol x3, then povidone-iodine x3, apply dressing. All others 2 mo of age or older, use ChloraPrep® x1, apply dressing.	Once a week if transparent dressing; q48h if gauze used and PRN. Use central line dressing kit. Do not use ChloraPrep® on infants <2 mo. NICU use povidone-iodine x3, then rinse with sterile saline solution, apply dressing. Non-NICU infants <2 mo, use alcohol x3, apply dressing. All others 2 mo or older, use ChloraPrep® x1, apply dressing.	Change access q7d and PRN. Dressing changes once a week with access changes; q48h if gauze used. Use central line dressing kit, new winged infusion set, 20 or 22 gauge, ¾ or 1 in needle as per patient.

Continued next page...

* as per individual policy

Table 23-5. Heparin Flush Table (Continued)

Intravenous Catheter and Central Line Catheter	Peripheral IV Catheter	Central Line Catheter	Percutaneous Inserted Central Line Catheter (PICC)	Tunneled Central Line Catheters Catheter	Implanted Port
Flush	Flush amounts for NICU by MD order. For all other patients: flush capped lines q8h and PRN Use 2.5 mL NS unless heparin flushes ordered, then use 2.5 mL 10 U/mL heparin	Flush amounts for NICU by MD order. For all other patients: flush all capped lumens q12h and PRN with 2.5 mL 10 U/mL heparin to each lumen. For blood withdrawal (for labs) discard 2 mL, withdraw specimens, flush with 5-10 mL NS, then heparin per above if capped	Never use anything smaller than 10 mL syringe on PICC and Groshong® catheter Flush amounts for NICU by MD order. For all other patients: PICC: 2.5 mL NS, then 2.5 mL 10 U/mL Heparin if <10 kg, 2.5 mL 100 U/mL if > 10 kg. q12h to each lumen. Groshong® PICC: 3-5 mL NS q8h when not in use, and after each use; 5-10 mL NS after blood infusion or withdrawal For blood withdrawal (for labs), only if PICC 3 Fr or larger, discard 2 mL, withdraw specimens, then flush with 5-10 mL NS, then heparin per above if capped	Hickman® or Broviac®: Flush amounts for NICU by MD order. For all other patients: 2.5 mL NS followed by 2.5 mL of 10 U/mL heparin q24h Groshong®: 5 mL NS q7 days when not in use; 5-10 mL NS after each use For blood withdrawal (for labs) discard 2 mL, withdraw specimens, then flush with 5-10 mL NS, then heparin per above if capped	Port-a-Cath® or Pas-Port®: Never use anything smaller than 10 mL syringe on ports. Flush daily with 2.5 mL NS, then 2.5 mL 10 U/mL heparin if <10 kg, 100 U/mL if >10 kg. At discharge and monthly, use 5 mL of 100 U/mL heparin to all ports. Groshong® port: 5-10 mL NS after each use; 10-20 mL after blood sampling or transfusion. If not in use, flush 1x mo with 10 mL NS. May require heparin if valve malfunctions, administer 5 mL heparin 100 U/mL For blood withdrawal (for labs) discard 3-5 mL, withdraw specimens, then flush with 5-10 mL NS, then heparin per above if capped

2. Ports

There are subcutaneous infusion systems with reservoirs that require the insertion of a needle through the skin to access the reservoir. The catheter port resides in a subcutaneous pocket in the upper chest, forming a small, palpable bulge under the skin. These catheters, typically Port-a-Cath® or Med-a-Port®, require a flush with anticoagulant only once a month or after completion of access. The risk of infection with this type of catheter is low when not in use (**Figure 23-13**)

Figure 23-13. Port-a-Cath®

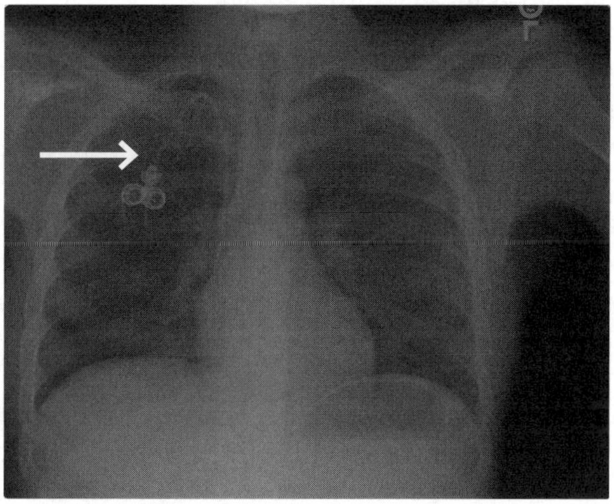

3. Peripherally Inserted Central Catheters

A peripherally inserted central catheter (PICC) or PIC line is a percutaneously placed catheter that is typically placed into the peripheral vein of the arm, such as the cephalic vein, basilic vein, or brachial vein, and threaded into a central (eg, subclavian) vein or the superior vena cava until the tip of the catheter rests near the cavo-atrial junction. PICCs are usually inserted with the use of local anesthesia or sedation. Typically, ultrasound or fluoroscopy is used to aid in their insertion and confirm proper placement. This catheter can be used for a prolonged period of time, typically for chemotherapy, extended antibiotic therapy, or parenteral nutrition (**Figure 23-14**).

Figure 23-14. Peripherally Inserted central catheter (PICC)

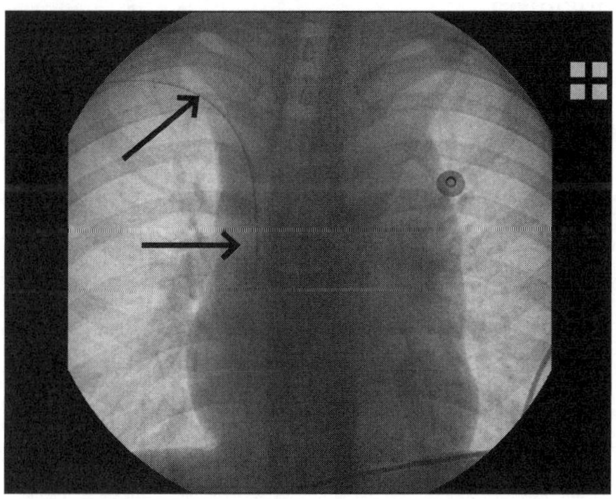

4. Complications

Potential complications associated with these catheters include occlusion, hemorrhage, thrombosis, infection, and phlebitis. These catheters may become displaced, disconnected dislodged, obstructed, or may simply fail. Children with displaced, dislodged, or disconnected, catheters may present with bleeding at the exit site. If the catheter is damaged or separated from an external connection, it may be possible to clamp the catheter near the exit site of the skin to prevent further bleeding. If the catheter is dislodged, direct pressure should be applied to the site, and ongoing assessment of the child's airway, breathing, circulation, and hemodynamics should be performed to assess for cardiorespiratory compromise.

The catheter may become obstructed by blood clots or crystals formed by medication or parenteral nutrition. The most serious risk of clot formation is the development of pulmonary embolism, which could lead to hypoxemia, respiratory distress, or shock. Signs and symptoms of emboli depend on the organ system affected and may include altered mental status, respiratory distress, cyanosis, dyspnea, chest pain, tachycardia, and shock. Air embolus is another serious risk for the child with indwelling venous access catheters. Signs and symptoms are the same as those for blood clot embolism. Treatment involves clamping the catheter, placing the child in a supine position with the left side down and head lower than the body, opening the airway, and administering 100% oxygen.

There is a risk for erosion or perforation of the catheter through the central vein, which may cause pneumothorax, hemothorax, or hydrothorax from the infusion of the intravenous solution. Prompt decompression may be necessary if these complications produce signs and symptoms. Erosion of the tip of the catheter through the right atrium can result in acute pericardial tamponade.

Infection is one of the most common complications associated with indwelling central access catheters, especially in a child who is immune compromised. Fever is a symptom of contamination and infection. The presence of swelling, erythema, tenderness, or bleeding at the exit site also may indicate infection. It is recommended to assess the hemodynamic status of the child, draw a blood culture from the catheter, and perform a complete blood count (CBC).

> **!** *Administration of broad-spectrum antibiotics is recommended until the source of infection can be determined.*

If the source of the infection is determined, the antibiotic spectrum should be narrowed to best treat the specific infectious organism.

E. Hemodynamic Monitoring Catheters

There are several types of catheters that may need to be inserted when a child is critically ill in order to monitor and assess hemodynamic status more closely and more accurately. These catheters include central venous access catheters and arterial catheters. The general trend over the past decade is not to insert pulmonary artery catheters or Swan-Ganz catheters in the pediatric patient.

F. Central Venous Catheters

Central venous cannulation can be defined as the percutaneous insertion of a vascular catheter within the lumen of a major high flow vein. The most common insertion sites for central venous catheter access include the internal jugular veins, subclavian veins, and femoral veins (**Table 23-6**). The femoral vein has become the most popular site for central venous cannulation in the pediatric patient. (**See Appendix 14.**) Central venous cannulation provides a more stable and reliable route of venous access than peripheral venous cannulation. Central venous access also allows hemodynamic monitoring and sampling of central venous blood for laboratory studies. A central venous catheter is a large bore catheter that allows for the rapid infusion of medications or large quantities of fluids. Central venous access eliminates the complications associated with administration of irritating or vasoconstrictive medications due to the lower risk of extravasation and the dilution of these medications by high-volume central venous blood flow. Indications for insertion of a central venous catheter include the following:

- Administration of fluids and medications to treat circulatory failure
- Administration of vasoactive medications
- Administration of hypertonic solutions
- Administration of caustic chemotherapy
- Measurement of venous vascular pressure (central venous pressure [CVP])
- Measurement of mixed venous blood gases
- Access for pacemaker or Swan-Ganz catheter placement
- Hemodialysis access
- Long-term vascular access

Table 23-6 Central Venous Catheter Sizes—Catheter Diameter (French)*

Age	Internal Jugular	Subclavian	Femoral
0-6 months	3	3	3
6 months-2 years	3	3	3-4
3 years- 6 years	4	4	4
7 years- 12 years	4-5	4-5	4-5
12 years and older	5-7	5-7	5-7

* Selection of catheter length is dependent upon operator's use for monitoring purposes or ability to infuse solutions rapidly.

Adapted from Lavelle J, Costarino A. Central venous access and central venous pressure monitoring. In: Henretig FM, King C, eds. *Textbook of Pediatric Emergency Procedures*. Baltimore, MD: Williams & Wilkins; 1997:251-278.

1. Complications

Complications of central venous catheterization occur more frequently in infants and children than adults (**Table 23-7**). Common complications include thrombosis, vascular/cardiac perforation, cardiac arrhythmia, air embolus, catheter fragment embolus, and catheter occlusion. Infection can occur with any method or site of central venous cannulation. Accidental entry of the guide wire into the central circulation is a rare complication that potentially requires removal by a surgeon or radiologist. This unusual complication can be avoided by always ensuring that the proximal end of the wire is secured at all times. The most common complications are thrombosis and suppurative thrombophlebitis. Proper cleansing of the insertion site and a sterile insertion technique will help to reduce the risk of complication. (**See Appendix 14.**)

Table 23-7. Complications of Central Venous Cannulation

Site	Complications
Internal jugular vein	Carotid artery puncture Carotid artery cannulation
Right subclavian vein	Pneumothorax Tension pneumothorax Thoracic duct puncture Decreased success rate with inexperience
Left subclavian vein	Pneumothorax Tension pneumothorax Thoracic duct puncture Decreased success rate with inexperience
Femoral Vein	Infection Arterial puncture Failure rate during hypotension/shock Inability to thread central catheter

Adapted from Fleck DA. Central venous catheter insertion(perform). In: Lynn-McHale DJ, Carlson K,eds. *AACN Procedure Manual for Critical Care.* 4th ed. Philadelphia, PA: W.B. Saunders; 2001:503-513.

G. Arterial Catheters

Arterial cannulation provides a direct means to continuously measure blood pressure and sample blood for evaluation of arterial oxygenation, carbon dioxide tension, and acid-base balance. Indications for insertion of an arterial catheter include the following:

- Hemodynamic monitoring
- Frequent arterial blood gas and laboratory sampling

An arterial catheter is the only method available for obtaining continuous beat-to-beat arterial blood pressure measurements. Noninvasive, indirect blood pressure measurements determined by auscultation of Korotkoff sounds distal to an occluding cuff consistently average 10 to 20 mm Hg lower than simultaneous direct arterial measurement.

The most common insertion sites for arterial catheters are the radial, femoral, axillary, posterior tibial, and dorsalis pedis arteries (**Table 23-8**). The site selection is based on palpable pulses, overall hemodynamic state, and other anatomic and physiologic factors unique to the individual patient. Because of the distance from the heart and the size of the vessel, the posterior tibial and dorsal pedis arteries are less reliable for hemodynamic pressure monitoring.

Table 23-8. Arterial Catheter Sizes by Site and Weight

	Infants <10 kg		10-40 kg		>40 kg	
Site	**Catheter Size**	**French Size***	**Catheter Size**	**French Size***	**Catheter Size**	**French Size***
Radial artery, posterior tibial artery, dorsalis pedis artery	Angiocath 22/24 gauge	2.5 F	Angiocath 22 gauge	2.5 /3.0 F	Angiocath 20/22 gauge	3.0 F
Femoral artery, axillary artery	Angiocath 18/20 gauge	3.0 /4.0 F	Angiocath 16/18 gauge	4.0/5.0 F	Angiocath 14/16/18 gauge	4.0/5.0 F

*Single lumen catheters are manufactured in standard French size and lengths. Only single lumen should be used for arterial vessel cannulation
Adapted from Torrey SB, Saladino R. Arterial puncture and catheterization. In: Henretig FM, King C, eds. *Textbook of Pediatric Emergency Procedures.* Baltimore, MA: Williams & Wilkins; 1997:783-795.

1. Complications

Arterial cannulation can produce complications. The complications include localized or generalized infection, proximal, distal air or particulate matter embolization, hematoma, blood loss, arterial thrombosis, and arterial pseudoaneurysm. Arterial thrombosis may result in tissue necrosis, tissue ischemia, and growth failure in the affected extremity. In children, the most common complications associated with radial artery cannulation are minor skin lesions, local necrosis, and radial artery occlusion. The potential for complication increases the longer the catheter remains in place.

Complications can be minimized by confirming adequate collateral circulation if performing a radial cannulation (Allen's test), performing a careful insertion, selecting an appropriately sized catheter for the artery involved, caring for the site, and implementing a continuous flush system. (**See Appendix 15**). The arterial waveform display on the monitor is a safety feature that will help detect inadvertent extravasation of blood through a catheter that has been accidently opened to the atmosphere. The extremity with the arterial catheter should be frequently assessed for evidence of ischemia.

> !
>
> *The catheter should be removed immediately at any sign of ischemia, such as blanching with flushing.*
>
> !

2. Measurements

The arterial pressure obtained from a properly assembled, positioned, and calibrated pressure monitoring system should be compared to the noninvasive cuff pressure. The hemodynamic waveform should be assessed. Several technical and anatomic factors may affect the accuracy of the pressures obtained from the arterial catheter system. The waveforms may display an under dampened or fling artifact, or over dampened wave.

Distortion of the arterial waveform signal may be caused by factors within the blood vessel, the hydraulic coupling of the transducer system, and system tubing compliance. Changes in the elasticity of the blood vessel wall, reflectance of the pulse waveform from the walls or tubing, small air bubbles in the system fluid column, small thrombi around or in the catheter, stiffness and length of the monitoring tubing, and other factors may cause an incorrect measurement of the true arterial blood pressure. The waveform must be assessed to ensure appropriate wave pattern. The arterial blood pressure should also be assessed in comparison to the noninvasive cuff pressure on a routine basis (**Figure 23-15**).

Figure 23-15. Arterial Wave Forms

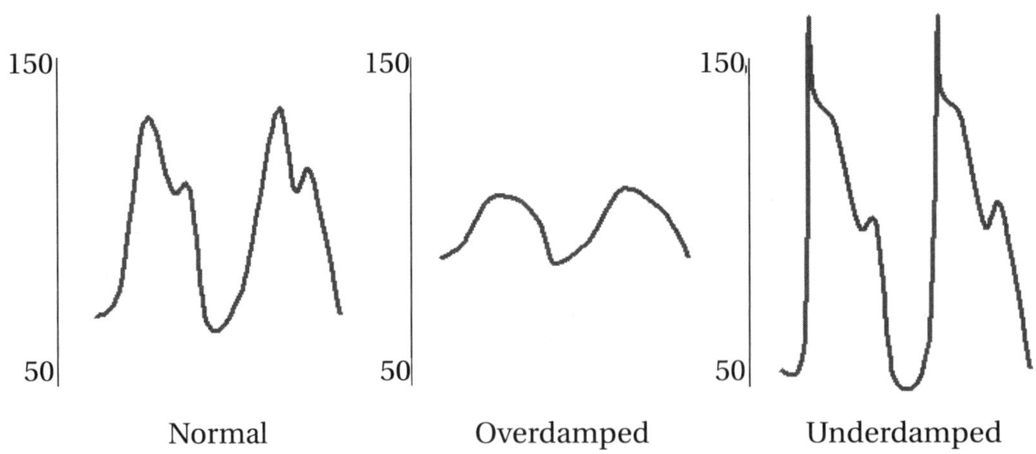

Key Points

Tubes, Lines and Shunts

■ Children should be assessed for the presence of devices, which must be evaluated to ensure proper functioning.

■ Insertion of hemodynamic monitoring catheters must be performed by individuals who have experience or expertise in the insertion techniques.

■ Any monitoring device requires that its users be thoroughly familiar with its operation and potential complications.

■ The two primary indications for insertion of an arterial catheter are the necessity of multiple arterial samples and continuous assessment of arterial blood pressure. Waveform analysis and troubleshooting are often required to ensure accuracy of measurement.

■ Management of abnormal pleural collections depends upon several factors: the etiology and size of the lesion, general condition of the patient, associated problems, need for patient transport, and need for mechanical ventilation or general anesthesia. Assessment of the need for tube thoracostomy needs to be performed. Not all pleural collections may require intervention or placement of a tube.

Suggested Reading

1. English LA, Maye JP, Dalton-Link MT. Hand ischemia associated with profound hypotension and radial artery catheterization in a pediatric patient: a case report. *AANA J.* 2003; 1:41-43.

2. Fiser DH, Graham J, Green JW, et al. Pediatric Vascular Access. In: Fuhrman BP, Zimmerman J, eds. *Pediatric Critical Care.* 3rd ed. Philadelphia, PA: Mosby; 2006:151-182.

3. Franklin C. The technique of radial artery cannulation. *J Critical Illn.* 1995; 10:424.

4. Hazinski MF, ed. *PALS Provider Manual.* Dallas, TX: American Heart Association, 2005.

5. Henretig FM, King C, eds. *Textbook of Pediatric Emergency Procedures.* Baltimore, MA: Williams & Wilkins; 1997.

6. Kovacevich DS, Papke LF. Guidelines for the prevention of intravascular catheter-related infections: Centers for Disease Control and Prevention. *Nutr Clin Pract.* 2003; 18:95-96.

7. Schindler E, Kowald B, Suess H, et al. Catheterization of the radial or brachial artery in neonates and infants. *Paediatr Anaesth.* 2005; 15:677.

8. Schwemmer U, Arzet HA, Trautner H, et al. Ultrasound-guided arterial cannulation in infants improves success rate. *Eur J of Anesthesiol.* 2006; 23:476-480.

9. Tegtmeyer K, Brady G, Lai S, et al. Placement of an arterial line. *NEJM.* 2006; 354:3.

Chapter 24:

HEMATOLOGY: COAGULATION AND TRANSFUSIONS

Objectives

- Identify coagulopathies and the proper management strategies.
- Evaluate therapeutic indications for the transfusion of blood products.
- Identify the signs and symptoms of adverse events frequently associated with blood transfusions.
- Determine apply therapeutic interventions for different adverse reactions.

Case Study

An 8-year-old, African-American female undergoing chemotherapy for acute lymphoblastic leukemia is in the clinic to receive her regular red blood cell (RBC) transfusion (q 3-4 weeks). After 30 minutes of the transfusion, she develops chills, fever, hypotension, gross hematuria, and extensive bleeding from her mucosal membranes. Her initial laboratory results show white blood cell (WBC) count of 32,000 (68% neutrophils, 20% bands, 12% lymphocytes), hemoglobin (Hgb) of 4.5 gm/dL, platelet count of 54,000/mm^3, prothrombin time (PT) at 38 sec, thromboplastin time (aPTT) at 58 seconds, fibrinogen of 50 mg/dL, and D-Dimer >10,000 ng/mL (0-230).

- What is the diagnosis?

- What is the immediate concern?

- What is the immediate treatment?

I. INTRODUCTION

Hemostasis is maintained through a delicate balance between pro-coagulant and antithrombotic factors. Severe deficiency of coagulation proteins can lead to bleeding or clotting. Clinically significant decreases in red blood cells, platelets, or coagulation factors require therapeutic intervention through transfusion medicine. Transfusion of blood products can assist in an oxygen carrying capacity, expanding the vascular volume, and improving coagulation and hemostasis. Packed red blood cells (PRBCs) are the most common blood component used, followed by platelets and fresh frozen plasma (FFP).

> !
>
> *Transfusion of blood products can assist in an oxygen carrying capacity, expanding the vascular volume, and improving coagulation and hemostasis.*
>
> !

II. COAGULOPATHIES

A. Consumptive Coagulopathies

Disseminated intravascular coagulation (DIC) due to malignancy, infection, or intravascular hemolysis can cause microangiopathy with hemolytic anemia and consumption of platelets and coagulation factors. DIC can result in life-threatening bleeding, large vessel thrombosis, or gangrenous limbs or digits. The main causes of DIC in children are infection (eg, meningococcemia), malignancy, massive tissue damage, and immunologic reaction. The focus of the treatment should be to treat the underlying condition and replace deficient coagulation factors and cellular elements with transfusions of FFP, cryoprecipitate, PRBCs, or platelets for bleeding symptoms. For this particular case, the transfusion needs to be stopped immediately, critical care support must be given, and depleted coagulation factors and RBCs should be replaced with FFP, cryoprecipitate, and PRBCs. Empiric antibiotics should be given to treat possible transfusion-associated bacterial infection.

Early recognition of the underlying cause of DIC will assist with the treatment and management of the patient. Conditions that are associated with consumptive coagulopathies are shown in **Table 24-1.**

Table 24-1. Diseases Associated With Consumptive Coagulopathies

Massive Tissue Damage: burns, shock, trauma, crush injury, brain injury, asphyxia
Malignancy: acute promyelocytic leukemia, solid tumors, metastatic malignancy
Vascular Disorders: aneurysm, vasculitis, hemangioma
Obstetric Complications: abruptio placenta, eclampsia, amniotic fluid emboli
Immunologic: anaphylaxis, transfusion reaction
Others: snake bite, hemorrhagic pancreatitis

DIC is a thrombotic disorder that may lead to thrombosis or hemorrhage. There are two primary manifestations in DIC: thrombin formation and hemorrhage. Patients often present with signs and symptoms of end-organ dysfunction secondary to microvascular fibrin formation or abnormal bleeding. The type of manifestation is dependent on the underlying problem.

Microthrombi can result in purpura fulminans or skin necrosis, organ failure, or gangrene. The thrombosis in the microvasculature results in a significant decrease in platelets and coagulation factors. The consumption of factors presents as purpura fulminans, mucosal bleeding, petechial hemorrhages, bleeding from central and peripheral lines, and possibly intracranial bleeding.

The diagnosis of DIC is made when the proper laboratory evidence and clinical findings are present. There is no specific test to diagnose DIC, however common laboratory findings in DIC consists of an elevated PT and aPTT, decreased fibrinogen, elevated D-dimer, decreased platelet count, decreased concentration of Factors V and VIII, and fragmented RBCs on the peripheral smear. These abnormalities are a reflection of the excessive thrombosis resulting in the consumption of platelets, coagulation factors, and fibrinolysis.

The most effective therapy of DIC begins with the treatment of the underlying illness, thus eliminating the catalysts of intravascular coagulation. Replacement therapy prior to the treatment of the underlying illness is important. In most critical care settings, treatment of the catalyst and replacement of factors is performed simultaneously. The replacement should begin with platelets and FFP. Transfusion of cryoprecipitate is required for the replacement of fibrinogen. Follow-up laboratory studies are necessary to monitor the correction of deficiencies.

> !
>
> *The most effective therapy of DIC begins with the treatment of the underlying illness.*
>
> !

Patients with large vessel thrombosis, purpura fulminans, or gangrene may benefit from anticoagulation therapy. The use of anticoagulation remains experimental and controversial and therefore should only be used in extreme circumstances by experienced practitioners.

B. Vitamin K Deficiency

Case Study

A full-term, appropriate-weight female is born after uncomplicated pregnancy and delivery. The mother is breastfeeding her child and refuses all immunizations and medications, including vitamin K. The baby is thriving until 5 weeks of age, when she has several days of watery diarrhea. The child presents to the emergency department with profuse rectal bleeding and scattered, large ecchymoses. She appears 5% dehydrated and has decreased capillary refill. Laboratory results show a low Hgb (6 g/dL) with normal platelet and WBC count. The PT and aPTT are both extremely elevated (>40 and >100 seconds, respectively), but the fibrinogen is normal (300 mg/dL). She is transferred to the critical care unit.

– What is the diagnosis?

– What is the treatment of choice?

This child most likely has late-onset hemorrhagic disease of the newborn (HDN) due to vitamin K deficiency and requires vitamin K administration and supportive care. Vitamin K is required for normal synthesis of Factors II, VII, IX, X, and Protein C and S.

The diagnosis of vitamin K deficiency is based on prolonged PT in the proper clinical context and correction of the PT with vitamin K administration. Patients have an elevated PT with a normal platelet count and normal fibrinogen levels. There will be a decrease in the vitamin K dependent factor levels (II, VII, IX, X, and Protein C and S). The diagnosis is made when the administration of vitamin K corrects the coagulopathy.

Deficiency of vitamin K may be due to malabsorption of fat-soluble vitamins, prolonged antibiotic use with decolonization of the gastrointestinal flora, or dietary insufficiency. Patients with vitamin K deficiency can be treated parenterally or orally depending on the clinical urgency. The decision of what method to use is based on the patient's state and the need for rapid correction. The use of oral vitamin K is best reserved for patients with dietary deficiencies. Patients that suffer from malabsorption should receive subcutaneous dosing or higher oral doses of 5 to 10 mg/day.

In severe cases where rapid correction is required, the vitamin K can be administered intravenously, although hypotension and anaphylaxis can occur. For warfarin reversal, a dose of 1 to 2 mg of vitamin K intravenously will reverse the effect. Patients with acute bleeding or those requiring emergency surgery should be given FFP every 6 hours until the PT normalizes.

C. Liver Disease

Case Study

A 15-year-old Hispanic boy has marked bruising. History suggests that this bruising involves all extremities, is usually small in size (1 x 1 cm), and sometimes spontaneous. The patient has a history of bleeding gums with tooth-brushing. There is no family history for any bleeding disorder. The patient had surgery in Central America for an abdominal problem about 10 years ago. Preliminary laboratory results show the following results: platelet count 80,000/mm^3, PT 25 seconds, aPTT 40 seconds, thrombin time 24 seconds (7 seconds prolonged), and fibrinogen 85 mg/dL. This patient had a previously undiscovered hepatitis B infection with liver disease and associated coagulopathy. The laboratory testing indicates liver disease manifested by abnormal coagulation in all screening parameters: slightly low platelet count; a more prolonged PT compared to the PTT, resulting also in a slightly low fibrinogen level and prolonged thrombin time; and the dysfibrinogen of liver disease.

– What is the diagnosis?

– What is the treatment?

Patients with liver disease have a multitude of hemostatic defects. The synthesis of coagulation factors and thrombopoietin, a regulator of thrombopoiesis, are produced primarily in the liver. The laboratory studies show a more prolonged PT compared to aPTT, Factor VII deficiency, increased Factor VIII, and usually, fibrinogen greater than 100 mg/dL. Patients with end-stage liver disease often have a fibrinogen level less than 100 mg/dL. Thrombocytopenia is a common finding secondary to platelet pooling from hypersplenism and decreased production from a decrease in thrombopoiesis.

In patients with coagulopathy from liver dysfunction, the platelet count should be maintained ≥100,000 cells/µL. The fibrinogen level should be maintained greater than or equal to 100 mg/dL by transfusing 5-10 mL/kg or 1 U per 5-10 kg of body weight of cryoprecipitate. For patients with active bleeding transfusing, FFP is indicated for prolonged PT/PTT and the replacement of clotting factors. Recombinant VIIa may be considered for liver disease associated coagulopathy if FFP is insufficient and the patient is bleeding, though it is not licensed for this indication.

III. BLOOD PRODUCTS

Case Study

A previously healthy 12-year-old female experiences decreased stamina, headache, and shortness of breath during exercise for the last several days. Her heart rate is 140/min, respiratory rate is 24/min, and blood pressure is 95/60 mm Hg. She is pale with cool skin. She has a flow murmur along the left sternal border. Preliminary laboratory results show a WBC of 3,000 (20% blasts), Hgb of 5.5 gm/dL, and platelet count of 54,000/mm^3.

– What is the diagnosis?

– What is the immediate concern?

– What is the immediate treatment?

The transfusion of blood products in newly diagnosed patients with leukemia is frequently a necessary treatment in the critical care setting. However, transfusing blood products is not without risk or complication. These complications arise from both infectious and noninfectious origins. Over the past 20 years, significant advances have been made in the screening of blood products, leading to a decrease in the incidence of infections. Still, the possibility continues to exist and must be carefully weighed. The decision to transfuse a patient should only be made when it is clinically indicated. Informed consent should always be obtained prior to the administration of blood products.

To decrease the chance of clerical error, all blood products drawn for typing and cross-match must be clearly labeled with the patient's identification. Prior to the transfusion of the blood products, the patient's identification band must be checked and blood type verified. The administration of the wrong blood products can result in serious consequences, including death.

Nucleic acid screening for human immunodeficiency virus types 1 and 2, hepatitis B and C, human T-lymphotropic virus types I and II, has virtually eliminated these infections from the blood supply, though there is a statistically calculable risk remaining. Bacterial infections still occur in up to 1 in 2,000 platelet transfusions and a smaller proportion of PRBC transfusions. Despite the improvements in screening, the risks have not been completely eradicated. Some of the pathogens transmitted by transfusions include *Bartonella* species, *Borrelia* species, *Brucella* species, *Leishmania* species, *Parvovirus*, plasmodia, rickettsia, *Toxoplasma* species, prions, and certain trypanosomas.

A. Red Blood Cells

Anemia is frequently encountered in the critical care setting. Red blood cells should only be administered with the consideration of clinical signs and symptoms (**Table 24-2**). A sudden loss of blood can compromise the cardiovascular system. Healthy, young individuals can tolerate a loss of approximately 30% of their blood volume. Unless there is rapid intervention, patients that lose 50% of their blood volume suffer from heart failure and death.

Patients with slow blood loss or chronic anemia are usually well-compensated. Subsequently, these patients may lack symptoms and do not seek medical attention immediately but may quickly decompensate if otherwise stressed. These patients often present with clinical signs and symptoms of anemia that include headache, fatigue, dyspnea, irritability, anorexia, and tachycardia.

Table 24-2. Clinical Signs and Symptoms of Anemia
General: Patients with sudden loss of blood can present with confusion and decreased responsiveness, as seen in patients with hypovolemic shock. Patients with a gradual onset of anemia have decreased stamina, headache, irritability, and anorexia.
Skin color: Check for pallor in the normal pink mucosa and nail beds, mottling, cool clammy skin, and delayed capillary refill. Prolonged iron deficiency can lead to softening and spooning of the fingernails.
Tachypnea: Rapid breathing and air hunger are important signs of anemia in infants and young children. Healthy adolescents tolerate moderately severe anemia with only dyspnea associated with exercise
Tachycardia: Patients with hypovolemic shock will have a rapid and thready pulse. Patients with prolonged anemia have an audible flow murmur on auscultation.

The underlying reason for anemia should be determined, and, when possible, corrected to avoid additional transfusions. Anemia can be caused by a number of factors, such as active bleeding, chronic inflammation, tumor infiltration of the bone marrow, bone marrow failure, nutritional deficiency, chemotherapy, and radiation therapy. The transfusion of PRBCs should be considered when the Hgb level falls below the 7 g/dL range. However, the decision to transfuse should be based on clinical parameters and context, and not solely on a laboratory value. The volume of PRBCs transfused in small pediatric patients who require less than 1 U should be based on body weight. As a general rule, 10 mL/kg of PRBCs will increase the recipient's Hgb by approximately 1.5 gm/dL. Severely anemic patients scheduled to undergo a surgical procedure or radiation therapy should be transfused prophylactically. Care should be taken not to rapidly transfuse a severely anemic patient, which may induce congestive heart failure. It is preferable to transfuse the severely anemic patient in smaller aliquots.

> !
>
> *Anemia can be caused by a number of factors, such as active bleeding, chronic inflammation, tumor infiltration of the bone marrow, bone marrow failure, nutritional deficiency, chemotherapy, and radiation therapy.*
>
> !

The current guidelines at the University of Texas M. D. Anderson Cancer Center utilizes: the "3, 4, 5 rule" for the initial transfusion. Patients with severe anemia (Hgb <5 g/dL), not secondary to acute hemorrhage, should be administered the amount/kg equal to the laboratory value of the Hgb. Transfuse 3 mL/kg for a Hgb of 3 g/dL; 4 mL/kg for a Hgb of 4 g/dL; and 5 mL/kg for a Hgb of 5 g/dL. Subsequent transfusions are administered at 10-15 mL/kg. This is performed to avoid heart failure.

One unit of PRBCs may contain 225 to 350 mL and, depending on the blood bank, may have a hematocrit of 55 to 80%. PRBCs are the product of choice to restore oxygen carrying capacity and RBC mass. PRBCs must be ABO and Rh(D) compatible to prevent a massive transfusion reaction. A cross-match is required to prevent transfusion of incompatible minor blood-group antigens. O-negative products should only be utilized in a life-threatening emergency.

The incidence of febrile reactions has decreased with the use of leukocyte filters. The utilization of leukocyte-depleted RBCs to reduce the incidence of febrile reactions and other cytokine-induced adverse events is standard practice in many institutions. The filters remove 99.9% of the leukocytes, which cause fever. Additionally, washed PRBCs effectively removes the unwanted cells, while still maintaining approximately 85% of the RBC mass. The use of irradiated blood is standard practice in cancer centers but is normally reserved for patients likely to undergo a bone marrow transplant. Indications for RBC transfusion are listed in **Table 24-3.**

Table 24-3. Indications for Red Blood Cell Transfusion

1. Infants less than 4 months old
    - **a.** Hgb level less than or equal to13 g/dL in neonates less than 24 hours old.
    - **b.** Hgb level less than or equal to 13 g/dL and presence of severe pulmonary disease, cyanotic heart disease or heart failure.
    - **c.** Acute blood loss of at least 10% of total blood volume.
    - **d.** Phlebotomy losses of at least 10% of the total blood volume.
    - **e.** Hgb level less than 9 g/dL in infants with clinical manifestations of anemia.
2. Patients 4 months of age or older
    - **a.** Symptomatic anemia.
    - **b.** Hgb less than or equal to 7 g/dL.
    - **c.** Hgb less than 8 g/dL in patients undergoing surgery or invasive procedures.
    - **d.** Intraoperative blood loss of 10% to 15% or more of total blood volume, postoperative Hgb level less than 8g/dL, and signs or symptoms of anemia.
    - **e.** Hgb less than or equal to 9 g/dL in patients with symptomatic anemia.
    - **f.** Hgb less than or equal to 10 g/dL in patients receiving radiation therapy.
    - **g.** Acute blood loss with hypovolemia unresponsive to crystalloid or colloid.
3. Patients with chronic congenital or acquired anemia and Hgb levels less than or equal to 8 g/dL with signs or symptoms of anemia.
    - **a.** Patients with sickle cell disease with an adequate reticulocyte count may tolerate Hgb levels of 6 to 7 g/dL.

B. Special Patients

1. Hemoglobinopathies

There is a high incidence of inherited defects in the globin structure in patients of African, Indian, Asian, and Mediterranean populations. The homozygous form of sickle cell anemia is a debilitating disease. Early in life, these patients present with severe hemolytic anemia and vasoocclusive disease. Patients with sickle cell anemia are at an increased risk of death secondary to sepsis or a thrombosis of the central nervous system (CNS). Patients with hemoglobinopathies, such as sickle cell disease, are at increased risk for vasoocclusive infarction of marrow, spleen, and renal medullary tissue. These patients often have recurrent painful crises.

Hypertransfusion therapy of PRBCs and maintaining the Hgb levels greater than 10 g/dL decreases production of sickle RBCs. This significantly decreases morbidity, the risk of other life-threatening events, and the frequency of painful crises. Patients with sickle cell disease have an increased risk of stroke and hyperviscosity, and, therefore, should not be transfused to a Hgb level above 12 g/dL.

Hypertransfusion is effective in minimizing the production of HgS. Because of the inherent risks with blood transfusions, prophylaxis transfusions are reserved for patients that are severely ill. Patients with a history of CNS thrombosis or transcranial doppler blood flow velocities greater than 200 cm/s in the middle cerebral or internal carotid arteries are recommended to undergo prophylaxis transfusions (**Table 24-4**).

Table 24-4. Indications in Sickle Cell Patients

Acute Transfusions	Prophylaxis Transfusion
Acute CNS thrombosis	Abnormal transcranial doppler
Acute chest syndrome	History of stroke
Aplastic crisis	Recurrent acute chest syndrome
Severe anemia	Uncontrolled pain crises
General anesthesia	
Multiorgan failure	

The use of exchange transfusion in sickle cell patients is also effective in reducing the amount of sickle cells. This modality of treatment is beneficial to patients with recurrent stroke, because there is no increase in hematocrit or blood viscosity. Exchange transfusions are also indicated in patients with hyperleukocytosis or hyperbilirubinemia. Considerations for exchange transfusions are listed in **Table 24-5.**

Table 24-5. Considerations for Exchange Transfusion

Considerations for Exchange Transfusion
Single volume exchange is an exchange of 80 ml/kg.
PRBCs are reconstituted in 5% albumin or normal saline solution to a Hgb of 10 g/dL for sickle cell patients.
Exchange equal aliquots and be certain that the final Hgb does not exceed 12 g/dL. This will help avoid the problem of hyperviscosity in children with sickle cell disease. The Hgb in children with hyperleukocytosis should not exceed 8 to 10 g/dL. In all cases, exchange transfusions require careful monitoring of Hgb level. Patients with sickle cell require monitoring of the percentage of HgA and Hgb S. Patients with hyperleukocytosis require monitoring of the white cell count.
Blood product preparation involves anticoagulation with calcium chelation. Therefore, patients administered large volume transfusions may develop hypocalcemia. Calcium gluconate should be administered in these situations.

2. Oncology Patients

It is not uncommon for pediatric oncology patients to be anemic at the time of diagnosis. In addition, patients are significantly anemic while undergoing chemotherapy. Patients undergoing treatment for malignancy are routinely transfused PRBCs. They are often anemic and are usually transfused if the Hgb level is less than or equal to 7 g/dL. Patients are transfused to maintain an Hgb level above 10 g/dL when receiving radiation therapy. All hematology-oncology patients should receive irradiated blood products to prevent transfusion-associated graft-versus-host disease.

3. Dosage

The dose of PRBCs is dependent on the desired Hgb or hematocrit, the rate of RBC destruction and the presence of blood loss. Patients with severe anemia and without ongoing blood loss that receive 10 mL/kg PRBCs will increase the Hgb level 1.5 g/dL (hematocrit increase of 3 to 4%).

C. Platelets

Platelets are instrumental in the role of hemostasis and coagulation. An adequate number of functional platelets are required for hemostasis. After vascular injury, the formation of the primary hemostatic plug subsequently prevents the flow of blood from small and medium-sized blood vessels. In addition, platelets release thromboxane A2, which mediates the change in vascular tone and platelet activation.

A healthy individual with functional platelets can withstand a platelet count of as low as 10,000/mm^3. Individuals with fever, infection, or who are acutely ill have a much higher risk of bleeding with platelet counts as high as 30,000/mm^3.

Clinical signs and symptoms of a reduced platelet count, known as thrombocytopenia, are nonspecific but primarily consist of gingival bleeding, epistaxis, hematuria, and petechial rash. The petechial rash is most commonly seen in the upper and lower extremities. Diagnosis of thrombocytopenia is based upon the platelet count.

The transfusion of platelets is used to prevent bleeding and to treat bleeding secondary to thrombocytopenia or platelet dysfunction. It is not indicated for patients with rapid destruction problems, such as immune thrombocytopenic purpura (ITP). In this circumstance, a platelet transfusion is only indicated if a life-threatening hemorrhage is present. Platelet transfusions are useful in the bleeding patient with a consumptive coagulopathy, such as DIC. Platelets are frequently administered in patients receiving chemotherapy or who have bone marrow infiltration. Indications for platelet transfusions are listed in **Table 24-6.**

Table 24-6. Indication for Platelet Tranfusions

Premature or Sick Infants
Platelet count less than 50,000/mm^3
Platelet count less than 100,000/mm^3 for infants hemodynamically unstable
Children
Platelet count less than 10,000 mm^3 with evidence of failure of platelet production
Active bleeding with a qualitative platelet defect
Platelet count less than 30,000/mm^3 with active bleeding
Platelet count less than 50,000/mm^3 with an anticipated minor invasive procedure and less than 100,000/mm^3 with an anticipated major surgery

continued nex page...

Table 24-6. Indication for Platelet Tranfusions (Continued)

Oncology
Platelet count less than 10,000/mm^3 without active bleeding and failure of platelet production
Platelet count less than 10,000/mm^3 when undergoing induction chemotherapy for acute lymphocytic leukemia
Platelet count less than 20,000/mm^3 when undergoing induction chemotherapy for acute myelogenous leukemia
Platelet count less than 30,000/mm^3 for patients with tumors in the central nervous system
Platelet count less than 20,000/mm^3 prior to spinal taps
Platelet count greater than 100,000/mm^3 in patients with a high risk of traumatic taps
Platelet count less than 50,000/mm^3 in a bleeding patient with normal coagulation studies
Platelet count less than 20,000/mm^3 prior to an intramuscular injection

1. Dosage

One unit of random platelets per 10 kg will increase the platelet count by approximately 50,000/mm^3 if there is no active consumptive process (fever, ITP, sepsis, alloimmunization, DIC) or sequestration. The platelet count should be checked 1 to 2 hours posttransfusion to identify refractory patients. A patient is refractory if 1 hour after transfusion, the platelet increase is less than 50-100,000/mm^3 on 2 separate transfusions.

A patient may have immune-mediated platelet refractoriness secondary to alloantibodies. Nonimmune causes of platelet refractoriness are common and include splenomegaly, fever, infection, DIC, and the use of amphotericin.

For refractory patients, a trial of cross-matched platelets should be given. Other possibilities for treatment (should this fail), include leukocyte-depleted human lymphocyte antigen (HLA) matched platelets, or massive transfusion with random donor platelets. Massive transfusion with random donor platelets will saturate the antibody concentration.

Pheresis platelets are harvested from a single donor and generally contain greater than 30,000/mm^3 platelets, which is equal to 6 to 8 U of random donor platelets. The volume is usually 250 to 300 mL. The use of single-donor apheresed platelets is indicated for patients who are frequently transfused or need multiple units in order to decrease donor exposure and the inherent risks.

D. Plasma Derivatives

1. Fresh Frozen Plasma

Patients with severe clotting deficiencies or undergoing a consumptive coagulopathy may require derivatives of plasma. FFP is a rich source for clotting factors. It contains a high concentration of fibrinogen, factor VIII, von Willebrand factor (vWF) and factor XIII. FFP is frequently used in patients unable to synthesize clotting factors due to liver disease or patients with a consumptive coagulopathy secondary to trauma.

FFP is plasma that has been harvested from whole blood. The whole blood is centrifuged, and the excess plasma is then frozen. The specimen must be frozen within 8 hours of collection and can be stored for 1 year at -20°C (-4°F). It is thawed at 37°C (98.6°F) for 30 to 60 minutes prior to transfusion. In order to increase the likelihood of the product remaining sterile and containing adequate levels of coagulation factors, FFP must be administered within 8 hours of being thawed. Additionally, the product must be ABO compatible with the patient's blood type.

Patients with a significantly prolonged PT and PTT have approximately 15 to 25% of their normal factor levels. Large amounts of FFP are required to increase the coagulation factor levels to greater than 30%. Each unit of FFP contains about 250 mL of plasma and yields only a 3% increase in coagulation factor levels. Indications for transfusion of FFP are listed in **Table 24-7.**

Table 24-7. Indications for Transfusion of FFP

Indications
Emergency reversal of coumadin anticoagulation
DIC
Thrombotic thrombocytopenic purpura
Prolonged PTT greater than 60 seconds
Prolonged PT greater than 18 seconds despite administration of vitamin K
Liver disease
Massive blood loss

FFP is dosed at 10 to 20 mL/kg and should be infused at a maximum rate of 0.5 mL/kg/min.

The use of FFP should be reserved for situations in which a concentrate of coagulation factors is not available. Generally FFP is no longer used for administration of factor VIII or IX.

2. Cryoprecipitate

The preparation of cryoprecipitate consists of flash freezing fresh plasma. It is then thawed at 4°C (39.2°F). The residual precipitate contains 150 to 200 mg of fibrinogen per 15 mL. Cryoprecipitate also contains factor VIII, factor XIII, vWF, and fibronectin at a much higher concentration then FFP. The use of cryoprecipitate is indicated when fibrinogen levels are less than 100 mg/dL. It should be transfused within 4 hours of thawing.

Cryoprecipitate is dosed 1 U per 5 to 10 kg of weight. One unit contains 10 to 15 mL of volume and will raise the fibrinogen level by 5 to 10 mg/dL. The therapeutic goal is a fibrinogen level >100 mg/dL.

IV. ADVERSE REACTIONS

Case Study

A 5-year-old female with sickle cell disease is in the emergency department to receive her regular RBC transfusion. Her trough Hgb prior to the transfusion is usually 6 to 7 g/dL. Twenty minutes into the transfusion, she develops chills, fever, hypotension, gross hematuria, and extensive bleeding from her mucosal membranes. Her initial laboratory results show WBC count of 32,000 (68% neutrophils, 20% bands, 12% lymphocytes), Hgb level is 4.5 gm/dL and platelet count is 54,000/mm^3.

– What is the diagnosis?

– What is the immediate concern?

– What is the immediate treatment?

The main cause of acute hemolytic reactions is ABO incompatibility. The focus of the treatment is to eliminate the catalyst and provide general supportive care. For this particular case, the transfusion needs to be stopped immediately and supportive care needs to be implemented. The lines need to be flushed with normal saline solution. This patient requires fluid resuscitation for the treatment of hypotension, antibiotics for possible infections, mannitol to maintain adequate diuresis, and FFP and matched RBCs for the replacement of the coagulation factors and RBCs. Once the patient is hemodynamically stable, mannitol may be needed to maintain adequate urine flow to prevent renal damage from hemoglobinuria.

> ! *The main cause of acute hemolytic reactions is ABO incompatibility.* !

The incidence of adverse reactions associated with the transfusion of blood products is about 5%. Most are mild urticarial reactions. These reactions can be treated with cessation of the transfusion for 30 minutes followed by the administration of antihistamines. If the symptoms subside, the transfusion can be restarted. All other reactions require stoppage of the transfusion. In addition, the transfused product and a blood sample from the patient must be sent to the blood bank for further evaluation.

A. Allergic Reactions

Severe allergic reactions can present with urticaria followed by laryngospasm and bronchospasm and angioedema. These patients require immediate cessation of the transfusion followed by intervention with steroids or possibly epinephrine. Anaphylaxis is a rare complication but, if not treated immediately, can result in the death of the patient. Most anaphylactoid reactions occur in patients with Ig-A deficiency. The transfusion should not be restarted after any severe reaction.

B. Febrile Nonhemolytic Reactions

Even after washing or filtering PRBCs, a percentage of leukocytes and cytokines remain present in blood products. The presence of leukocytes results in the release of cytokines during transfusion in patients with antibodies that react with alloantigens in the blood product. This often results in fever, chills, or diaphoresis. These symptoms can also occur if the blood product is contaminated with bacteria. Patients that have chronic transfusions should receive leukocyte-depleted blood products. This will help minimize the development of antibodies that react with foreign WBCs.

The treatment for febrile nonhemolytic reactions consists of stoppage of the transfusion. The patient should receive a physical examination and their vital signs should be monitored. Symptoms should be treated with antipyretics and, possibly, antibiotics. The transfused product should be evaluated with culture data and cross-matched again.

C. Acute Hemolytic Transfusion Reactions

Transfusion of ABO-incompatible blood products results in acute hemolytic transfusion reactions. This is usually a result of mislabeled blood products or the administration of blood products to the wrong patient. This results in the immunologic destruction of the transfused RBCs.

Clinical signs and symptoms of acute hemolytic reactions consist of fever, chills, urticaria, dyspnea, tachycardia, nausea, abdominal or lower back pain, hyper- or hypotension, jaundice, hemoglobinuria (port wine colored urine), and shock. The hemoglobinuria leads to oliguria and, eventually, renal failure. Laboratory evaluation should include a complete blood count (CBC), coagulation studies, urine analysis, and a direct Coombs test. Significant laboratory findings may include anemia, DIC and hemoglobinuria, and a positive Coombs test.

Therapy for acute hemolytic transfusion reactions involves immediate cessation of the transfusion and fluid support with diuretics (mannitol) to maintain adequate renal blood flow and cardiovascular tone. The urine output should be maintained at approximately 1 to 2 mL/kg/h. Vasopressors and inotropes may be required to maintain hemodynamic stability. The use of steroids is indicated in the management of acute hemolytic reaction transfusions because of its effectiveness in suppressing the inflammatory reaction.

D. Delayed Hemolytic Transfusion Reactions

There are two different types of delayed hemolytic transfusion reactions: primary immunization and anamnestic response. The primary immunization type is characterized as a mild reaction tending to occur weeks after the administration of blood products. This type of reaction rarely leads to significant hemolysis. Laboratory evaluation will usually demonstrate a decrease in hemoglobin level 2 to 4 weeks after transfusion.

The anamnestic response tends to occur in patients with a previous history of sensitization to minor blood group antigens secondary to pregnancy or a previous blood transfusion. This reaction can result in a severe drop in hemoglobin over 3 to 10 days. The clinical signs and symptoms are not as severe as in hemolytic anemias secondary to ABO incompatibility. As with all hemolytic reactions, the diagnosis is confirmed with a positive Coombs test and the identification of alloantibodies in the patient's RBCs. The management of delayed hemolytic transfusion reactions is nonspecific, because the symptoms are usually mild. Symptom control is usually sufficient.

E. Transfusion Related Acute Lung Injury (TRALI)

This is a clinical syndrome that presents with dyspnea, hypoxemia, cyanosis, hypotension, fever, chills, and the non-cardiogenic pulmonary edema. This is a severe and sometimes fatal reaction. It is the third most frequent cause of transfusion-related mortality. The symptoms ordinarily begin 1 to 4 hours after the transfusion of blood products. The pathophysiology is secondary to the transfusion of HLA-specific antibodies. The passive transfer of these antibodies results in increased capillary permeability and microvascular pulmonary damage. The treatment is respiratory supportive care (**Table 24-8**).

Table 24-8. Treatments for Transfusion Reactions

Article I Drug	Article II Dosage	Article III Indications
Diphenhydramine	0.5-1 mg/kg IV (max dose 50 mg)	Urticaria and hives
Acetaminophen	10-15 mg/kg po (max dose 1000 mg)	Fever and chills
Hydrocortisone	1-2 mg/kg IV (max dose 100 mg)	Severe urticaria, diaphoresis, rigor, or pallor
Epinephrine (1:1000)	0.01 mL/kg SQ (max dose 0.5 ml/dose)	Shock*, bronchospasm, and hypotension
Furosemide	1-2 mg/kg/ IV (infants) 0.5-1 mg/kg (older children and adolescents; max dose 40 mg)	Acute hemolytic reaction-maintain urine flow greater than 1 ml/kg/h
Oxygen	100% via non-rebreather face mask	

*Patients with shock may require additional therapeutic interventions including fluids, advanced airway management protection, and vasoactive medications.

V. TRANSFUSION-TRANSMITTED DISEASES

Significant advances in the screening of blood products have led to a decrease in the incidence of infections. The common serious culprits of transfusion-related diseases are hepatitis C (HCV), hepatitis B (HBV), human immunodeficiency virus (HIV), and cytomegalovirus (CMV). Blood donations are routinely screened for HBV, HCV, and HIV. However, donors who have been recently infected can go undetected. Transfusion recipients may also be at risk for parvovirus B19 and various parasitic infections.

A. Posttransfusion Hepatitis

The current estimated risk of posttransfusion HBV infection is 1 in 63,000 U transfused. HBV is symptomatic in 50% of adults infected. Approximately 5 to 10% become chronic carriers. This is in stark contrast to the pediatric population, where patients are usually asymptomatic but roughly 70% become chronic carriers.

The current estimated risk of posttransfusion HCV infection is 1 in 103,000 U transfused. Pediatric patients infected with HCV have a 30 to 50% chance of spontaneous clearance of the virus. Approximately 20% develop signs of cirrhosis after 18 years of age.

B. Cytomegalovirus

Patients with a transfusion-associated CMV infection exhibit signs and symptoms of a mild mononucleosis approximately 4 weeks after the transfusion. Transfusion associated CMV infection in an immunocompromised patient who has not been previously exposed to CMV can result in life-threatening illness. All immunocompromised patients (bone marrow transplant recipients, organ transplant recipients, and high-risk neonates) without serologic evidence of CMV require CMV-negative or leukodepleted PRBCs.

C. Human Immunodeficiency Virus

The current risk for HIV infection is approximately 1 in 675,000 U of blood transfused. Routine screening of anti-HIV antibody and HIV-antigen has significantly decreased the incidence of transfusion-associated HIV infection.

D. Parvovirus B19

Antibodies to parvovirus B19, a single-stranded DNA virus, are present in about 30 to 60% of blood donors. The presence of antibodies indicates immunity. It is rare for patients with parvovirus B19 to be chronic carriers, and the virus is estimated to be present in as few as 1 in 20,000 blood donors. However, if the virus is present in any plasma derivative, it can be transmitted to blood product recipients. The virus lacks a lipid envelope and, consequently, is not inactivated by heat or solvent/detergent treatment. Transfusion-associated parvovirus B19 infection in an immunocometent patient often is asymptomatic.

E. Parasitic Infections

Malaria remains the most common transfusion-transmitted parasitic infection. Malaria is an intraerythrocytic parasite. Therefore, any blood product with the presence of RBCs can transmit the parasite. Patients with a transfusion-associated malaria infection often present with nonspecific signs and symptoms 1 week after transfusion. Symptoms may include fever, chills, headache, and hemolysis.

Currently, there is no effective blood donor-screening device approved for malaria in the United States. Donors that are identified in the questionnaire as high-risk for transmitting malaria should be excluded from donating.

Key Points

Hematology: Coagulation and Transfusions

- Decreased stamina, the presence of headaches, dyspnea, and pallor are signs of anemia.
- The treatment of DIC focuses on the elimination of the catalyst.
- DIC replacement therapy consists of the use of platelets, FFP, and cryoprecipitate. Follow-up laboratory studies are necessary to monitor the correction of deficiencies.
- The use of anticoagulation and antifibrinolytics in patients with severe DIC remains controversial.
- For rapid correction of severe vitamin K deficiency, administer vitamin K intravenously.
- The use of recombinant factor VIIa has been used with some degree of success in patients with coagulopathies secondary to liver failure.
- When possible, the underlying reason for anemia should be determined and corrected to avoid additional transfusions.
- The standard dose of PRBCs is 10 to 15 mL/kg administered over a 2- to 4-hour period to avoid congestive heart failure. The rapid replacement of PRBCs is indicated in cases of acute blood loss or shock.
- Patients suffering from severe anemia without ongoing blood loss who receive 10 mL/kg PRBCs will increase the Hgb 1.5 g/dL.
- One unit of random platelets per 10 kg will increase the platelet count by approximately 50,000/mm^3, provided there is no active consumptive process (fever, ITP, sepsis, alloimmunization, DIC) or sequestration.
- Fresh frozen plasma is dosed at 10-20 mL/kg and should be infused at a maximum rate of 0.5 mL/kg/min.
- Transfusion-related lung injury is a clinical syndrome and presents with dyspnea, hypoxemia, cyanosis, hypotension, fever, chills, and noncardiogenic pulmonary edema. It requires respiratory support.
- Malaria remains the most common transfusion-transmitted parasitic infection.

Suggested Readings

1. Consumptive coagulopathies. In: Hillman RS, Ault KA, Rinder HM. *Hematology in Clinical Practice.* 4th ed. New York, NY: McGraw Hill; 2005:387-392.

2. Hemoglobinopathies. In: Hillman RS, Ault KA, Rinder HM. *Hematology in Clinical Practice.* 4th ed. New York, NY: McGraw Hill; 2005:80-93.

3. Kreuz WD. Treatment of consumption coagulopathy with antithrobin concentrate in children with acquired Antithrombin deficiency: A feasibility pilot study. *Eur J Pediatr.* 1999; 158:S187-S191.

4. Lusher JM. Clinical and laboratory approach to the patient with bleeding. In: Nathan DG, Orkin SH, Look AT, Ginsberg D. *Hematology of Infancy and Childhood.* 6th ed. Philadelphia, PA: W.B. Saunders; 2003:1515-1526.

5. Mattay MA. Severe sepsis: A new treatment with both anticoagulant and anti-inflammatory properties. *N Engl J Med.* 2001; 344:759-562.

6. M.D. Anderson Children's Cancer Hospital clinical practice guidelines for blood/blood product transfusion in non-neonatal pediatric hematology-oncology patients. The University of Texas; February 2007.

7. Sloan SR, Benjamin RJ, Freidman DF, et al. Transfusion medicine. In: Nathan DG, Orkin SH, Look AT, Ginsberg D. *Hematology of Infancy and Childhood.* 6th ed. Philadelphia, PA: W.B. Saunders; 2003:1709-1756.

8. Transfusion medicine blood component therapy. In: Hillman RS, Ault KA, Rinder HM. *Hematology in Clinical Practice.* 4th ed. New York, NY: McGraw Hill; 2005:431-440.

9. Wong ECC, Perez-Albuerne E, Moscow JA, et al. Transfusion management strategies: A survey of practicing pediatric hematology-oncology specialists. *Pediatr Blood Cancer.* 2005; 44:119-127.

Appendix 1:

The Role of the Rapid Response Team

I. What is a Rapid Response Team?

A. The rapid response team (RRT) is a team of skilled providers who can be called into action by any concerned person who notice abnormalities in patient presentation or whenever there is a concern that a patient appears at risk.

B. The primary strategy is to rapidly evaluate and intervene for patients prior to the development of a cardiopulmonary arrest or other sentinel event.

C. There are many different names for RRTs, including Medical Emergency Teams (METs), Pre-Code Blue Teams, etc. Whatever the name, the common theme is the focus on detection and management of signs and symptoms of deterioration.

II. Why a Rapid Response Team?

A. Hospitalized patients can experience adverse outcomes as a result of their disease process or its treatment. Brennan and colleagues reported that adverse outcomes affected 4% of all admissions in United States hospitals, 13.6% of which lead to death.[1] Similar studies in Europe and Australia yielded similar results. Many of these adverse events are preventable.

B. The Institute for Healthcare Improvement (IHI) launched the 100,000 Lives Campaign in December 2004, and the 5 Million Lives Campaign in 2007, to bring awareness to sentinel events, which occur all too frequently, and with the goal of reducing preventable morbidity and mortality in (United States) hospitals through 6 patient safety strategies.

C. Deployment of a RRT was one of the key initiatives identified to improve patient outcomes and prevent avoidable injuries or deaths as well as reducing costs.[2]

D. Pioneered in Australia and the United Kingdom, RRTs have been deployed in more than 950 United States hospitals participating in the IHI 100,000 Lives Campaign.

III. The Role of RRT in Pediatrics

A. Several studies have demonstrated that patients often have signs and symptoms of clinical deterioration for several hours before a crisis event occurs.

1. Tibballs and Kinney reported 1.06 cardiac arrests, and 0.34 respiratory arrests per 1,000 admissions.[4] Only 36 % of those children with cardiac arrest were discharged from the hospital, while only 34% were alive at 1 year. The 1-year survival for respiratory arrest was 97%.
2. Buist and colleagues reported patients having circulatory or respiratory systems deterioration for at least 1 hour prior to unexpected cardiac arrests; unplanned intensive care unit admissions occurred in three-quarters of the subjects that were studied.
3. Weil and Fries showed that early recognition of signs and symptoms of clinical instability, coupled with intensive patient monitoring, reduced the need for cardiopulmonary resuscitation.

B. There are few reports in the medical literature on the incidence and outcomes of pediatric in-hospital arrest. Poor outcomes are reported and most in-hospital pediatric cardiac arrests result from unidentified or unsuccessfully managed respiratory compromise.

C. Detection and intervention are the essential elements of a RRT.

1. Brings additional experienced providers with more advanced monitoring tools to the patient's bedside
2. Provides a pathway for immediate interventions and advanced therapies to every bedside
3. Facilitates rapid transfer (if necessary) to a higher level of care

IV. The Composition and Function of the RRT

A. The most successful RRTs have developed the team by leveraging existing resources in the hospital targeted at their at-risk patient population.

1. Multidisciplinary, physician-led teams are more prevalent in academic centers with training programs.
2. Nurse-led or nurse-respiratory therapist teams with physician back-up (or medical control similar to the Emergency Medical Services model) are more often found in community hospitals without training programs.

B. The implementation of standardized protocols or standing orders allows the team to use evidence-based best practice to address commonly identified clinical issues, especially in circumstances where there is difficulty contacting the responsible physician.

V. Activation of the Team

A. RRT activation can be triggered by acute changes in physiology, observable organ system abnormalities, or events

   1. Acute changes in physiology can include changes in vital signs that exceed predefined limits appropriate for pediatric patients like tachycardia, tachypnea, hypotension, and oliguria.
   2. The detection of one or more indicators of organ system dysfunction may trigger activation of the RRT.
   3. The use of a scoring system in the evaluation and management of the at-risk patient can provide an assessment of clinical status, feedback regarding the effectiveness of interventions, and can facilitate decision-making.
      1. Aggregate of points assigned to various results for symptoms, vital signs, and laboratory studies
      2. The farther from normal the signs, the greater the point value..
   4. As there are no validated scoring systems for pediatric RRTs, evaluation should be targeted to the specific age ranges and patient population served.

B. The most important activation criterion is the bedside staff's and/or family member's concern that something is wrong, even if the other indicators are within acceptable limits. This clinical intuition is often quite sensitive and warrants additional assessment.

VI. Education, Communication and Evaluation

A. RRT members will need ongoing training in the management of common indicators of at-risk patients, effective interventions, and communication strategies.

   1. The mentoring of bedside nursing staff in critical assessment skills and effective communication skills is a primary team education objective.
   2. High-fidelity simulation in a simulation center and /or low-fidelity simulations with mock medical emergency scenarios or table-top exercises are very effective .

B. Targeted education activities may include regularly scheduled topical presentations, RRT case reviews, SBAR (Situation, Background, Assessment, Recommendations, Interventions) practice sessions, and mock event drills.

   1. Regularly scheduled staff in-services and mock event drills are effective in maintaining competencies in identifying the at-risk patient.
   2. Public posting and discussion of activation criteria can further enhance the use of RRT services and reduce patient clinical crises.
   3. Each call, whether or not the patient is actually in crisis, should be treated as a teachable moment. Success of the program depends on the effective dialogue that ensues between all providers.

C. The RRT members and the bedside nursing staff have to gain an understanding of when and how to activate the team, and the scope of team capabilities.

   1. Effective communication and accurate documentation is essential for safe and accurate interventions.
   2. Communication between all providers must be mutually respectful and designed to promote safety and quality for all patients while mentoring staff as to assessment and interventions.
   3. Communication strategies, like SBAR are essential to the early detection and management of at-risk patients.

D. The equipment and supplies carried by the RRT should be tailored to the needs of the patient population served, but then standardized to ensure that the appropriate resources reach the bedside with each call.
   1. RRTs should have portable cardiac, respiratory, and hemodynamic monitors.
   2. Other equipment and supplies are dictated by the patient population served and the team composition.
   3. Equipment and supplies should be reviewed frequently to ensure that only what is useful and needed is carried.

E. Evaluation of activation process, response and equipment use should be reviewed as part of the quality improvement program.

F. Collection and analysis of aggregate scores in patients receiving the RRT services can be used for quality improvement efforts, such as evaluation of standing orders, event cluster identification, and resource utilization.

G. Data collection should be embedded into the clinical workflow to facilitate monitoring of clinical and service outcomes.

VII. Summary

A. Important factors in the successful implementation of a RRT include:
   1. Appropriate team composition
   2. Concise activation criteria based on acute changes in physiology, organ system specific changes, and event triggers
   3. The use of scoring systems to risk stratify at-risk patients
   4. Effective communication strategies like SBAR
   5. Ongoing education to enhance detection and management of potential clinical crises
   6. Appropriate advanced clinical monitors, equipment, and medications to conduct the RRT activities

B. The team should be empowered by the support of leadership to activate the RRT according to established criteria.

Table A1-1. Clinical Assessment Clues for Rapid Response Activation: Acute Physiologic Criteria Model

Clinical Changes	Infant	Child	Adolescent
Acute changes in heart rate	< 80 or > 180	< 60 or >180	< 60 or > 100
Acute changes in systolic blood pressure (mmHg)	< 60 or > 130	< [70 + (2 x age in years)] or > 130	< than 90 or > 130
Acute changes in urine output over 4 consecutive hours	< 1 cc/kg/hour	< 1 cc/kg/hour	< 1 cc/kg/hour
Acute changes in respiratory rate	< 14 or > 40	< 10 or > 30	< 10 or > 30
Acute changes in pulse oximetry (despite supplemental O_2)	< 90%	< 90%	< 90%
Acute changes in level of consciousness	Unusual irritability, lethargy or decreased response to parents and/or painful stimuli	Unusual irritability, lethargy, or decreased response to parents and/or painful stimuli	Lethargy, or decreased response to painful stimuli

*Qualitative deterioration in clinical status

Table A1-2. Organ System Specific Criteria Model

Airway

- Respiratory distress (Nasal flaring, retractions, grunting, increased oxygen requirement)
- Threatened airway

Breathing

- Tachypnea
- Bradypnea
- New stridor or retractions
- SpO2 <90% on oxygen
- Difficulty speaking in verbally communicative children

Circulation

- Hypotension despite treatment
- Tachycardia

Neurology

- Any unexplained change in mental status in the level of consciousness
- Agitation or delirium
- New or increased seizure activity

Other

- Significant or ongoing blood loss
- Concern about the patient
- Uncontrolled pain
- Failure to respond to treatment
- Unable to obtain prompt assistance

Table A1-3. SBAR Communication Tool (Situation, Background, Assessment, Recognition)

Rapid Response Team Call Record

Patient Label

Code Status:
Responsible Physician:
Attending Physician:
Patient Location:

Event Date: Time called: Arrival time: End time:

RRT members:

Primary Reason for RRT Call

Respiratory change HR change LOC change BP change Rhythm change

Spo_2 change Chest Pain SOB UOP low Staff concern

Delayed response from pediatric medical/surgical team Event: ____________________

History/HPI:
Vital Signs: T P RR BP Spo_2
Exam:
Labs:

Situation:

What is happening with the patient?

Background:

What is the clinical background or context?

Assessment:

What do I think is the problem?

Recommendation/Interventions:

What would I do to evaluate and correct it?

PLAN:

Disposition: Stay on Floor Transfer to ICU Code Blue: survived expired

Follow-up within 12 hours after event:

Attending Physician Notified (name)____________________ Time: ____________

By Whom: ____________________

Signature: ____________________

Suggested Readings

1. Brennan TA, Leape LL, Laird N, et al. Incidence of adverse events and negligence in hospitalized patients: Results of the Harvard Medical Practice Study I. *N Eng J Med.* 1991;324:370-376.

2. Bristow PJ, Hillman KM, Chey T, Daffurn K, et al. Rates of in-hospital arrests, deaths and intensive care admissions: The effects of a Medical Emergency Team. *Med J Aust.* 2000;173:236-240.

3. Buist MD, Moore GE, Bernard SA, Waxman BP, Anderson JN, Nguyen TV. Effects of a Medical Emergency Team on reduction of, incidence of, and mortality from unexpected cardiac arrest in hospital: A preliminary study. *BMJ.* 2002;324:387-390.

4. DeVita MA, Hillman K, Bellomo R, eds. *Medical Emergency Teams: Implementation and Outcome Measurement.* New York, NY: Springer Science + Business Media, Inc; 2006.

5. Leonard M, Graham S, Bonacum D. The human factor: the critical importance of effective teamwork and communication in providing safe care. *Qual Saf Health Care.* 2004;13(suppl 1):i85-i90.

6. Subbe CP, Kruger M, Rutherford P, Gemmel L. Validation of a modified Early Warning Score in medical admissions. *Q J Med.* 2001;94:521-526.

7. Tibballs J, Kinney S. A prospective study of outcome of in-patient pediatric cardiopulmonary arrest. *Resuscitation.* 2006;71(3): 310-318.

8. Weil MH, Fries M. In-hospital cardiac arrest. *Crit Care Med.* 2005;33:2825-2830.

Web Sites

1.International Conference on Medical Emergency Team Response. www.metconference.com

2. Rapid response team: The care for early intervention. Institute of Healthcare Improvement: http://www.ili.org

Event Trigger Model

1. Unscheduled naloxone dose administered
2. Increase in oxygen requirement
   - Any change to a 100% reservoir bag oxygen mask
   - Any change in FIO_2 delivery by ≥ 20%
3. After 3 unanticipated pages to pediatric medical/surgical team for any patient in a shift
4. Greater than 30 minute response time to pediatric medical/surgical team page
5. Family concern about patient status
6. Any falls, or traumatic injuries
7. Pain score ≥ 4/10 more than 30 minutes after highest ordered dose of analgesic administered
8. Persistent nausea/vomiting more than 30 minutes after highest dose of antiemetic administered

Appendix 2:

Pediatric Normal Values

Table A2-1. Pediatric Laboratory Values

	Conventional Unit	SI Unit
Acid Phosphatase		
Newborn	7.4-19.4 U/L	7.4-19.4 U/L
2-13 years	6.4-15.2 U/L	6.4-15.2 U/L
Alanine Aminotransferase (ALT)		
Infant	<54 U/L	<54 U/L
Child/Adult	1-30 U/L	1-30 U/L
Albumin		
Newborn	3.2-4.8 g/dL	
1 day – 1 month	2.5-5.5 g/dL	
1-3 months	2.1-4.8 g/dL	
4-6 months	2.8-5.0 g/dL	
7-12 months	3.2-5.7 g/dL	
13-24 months	1.9-5.0 g/dL	
25-36 months	3.3-5.8 g/dL	
3-5 years	2.9-5.8 g/dL	
6-8 years	3.3-5.0 g/dL	
9-11 years	3.2-5.0 g/dL	
12-16 years	3.2-5.1 g/dL	
Alkaline Phosphatase		
Infant	150-420 U/L	150-420 U/L
2-10 years	100-320 U/L	100-320 U/L
11-18 years, boy	100-390 U/L	100-390 U/L
11-18 years, girl	100-320 U/L	100-320 U/L
Ammonia		
Newborn	90-150 µg/dL	64-107 µmol/L
0-2 weeks	79-129 µg/dL	56-92 µmol/L
>1 month	29-70 µg/dL	21-50 µmol/L
Amylase		
Newborn	0-44 U/L	5-65 U/L
Adult	0-88 U/L	0-130 U/L

continued next page...

Table A2-1. Pediatric Laboratory Values (continued)

		Conventional Unit	SI Unit
Aspartate Aminotransferase (AST)			
Newborn/ Infant		20-65 U/L	20-65 U/L
Child/Adult		0-35 U/L	0-4350 U/L
Bicarbonate			
Preterm		18-26 mEq/L	18-26 mmol/L
Full term		20-25 mEq/L	20-25 mmol/L
>2 years		22-26 mEq/L	22-26 mmol/L
Bilirubin (Total)			
0-1 day	Preterm	<8 mg/dL	<137 µmol/L
	Term	<6 mg/dL	<103 µmol/L
1-2 days	Preterm	<12 mg/dL	<205 µmol/L
	Term	<8 mg/dL	<137 µmol/L
3-5 days	Preterm	<16 mg/dL	<274 µmol/L
	Term	<12 mg/dL	<205 µmol/L
Thereafter	Preterm	<2 mg/dL	<34 µmol/L
	Term	<1 mg/dL	<17 µmol/L
Bilirubin (Conjugated)			
All ages		0-0.4 mg/dL	0-8 µmol/L
Calcium (Total)			
Preterm <1 week		6-10 mg/dL	1.5-2.5 mmol/L
Full term <1 week		7-12 mg/dL	1.75-3 mmol/L
Child		8-10.5 mg/dL	2-2.6 mmol/L
Calcium (Ionized)			
Newborn < 48 hour		4-4.7 mg/dL	1-1.18 mmol/L
Adult		4.52-5.28 mg/dL	1.13-1.32 mmol/L
Carbon Dioxide (CO_2 Content)			
Infant/ Child		20-24 mEq/L	20-24 mmol/L
Carbon Monoxide (Carboxyhemoglobin)			
Nonsmoker		0-2% of total hemoglobin	
Chloride (Serum)			
Pediatric		99-111 mEq/L	99-111 mmol/L
C-Reactive Protein			
All ages		0-0.5 mg/dL	
Creatine Kinase (Creatine Phosphokinase)			
Newborn		10-200 U/L	10-200 U/L
Adult Woman		10-55 U/L	10-55 U/L
Adult Male		12-80 U/L	12-80 U/L

continued next page...

Table A2-1. Pediatric Laboratory Values (continued)

	Conventional Unit	SI Unit
Creatinine (Serum)		
Newborn	0.3-1 mg/dL	27-88 µmol/L
Infant	0.2-0.4 mg/dL	18-35 µmol/L
Child	0.3-0.7 mg/dL	27-62 µmol/L
Adolescent	0.5-1 mg/dL	44-88 µmol/L
Fibrinogen		
All ages	200-400 mg/dL	2-4 g/L
γ-Glutamyltransferase (GGT)		
Preterm	56-233 U/L	56-233 U/L
0-3 weeks	0-130 U/L	0-130 U/L
3 weeks-3 months	4-120 U/L	4-120 U/L
>3 months, boy	5-65 U/L	5-65 U/L
>3 months, girl	5-35 U/L	5-35 U/L
1-15 years	0-23 U/L	0-23 U/L
Glucose (Serum)		
Preterm	45-100 mg/dL	1.1-3.6 mmol/L
Full term	45-120 mg/dL	1.1-6.4 mmol/L
1 week- 16 years	60-105 mg/dL	3.3-5.8 mmol/L
Iron		
Newborn	100-250 µg/dL	18-45 µmol/L
Infant	40-100 µg/dL	7-18 µmol/L
Child	50-120 µg/dL	9-22 µmol/L
Ketones (Serum)		
Qualitative	Negative	
Quantitative	0.5-3 mg/dL	5-30 mg/L
Lactate		
Capillary blood		
Newborn	<27 mg/dL	0-3 mmol/L
Child	5-20 mg/dL	0.5-2.2 mmol/L
Venous	5-20 mg/dL	0.5-2.2 mmol/L
Arterial	5-14 mg/dL	0.5-1.6 mmol/L
Lactate Dehydrogenase (at 37° C)		
Neonate	160-1500 U/L	160-1500 U/L
Infant	150-360 U/L	150-360 U/L
Child	150-300 U/L	150-300 U/L
Lead		
Child	<10 µg/dL	<48 µmol/L
Lipase		
All ages	4-24 U/dL	

continued next page...

Table A2-1. Pediatric Laboratory Values (continued)

		Conventional Unit	SI Unit
Magnesium			
All ages		1.3-2.0 mEq/L	0.65-1.0 mmol/L
Methemoglobin			
All ages		0-1.3% total hemoglobin	
Osmolality			
All ages		285-295 mOsm/kg	285-295 mmol/kg
Phosphorus			
Newborn		4.2-9.0 mg/dL	1.36-2.91 mmol/L
0-15 years		3.2-6.3 mg/dL	1.03-2.1 mmol/L
Potassium			
<10 days		4-6 mEq/L	4-6 mmol/L
>10 days		3.5-5 mEq/L	3.5-5 mmol/L
Prealbumin			
Newborn – 6 weeks		4-36 mg/dL	
6 weeks – 16 years		13-27 mg/dL	
Protein (Total)			
Newborn- 1 month		4.4-7.6 g/dL	
1-3 months		3.6-7.4 g/dL	
4-6 months		4.2-7.4 g/dL	
7-12 months		5.1-7.5 g/dL	
13-24 months		3.7-7.5 g/dL	
25-36 months		5.3-8.1 g/dL	
3-5 years		4.9-8.1 g/dL	
6-16 years		6.0-7.9 g/dL	
Pyruvate			
All ages		0.3-0.9 mg/dL	0.03-0.1 mmol/L
Sodium			
Preterm		130-140 mEq/L	130-140 mmol/L
Older		135-148 mEq/L	135-148 mmol/L
Triglycerides (Fasting)			
Male			
	0-5 years	30-86 mg/dL	0.3-0.86 g/L
	6-11 years	31-108 mg/dL	0.31-1.08 g/L
	12-15 years	36-138 mg/dL	0.36-1.38 g/L
Female			
	0-5 years	32-99 mg/dL	0.32-0.99 g/L
	6-11 years	35-114 mg/dL	0.35-1.14 g/L
	12-15 years	41-138 mg/dL	0.41-1.38 g/L

continued next page...

Table A2-1. Pediatric Laboratory Values (continued)

	Conventional Unit	SI Unit
Troponin		
All ages	0.03-0.15 ng/mL	
Urea Nitrogen (BUN)		
All ages	7-22 mg/dL	2.5-7.9 mmol/L
Uric Acid		
0-2 years	2.4-6.4 mg/dL	0.14-0.38 mmol/L
2-12 years	2.4-5.9 mg/dL	0.14-0.35 mmol/L
12-14 years	2.4-6.4 mg/dL	0.14-0.38 mmol/L

Adapted from Robertson J. Blood Chemistries and body fluids. In: Robertson J, Shilkofski N, eds. *The Harriet Lane Handbook*. 17th ed. Baltimore, MD, 2005, Elsevier-Mosby.

Table A2-2. Normal Respiratory Rates

Age	Respiration (breaths/min)
Newborn	30-60
6 months	25-40
1-3 years	20-30
6 years	18-25
10 years	15-20

Table A2-3. Normal Heart Rates in Children

Age	Heart Rate (beats/min)
Newborn	80-200
<2 years	80-180
2 - 10 years	60-150
>10 years	60-100

Table A2-4. Lower Limit of Systolic Blood Pressure by Age

Age	Systolic Blood Pressure (mm Hg)
Newborn	60
<1 year	70
1 - 10 years	70 + (age in years x 2)
>10 years	90

Appendix 3:

Acid-Base Balance and Arterial Blood Gas Analysis

Acid-base disorders are common in critically ill children and are due to metabolic and/or respiratory compromise. The arterial blood gas measurement is an important laboratory test in the evaluation of a child's acid-base status.

I. Blood Gas

A blood gas is composed of four basic parts:

A. pH is derived from the logarithmic expression of the hydrogen ion concentration (H^+) and is a measure of acidosis or alkalosis. A normal pH is 7.4 ± 0.05. A pH >7.45 is indicative of alkalosis and a pH <7.35 indicates acidosis. Respiratory and metabolic processes contribute to the pH as described below.

B. $Paco_2$ represents the partial pressure of CO_2 in arterial blood and is a measure of the adequacy of minute ventilation. It has a significant effect on pH in that for every 10 mm Hg change in $Paco_2$ from the baseline of 40 mm Hg, there is a corresponding change in the opposite direction by 0.08 in the pH. Hence, looking at an arterial blood gas sample, one can determine whether the pH is attributable solely to the Pco_2 level.

For example, if a patient has a pH of 7.32 and a $Paco_2$ of 50 mm Hg, then this is entirely due to the contribution of the respiratory acidosis (elevated $Paco_2$). However, if the pH is 7.28 and the $Paco_2$ is 50 mm Hg, the $Paco_2$ is only partly responsible for the acidosis and so the patient likely has a mixed/combined respiratory and metabolic acidosis.

C. Pao_2 represents the partial pressure of oxygen in the arterial blood. This provides an assessment of the patient's oxygenation and should be within the range of 80 to 100 mm Hg for a patient breathing room air and with no intracardiac right-to-left shunt. However, in cases of lung disease, hypoxemia might ensue and Pao_2 levels may decline despite supplemental oxygen.

D. Bicarbonate level (HCO_3) is a measure of the presence of metabolic acidosis or alkalosis. Assuming a $Paco_2$ of 40 mm Hg, a change in the bicarbonate level for every 10 mEq/L above or below the normal of 24 mEq/L is associated with a change in the pH of 0.15 in the same direction. This allows an assessment of the contribution of the metabolic component to the acid-base (pH) status.

Another corollary that can be drawn from this is the calculation of the base excess (metabolic alkalosis) or base deficit (metabolic acidosis).

Since the volume of distribution of bicarbonate is 0.3 L/kg body weight, the total body HCO_3 deficit = (calculated base deficit X 0.3 X weight [kg]) mEq.

II. How to Evaluate an Arterial Blood Gas

When analyzing an arterial blood gas:

A. First look at the pH. Determine if the pH is normal (7.35-7.45), low (i.e., acidosis; <7.35), or high (i.e., alkalosis; >7.45)

B. Next evaluate the $Paco_2$. Determine if the $Paco_2$ is high (>45 mm Hg) or low (<35 mm Hg). When **high**, think respiratory acidosis if the corresponding pH is low.

C. Next look at the bicarbonate level. If it is low (<22 mEq/L) and the pH is low, think metabolic acidosis. If the bicarbonate level is high (>26 mEq/L) and the pH is high, think metabolic alkalosis.

Table A3-1. Arterial Blood Gas Analysis

Acidosis	Alkalosis	Metabolic	Respiratory	pH (7.35-7.45)	$Paco_2$ (35-45 mm Hg)	HCO_3 (22-26 mEq/L)
X			X	< 7.35	>45	normal
X		X		< 7.35	normal	<22
	X		X	> 7.45	<35	normal
	X	X		> 7.45	normal	>26

These examples primarily pertain to acute acidosis and acute alkalosis. If the conditions have been present for several hours or longer, the body attempts to compensate for these abnormalities. Hyperventilation occurs to compensate for the profound metabolic acidosis as seen in diabetic ketoacidosis; alternately renal compensation ensues in cases of chronic respiratory acidosis (seen in chronic lung disease/bronchopulmonary dysplasia). In addition, many times the abnormalities are mixed, meaning they have components of each.

We have discussed arterial blood gas analysis because this is the “gold standard” for measuring acid-base status. In patients with indwelling lines with a free flow of blood, venous blood gas analysis remains of some benefit, but is different; Pvo_2 levels might not reflect hypoxemia but might give an idea of the circulatory status. If the Pvo_2 level is <25 mm Hg, it indicates that cardiac output is low. Capillary blood gas analysis is not as helpful due to the potential for hemolysis during sample collection from a heel stick, and the oxygen levels are not predictive of hypoxemia.

Appendix 4:

Airway Adjuncts

I. Oxygen Delivery Devices

A. The *simple oxygen mask* is a low flow device that delivers oxygen with a flow rate of 6 to 10 L/min. The oxygen concentration delivered to the patient can reach a maximum of 60% because of entrainment of room air through the exhalation ports of the mask. It is important to maintain an oxygen flow rate of at least 6 L/min to sustain an optimal inspired oxygen concentration and prevent rebreathing of exhaled carbon dioxide.

B. A *partial rebreathing mask* consists of simple facemask with reservoir bag. It provides oxygen concentrations of 50-60%. During inspiration the patient draws gas predominantly from the fresh oxygen inflow and the reservoir bag, so entrainment of room air through the exhalation ports is minimized. An oxygen flow rate of 10-12 L/min is usually required.

C. A *non-rebreathing mask* consists of a facemask and reservoir bag with a valve incorporated into one or both exhalation ports to prevent entrainment of room air during inspiration. Another valve is placed between the reservoir bag and mask to prevent flow of exhaled gas into the reservoir. An inspired concentration of 95% can be achieved with an oxygen flow rate of 10-15 L/min and use of well-sealed mask.

D. A *face tent* is a high flow soft plastic bucket that is often better tolerated by children than a facemask. Even with a high oxygen flow rate, inspired oxygen concentrations over 40% cannot be reliably provided. A face tent permits access to the face without interrupting oxygen flow.

E. A *nasal cannula* is a low flow oxygen delivery system that is useful when low levels of supplemental oxygen are required. The net F_{IO_2} depends on the child's respiratory effort, size, and minute ventilation in comparison with the nasal cannula flow.

II. LARYNGEAL MASK AIRWAY (LMA)

A. Indications
1. Provide an airway and ventilation when bag-mask ventilation is difficult
2. Provide a temporizing airway when endotracheal intubation is unsuccessful

B. Equipment
1. Bag-mask resuscitation unit with oxygen supplementation
2. Pulse oximeter
3. Electrocardiographic monitor
4. Blood pressure monitoring
5. Gloves, mask, eye protection
6. Laryngeal mask airway of appropriate size (**Table A4-1**)
7. Syringe for cuff inflation
8. Water-soluble lubricant
9. Qualitative CO_2 detector or CO_2 monitor
10. Resuscitation cart

C. Preparation for insertion
1. Don gloves, mask, eye protection
2. Assure patent airway and optimal oxygenation and ventilation
3. Assure IV access
4. Apply pulse oximeter, electrocardiographic and blood pressure monitor
5. Select appropriate size LMA
6. Check cuff integrity by inflating and fully deflating
7. Lubricate only the posterior aspect of the deflated mask with a water-based lubricant
8. Preoxygenate with 100% oxygen for 2 to 3 minutes if time permits

Table A4-1. Laryngeal Mask Airway Size and Cuff Inflation

LMA Size	Patient Size	Maximum Cuff Volume	Largest ETT ID (mm)*
1	Neonate/infant to 5 kg	Up to 4 mL	3.5
1.5	5-10 kg	Up to 7 mL	4.0
2	10-20 kg	Up to 10 mL	4.5
2.5	20-30 kg	Up to 14 mL	5.0
3	>30 kg/small adult	Up to 20 mL	6.0 cuffed
4	Average adult	Up to 30 mL	6.0 cuffed
5	Large adult	Up to 40 mL	7.0 cuffed

* Largest endotracheal tube size (ETT ID) that will fit through LMA tube lumen.

D. Technique **(Figure A4-1)**

1. The cuff is deflated completely so that it forms a spoon shape and there are no folds in the mask.
2. The operator stands behind the head of the bed, and the bed is raised to a position of comfort for the operator.
3. The patient is placed in the sniffing position (ie, head extended, neck flexed), unless potential or definite cervical spine injury prevents neck flexion/extension.

Figure A4-1. Insertion technique for laryngeal mask airway

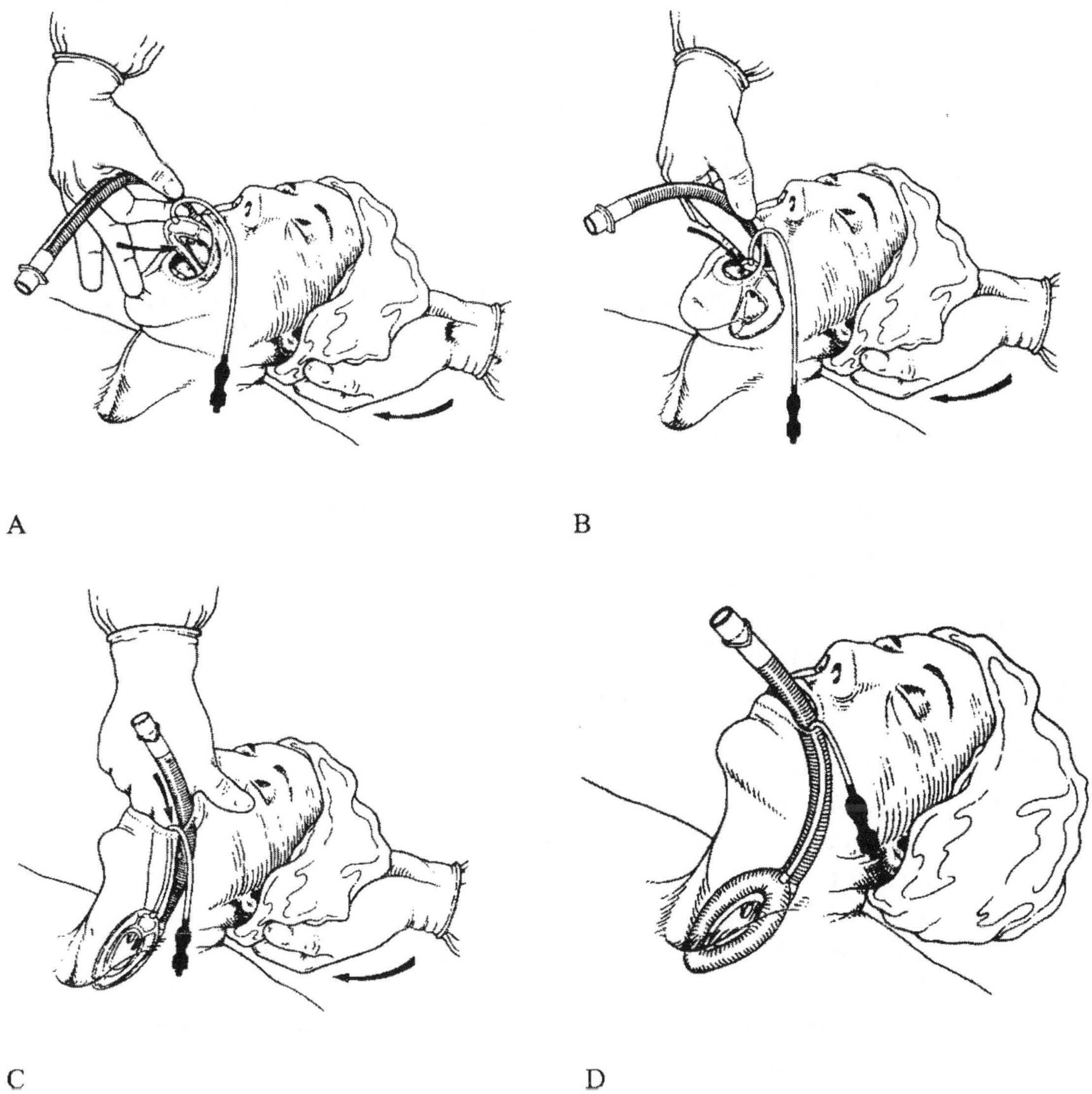

A) Insert lubricated and deflated mask into the open mouth with the bowl facing anterior. (B) Hold the device like a pencil, pressing against the palate and pharyngeal wall with the index finger. (C) Continue inserting the cuff behind the tongue into the hypopharynx until definite resistance is felt. (D) Without holding the device, inflate cuff with enough air to obtain a seal. Attach manual ventilation device and ensure chest movement. Adapted from Brain AIJ. *The Intravent Laryngeal Mask Instruction Manual.* Berkshire, UK: Brain Medical, 1992.

4. Cricoid pressure is not recommended during placement of the LMA because it may interfere with correct placement.
5. The mask is positioned with the bowl facing anteriorly. Hold the device like a pencil, with the index finger of the dominant hand at the junction of the bowl and tube, pressing against the palate and pharyngeal wall with the index finger.
6. The cuff is inserted into the hypopharynx until definite resistance is felt.
7. Without the operator holding the device, the cuff is inflated with enough air to obtain a seal around the laryngeal inlet. This step results in an outward movement of the tube.
8. The cuff is inflated with enough air to obtain a seal (intracuff pressure of approximately 60 cm H_2O. Maximum volumes are listed in **Table A4-1**, but lesser volume may provide an adequate seal.
9. A manual ventilation device is attached, and chest movement and breath sounds are verified in both lung fields. Correct position should be confirmed with a qualitative or quantitative end-tidal CO_2 detector.
10. If chest movement is inadequate, or if a large air leak is present, the device should be removed and reinserted.
11. When the LMA is positioned appropriately, the tube is secured with tape.

III. ESOPHAGEAL-TRACHEAL DOUBLE-LUMEN AIRWAY DEVICE

A. Indications
   1. Cardiorespiratory arrest and inability to provide an airway by other means

B. Equipment
   1. Bag-mask resuscitation unit with oxygen supplementation
   2. Pulse oximeter
   3. Electrocardiographic monitor
   4. Blood pressure monitoring
   5. Gloves, mask, eye protection
   6. Esophageal-tracheal double-lumen device
   7. Syringe for cuff inflation
   8. Water-soluble lubricant
   9. Qualitative CO_2 detector or CO_2 monitor
   10. Resuscitation cart

C. Preparation for insertion
   1. Don gloves, mask, eye protection
   2. Assure patent airway and optimal oxygenation and ventilation
   3. Assure IV access
   4. Apply pulse oximeter, electrocardiographic and blood pressure monitor
   5. Select appropriate size device
   6. Check integrity of both cuffs by inflating and fully deflating
   7. Preoxygenate with 100% oxygen for 2 to 3 minutes if time permits

D. Technique

1. The cuffs should be deflated completely.
2. The operator stands behind the head of the bed, and the bed is raised to a position of comfort for the operator.
3. The patient is placed in a neutral or sniffing position (ie, head extended, neck flexed), unless potential or definite cervical spine injury prevents neck flexion/extension.
4. The patient's tongue and jaw are grasped between the thumb and index finger, and the device is inserted blindly. It is advanced until the placement ring markers on the tube are positioned as indicated by the manufacturer. Do not force the tube if resistance is met. A laryngoscope can be used to assist with placement.
5. The pharyngeal cuff is inflated first to seal the posterior pharynx.
6. The distal cuff is then inflated.
7. Ventilation should be attempted first through the pharyngeal lumen, and the chest should be auscultated for breath sounds and observed for movement. The tube enters the esophagus approximately 95% of the time.
8. If breath sounds are absent, ventilation should be attempted through the tracheal lumen while auscultating for breath sounds.
9. Use of the correct lumen for ventilation should be confirmed with a qualitative/quantitative end-tidal CO_2 or esophageal detector device.
10. When the device is positioned appropriately, the tube is secured with tape.

Suggested Readings

1. Danks RR, Danks B. Laryngeal mask airway: review of indications and use. *J Emerg Nurs.* 2004;30:30-35.

2. Krafft P, Schebesta K. Alternative management techniques for the difficult airway: esophageal-tracheal Combitube. *Curr Opin Anaesthesiol.* 2005;17:499-504.

3. Mace SE. The laryngeal mask airway: guidelines for appropriate usage. *Resid Staff Physician.* 2001;47:30.

Appendix 5:

Endotracheal Intubation

I. Indications

A. Loss of protective airway reflexes
B. Alteration or absence of neuronal respiratory drive
C. Increased work of breathing resulting in respiratory distress
D. Airway obstruction to gas flow
E. Alteration in patient's level of consciousness
F. Elective intubation for procedural or operative procedure

II. Equipment

A. Bag-valve-mask resuscitation unit with oxygen supplementation – size appropriate
B. Airway mask – size appropriate
C. Towel roll or pad for occipital elevation
D. Medication for analgesia/anesthesia, sedation, and neuromuscular blockade
E. Gloves, gown, mask, protective eye gear
F. Blood pressure device
G. Pulse oximeter
H. Electrocardiography monitor
I. Laryngoscope handle and blade(s)
J. Endotracheal tubes – consider one size smaller, one size appropriate, and one size larger
K. Stylet – size appropriate: small, pediatric, adult
L. Yankauer and tracheal suction catheters and suction device – size appropriate
M. 10-mL syringe to inflate cuff, if appropriate
N. Water-soluble lubricant
O. Qualitative CO_2 detector, CO_2 monitor, or esophageal detector device
P. Tape or tracheal tube stabilization device
Q. Intravenous tubing and fluid
R. Resuscitation cart

III. Orotracheal Intubation via Direct Laryngoscopy

A. Preparation

1. Assemble all equipment and ensure proper working order
2. Don gloves, gown, mask, and eye protection
3. Explain the procedure to the patient and/or parent
4. Assure patent airway
5. Assure optimal oxygenation and ventilation
6. Assure intravenous access
7. Apply pulse oximeter, electrocardiograph, and blood pressure devices
8. Prepare the endotracheal tube
    a. If cuffed tube, check integrity by inflating and fully deflating cuff
    b. Insert stylet into endotracheal tube, bend to configuration predicted to assist glottic entry
    c. Apply water-soluble lubricant to the cuff end of the tube per preference
9. Connect laryngoscope blade to handle
    a. Blade selection (operator's choice): The larynx of the infant or small child is cephalad, appearing anterior; most clinicians do not use curved blades in infants
        i. Straight blade – used to elevate the epiglottis anteriorly
        ii. Curved blade – inserted into the vallecula
    b. Select blade length: The blade length must be long enough to reach the epiglottis
    c. Assure that light from bulb is bright
10. Place the patient in the proper head position. A towel placed under the shoulders is usually needed to achieve the sniffing position in infants; Older children and adults may require a towel roll under the head to achieve the sniffing position (if cervical spine injury is not suspected)
11. Pre-oxygenate with 100% oxygen for 2-3 minutes, to assure adequate oxygenation and assure ability of operator to maintain effective ventilation, if time permits
12. Proceed with analgesia, sedation, and neuromuscular blockade as necessary

B. Technique

1. The operator stands at the head of the patient and the bed is raised to a position of comfort for the operator. The head of the bed may be flat or raised slightly per operator preference.
2. When no cervical spine injury is suspected, place the patient in the sniffing position and gently extend the neck (**Figure A5-1**). When cervical spine injury is suspected, these steps are omitted, and the neck is stabilized by an assistant and the anterior portion of the cervical collar is removed.
3. Regardless of the operator's dominant hand, the laryngoscope is always held in the left hand.
4. Cricoid pressure should be gently but firmly applied by an assistant as soon as consciousness is lost and should be sustained until endotracheal tube placement is confirmed and the cuff is inflated, if indicated.
5. Mouth opening in the sedated/relaxed patient may be assisted by a cross-finger technique, wherein the thumb of the right hand is placed on the front lower teeth or gum of the mandible and the first finger on the upper teeth/gum of the maxilla. The mouth is gently opened by a "reverse scissor" movement of the fingers and the laryngoscope is introduced into the mouth.

6. The tip of laryngoscope blade is inserted into the right side of the patient's mouth (**Figure A5-2**); the blade is advanced to the base of the tongue.
7. The tongue is swept to left; proper tongue control is key to laryngeal visualization.
8. The blade is gently advanced further to its proper position. A straight blade is placed beneath the epiglottis; a curved blade is placed into the vallecula above the epiglottis.
9. Traction should be applied only along the long axis of the laryngoscope handle as the laryngoscope lifts the tongue upward away from the larynx, revealing the glottic opening. A rocking or rotating motion of the blade and handle may damage teeth, gingiva, or lips. The base of the laryngoscope blade should never contact the upper teeth.

Figure A5-1. Positioning for Orotracheal Intubation.

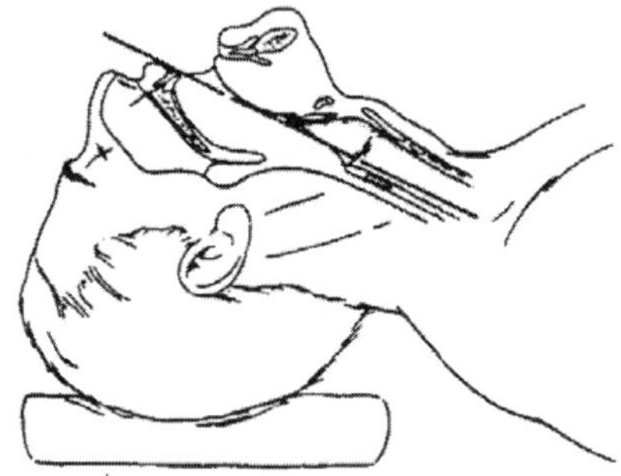

To visual the trachea, the axial planes of the oral, pharyngeal, and tracheal axes must be aligned. This alignment can be accomplished by flexing the neck at the level of the cervical spine and extending the head at the atlanto-occipital joint. Illustration © by Robert Margulies and reproduced with permission from the artist and *The Journal of Critical Illness.*

Figure A5-2. Insertion of Laryngoscope.

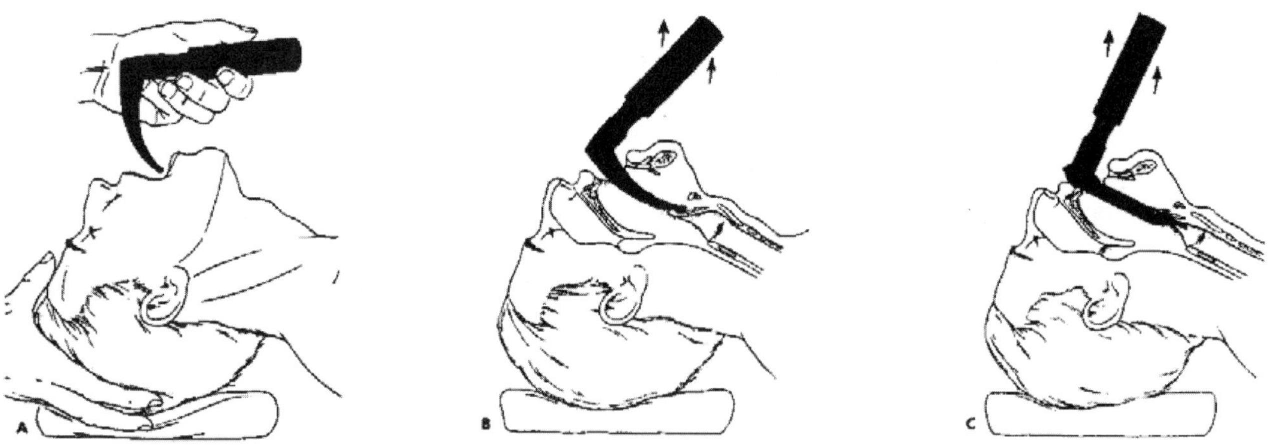

(A) The blade of the laryngoscope is inserted into the patient's mouth and pushes the tongue to the left. (B) The straight blade is inserted beneath the epiglottis, and (C) the curved blade follows the base of the tongue and is inserted into the vallecula. Illustration © by Robert Margulies and reproduced with permission from the artist and *The Journal of Critical Illness.*

10. The vocal cords and glottic opening should be visualized.
11. If the vocal cords and glottis cannot be visualized, it may be helpful for an assistant to grasp the thyroid cartilage between the thumb and index finger and exert pressure in the following sequence: Pressure is applied backward against the cervical vertebrae and then in an upward direction to shift the larynx superiorly. Additional pressure is applied to shift the thyroid cartilage no more than 2 cm to the right side of the patient's neck.
12. The endotracheal tube gently is inserted through the vocal cords (**Figure A5-3**), holding the tube/stylet with the right hand. The proper depth of insertion in centimeters can be estimated by multiplying the internal diameter of the endotracheal tube by 3 (e.g., internal diameter = 4.0; depth of insertion = 4 x 3 = 12 cm).
13. The stylet and laryngoscope should be removed carefully. The operator must continue to hold the endotracheal tube firmly.
14. The cuff is inflated, if indicated.
15. To ensure proper position of the tube:
    a. Inspect and auscultate the chest to assure equal bilateral gas entry
    b. Use a qualitative CO_2 detector, monitor, or esophageal detector device. Lack of color change with a qualitative CO_2 detector or low exhaled CO_2 may occur with a correctly placed endotracheal tube in the patient with poor pulmonary perfusion
    c. Observe for condensation in the endotracheal tube during exhalation
    d. Listen for breath sounds through the endotracheal tube as the patient is breathing spontaneously or with bag-valve-mask assistance.
    e. Obtain chest radiograph. Tube tip should be seen 2 to 3 cm above carina.
16. The endotracheal tube should be secured with tape or a tube stabilization device.

Figure A5-3. Placement of Endotracheal Tube.

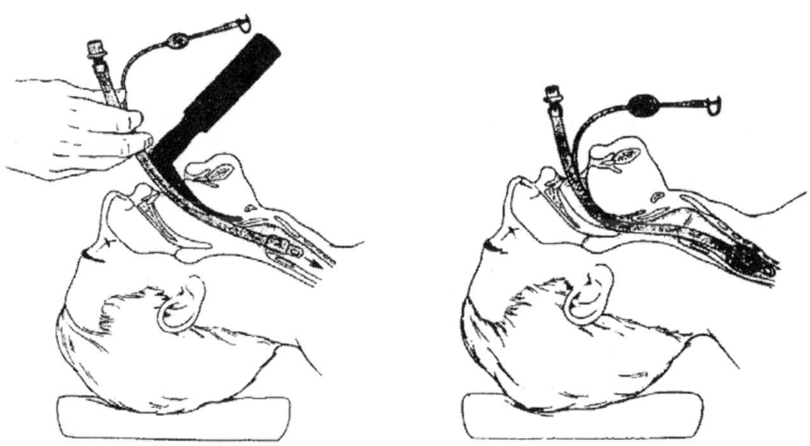

A B

(**A**) The endotracheal tube is inserted through the vocal cords until the distal end rests approximately 2 to 3 cm above the carina. (**B**) Once the endotracheal tube is in proper position, the laryngoscope and stylet are removed and the cuff is inflated. Illustration © by Robert Margulies and reproduced with permission from the artist and *The Journal of Critical Illness.*

IV. Pediatric Considerations

A. Anatomic differences between adults and children

1. The larynx is more cephalad in infants than in adults, making it appear more anterior and resulting in a more difficult visualization during laryngoscopy.
2. Cricoid pressure is valuable during laryngoscopy because of the position of the larynx and assists in preventing aspiration.
3. In young children, the narrowest part of the airway is at the level of the cricoid cartilage, not at the larynx, making an anatomic "cuff" below the vocal cords.
4. In general, the diameter of the small finger approximates the proper size of the endotracheal tube. A full-term neonate can accept a 3.5-mm inner-diameter tube.
5. Cuffed tubes are usually limited to use in children > 8 years of age (endotracheal tube size >6.0 mm internal diameter); uncuffed tubes are generally used in younger children. Consideration of a cuffed tube in a younger child may be necessary when a prolonged course of mechanical ventilation or positive pressure ventilation is anticipated.

V. Precautions/Complications

A. Hypoxia, hypercapnia during procedure
B. Cardiovascular compromise during and immediately after procedure
C. Damaged teeth, lips, gingiva
D. Malpositioned tube (right or left mainstem bronchus, esophagus)
E. Pharyngeal, laryngeal, tracheal damage
F. Gastric distension and aspiration of gastric contents
G. Bronchospasm

Suggested Readings

1. Balk RA. The technique of orotracheal intubation. *J Crit Illn.* 1997;12:316.

2. Gerardi MJ, Sacchetti AD, Cantor RM, et al. Rapid-sequence intubation of the pediatric patient. Pediatric Emergency Medicine Committee of the American College of Emergency Physicians. *Ann Emerg Med.* 1996;28:55-74.

3. McLean B, Zimmerman JL, eds. *Fundamental Critical Care Support.* 4th ed. Mount Prospect, IL: Society of Critical Care Medicine; 2007.

4. Tobias JD. Airway management for pediatric emergencies. *Pediatr Ann.* 1996;25: 317-320, 323-328.

Appendix 6:

Difficult Airway Algorithm

Approach to difficult and failed intubation.

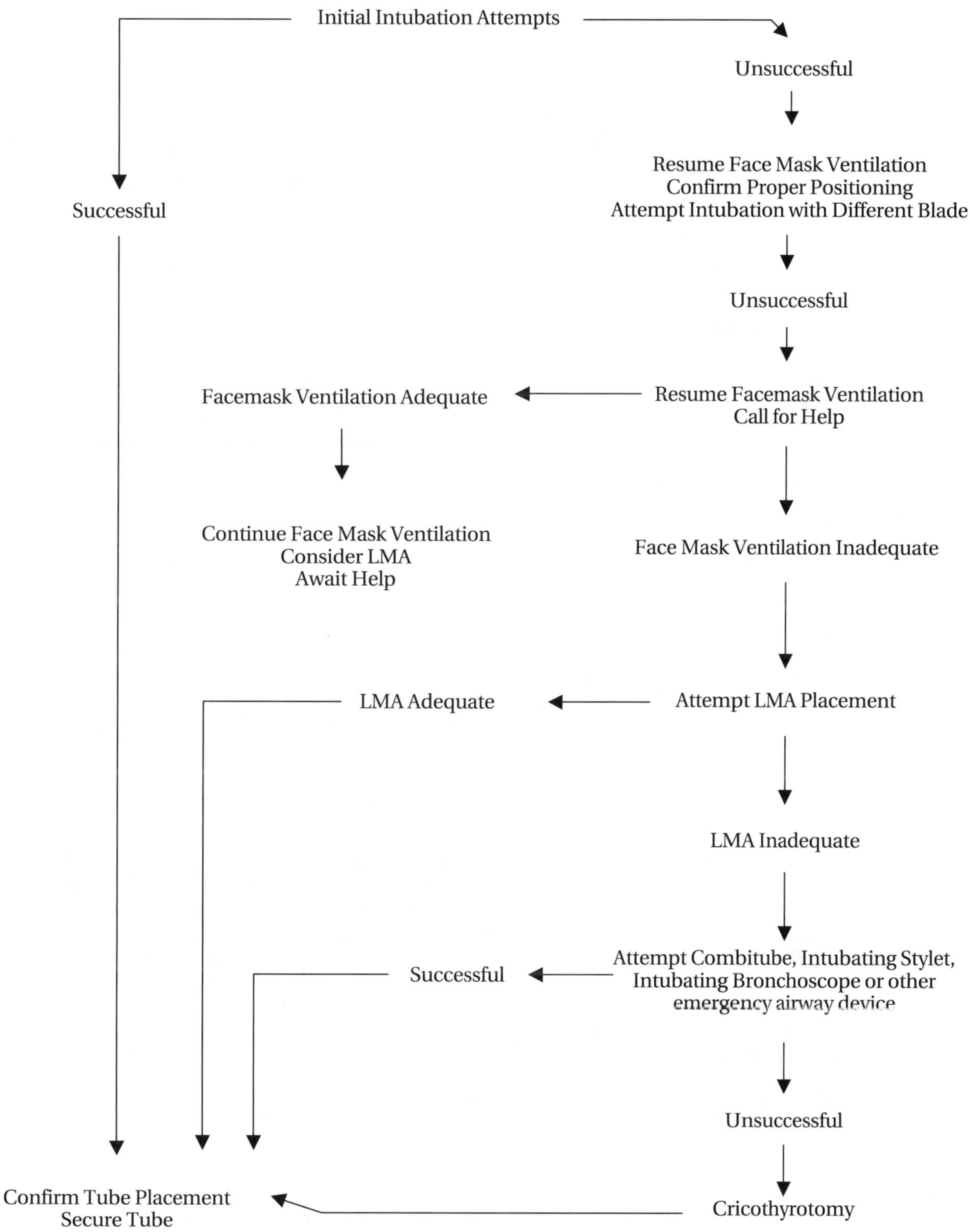

Appendix 7:

ADVANCED LIFE SUPPORT ALGORITHM

Figure A7-1. Pulseless Arrest Algorithm

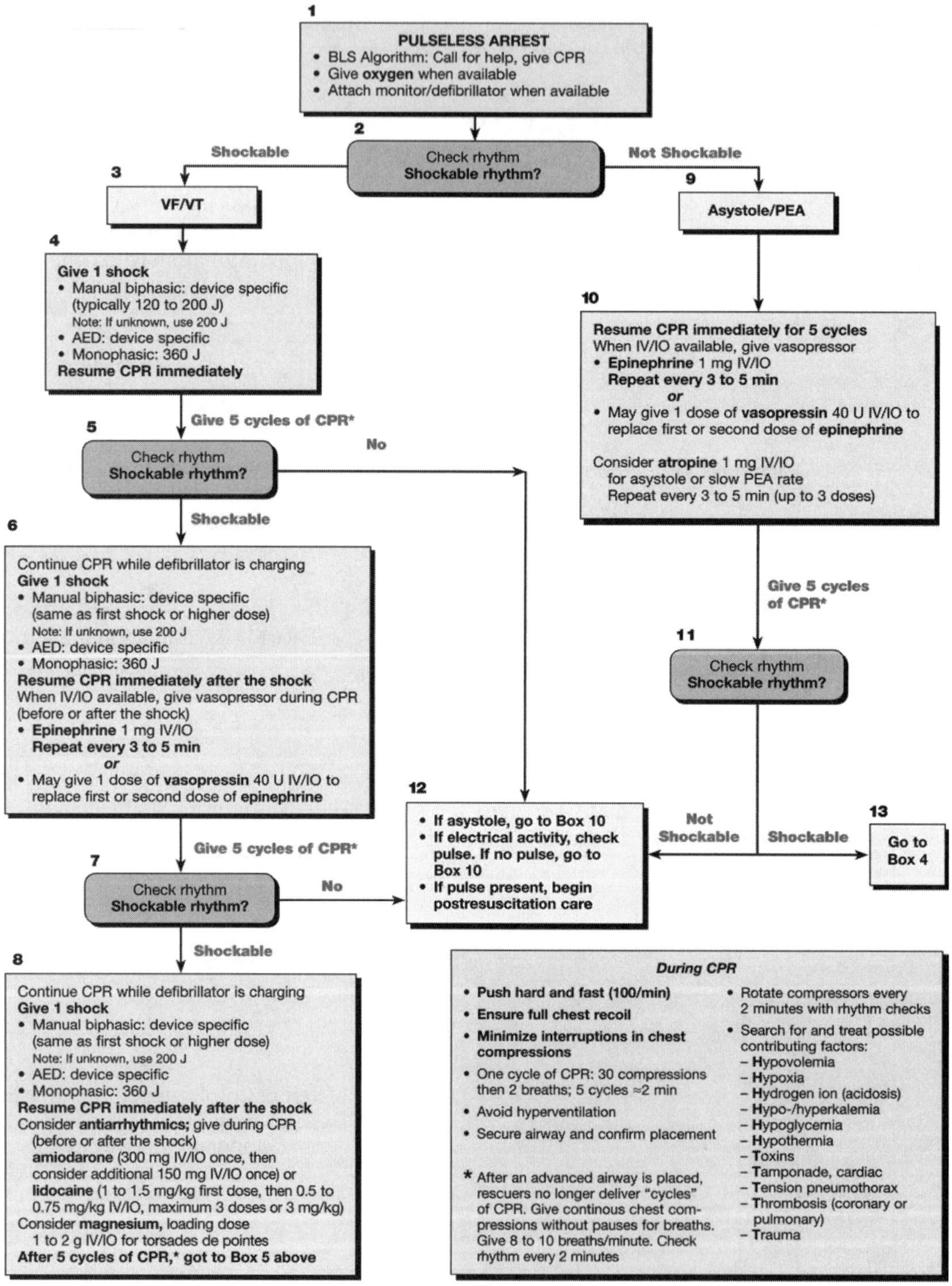

Figure A7-2. Bradycardia Algorithm

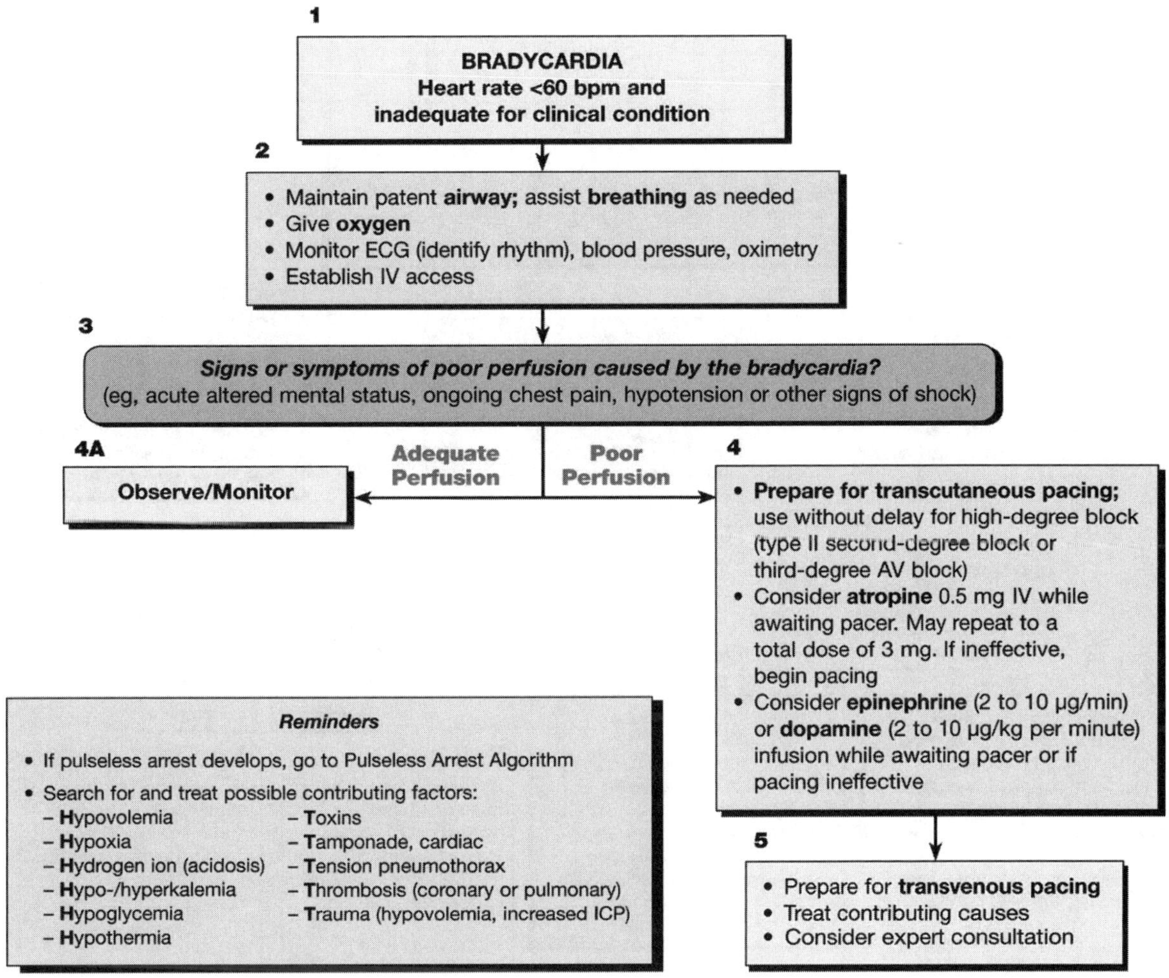

Reproduced with permission from The American Heart Association in Collaboration with the International Liaison Committee on Resuscitation (ILCOR): 2005 American Heart Association Guidelines for Cardiopulmonary Resuscitation and Emergency Cardiovascular Care. *Circulation* 2005;112:IV67-IV77.

Figure A7-3. Tachycardia Algorithm

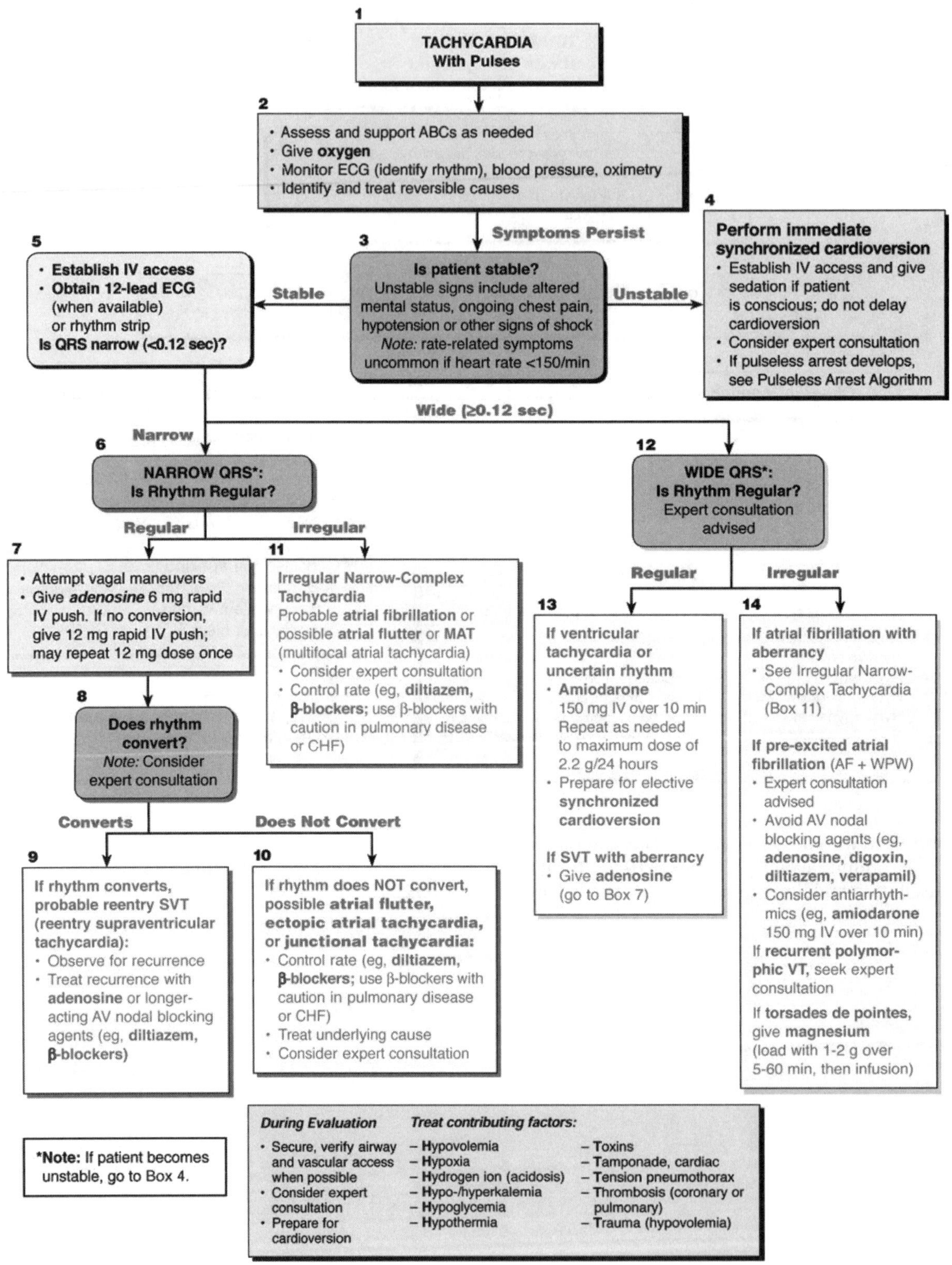

Figure A7-4. Pediatric Pulseless Arrest Algorithm

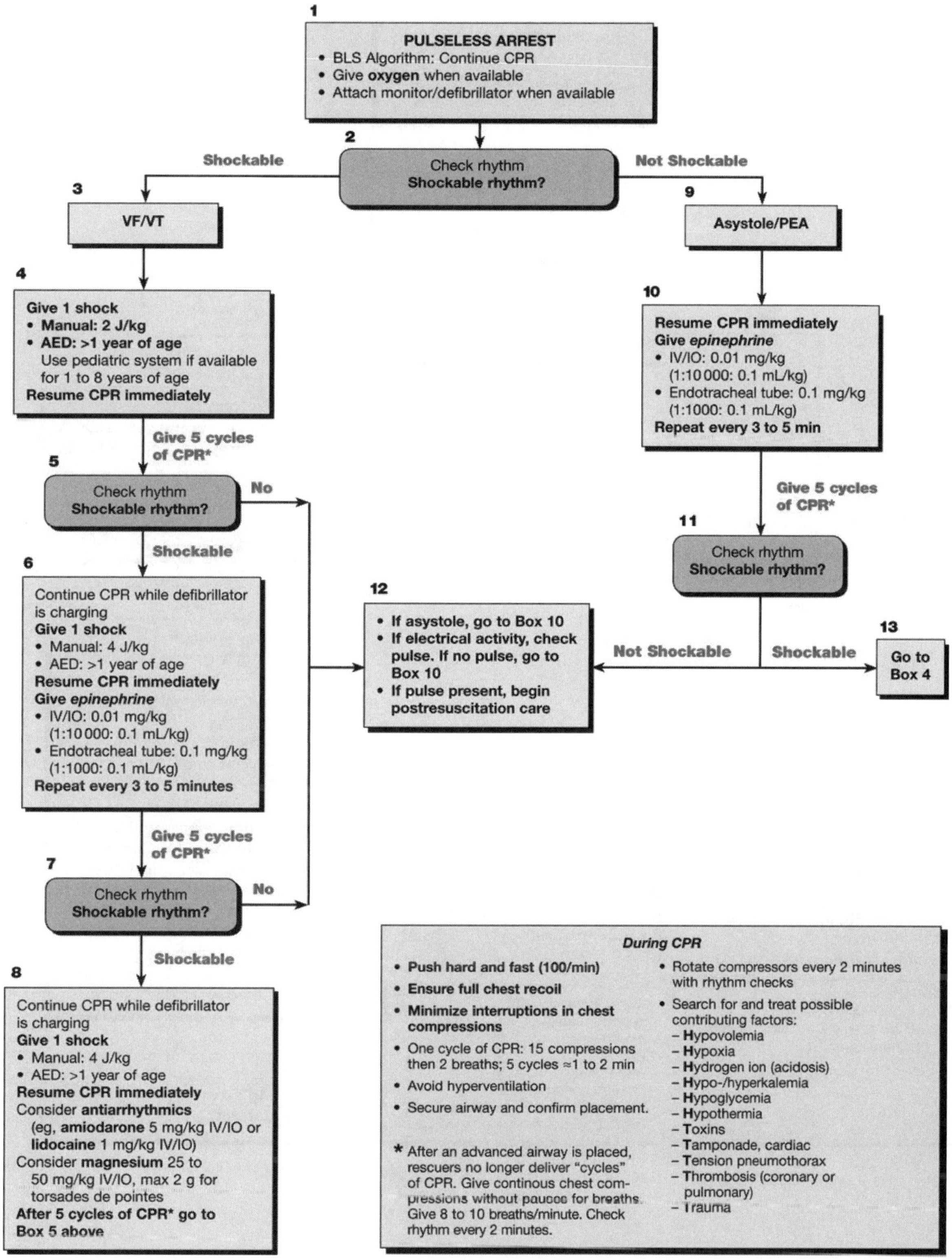

Reproduced with permission from The American Heart Association in Collaboration with the International Liaison Committee on Resuscitation (ILCOR): 2005 American Heart Association Guidelines for Cardiopulmonary Resuscitation and Emergency Cardiovascular Care. *Circulation* 2005;112: IV167-IV187.

Figure A7-5. Pediatric Bradycardia Algorithm

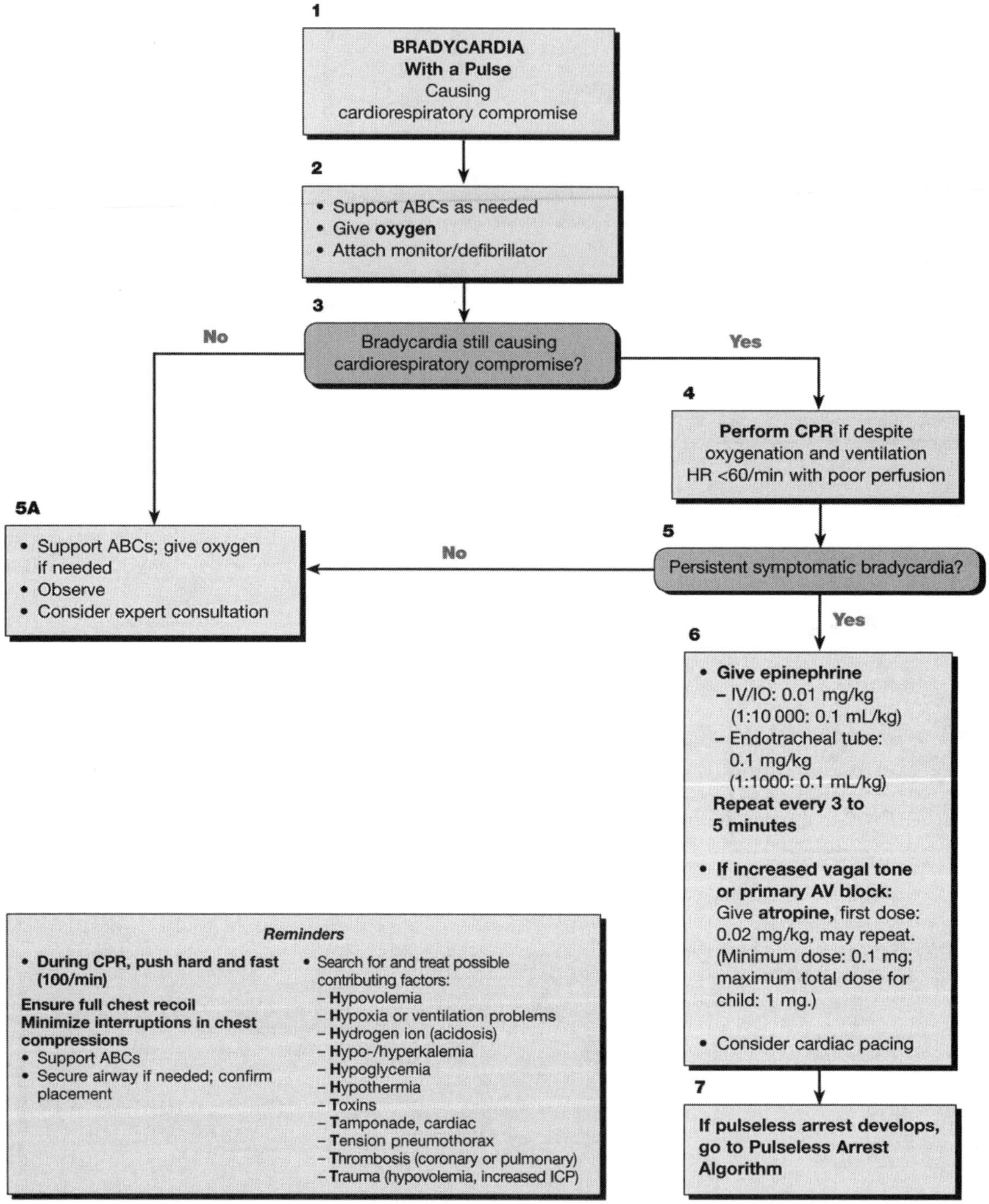

Reproduced with permission from The American Heart Association in Collaboration with the International Liaison Committee on Resuscitation (ILCOR): 2005 American Heart Association Guidelines for Cardiopulmonary Resuscitation and Emergency Cardiovascular Care. *Circulation* 2005;112: IV167-IV187.

Figure A7-6. Pediatric Tachycardia Algorithm

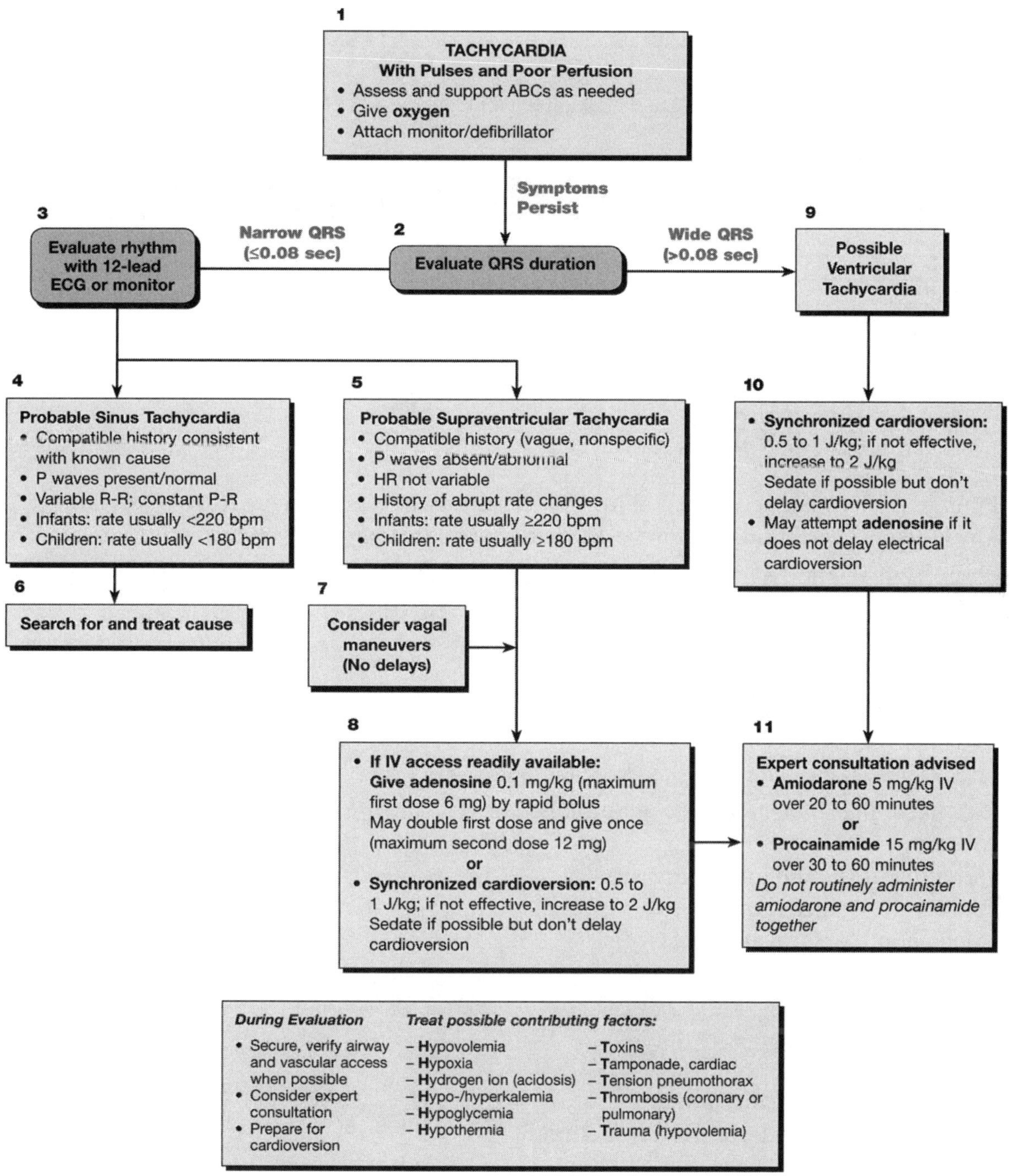

Reproduced with permission from The American Heart Association in Collaboration with the International Liaison Committee on Resuscitation (ILCOR): 2005 American Heart Association Guidelines for Cardiopulmonary Resuscitation and Emergency Cardiovascular Care. *Circulation* 2005;112: IV167-IV187.

Appendix 8:

Intraosseous Needle Insertion

I. INDICATIONS

A. Emergency vascular access in children if intravenous access is delayed
B. Any fluid or medication that can be given intravenously can be given by the intraosseous route in the same dosages

II. EQUIPMENT

A. Conductive gel or self-adhesive defibrillation pads
B. Sternal or iliac bone marrow aspiration needle (15- to 18-gauge) or disposable intraosseous needle
C. Sterile syringes and infiltrating needles
D. Sterile 4 × 4 gauze sponges
E. Medication for local anesthesia
F. Gloves, sterile drapes
G. Skin disinfectant
H. Supplemental oxygen
I. Pulse oximeter
J. Electrocardiography monitor
K. Intravenous tubing, T-connector, and fluid

III. SITE SELECTION

A. Young children

1. In neonates, proximal tibia, just below the growth plate, distal to the tibial tubercle; in infants 6 to 12 months old, insert 1 cm distal to tibial tuberosity; in children > 1 year of age, insert 2 cm distal to the tibial tuberosity

B. Child

1. Proximal tibia
2. Proximal humerus
3. Distal tibia above the medial malleolus
4. Lateral or medial malleolus
5. Distal radius and distal ulna
6. Distal femur

C. Alternate sites

1. Anterior-superior iliac spine

IV. TECHNIQUE (TIBIAL SITE)

A. Apply oxygen, monitor pulse oximeter and electrocardiography
B. Restrain leg with a small sandbag or intravenous fluid bag behind the knee for support
C. Create sterile field
D. Infiltrate local anesthetic if clinical situation permits
E. Use proximal anterior tibia, midpoint of the medial flat surface, 1 to 3 cm below the tibial tuberosity (**Figure A6-1**)
F. Insert the needle at 60° to 90° to the skin away from the growth plate; advance with a screwing motion

Figure A6-1. Intraosseus Needle Insertion

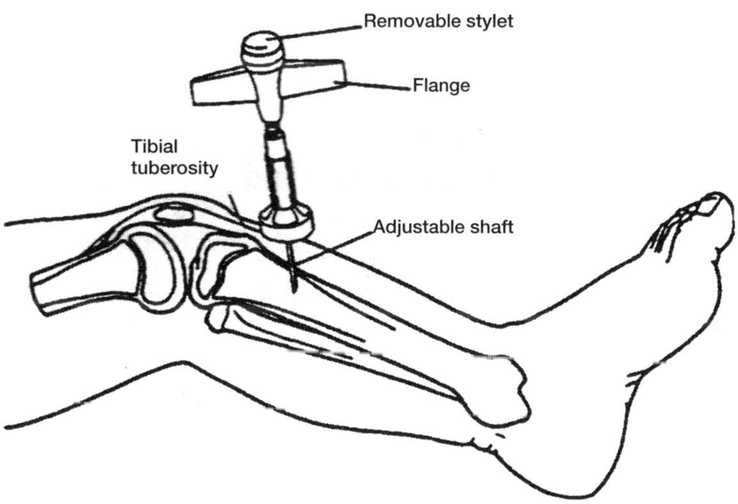

Approach to puncture of the proximal anterior tibia. Reprinted with permission from Fiser HD. Intraosseous infusion.. *N Engl J Med* 1990; 322:1579-1581.

G. Use the distal tibia only if the proximal tibia is impenetrable (just proximal to the medial malleolus and posterior to the saphenous vein)
H. Confirm entry into the marrow space by noting a lack of resistance after the needle has passed through the cortex
I. Aspirate marrow into the syringe; this should be accomplished easily, but failure to do so does not necessarily indicate improper placement
J. Infuse fluids; fluids should flow freely
K. Secure needle by taping flanges to the skin (may require support of external portion of the needle)
L. Consider flushing with heparin-saline solution
M. Infuse intravenous fluids
N. Observe for infiltration of fluids
O. Continue attempts to place intravenous catheter(s)
P. Discontinue intraosseous infusion and withdraw needle after intravenous access is established (preferably within 1 to 2 hours)
Q. Apply pressure to puncture site for approximately 5 minutes
R. Apply sterile dressing

V. PRECAUTIONS/COMPLICATIONS

A. Inability to place needle (approximately 20% of patients)
B. Subcutaneous and/or subperiosteal infiltration of fluid
C. Tibial fracture
D. Compartment syndrome
E. Clotting of marrow within the needle
F. Cellulitis, subcutaneous abscess
G. Osteomyelitis (0.6%)
H. Pain (usually minor))

Suggested Readings

1. 2005 American Heart Association Guidelines for Cardiopulmonary Resuscitation and Emergency Cardiovascular Care: Pediatric advanced life support. *Circulation.* 2005;112:IV-167--IV187. Available at www.circulationaha.org.

2. Fiser HD. Intraosseous infusion. *N Engl J Med.* 1990;322:1579-1581.

3. Fiorito BA, Mirza F, Doran TM, et al. Intraosseous access in the setting of pediatric critical care transport. *Pediatr Crit Care Med.* 2005;6:50-53..

4. The International Liaison Committee on Resuscitation (ILCOR) consensus on science with treatment recommendations for pediatric and neonatal patients: Pediatric basic and advanced Life support: *Pediatrics.* 2006;117:e955-e977.

Appendix 9:

Defibrillation/Cardioversion

I. INDICATIONS

A. Defibrillation/unsynchronized cardioversion
   1. Ventricular fibrillation
   2. Pulseless ventricular tachycardia
   3. Polymorphic ventricular tachycardia

B. Synchronized cardioversion
   1. Unstable or stable ventricular tachycardia with a pulse
   2. Unstable or stable supraventricular tachycardia, atrial fibrillation, or atrial flutter

II. EQUIPMENT

A. Conductive gel or self-adhesive defibrillation pads
B. Defibrillator/cardioverter
C. Connecting cable, leads, and electrodes
D. Medication for sedation
E. Supplemental oxygen with bag-mask oxygen delivery device
F. Emergency suction and intubation equipment
G. Pulse oximeter
H. Electrocardiography and blood pressure monitor
I. Intravenous catheter, infusion pump, tubing, fluids
J. Resuscitation cart

III. TECHNIQUE

A. Recognize cardiac rhythm, determine severity of its physiologic effect
B. In patients with unstable rhythms or adverse physiologic effects on systemic perfusion, begin immediate defibrillation/cardioversion, after initiation of cardiopulmonary resuscitation
C. Recognize that time delays under the above circumstances decrease the likelihood of conversion to a stable rhythm
D. Inform and prepare patient as clinical situation dictates; sedate if necessary
E. Assure intravenous access
F. Provide supplemental oxygen

G. Monitor pulse oximeter and electrocardiography
H. Turn on defibrillator/cardioverter
I. Attach monitoring electrodes (if needed)
J. Apply conductive gel to paddles or apply conductive pads to chest wall
   1. Male patients with a hirsute chest may require rapid shaving to ensure adequate contact
K. Paddle/electrode placement
   1. Anterolateral
      a. One paddle/electrode to right of upper sternum below clavicle
      b. One paddle/electrode to left of nipple with center in midaxillary line
   2. Anteroposterior
      a. One paddle/electrode anteriorly over left precordium, below clavicle
      b. One paddle/electrode posteriorly in left infrascapular location, left of thoracic spine
   3. Avoid placement over permanent pacer or implantable cardioverter-defibrillator
L. Paddle pressure (if used)
   1. Adult — approximately 25 lb of pressure to each paddle
   2. Pediatric — ensure good contact with chest wall
M. Activate appropriate switch for synchronized cardioversion or unsynchronized defibrillation
N. Set energy level of electrical discharge (in accordance with recommendations of the American Heart Association)
   1. Manual Defibrillator
      a. Appropriate paddle size is important; use the largest paddle size possible, assuring good chest contact over its entire area and good separation between the two paddles (about 3 cm)
         i. Infants (< 10 kg) — 4.5-cm paddles usually used
         ii. Children (>10 kg) — 8.0- to 13-cm paddles usually used
      b. Paddle placement is similar to that for adults
      c. Be sure that the defibrillator/cardioverter provides a low-dose range for infants. Some defibrillators do not go below 10 joules and therefore should not be used for converting infants/children weight <20 kg (5 to 6 yrs of age)
      d. Pediatric defibrillation
         i. 2 joules/kg (initial)
         ii. Advance to 4 J/kg if rhythm persists
         iii. Use adult energy levels in children ≥ 50 kg
      e. Pediatric cardioversion
         i. Stable or unstable ventricular tachycardia: 0.5 to 1.0 J/kg
         ii. Stable or unstable supraventricular tachycardia: 0.5 to 1.0 J/kg
         iii. Advance to 2 J/kg if unsuccessful
   2. AED (Automatic external defibrillator)
      a. > 25 kg (8 years old): Use standard adult AED with adult pad-cable system
      b. < 25 kg (>1 year old but < 8 years old): Use attenuated dose if a pediatric system is available. Use adult system if pediatric system is not available
      c. < 1 year old. There is currently insufficient evidence to recommend for or against the use of an AED

O. Ensure electrical safety (all personnel clear of contact with the patient, bed, and equipment)
P. Charge capacitors through defibrillator/cardioverter
Q. Depress discharge button(s) on the device or simultaneously on the defibrillator/paddles (with synchronized cardioversion, the discharge buttons must remain depressed until the energy is released)
R. If defibrillation performed, immediately resume chest compressions; if cardioversion performed, assess patient (respiration, pulse, and rhythm)
S. If unsuccessful, repeat process, following standard Pediatric Advanced Cardiovascular Life Support protocols

IV. PRECAUTIONS/COMPLICATIONS

A. During procedure
1. Skin burn may occur if insufficient gel or improper pads are used, poor contact with the chest wall occurs during discharge, or if the pads/paddles are too close to each other.
2. All metal objects should be removed from the patient to avoid skin burns.
3. Patient's environment and chest must be dry to avoid current traveling across water, resulting in a decreased amount of delivered energy.
4. Transdermal patches should be removed as they may impede transmission of current.
5. Medical personnel may sustain electrical shock or burn if safety precautions are not followed.

B. After procedure
1. Arterial embolization
2. Pulmonary edema
3. Postcardioversion arrhythmias; be prepared to institute cardiopulmonary resuscitation
4. Post-shock syndrome (myocardial damage)

Suggested Readings

1. American Heart Association. *Advanced Cardiovascular Life Support: Provider Manual.* Dallas, TX: American Heart Association; 2006.

2. 2005 American Heart Association Guidelines for Cardiopulmonary Resuscitation and Emergency Cardiovascular Care. Electrical Therapies: Automated external defibrillators, defibrillation, cardioversion, and pacing. *Circulation.* 2005;112(suppl IV):IV-35-IV-46. Available at www.circulationaha.org

3. Wiegand D, Carlson, K. *AACN Procedure Manual for Critical Care.* 5th ed. St. Louis, MO: Elsevier Saunders; 2005.

Appendix 10:

Temporary Transcutaneous Cardiac Pacing

I. INDICATIONS/CONTRAINDICATIONS

A. Indications
   1. Symptomatic bradycardia (hypotension, chest pain, syncope, altered mental status, heart failure, etc) unresponsive to pharmacologic management
   2. Overdrive pacing of tachycardias, refractory to drug therapy or electrical cardioversion

B. Contraindications
   1. Severe hypothermia
   2. Not recommended for asystole

II. EQUIPMENT

A. Cardiac pacing electrode pads
B. Pulse generator
C. Connecting leads
D. Medication for sedation and/or analgesia, if necessary
E. Supplemental oxygen (cannula, mask, other as necessary)
F. Pulse oximeter
G. Electrocardiography monitor
H. Intravenous catheter, tubing, fluids
I. Resuscitation cart with pediatric and adult sized equipment

III. TECHNIQUE

A. Recognize cardiac rhythm, determine severity
B. Prepare patient
C. Obtain intravenous access if not done previously
D. Apply oxygen; monitor pulse oximeter and electrocardiogram
E. Attempt pharmacologic management, including atropine, epinephrine, and/or dopamine when appropriate (follow Pediatric Advanced Cardiovascular Life Support guidelines)
F. Assemble equipment

G. Apply electrode pads
  1. Anteroposterior
    a. One electrode anteriorly over left precordium as close as possible to maximal cardiac impulse, below clavicle
    b. One electrode posteriorly in left infrascapular location directly behind anterior electrode, left of thoracic spine
  2. Anterolateral
    a. One electrode to right of upper sternum below clavicle
    b. One electrode to left of nipple with center in midaxillary line
  3. Shaving of excessive body hair may be required to ensure good contact

H. Administer sedation or analgesia as necessary and tolerated by patient

I. Connect leads to pulse generator

J. Turn on pulse generator and monitor

K. Set rate to 100 beats/min; adjust as needed, based on clinical response

L. Adjust pulse generator output (mA) upward until electrical and mechanical ventricular capture (threshold) occurs (usually 20 to 60 mA). Set output 2 mA above threshold to allow for safety margin. In the setting of severe symptoms or bradyasystolic arrest, it may be appropriate to start at the maximal output and then decrease if capture is achieved.

M. Criteria for proper electrical capture
  1. Pacer spike followed by a ventricular complex 100% of the time
  2. Wide QRS complex
  3. T-wave in an opposite deflection from baseline as the QRS complex

N. Assess efficacy of mechanical capture — obtain blood pressure and palpate pulse. Palpate pulse distal to carotid site as electrical stimulation from the pacemaker may mimic a carotid pulse.

O. Arrange for temporary or permanent transvenous pacemaker as necessary

IV. SPECIAL CONSIDERATIONS

A. Bradycardia in children is most often secondary to hypoxemia

B. Pacing for bradycardic rhythms secondary to hypoxemic insult may be considered after airway management, oxygenation, ventilation, chest compressions, epinephrine bolus (0.01 mg/kg, 1:1,000 concentration) and infusion, and possibly atropine bolus (0.02 mg/kg, may repeat; minimum dose 0.1 mg and maximum total dose for child 1 mg) have been accomplished

C. The effectiveness of cardiac pacing in this setting is unproven

D. Even if electrical capture of the heart is accomplished, contractility and myocardial blood flow may not improve without mechanical capture

E. It is recommended to use the largest available paddles or self-adhering electrode pads that will fit on the chest wall without touching (allow at least 3 cm between paddles or pads).
  1. For children > 10 kg (> 1 year of age) use large adult paddles.
  2. For children < 10 kg (< 1 year of age) use small infant paddles (4.5 cm)

V. PRECAUTIONS/COMPLICATIONS

A. Inability to capture (~20% of patients), usually related to delay in attempting to pace
B. Painful skeletal muscle contraction
C. Skin or tissue damage
D. Temporizing measure only, prior to transvenous pacing

Suggested Readings

1. American Heart Association. *Advanced Cardiovascular Life Support: Provider manual.* Dallas, TX: American Heart Association; 2006.

2. Hazinski MF, Nadkarni VM, Hickey RW, O'Connor R, Becker LB, Zaritsky A. Major changes in the 2005 AHA Guidelines for CPR and ECC: reaching the tipping point for change. *Circulation.* 2005;112(24 suppl):IV206-IV211.

3. Wiegand D, Carlson K. *AACN Procedure Manual for Critical Care.* 5th ed. St. Louis, MO: Elsevier Saunders; 2005.

Appendix 11:

Thoracostomy

I. Indications/Contraindications

A. Indications
1. Tension pneumothorax
2. Large simple pneumothorax
3. Penetrating thoracic wound with concurrent need for positive-pressure ventilation
4. Hemothorax
5. Symptomatic pleural effusion (recurrent, following thoracentesis)
6. Empyema
7. Chylothorax

B. Contraindications
1. Coagulopathy
    a. Correct prior to nonemergent thoracostomy.
    b. Risk of hemorrhage must be accepted with tension pneumothorax.
2. Inability to aspirate fluid or air to confirm a patent pleural space
    a. This dictum holds in all circumstances except a penetrating thoracic wound with need for positive-pressure ventilation.
    b. Attempted tube placement in the presence of an obliterated pleural space risks pulmonary injury and potentially fatal hemorrhage.
    c. Aspiration is performed most conveniently through the thoracostomy incisional wound immediately before tube placement.
    d. Aspiration is most important when an apparent effusion presents as "whiteout" on chest radiograph, and its free-flowing nature cannot be confirmed radiographically. Such an apparent effusion in reality may be solid tumor; blunt dissection into such tumor may have devastating hemorrhagic consequences.

II. Equipment

A. Needle thoracostomy
   1. 14- to 16-gauge catheter over needle
   2. 23-gauge butterfly needle (infants)

B. Tube thoracostomy
   1. Sterile gloves, gown, eye protection, mask, cap, and drapes
   2. Intravenous catheter, tubing, and fluid
   3. Supplemental oxygen
   4. Monitors (echocardiographic, pulse oximeter)
   5. Skin disinfectant
   6. Sterile syringes and infiltrating needles
   7. Local anesthetic
   8. Scalpel with #10 or #15 blade
   9. Forceps
   10. Curved clamp
   11. Thoracostomy tubes for infants and children are listed in **Table A11-1**.
       a. 32- to 40-French thoracostomy tubes are placed in trauma settings to evacuate an acute hemothorax that potentially contains clots. The largest diameter tube accommodated by the intercostal space is used in this circumstance.
   12. Water-seal drainage system
   13. Needle holder
   14. 0-silk or 0-polypropylene suture on cutting needle
   15. Suture scissors
   16. 1/4-inch-wide adhesive tape strips or "cable ties" with applicator
   17. Sterile 4 × 4 gauze sponges
   18. Petroleum jelly gauze
   19. Antiseptic ointment
   20. 4-inch-wide impervious tape strips
   21. 1-inch-wide adhesive tape
   22. Resuscitation cart

Table A11-1. Approximate Sizes for Pediatric Thoracostomy Tubes by Age and Weight*

Age	Approximate Weight (kg)	Tube Size (French)
Newborn to 9 months	3.5-8	12-18
10 to 17 months	10	14-20
18 months to 3 years	12-15	14-24
4 to 7 years	17-22	20-32
8 years	28	28-32
≥9 years	≥35	28-38

* Needle thoracostomy can usually be accomplished on infants with a 23-gauge butterfly needle.

III. Technique

A. Analgesia/Sedation

1. Tube thoracostomy is a painful procedure. In nonemergent and semi-urgent circumstances, intravenous narcotic analgesia and a benzodiazepine should be titrated to effect as hemodynamic and respiratory status allow. Local anesthetic should be infiltrated generously throughout the tube thoracostomy tract.

B. Preliminary needle thoracostomy (**Figure A11-1**)

1. Indication: before tube thoracostomy for rapid temporizing treatment of tension pneumothorax.
2. Site
    a. Midclavicular line at the second intercostal space; necessitates that the pectoralis major muscle and possibly breast tissue be penetrated before the intercostal space.
    b. Midaxillary line at the fifth intercostal space; placed in the auscultatory triangle posterior to the pectoralis and anterior to latissimus dorsi muscles where only the thin serratus anterior muscle need be penetrated prior to the intercostal space.
3. Don cap, mask, eye protection and sterile gloves.
4. Quickly prepare the access site with povidone-iodine solution.
5. Advance 14-gauge catheter over needle with attached syringe immediately over the superior aspect of the rib while aspirating.
6. When air is aspirated, advance catheter completely, and withdraw needle and syringe. Withdraw catheter following completion of tube thoracostomy.
7. Note: 1 mL of saline in the aspirating syringe allows access of intrapleural air to be recognized as bubbles.

Figure A11-1. Sites for needle thoracostomy.

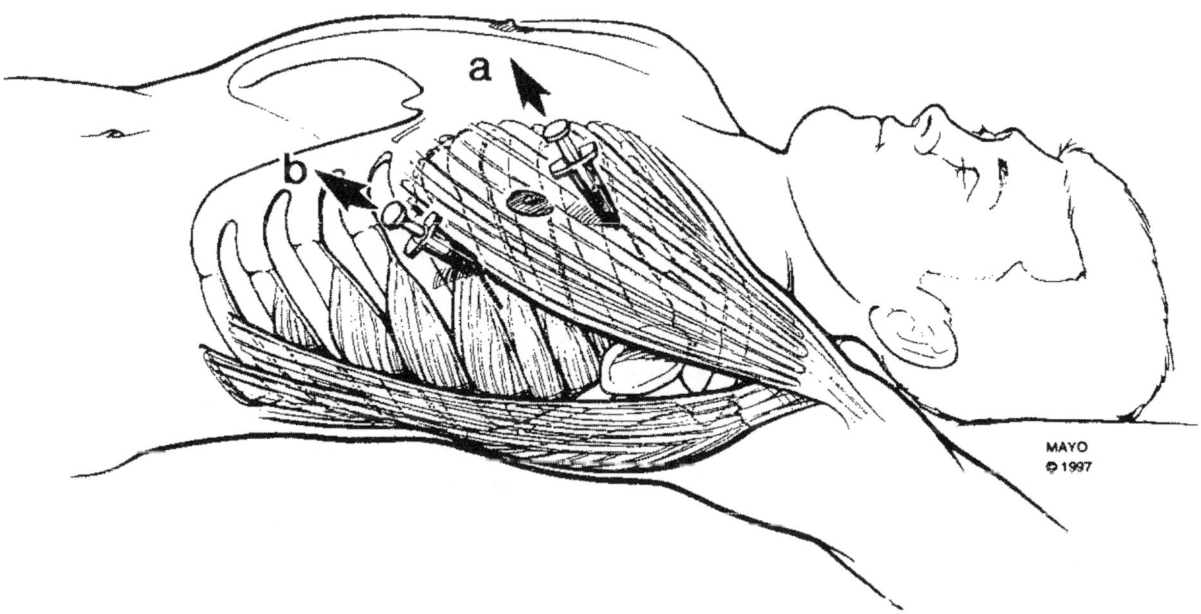

(A) Second intercostal space, midclavicular line. (B) Fifth intercostal space, midaxillary line. The latter is also the incision site for placement of a thoracostomy tube and necessitates transgression of much less chest wall musculature and no breast tissue. Reprinted with permission of the Mayo Foundation.

C. Preparation for tube thoracostomy

1. Provide supplemental oxygen.
2. In nonemergent circumstances, establish intravenous access, electrocardiographic monitoring, and pulse oximetry.
3. Assemble the following nonsterile materials: water-seal drainage system, 1/4-inch-wide strips of adhesive tape or cable ties to secure thoracostomy tube to drainage system, 4-inch-wide impervious tape strips to secure dressing.
4. Ensure adequate lighting.
5. Place patient in supine position with ipsilateral arm extended.
6. Don cap, mask, eye protection, and sterile gloves.
7. Paint patient's anterior and lateral chest wall with antiseptic solution. Remove gloves.
8. Don sterile gown and gloves.
9. On a sterile work space, lay out, from left to right, the following sterile instruments and materials in sequence: syringe with infiltrating needle loaded with local anesthetic, scalpel with blade, forceps, curved clamp, thoracostomy tube, needle holder loaded with suture, suture scissor, dressing comprised of gauze 4 × 4 sponges, petroleum jelly gauze, and antiseptic ointment. These instruments and materials will be used in this sequence.

D. Insertion

Instrument	**Maneuver**
1. Syringe and needle with local anesthetic	a. Raise cutaneous wheal at incision site. b. Deeply infiltrate underlying subcutaneous tissue.
2. Scalpel	a. 3-cm incision at position *B* in **Figure A11-1** through the skin and subcutaneous tissue of the fifth intercostal space. b. Deepen incision to level of chest wall musculature. Note: The skin incision parallels the intercostal space. It should be placed one interspace below the intended level of pleural entry so that a tract deep to subcutaneous tissue can be created for the tube. This tract closes spontaneously upon tube removal.
3. Syringe and needle with local anesthetic	a. Through wound, infiltrate subcutaneous tissue cephalad to incision.
4. Forceps	a. Using left hand, retract subcutaneous tissue cephalad away from chest wall to create tension at junction of subcutaneous tissue and chest wall musculature (**Figure A11-2**).
5. Curved clamp	a. Continue to apply above traction with forceps. b. With curved clamp in right hand, spread at junction of subcutaneous tissue and chest wall musculature to open this plane (**Figure A11-2**).
6. Syringe and needle with local anesthetic	a. Through incisional wound, infiltrate musculature and pleura of fourth intercostal space. b. Advance needle into pleural space while aspirating syringe. c. Confirm presence of air or fluid in the pleural space.

7. Curved clamp	a. With curved clamp in right hand, hold tips against superior aspect of fifth rib with concavity of clamp facing pleural space. b. Intercostal dissection must be performed immediately superior to a rib to avoid injury to the neurovascular bundle that lies inferior to each rib. c. Advance curved clamp through musculature (serratus anterior and intercostal muscles) and pleura into the pleural space **(Figure A11-3)**. Note: This maneuver may need to be forceful but must always be restrained. A dramatic loss of resistance will signal entry into the pleural space and will be followed by egress of fluid and/or air. d. Ensuring that the tips of the clamp remain on the superior aspect of the fifth rib, widely separate the jaws of the clamp to create a generous opening through the serratus anterior muscle, intercostal muscles, and pleura. e. Insert the left index finger into the pleural space as the clamp is withdrawn. Palpation of the smooth pleura confirms the intrapleural location. Sweep the finger through 360° to ensure the absence of adhesions between parietal and visceral pleura. Such adhesions and obliteration of the pleural space would predispose to pulmonary injury during tube insertion.
8. Thoracostomy tube	a. Keep the left index finger in the pleural space. b. With the right hand, advance the thoracostomy tube over the tip of the left index finger into the pleural space **(Figure A11-4)**. Passage of the tube over the tip of the intrapleural index finger ensures intrapleural placement of the tube. c. Advance the tube until resistance is encountered (approximately 15 to 25 cm). The last side hole of the tube should reside 2 cm within the pleural cavity. Ideally, the tip of the tube lies at the pleural apex.
9. Water-seal drainage system	a. Connect the thoracostomy tube to the drainage system.
10. Needle holder and suture	a. Place a suture of 0-nonabsorbable material through the wound on either side of the thoracostomy tube. b. Tie each suture to close the wound. c. Tie each suture about the thoracostomy tube to secure it. d. Place additional sutures as necessary to close the wound.

11. 1/4-inch adhesive tape or cable ties	a. Secure connection between chest tube and drainage system tubing (**Figure A11-5**). b. Tape should never be placed in such a manner as to obscure the connection from view. One must be able to see that the connections are intact at all times.
12. Dressing of gauze, 4 x 4 sponges, petroleum jelly gauze, antiseptic ointment, and impervious tape	a. Place dressing over thoracostomy site. b. Secure dressing with impervious tape.
13. 1-inch adhesive tape	a. Secure chest tube and drainage system tubing to patient's trunk.

Figure A11-2. Blunt Dissection for Thoracostomy

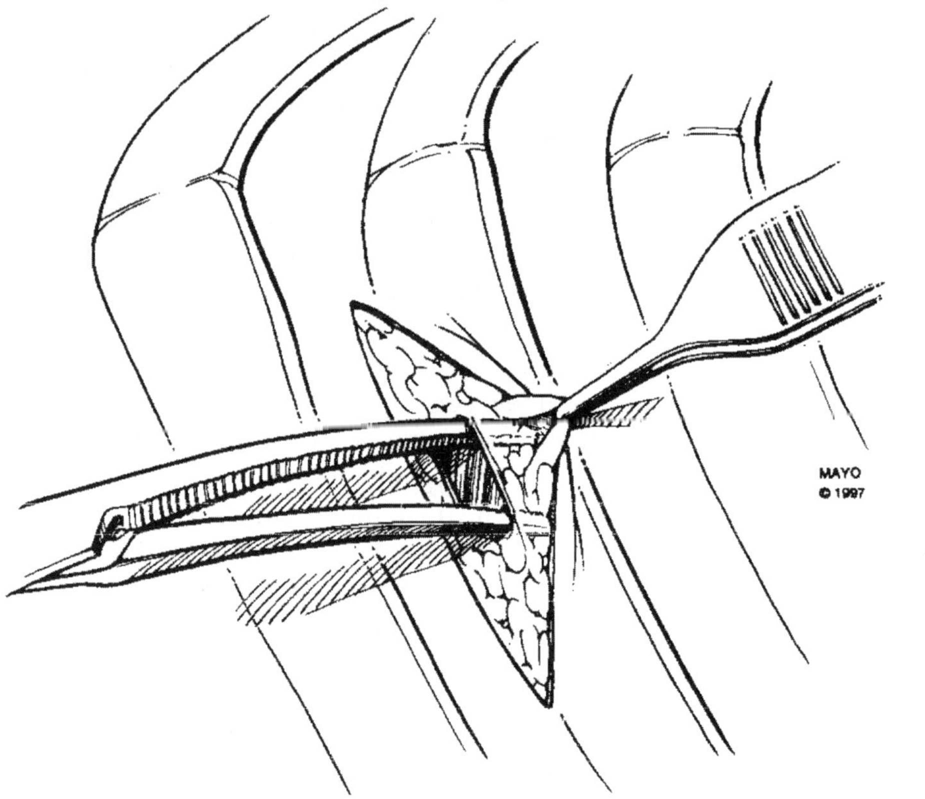

Retraction of skin and subcutaneous tissue with blunt dissection of subcutaneous tissue from chest wall musculature superior to incisional wound. Reprinted with permission of the Mayo Foundation.

Figure A11-3. Creation of Pleural Opening

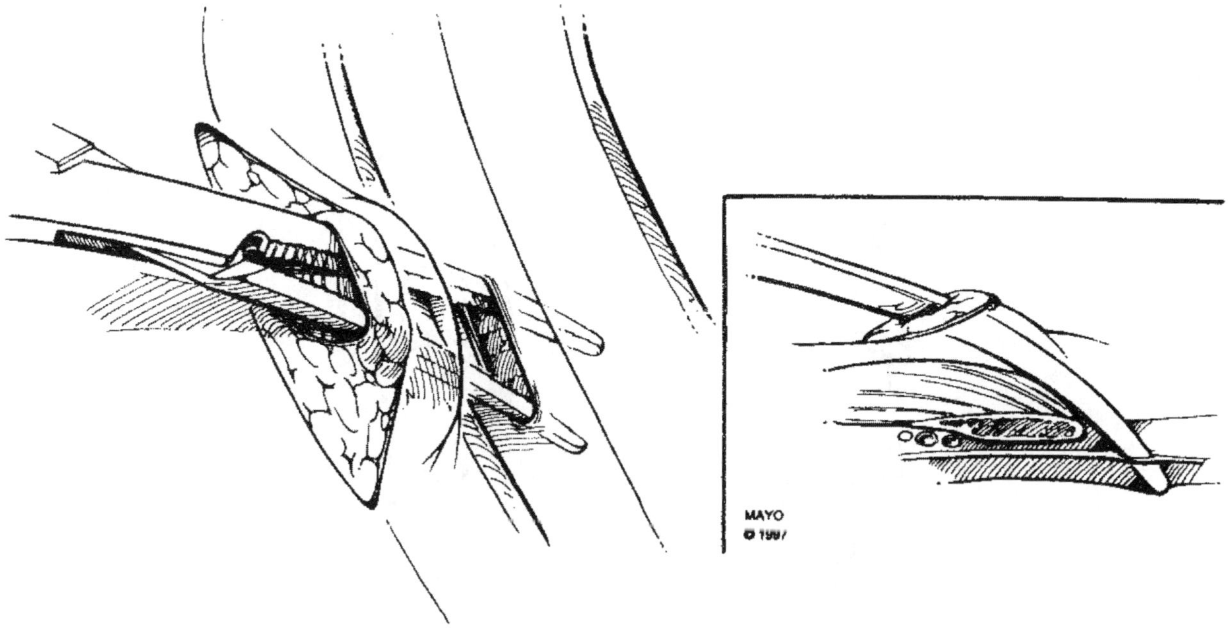

The curved clamp has been advanced into the superior aspect of the incisional wound and advanced through the intercostal musculature and pleura at the superior margin of the fifth rib. The jaws of the clamp are then spread to create a pleural opening. The opening should be generous enough to simultaneously admit a finger and the thoracostomy tube. Insert shows the path of the curved clamp in cross-section. Reprinted with permission of the Mayo Foundation.

Figure A11-4. Placement of Thoracostomy Tube

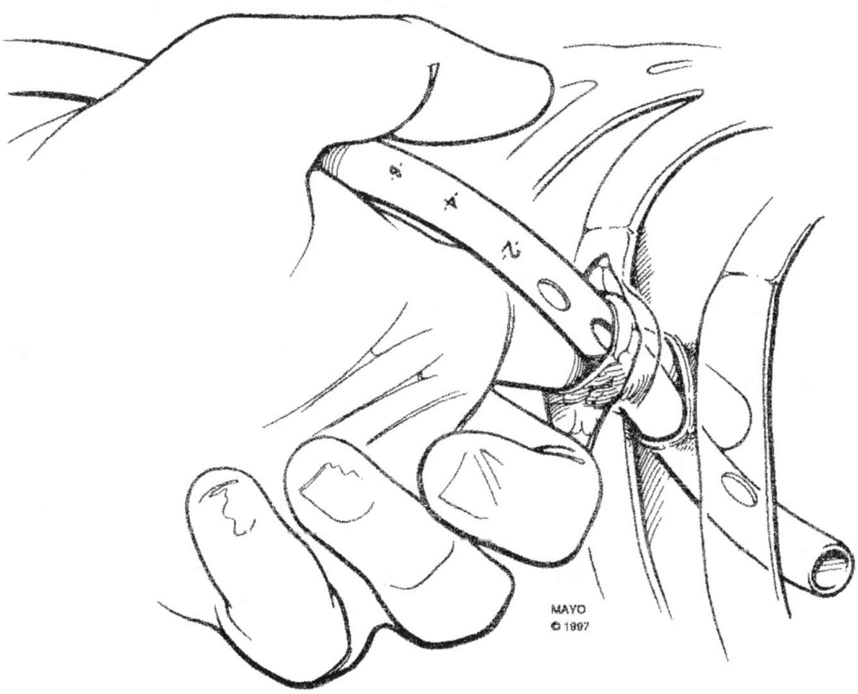

The left index finger replaces the curved clamp and remains within the pleural space as the thoracostomy tube is advanced over the tip of the finger, ensuring intrapleural location. Reprinted with permission of the Mayo Foundation.

Figure A11-5. Connection of Thoracostomy Tube

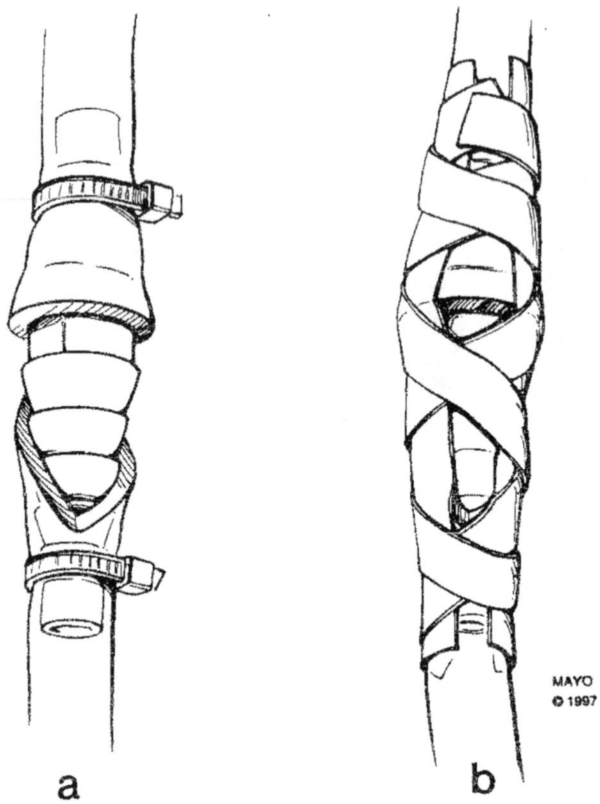

The thoracostomy tube and tubing from the draining system are secured about a conical connecting adaptor with "cable ties" (a) or strips of adhesive tape placed longitudinally and in a spiral fashion (b). Reprinted with permission of the Mayo Foundation.

E. Pleural decompression
   1. Adjust suction to 20 cm H_2O.
   2. Consider prophylactic antibiotic coverage.

F. Thoracostomy tube monitoring
   1. A thoracostomy tube should be monitored frequently with portable chest radiography to ensure appropriate tube placement and the absence of iatrogenic pneumothorax. The last side hole of the thoracostomy tube lies on a radiopaque line and thus is visible on the radiograph as a gap in this line; the gap should always appear well within the pleural space.
   2. Patency of the chest tube is assured by the presence of a to-and-fro movement of fluid with respiration (respiratory variation). This may be detected within the thoracostomy tube, the tubing of the collection device, or the water-seal chamber. As the pleural space is definitively decompressed, the thoracostomy tube will become loculated from the general pleural space by adhesion of visceral and parietal pleura around it; respiratory variation will then be lost.
   3. The character and volume of pleural drainage must be assessed frequently. The significance of diminished drainage volume can only be determined in light of concurrent chest radiographic findings. For example, diminishing sanguineous drainage

may mean cessation of bleeding or occlusion of the thoracostomy tube by clot; the chest radiograph will reveal increasing effusion/hemothorax in the latter circumstance, but not the former.

4. Air leaks are apparent as air bubbling through the water seal (not the suction regulator). Small air leaks will demonstrate bubbling only during spontaneous expiration or mechanical inspiration. Large air leaks will demonstrate bubbling through both phases of the respiratory cycle. These continuous air leaks may indicate a bronchopleural fistula or tracheobronchial laceration.

G. Thoracostomy tube removal
1. General criteria for thoracostomy tube removal
   a Complete radiographic expansion of the lung
   b. Absence of air leak for 24 hours
   c. Drainage volume <100 mL over 24 hours
2. Prepare a dressing of impervious tape, gauze 4 × 4 sponges, petroleum jelly gauze, and antiseptic ointment.
3. With a sterile scissors, divide the sutures securing the thoracostomy tube.
4. Instruct the patient to take a full inspiration, hold the breath, and perform a Valsalva maneuver. Practice this sequence several times.
5. Repeat the above sequence, briskly withdraw the thoracostomy tube with the patient performing a Valsalva maneuver at full inspiration, and immediately apply the occlusive dressing to the thoracostomy wound.
6. Do not close the thoracostomy site with suture or other material.
7. Obtain an immediate portable chest radiograph to ensure the absence of pneumothorax.

IV. Precautions/Complications

A. Possible injury to intercostal artery, vein, or nerve
B. Extrapleural tube position
C. Subcutaneous emphysema
D. Break in water seal, resulting in pneumothorax
E. Chest wall hematoma/ecchymosis
F. Chest wall or intrapleural hemorrhage
G. Infection
1. Insertion-site cellulitis
2. Tract infection
3. Empyema

H. Laceration of diaphragm or intrathoracic/intra-abdominal viscera
I. Recurrence of pneumothorax (upon removal, secondary to entrained room air or rupture of pulmonary bulla/bleb).
J. Clamping a chest tube in the presence of an air leak may result in life-threatening tension pneumothorax.

Suggested Readings

1. Etoch SW, Bar-Natan MF, Miller FB, Richardson JD. Tube thoracostomy. Factors related to complications. *Arch Surg.* 1995;130:521-525.

2. Martino K, Merrit S, Boyakye K, et al. Prospective randomized trial of thoracostomy removal algorithms. *J Trauma* 1999;46:369-371.

3. Richardson JD, Spain DA. Injury to the lung and pleura: In: Mattox KL, Feliciano DV, Moore EE, eds. *Trauma.* 4th ed. New York, NY: McGraw-Hill, 2000; 523-543.

4. Warren WH. Chest tube thoracostomy. In: Parrillo JE, Dellinger RP, eds. *Critical Care Medicine.* 2nd ed. St. Louis, MO: Mosby, Inc., 2001; 238-248.

Pediatric Transport Form

Date:_______________ Time:_____________________

NAME: ______________________________ AGE:__________ WEIGHT:_____________

DIAGNOSIS: ____

REFERRAL HOSPITAL: ____

REFERRAL MD: __________________________ REFERRAL HOSPITAL PHONE:___________

ACCEPTING MD: ____

MEDICAL CONTROL MD: ____

HISTORY/PE:
VITAL SIGNS: T: _____ HR: ______ RR: _____ BP: _______ SpO_2: ________ FIO_2_________________

Hx:

PE:

Labs:

THERAPY/RECOMMENDATIONS:
Discuss possible interventions:

Discussion with transport team:

Medical Control MD:

BED CONTROL: Time contacted _________ Approved by____________ Time__________
(Name)

TIME TEAM DISPATCHED: ___________ ☐Helicopter ☐ Fixed Wing ☐ Ground Ambulance

☐ Pediatric/NICU Specialty Team ☐ACLS Ambulance

TIME ACCEPTED: _________________ for admission to ☐ PICU ☐ ER ☐ PEDS FLOOR ☐ NICU

TIME ACCEPTING MD NOTIFIED OF ETA____

Appendix 13:

Common Medications

Table A13-1. Analgesics and Sedatitves

Agent	Dosing	Onset and Duration	Benefits	Cautions
Fentanyl	1-2 µg/kg/dose IV every 2 min, titrate to effect	Onset: Immediate Duration: 30-60 min	- Rapid onset of action - Short acting - Reversible - Relatively stable hemodynamic profile	- Rigid chest syndrome - Respiratory depression - Lacks amnestic properties
Morphine	0.05- 0.1 mg/kg IV	Onset: 5 min Duration: 2 h	- Useful for acute and chronic pain	- Respiratory depression - Histamine release - Hypotension
Midazolam	0.2 mg/kg/dose IV every 5 min, titrate to effect	Onset: 1-5 min Duration: 20-30 min	- Rapid onset - Short acting - Provides amnesia - Reversible	- Lacks analgesic properties - Respiratory depression - Hypotension and bradycardia
Lorazepam	0.05- 0.1 mg/kg IV	Onset: 15- 30 min Duration: 8-12 h	- Useful for sedation and status epilepticus	- Respiratory depression, apnea - Bradycardia, hypotension
Ketamine	1 mg/kg/dose IV every 5 min, titrate to effect	Onset: 1-2 min Duration: 10-30 min	- Rapid onset - Airway protective reflexes remain intact - No hypotension or bradycardia	- Increases airway secretions and laryngospasm (blunted with atropine) - Elevates intracranial and ocular pressure - Emergence reactions (blunted with benzodiazepines)
Etomidate	0.3 mg/kg/dose IV every 5 min, titrate to effect	Onset: 10-20 sec Duration: 4-10 min	- Rapid onset - Short acting - Stable hemodynamic profile	- Potential for adrenal insufficiency
Thiopental	2-3 mg/kg/dose IV, repeat as needed	Onset: 30-60 sec Duration: 5-30 min	- Ultra-short acting barbiturate - Decreases intracranial pressure	- Cardiovascular and respiratory depression
Pentobarbital	1-3 mg/kg IV 2-6 mg/kg IM and PO	Onset IV: 1 min Duration IV: 15 min	- Rapid onset IV - Useful in status epilepticus and increased intracranial pressure	- Laryngospasm and respiratory depression - Bradycardia and hypotension
Dexmedetomidine	Initial load of 1 µg/kg over 10 min IV 0.2-0.7 µg/kg/h		- Provides both sedation and analgesia	- Can cause hypotension and bradycardia
Propofol	1-3 mg/kg/dose IV, repeat as needed	Onset: 30-60 sec Duration: 5-10 min	- IV general anesthetic - Rapid onset and recovery	- Cardiovascular and respiratory depression - Contraindicated in egg allergy
Chloral hydrate	25-75 mg/kg PO 30 min before procedure	Onset: 30-60 min Duration: 4-8 h	- Short-term sedative and hypnotic for diagnostic procedures	- May cause "hangover" effect

IV, intravenous; IM, intramuscular; PO, by mouth; PR, by rectum; NSAID, nonsteroidal anti-inflammatory drug

Table A13-2. Nonsteroidal Anti-inflammatory Drugs (NSAIDs) - Recommended doses (< 50 Kg)

*These doses have a ceiling effect and maximum dose should not be exceeded.

Agent	Dosing	Onset and Duration	Benefits	Cautions
Acetaminophen	PO: 10-15 mg/kg every 3-4 h PR: 15-20 mg/kg every 4 h	Onset: 10-60 min Duration: 1-3 h	- Analgesic - Anti-inflammatory agent - Antipyretic - NSAID	Maximum dose, 75 mg/kg/day
	Newborn dose (< 6 kg or < 6 mo): PO: 10-15 mg/kg every 4-6 h PR: 20-25 mg/kg every 4-6 h	newborn dosing, 2-5 h		
Ketorolac	IM/IV: 0.5 mg/kg every 6 h Max dose 30 mg/dose	Onset: 30 min Duration: 4-6 h	- Analgesic - Anti-inflammatory agent - Antipyretic - NSAID	Maximum 5 days of therapy
Ibuprofen	PO: 10 mg/kg every 6-8 h	Onset: 60- 120 min Duration: 6- 8 h	- Analgesic - Anti-inflammatory agent - Antipyretic - NSAID	Should not be used with platelet count < 50,000/mm^3
Aspirin	PO: 10-15 mg/kg every 4 h	Onset:15-20 min Duration: dose dependent, ranging from 3 h to 10 h with higher doses (> 1 g)	- Analgesic - Anti-inflammatory agent - Antipyretic - NSAID	Contraindicated in children with low platelet counts, or in the presence of fever or other viral illness

IV, intravenous; IM, intramuscular; PO, by mouth; PR, by rectum; NSAID, nonsteroidal anti-inflammatory drug

Table A13-3. Neuromuscular Blockade Agents

Agent	Dosing	Onset and Duration	Benefits	Cautions
Succinylcholine (depolarizing neuromuscular blockade)	1 mg/kg IV	Onset: 30-60 sec Duration: 4-6 min	- Rapid onset - Short duration	- Causes muscle fasciculations (blunted with low dose non-depolarizing neuromuscular blocker) - Potentiates hyperkalemia (contraindicated in head trauma, crush injury, burns, hyperkalemia) - May induce neuroleptic malignant syndrome
Vecuronium (non-depolarizing neuromuscular blockade)	0.1 mg/kg IV	Onset: 1-3 min Duration: 30-40 min	- No fasciculations	- Slower onset - Longer duration of action
Rocuronium (non-depolarizing neuromuscular blockade)	0.6-1.0 mg/kg IV	Onset: 30-60 sec Duration: 30-40 min	- No fasciculations	
Cisatracurium (non-depolarizing neuromuscular blockade)	0.1-0.2 mg/kg IV	Onset: 2-3 min Duration: 35-45 min	- Can be used in renal failure - Metabolized through Hoffman elimination	- Potential histamine release
Atracurium (non-depolarizing neuromuscular blockade)	0.3-0.5 mg/kg	Onset: 3 -5 min Duration: 20-35 min	- Can be used in renal failure - Metabolized through Hoffman elimination	- Potential histamine release

IV, intravenous; IM, intramuscular; PO, by mouth; PR, by rectum; NSAID, nonsteroidal anti-inflammatory drug

Appendix 14:

Central Venous Catheter Insertion

I. Indications

A. Poor peripheral venous access
B. Need for administration of multiple incompatible medications
C. Administration of vasoactive, irritating, caustic, or hypertonic solutions
D. Hemodynamic monitoring
E. Insertion of a transvenous cardiac pacing catheter
F. Support of rapid infusion of resuscitation fluids
G. Support of frequent blood sampling; minimize repeated venipuncture
H. Support hemodialysis

II. Equipment

A. Sterile central venous catheter (antibiotic impregnated catheter is recommended); guide wire; 18-, 22- or 25-gauge needle, according to catheter size; or central venous catheter kit (single lumen or multilumen central venous catheter)
B. Syringe, scalpel, dilator, suture or securement device, infiltrating needles
C. Saline or heparinized saline solution
D. Semitransparent dressing
E. Chlorhexidine impregnated patch for patients ≥2 months, per institution-specific protocol
F. Sterile 2x2 and 4x4 gauze sponges
G. Medication for local anesthesia and sedation
H. Sterile gloves, gown, mask, protective eye gear, hat, drapes
I. Chlorhexidine for children ≥2 months of age and povidone iodine for infants <2 months of age
J. Supplemental oxygen
K. Pulse oximeter
L. Electrocardiographic monitor
M. Intravenous tubing and fluid
N. Resuscitation cart available

III. Technique

A. Modified Seldinger technique

1. Obtain consent
2. Inform the patient using appropriate developmental approach
3. Notify licensed provider for appropriate timing of sedation
4. Choose catheter size and site, gather equipment
5. Ensure appropriate cardiorespiratory monitoring
6. Conduct final patient verification process
7. Assure patent peripheral intravenous access or intraosseous access, if possible
8. Put on hat, mask, and protective eye gear
9. Wash hands
10. Position the patient and identify anatomical landmarks (**Table A14-1**)
11. Wash hands

Table A14-1. Insertion Site and Patient Positioning

Internal Jugular Site	Subclavian Site	Femoral Site
Patient position: Trendelenburg	Patient position: Trendelenburg	Patient position: Supine with hip abduction and leg in external rotation on side of cannulation
1. Turn patient's head to side opposite of insertion site	1. Turn patient's head to side opposite of insertion site	Place roll under hip side to be cannulated
2. Extend the neck and head by placing a towel under the shoulder on the side of the insertion site if no cervical spine injury is present	2. Place shoulder roll under and parallel along spine and hyperextend neck, if no cervical spine injury is present	

Table A14-1. Insertion Site and Patient Positioning (Continued)

Internal Jugular Site Landmark	Subclavian Site Landmark	Femoral Site Landmark
1. Medial and lateral bellies of the sternocleidomastoid muscle form a triangle with the clavicle at the base	Palpate the clavicle bone	1. Palpate the anterior superior iliac spine and pubic tubercle that delineate the course of the inguinal ligament
2. The internal jugular vein lies within the carotid sheath just beneath the apex of this triangle		2. Palpate the femoral artery that runs beneath the inguinal ligament
3. The carotid artery also lies within the carotid sheath just medial and deep to the internal jugular vein		3. The femoral vein lies ~1 cm medial and parallel to the femoral artery

12. Put on sterile gown and gloves
13. Create sterile field
14. Open sterile central venous catheter kit
15. Prep the area for cannulation using povidone iodine for infants <2 months of age and chlorhexidine for infants and children ≥2 months of age; allow area to dry
16. Administer local anesthetic
17. Flush the needle and catheter with sterile saline or heparinized saline solution according to manufacturer's recommendations
18. Insert needle with attached syringe into selected site at the specified angle and depth while gently aspirating on the syringe (**Table A14-2** and **Figure A14-1**)
19. When back flash of nonpulsatile dark blood is noted, stabilize the needle, disconnect the syringe, and cover the needle hub with your gloved finger
20. Remove needle and hold pressure for 5 minutes, if pulsatile bright red blood return is obtained on needle insertion
21. Insert the guide wire through the needle during positive pressure breath or spontaneous exhalation; minimal-to-no resistance should be met
22. Monitor cardiac rhythm for ectopy when inserting the guide wire, because it may be long enough to reach the heart
23. Make a small incision with the scalpel adjacent to the needle to slightly enlarge the puncture site and more easily accommodate the dilator and catheter
24. Remove the needle, while maintaining control of the guide wire
25. Pass the dilator over the needle to gently dilate the skin and subcutaneous tissue
26. Remove the dilator while maintaining control of the guide wire
27. Pass the catheter over the guide wire and advance the catheter to the predetermined landmark, while maintaining control of the guide wire
28. Remove the guide wire
29. Aspirate blood from all ports of the catheter
30. Once blood return is confirmed, flush ports

Table A14-2. Angle of Insertion Based on Anatomical Insertion Site

Internal Jugular Site	Subclavian Site	Femoral Site
Angle of Insertion	Angle of Insertion	Angle of Insertion
Anterior Route: Aiming toward the ipsilateral nipple, insert needle at the midpoint of the anterior margin of the sternocleidomastoid muscle at a 30° angle posteriorly. Central Route: Aiming toward the ipsilateral nipple, insert needle at the apex of the triangle formed by the sternoclavicular heads of the sternocleidomastoid muscle and the clavicle at a 30° angle. Posterior Route: Aiming toward the suprasternal notch, insert needle under the posterior border of sternocleidomastoid muscle approximately halfway between the mastoid process and clavicle.	Insert the needle under the clavicle bone at the junction of the medial and middle thirds of the clavicle, aiming toward the suprasternal notch at a 45° angle. Needle should be parallel to the frontal plane, directed medially and slightly cephalad, beneath the clavicle bone toward posterior aspect of the sternal end of the clavicle.	Insert the needle one finger's width below inguinal ligament and medial to the femoral artery at a 30° angle, aiming toward the umbilicus.
Depth of Insertion	Depth of Insertion	Depth of Insertion
Approximately 1-2 cm	Approximately 2-3 cm	Approximately 1-2 cm

Figure A14-1. Modified Seldinger technique.

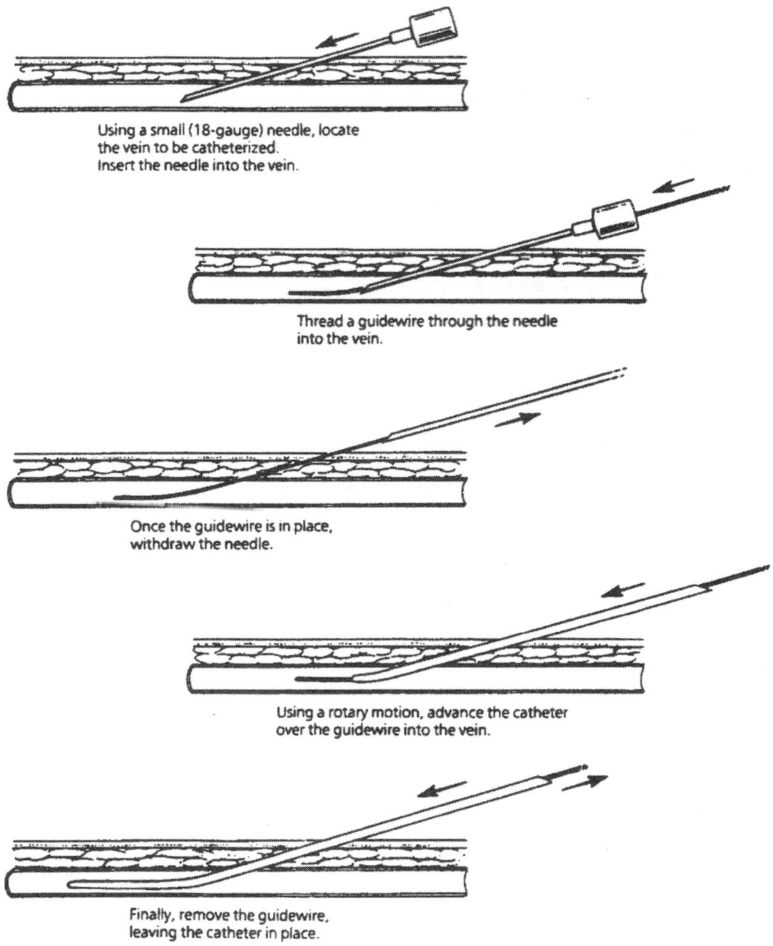

Illustration © by Robert Margulies and reproduced with permission from the artist and *The Journal of Critical Illness.*

31. Connect distal port to monitor to confirm central venous position waveform (nonpulsatile)
32. Suture catheter or use other securement device as appropriate
33. Apply chlorhexidine-impregnated patch for infants and children ≥2 months of age
34. Apply sterile occlusive dressing
35. Obtain chest or abdominal radiograph to confirm proper positioning of catheter
36. Attach IV fluids

IV. Precautions/Complications

A. Hemothorax
B. Pneumothorax
C. Chylothorax
D. Bleeding/hemorrhage
E. Venous thrombosis
F. Arterial puncture
G. Heart perforation
H. Air embolism
I. Infection
J. Dysrhythmias
K. Catheter or guide wire embolism
L. Local subcutaneous tissue, nerve, artery, or vein damage.

Appendix 15:

Arterial Catheter Insertion

I. Indications

A. Hypertension, hypotension, labile blood pressure
B. Continuous assessment of systolic, diastolic, and mean blood pressure
C. Use of vasoactive agents (vasopressors, vasodilators, or other cardioactive medications)
D. Frequent sampling of laboratory specimens (arterial blood gases or otherwise)

II. Equipment

A. Arterial catheter kit with appropriate-sized safety cannula over needle *or* procedure tray with catheter over guide wire (generally 22- to 24-gauge for radial and 20-gauge for femoral)
B. 2% chlorhexidine, 10% povidone-iodine, or 70% alcohol
C. Sterile towels, gloves, and gown
D. Mask
E. Protective eyewear
F. Surgical hat
G. Tape
H. Gauze sponges (2x2 and 4x4)
I. Armboard, if radial artery is being used
J. 3.0 or 4.0 suture and needle driver or other securement device, such as StatLock™ (if not included in arterial catheter kit)
K. Transparent semipermeable dressing
L. Local anesthetic, such as lidocaine
M. Medication for sedation, if necessary
N. Pressure transducer, tubing, and pressure monitor

III. Technique

A. Ensure that child and family understand procedure and all questions are answered
B. Gather supplies
C. Assure intravenous access
D. Wash hands
E. Perform final patient identification process per institution specific policy (ie, time-out)
F. Ensure appropriate cardiorespiratory monitoring
G. Perform modified Allen's test (see **Table A15-1**), if using radial artery
H. Use armboard for immobilization, if using radial artery
I. Administration of analgesia and/or sedation, as appropriate
J. Position patient appropriately (**Figure A15-1 and Table A15-2**)

Figure A15-1. Catheter-over-needle technique

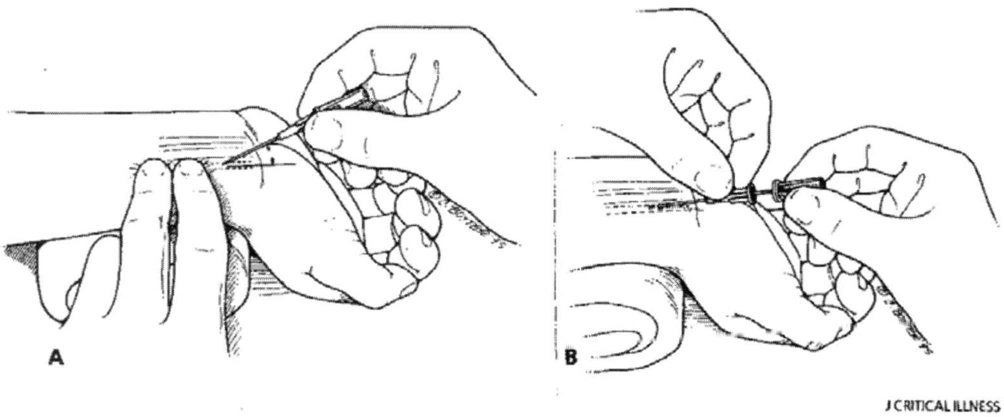

(A) After extending and immobilizing the wrist, the radial artery is localized by palpation. The needle is inserted at a 20° to 45° angle. (B) After the artery is entered, the catheter is advanced over the needle and the needle is withdrawn. Illustration © by Charles H. Boyter and reproduced with permission from the artist and *The Journal of Critical Illness.*

Table A15-1. Allen's Test

Allen's Test is used to test blood supply in the hand. It is performed prior to radial artery blood sampling or cannulation.

1. The hand is elevated and a fist is made for approximately 30 seconds.
2. Pressure is applied over the ulnar and radial arteries so as to occlude both of them simultaneously.
3. While elevated, the hand is opened. It should appear blanched.
4. Ulnar pressure is released and the color to the hand should return in approximately 7 seconds.
5. If color does not return or returns > 7 seconds, then the ulnar artery supply to the hand is not sufficient and the radial artery cannot be safely punctured.

Table A15-2. Anatomical Position for Insertion*

Radial Artery	Femoral Artery
Position patient appropriately	Position patient appropriately
• Dorsiflex wrist 45-60 degrees using small roll under the wrist	• Place towel or blanket under hips and place in frog-leg position

* Axillary, dorsalis pedis, posterior tibial and umbilical artery catheterizations have been described but will not be discussed here.

K. Don mask, cap, gown, and sterile gloves
L. Prepare site using 2% chlorhexidine for infants >2 months of age, 10% povidone-iodine, or 70% alcohol
M. Scrub site with back and forth motion using friction; allow area to air dry
N. Prepare sterile field
O. Identify landmarks; palpate artery
P. Infiltrate area with local anesthetic
Q. Puncture anatomical insertion site (**Tables A15-3, A15-4 and Figure A15-2**)

Table A15-3. Anatomical Insertion Site

Radial Artery	Femoral Artery
• Puncture skin at a 30 angle, directing the safety catheter or needle toward the underlying artery	• Puncture skin at 45 angle, needle bevel up, below the inguinal crease and a few centimeters distal to palpable pulse
• Advance the needle slowly, while watching for flashback	• Enter through skin, advancing introducer needle into femoral artery
• When blood is obtained, remove syringe and bring needle down against skin	• When blood is obtained, remove syringe and bring needle down against skin

Table A15-4. Insertion Technique

Catheter Over Needle	Modified Seldinger Technique
Advance the catheter using a rotating motion to the hub and remove needle	• Immobilize needle with free hand • Advance guide wire through needle slowly; do not force wire in if resistance is met • Remove needle and wire if unable to remove wire from needle during insertion attempts • Remove needle while holding guide wire in place • Pass catheter over guide wire, while inserting catheter to the hub; do not force catheter in if resistance is met • Remove guide wire

Figure A15-2. Modified Seldinger technique

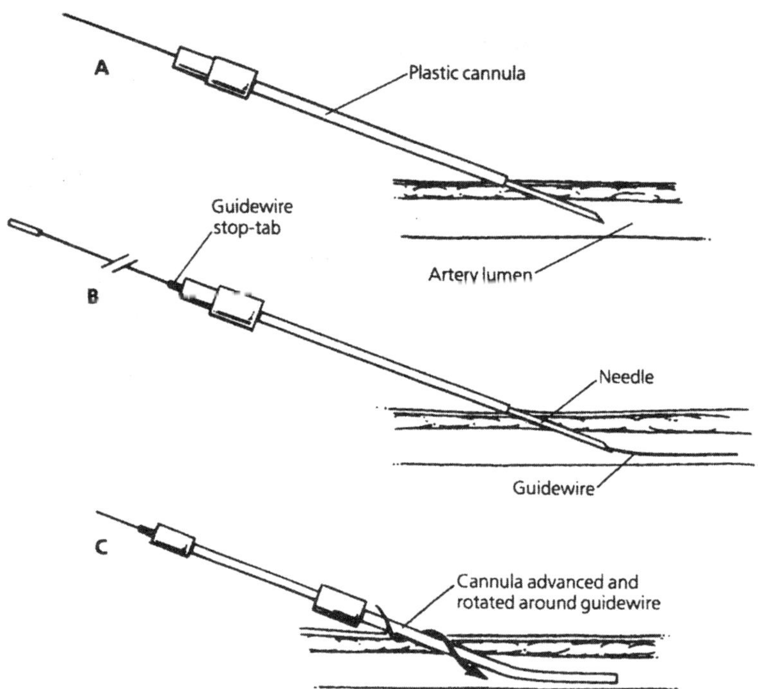

(A) The needle is inserted into the artery. (B) The guidewire is advanced until the stop-tab reaches the needle hub. (C) The catheter is advanced over the guidewire into the artery. Illustration © by Robert Margulies and reproduced with permission from the artist and *The Journal of Critical Illness.*

R. Attach catheter to transducer to observe for presence of arterial waveform and for ease of flushing and aspirating of blood from catheter
S. Secure with suture or sutureless securement device
T. Surround site with chlorhexidine impregnated sponge, per institution-specific protocol
U. Cover site with semipermeable transparent dressing, per institution-specific protocol
V. Dispose of supplies appropriately
W. Remove personal protective equipment
X. Assess circulation to distal extremity
Y. Wash hands
Z. Documentation of procedure may include the following:
    1. Type of procedure
    2. Informed consent
    3. Risks/Benefits
    4. Skin preparation
    5. Insertion site
    6. Use of local anesthetic or systemic sedation/analgesia
    7. Condition of child at end of procedure
    8. Unexpected outcomes

IV. Validation of Measures and System Characteristics

A. Systolic return-to-flow blood pressure assessment (**Figure A15-3**)
    1. Observe arterial waveform
    2. Place a manual blood pressure cuff on the same extremity as the arterial catheter and inflate until the arterial waveform flattens
    3. Release pressure in cuff slowly until the first evidence of pulsatile waveform is again observed, and note pressure on sphygmomanometer
    4. Sphygmomanometer pressure is the "true" systolic blood pressure and should correlate with pressure measured through arterial catheter
B. Square wave test
    1. Use to test system characteristics of tubing (eg, length, stiffness, presence of bubbles)
    2. Rapidly flush the arterial line tubing (**Figure 15-4**)
    3. Observe wavefrom for underdamping or overdamping (**Figures A15-5 and A15-6**)
C. Factors that may interfere with monitoring accuracy
    1. Connections of stopcocks and interface
    2. Constant pressure application (300 mm Hg)
    3. Elasticity alterations of the blood vessel wall
    4. Reflectance of the pulse wave from the walls or tubing
    5. Air bubbles in the fluid column throughout the system
    6. Thrombi around or in the catheter
    7. Stiffness and length of the plastic tubing

Figure A15-3. Instructions for obtaining systolic return-to-flow blood pressure

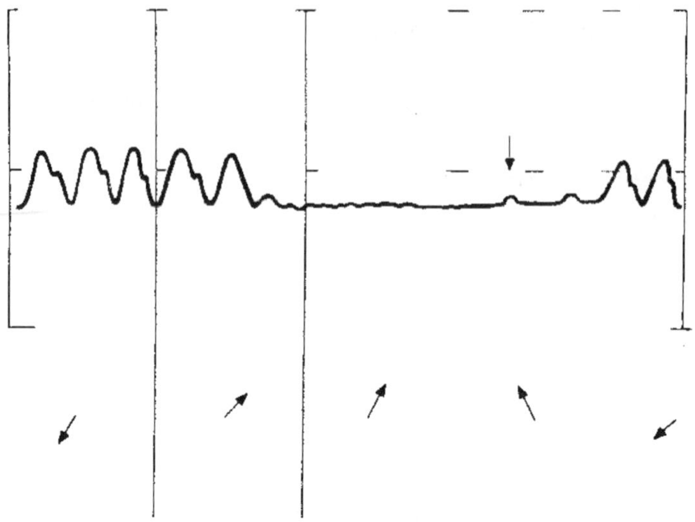

(A) Observe arterial waveform. (B) Place a manual blood pressure cuff on the same extremity as the radial or dorsalis pedis arterial catheter and inflate it. Arterial waveform flattens as the manual blood pressure cuff is inflated. (C) Release pressure in cuff slowly until the first evidence of pulsatile waveform is again observed, at which point the pressure on the sphygmomanometer is noted. This sphygmomanometer pressure is the return-to-flow or "true" systolic blood pressure.

Figure A15-4. Square Wave Test

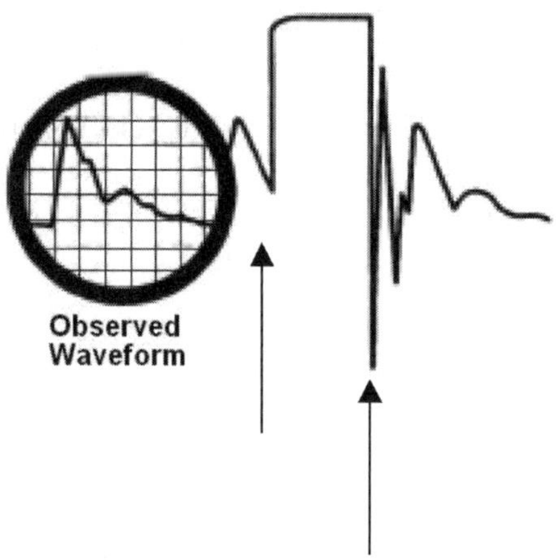

Application of a rapid in-line flush and the correlating evaluation of the monitoring system. First arrow indicates flush applied and second arrow indicates the rapid frequency response when released. Reprinted with permission from Edwards Lifesciences.

Figure A15-5. Overclamping

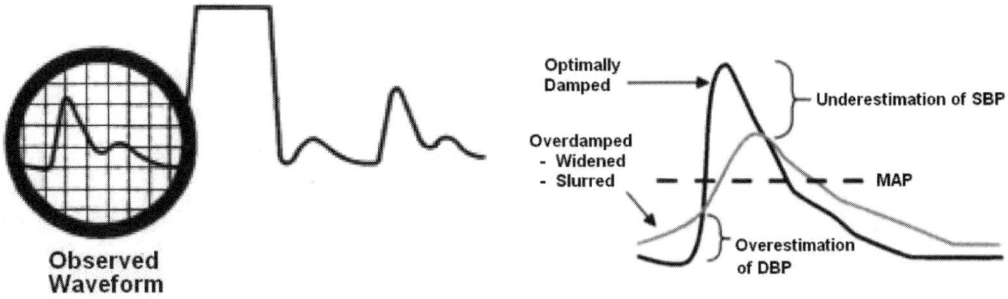

An overdamped signal indicates loss of signal related to loose connections, air bubbles in the system, and/or inadequate fluid and pressure applied. SBP, systolic blood pressure; MAP, mean arterial pressure; DBP, diastolic blood pressure. Reprinted with permission from Edwards Lifesciences.

Figure A15-6. Underclamping

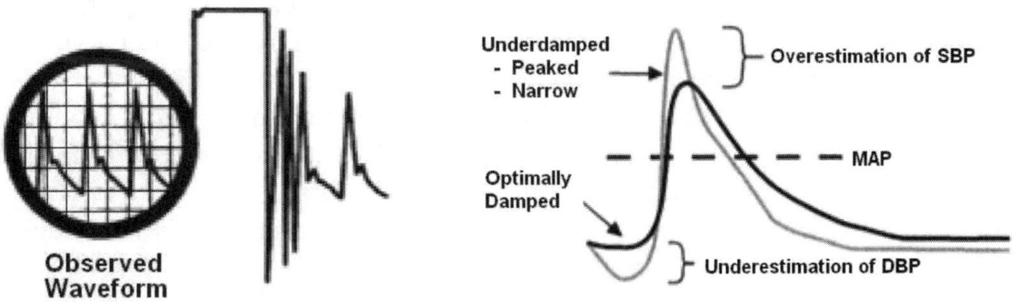

An underdamped signal indicates significant increase in frequency response and is in general related to loss of calibration of the transducer, requiring a transducer change. SBP, systolic blood pressure; MAP, mean arterial pressure; DBP, diastolic blood pressure. Reprinted with permission from Edwards Lifesciences.

V. Complications

A. Compromised circulation/ischemia to extremity at insertion site and distal to insertion site
B. Infection
C. Hemorrhage
D. Arterial air embolism
E. Arteriovenous fistula
F. Arterial aneurysm

VI. Precautions/Contraindications

A. Ischemia of the extremity
B. Infection at the puncture site
C. Raynaud's disease
D. Prior vascular surgery or cutdown procedure involving the artery to be punctured

Appendix 16:

Hospitalists and the Critically Ill Child

I. What is a Hospitalist?

A. The Society of Hospital Medicine defines hospitalists as "physicians whose primary professional focus is the general medical care of hospitalized patients. Their activities include patient care, teaching, research and leadership related to hospital care."

B. Improvements in cost of care and length of stay have been documented for both hospitalists and intensivists in their respective environments. Hospitalists have also been shown to improve outcomes of pediatric patients in intensive care units.

C. It is estimated that there will be 30,000 hospitalists in North America by 2010. Pediatric hospitalists comprise 8-10% of this total.

II. Pediatric Hospitalist Practice Environment

A. Pediatric ICUs should be under the distinct control of Board Certified/Board Eligible pediatric intensivists.

B. Pediatric hospitalists may provide intermediate level services without the formal involvement of intensivists in appropriate settings.

C. In an institution that does not have a formal Pediatric Intensive Care Unit (PICU), pediatric hospitalists may provide intermediate levels of care on a general pediatric ward.

III. Scope of Practice

A. Hospitalists who work in the PICU must assure their scope of practice complies with hospital and state regulations.

B. The AAP Policy statement "Levels of Pediatric Critical Care" states that

1. Level I PICU: essential to have a Resident or training physician post-graduate year (PGY) 2 available in the PICU 24/7, a PGY3 or above (in pediatrics or anesthesia) in-house 24/7, and a pediatric intensivist available in 30 minutes or less 24/7.
2. Level II PICU: essential to have a PGY2 or higher available in the PICU 24/7, optional to have a PGY3 or higher pediatrician or anesthesiologist in the hospital 24/7, and desirable to have a pediatric intensivist available within 30 minutes 24/7.

C. Hospitalists are physicians who have elected to concentrate their practice in the acute care environment found within the hospital setting. Many hospitalists are planning a lifetime career in hospital medicine.

D. When a hospitalist is working under the supervision of an intensivist, the standards of care required are comparable to those of the intensivist, similar to standards expected in the situation of a resident working under the supervision of an intensivist.

E. With consistent presence in a PICU, and when an appropriate investment is made in the training and education of the hospitalist, a hospitalist can accumulate cognitive and procedural experience that far surpasses a resident rotating on a 30-day basis.

IV. Relationship between Intensivist, Team Members and Hospitalist

A. While the hospitalist has a secondary role in terms of critical care knowledge and experience compared to the intensivist, the relationship should be more collegial and less hierarchical when it comes to the professional interaction between the two parties than the relationship between physician-in-training and the intensivist.

B. Trust is developed over time and depends on the foundation of carefully developed guidelines outlining the scope of practice for the hospitalist, an appropriate orientation program with on-going training and feedback, and graduated responsibility for patient care in the PICU.

1. The intensivist must trust the hospitalist to call for help early rather than late.
2. The hospitalist must trust the intensivist to give phone advice when appropriate, and to come in when appropriate.

C. A hospitalist working in the PICU must recognize their own limitations as well as the expertise and limitations of others.

1. It is up to the individual hospitalist to recognize when their limitations are being stretched, and ask for additional resources and help.
2. Mutual trust and confidence are enhanced when nurses, therapists, pharmacists and others are engaged as resources and collaborators.

V. Logistics of Integrating Hospitalists into the Critical Care Team

A. During the initial orientation/supervision period, there is value to concentrating the hospitalist's experience in the PICU for the hospitalist to gain expertise, efficiency and familiarity. This period may be 1-3 months, depending upon the hospitalist's level of expertise and the acuity of patients in the unit.

B. Many programs use hospitalists in an after-hours role as part of the 24/7 coverage model, and do not use hospitalists during the day when physician staffing is otherwise adequate.

1. It is recommended that hospitalists have regular daytime exposure in the PICU initially for orientation purposes and thereafter on a regular basis to maintain consistency and proficiency.

2. It is not anticipated new hospitalists providing daytime coverage in the PICU to develop minimal proficiency until at least a month of working in the PICU alongside attending intensivist(s).
3. Regular rotation during the day on a quarterly basis at minimum minimizes division between the two services.

C. After initial orientation and evaluation, individual programs, with the input of the attendings and hospitalists, must determine what the needs of the PICU are and how best to integrate the hospitalist into the structure and schedule over the course of the year.

D. During orientation and ICU assignment:

Daily rounds

1. Work Rounds with hospitalists does not differ from rounds with a teaching team of residents, fellows or allied professionals.
2. Provides a rich environment for discussing clinical considerations, pathophysiology, diagnostic and treatment approaches, as well as institutional policies and personal style.
3. With a stable cohort of hospitalists, basic lectures give way to more advanced and focused topics.
4. Where there is a regular schedule of residents or training physicians who need core PICU lectures, the hospitalists may be able to perform this function.

VI. Critical Care Training for the Hospitalist

A. Procedural competency:

1. Hospitalists must demonstrate competency in performing a procedure in order to be credentialed to perform that procedure at a given institution.
2. The expected range of procedures performed by pediatric hospitalists will vary from institution to institution and from hospitalist to hospitalist.
3. Essential procedures for all pediatric hospitalists include PALS procedures, peripheral venous access, arterial puncture, venipuncture, lumbar puncture, bladder catheterization and bag-valve- mask ventilation.
    a. Hospitalists should be proctored until they demonstrate competence in these procedures.
    b. While there are recommendations for the types of procedures that might be needed (*Crit Care Med*; 32: 263-272), there are insufficient data to recommend a universally applied number of procedures required for certification or credentialing of individuals.
    c. A program that expects hospitalists to perform invasive procedures on a regular basis should provide procedural training and experience similar to that provided to a PICU fellow.
    d. Hospitalists must know their limitations. Outside of a cardiopulmonary arrest, one can usually wait for backup before performing an invasive procedure.
        i. In –house anesthesiologists may provide support for the hospitalist to perform a planned intubation.
        ii. Preparation for a central line insertion may occur while waiting for an intensivist or surgeon.

B. Ongoing education (CME) for the pediatric hospitalist
   1. Programs where hospitalists routinely work in the PICU should develop C ms internally to promote the most relevant continued professional education alists (and intensivists).
   2. CME activity focused on critical and intermediate care should be included privileging requirement for all hospitalists who provide intermediate and/c care services.
      a. Pediatric advanced life support training is mandatory for hospitalist, in a PICU.
   3. Hospitalists should be included in M&M conferences, QI committees, journa ase presentations, and guideline and protocol development within the departme

VII. Business Plan

A. Should include estimates of the initial and on-going costs to orient new hospitalists an maintain credentials.
B. Orientation related activities required in a PICU hospitalist program should be include budget and schedule for all participants.
C. In situations where a hospitalist is supervised by another physician or member of anoth up when performing the procedure, it is appropriate to document the supervising role playe the other physician and for this supervising physician to submit the bill for the service as he legal regulations of the practice environment.
D. Guidelines for practice and integration should include (but not be limited to) the items in **Table A16-1**.
E. Billing and Coding for practice in the United States
   1. Current Procedural Terminology (CPT) codes define critical care as "the direct deliv by a physician, of medical care for a critically ill or critically injured patient" (CPT 20 Critical care is defined by the severity of illness and intensity of care provided; it is nc defined by the location of care and is not restricted to intensivists. Any physician, in location, can bill for critical care services as long as the severity of illness and intensity f services provided warrant it.
   2. There are 2 major types of critical care codes, time based codes for children two years age or older (including adults), and global codes for children younger than 2 years.
   3. The billable and included procedures are detailed in the American Medical Association's CPT Code Book.

1. Components of the orientation program for the PICU

nd knowledge of clinical guidelines, policies and
including order sets, nursing protocols, and/or
es.
ion order sets and clinical pathways
or FAST team responsibilities
ter plans
ult Process and expectations.
tion Team.
oonsibilities to surgical subspecialty patients

ters/Medical Information Systems (if in use)
sician order entry
s
aging

ting
dside flow sheets
&P, progress notes, transfer summaries, discharge
mmaries, dictations
illing

edules
Daily rounds
Multi-disciplinary meetings
Sign-out
Schedule including weekend and overnight obligations, CME and vacation requests, and process for changing schedule

nvironment Logistics
. Office space, call room, lockers
. Keys, access codes, ID
. Phone numbers and pagers

Communication with other providers
a. Expected frequency and style of communication with referring MDs, consulting physicians, co-managing physicians
b. Role of Primary care physician for patients hospitalized in the PICU
c. Rules of engagement with other Services

7. QI and Patient safety efforts
   a. Protocols in use
   b. Institution specific projects
8. Ancillary Support
   a. Nursing leadership and nursing staff
   b. Respiratory Therapy
   c. Pharmacy
   d. Social Work
   e. Case Management
   f. Child Life
   g. Additional services (eg Housekeeping, Transport, etc)
9. Education (Institution or Unit specific)
   a. House staff rotation
   b. Fellowship program
   c. Division and Department meetings
   d. Electronic and print libraries/references.
10. Research/Data Collection (Institution or Unit specific)
    a. Database for PICU patients
11. Transport (Institution or Unit specific)
    a. Intake from referring hospital
    b. Triage process
    c. Transport personnel
    d. Hospitalist role
12. Facility
    a. Location of ER including pediatric resuscitation room
    b. Imaging facilities
    c. Cafeteria
    d. Parking
13. Compensation (Institution or Unit specific)
    a. Timesheet if required
    b. Payroll and direct deposit
    c. CME, Paid time off, sick leave, holiday policies
    d. Expense reimbursement process (license, CME, etc)
    e. Health insurance, disability, flexible spending

VIII. Considerations for community hospitals without a PICU

A. Hospitalists in community hospitals without a PICU or Pediatric Emergency Department often must provide initial resuscitation, stabilization and management beyond that customarily required of a "floor" hospitalist in a tertiary care setting.

B. There is value for hospitalists in both community and tertiary institutions to possess fundamental knowledge and familiarity with pediatric critical care services.

C. Experienced hospitalists in community hospitals may provide intermediate care services to transiently ill, improving patients on a general ward who might be transferred to a step-down unit in a tertiary care institution.

D. Community pediatric hospital medicine programs should track all patients and outcomes to monitor both their individual program statistics and to contribute to the pediatric hospital medicine body of knowledge as a whole.
   1. Programs should monitor lengths of stay and complication rates for specific diseases to compare to national benchmarks for specific populations.
   2. Hospitalist groups that infrequently provide intermediate or critical care services may choose to perform individual chart review on each patient who meets this threshold.
   3. The minimal metrics for all pediatric hospital medicine programs providing critical and intermediate care services:
      a. Diagnosis and age of all patients who receive intermediate level of services.
      b. Diagnosis and age of all patients who are transferred out of the ward to another institution or to a higher level of care (e.g., PICU).
      c. Diagnosis, age and clinical scenario for all cardiopulmonary arrests that occur on the pediatric ward.

IX. Role of the Hospitalist

Generally trained pediatricians concentrating their practice in the inpatient arena can significantly contribute to the care, not only of general pediatric patients, but of critically ill children as well.

A. Hospitalists' involved in patient care around the clock, their clinical knowledge, procedural skill set, communication abilities, systems oriented mindset, and enthusiasm for the care of hospitalized children are a natural fit with intensive care

B. Collaboration between intensivists and hospitalists facilitates fluidity between general wards and the PICU, and may allow earlier transfer out of the PICU to promote optimal bed utilization.

C. The additional expertise acquired working in the PICU, allows hospitalists to recognize early signs of deterioration and either avert a transfer to PICU, or facilitate transfer in a more controlled manner.

D. The successful implementation of the hospitalist role requires clear identification of the expectations and limitations for the hospitalist and intensivist, ready availability of appropriate backup, continued education and training, and a collegial, mutually respectful relationship.